Healing

with

Vitamins

STRAIGHT FROM NATURE, BACKED BY SCIENCE

Healing
with
Vitamins

The Best Nutrients to Slow, Stop, and Reverse Disease

BY THE EDITORS OF
RODALE HEALTH BOOKS

RODALE

This book is intended as a reference volume only, not as a medical manual. The information given here is designed to help you make informed decisions about your health. It is not intended as a substitute for any treatment that may have been prescribed by your doctor. If you suspect that you have a medical problem, we urge you to seek competent medical help.

Mention of specific companies, organizations, or authorities in this book does not imply endorsement by the author or publisher, nor does mention of specific companies, organizations, or authorities imply that they endorse this book, its author, or the publisher.

Internet addresses and telephone numbers given in this book were accurate at the time it went to press.

Rodale books may be purchased for business or promotional use for special sales. For information, please write to: Special Markets Department, Rodale Inc., 733 Third Avenue, New York, NY 10017

Printed in the United States of America
Rodale Inc. makes every effort to use acid-free ♾, recycled paper ♻.

Contributing writers: Elizabeth Shimer Bowers, Sandra Salera-Lloyd, Wyatt Myers, and Marie Suszynski
Book design by Christopher Rhoads

Library of Congress Cataloging-in-Publication Data

Healing with vitamins : straight from nature, backed by science—the best nutrients to slow, stop, and reverse disease / by the editors of Rodale Health Books. — Rev. ed.
    p.   cm.
   Includes index.
   ISBN-13 978–1–59486–760–6 hardcover
   ISBN-10 1–59486–760–7 hardcover
   ISBN-13 978–1–59486–806–1 paperback
   ISBN-10 1–59486–806–9 paperback
   1. Vitamin therapy.   2. Minerals—Therapeutic use.   I. Title: Healing with vitamins.
RM259.P74   2008
615'.328—dc22
                                         2007046153

Distributed to the trade by Macmillan

6 8 10 9 7   hardcover
2 4 6 8 10 9 7 5 3 1   paperback

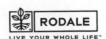

RODALE
LIVE YOUR WHOLE LIFE™

We inspire and enable people to improve their lives and the world around them

For more of our products visit **rodalestore.com** or call 800-848-4735

CONTENTS

Introduction / Tapping Into Nature's Vital Healing Power　　ix

PART ONE
VITAMINS AND MINERALS FOR HEALTH

Beta-Carotene 3

Biotin .4

Calcium. 5

Folic Acid 7

Iron. 9

Magnesium. 10

Niacin 12

Pantothenic Acid 14

Phosphorus 15

Potassium. 16

Riboflavin 18

Sodium. 20

Sulfur .21

Thiamin 22

Trace Minerals. 23

Vitamin A 36

Vitamin B_6 38

Vitamin B_{12} 40

Vitamin C 42

Vitamin D 46

Vitamin E 48

Vitamin K 50

Zinc. 52

PART TWO
THERAPEUTIC PRESCRIPTIONS FOR HEALING

Age Spots / Going, Going, Gone. 61

Aging / A Radical Solution. 66

Alcoholism / Repairing Nutritional Damage. 72

Allergies / Nutrients That Ease the Sneeze. 79

Alzheimer's Disease / Fighting the Memory Thief. 84

Anemia / Getting Back in the Pink 91

Angina / Easing the Squeeze 97

Asthma / Opening Up for Easier Breathing. 102

Bedsores / Nourishing Skin under Pressure. 109

Beriberi / Getting Enough Thiamin 112

Birth Defects / Eating Right for Two. 114

Bladder Infections / Flushing Out Trouble 119

Bruises / Fading Out the Black and Blue. 123

Burns / Repairing the Damage. 127

Cancer / Prevention Starts on Your Plate 132

Canker Sores / Soothing a Sore Mouth. 151

Cardiomyopathy / Heart-Protecting Nutrients. 155

Carpal Tunnel Syndrome / Opening Up to Relief. 161

Cataracts / Chasing Away the Clouds. 166

Celiac Disease / Fighting to Absorb Enough Nutrition 171

Cervical Dysplasia / Getting Your Cells in Line. 174

Chronic Fatigue Syndrome / Building Energy with Nutrients. 179

Colds / Common Nutrients for a Common Condition 187

Cold Sores / Minor Miracles for Your Mouth 193

Cystic Fibrosis / Nutrition for a Life-Threatening Condition. 197

Depression / Dispelling the Darkness. 202

Dermatitis / Supplements to Save Your Skin 208

Diabetes / Helping the Body Handle Sugar 213

Diarrhea / Foods That Can Stop the Flow. 223

Eating Disorders / Mending the Mind-Body Connection 226

Endometriosis / Living without Pain 233

Epilepsy / Quieting a Short-Circuited Brain. 240

Fatigue / Put the Pep Back in Your Step 247

Fibrocystic Breasts / Lessening the Lumps. 251

Fingernail Problems / Beating Brittle Nails 257

Gallstones / Healthy Ways to Prevent the Pain 259

Genital Herpes / Put a Stop to the Sores 263

Gingivitis / Nutritional Secrets to Healthy Gums 268

Glaucoma / Easing Eye Pressure Naturally 271

Gout / Fight Foot Pain with Food 275

Hair Loss / Keeping What You Have 280

Heart Arrhythmia / Subduing the Electrical Storms of the Heart 284

Heart Disease / Keeping Your Heart's Pathways Clear 290

High Blood Pressure / Mineral Magic Can Bring It Down 301

High Cholesterol / Protecting Yourself from the Bad Stuff,
Getting Enough of the Good 309

HIV / Aggressive Nutrition Prolongs Life 314

Immunity / Fortifying the Troops 324

Infertility / Improving Your Chances 332

Insomnia / Resetting the Sleep Clock 339

Intermittent Claudication / Improving Circulation 345

Kidney Stones / Dissolving a Painful Problem 349

Leg Cramps / Stopping the Squeeze 355

Lou Gehrig's Disease / A Potentially Radical Solution 359

Lupus / Fighting Off an Immune System Attack 362

Macular Degeneration / Protecting Vision into the Later Years 367

Memory Loss / Helping Your Brain Work Better 373

Ménière's Disease / Stopping the Spinning 380

Menopausal Problems / Reinventing the Change of Life 385

Menstrual Problems / Nutrients to Ease Monthly Distress 393

Migraines / Ending the Pain 399

Mitral Valve Prolapse / Easing Symptoms of a Troubled Heart 404

Morning Sickness / Taming the Turbulent Tummy 409

Multiple Sclerosis / Slowing a Nerve-Racking Disease 411

Night Blindness / Eyes Need Vitamin A 417

Osteoarthritis / Slowing Joint Wear and Tear 421

Osteoporosis / Walking Tall into Your Golden Years **427**

Overweight / Nourishing Yourself Thin **438**

Parkinson's Disease / Smoothing Out the Tremors **447**

Pellagra / Decoding a Turn-of-the-Century Mystery **453**

Phlebitis / Staying Out of Deep Trouble **456**

Premenstrual Syndrome / Putting an End to Monthly Discomfort **460**

Prostate Problems / Dealing with a Common Condition **467**

Psoriasis / Prescription Vitamin D Delivers Hope **472**

Raynaud's Phenomenon / Defrosting Frigid Digits **477**

Restless Legs Syndrome / When Your Legs Have a Life of Their Own . . . **481**

Rheumatoid Arthritis / Cooling Down the Inflammation **487**

Rickets / Building Strong Bones **496**

Scleroderma / Softening Rock-Hard Skin **499**

Scurvy / Solved with Vitamin C **503**

Shingles / Chickenpox Revisited **507**

Smog Exposure / Protection from Pollution **512**

Smoking / Controlling Damage while Kicking the Habit **517**

Sunburn / Protecting Yourself from Harmful Rays **525**

Surgery / Minding Your Mending **531**

Taste and Smell Problems / Sense-sational Nutrition **539**

Tinnitus / Silencing the Ring **542**

Varicose Veins / Winning an Uphill Battle **549**

Water Retention / Beating the Bloat **554**

Wilson's Disease / Neutralized by Zinc **559**

Wrinkles / Smoothing Out the Lines **563**

Yeast Infections / Ditching the Itch **568**

Index **575**

TAPPING INTO NATURE'S VITAL HEALING POWER

Vitamins are not magic pills. But let's face it: It's really tempting to think of them that way. Anything that can help you live longer, look younger, enhance your immune system, fight illness, and boost your energy certainly sounds pretty miraculous or magical.

A few decades ago, when word started to spread about the healing potential of vitamins and minerals, the general public went wild for bottled nutrients. So did health writers and even some doctors. For a while, it was starting to sound like megadoses of vitamins could cure anything.

Well, that bubble burst soon enough. Of course, vitamins and minerals can't cure everything. But they can do a lot. Research breakthroughs over just the past few years are making interest in the topic heat up all over again. Some of the things that scientists have discovered about the healing power of these vital nutrients all but boggle the mind.

As more and more rigorous scientific studies accumulate showing spectacular health benefits from vitamins and minerals, we're all back where we were a few decades ago: eager to take advantage of all of this healing potential—and thoroughly confused. While the reasons for taking vitamins and minerals are now based on solid science, shopping for nutrients is still nothing less than overwhelming.

You know what happens when you make a trip to your local pharmacy or supermarket to buy nutrients. You're faced with overwhelming choices. Shelf after shelf in aisle after aisle offers nothing but confusion. Letters and numbers, single nutrients and combinations, capsules and tablets, bottles in different sizes and colors from different companies, covered with enticing claims that compete for your attention and your precious consumer dollar.

What's a person who wants to take vitamins and minerals in a safe and responsible manner supposed to do? All you really want to know, after all, is what really works.

Well, search no more. That's what this book is all about.

To write it, we've interviewed the nation's top doctors and researchers, asking exactly those questions that you want answered: Which vitamins and minerals can you take to prevent, cure, or ameliorate specific diseases? How much of the nutrients do you take? Are they safe? What kinds of results can you expect? We've also scanned the scientific literature to answer these questions. And we've put it all together in one easy-to-use volume, which you're holding in your hands right now. If you want to know which nutrients to take and in what amounts, simply look up the disease you want to know about.

Along with the scoop on how to use nutrients to fight disease, we've made several important discoveries during the course of our research.

One is that supplements are not a substitute for good nutrition. It will come as no surprise to anyone who pays attention to natural healing and prevention that scientists can't beat nature when it comes to packaging healing therapies.

And that's why, so often in this book, you'll find doctors and researchers saying that you should get your healing vitamins and minerals from foods whenever you can. At the same time, doctors and researchers in this book often recommend taking supplements—at least a multivitamin for what they call insurance. Why is that?

It's often not practical to get adequate therapeutic amounts of vitamins and minerals from foods. That's right, therapeutic. Large doses of some nutrients have such powerful effects on the body that they act like drugs.

That brings us to the second important discovery that we've made: Vitamin and mineral supplements should be treated with the same care and concern for safety that you reserve for prescription and over-the-counter medications.

Large doses of certain nutrients can be toxic. They can cause side effects. They can interact with medications that you might be taking. So there are a few rules to follow when using this book.

Please take the Medical Alerts seriously. They are there for your safety. If you are under a doctor's care for a serious disease, you should talk to him about your interest in using nutrients as part of your treatment. With all of the scientific breakthroughs in this area, doctors are increasingly open to nutritional therapy. You may be pleasantly surprised to find your doctor willing to work with you to find the right dosages and monitor your progress.

And if you're pregnant or nursing a baby, make sure you mention any supplements you're taking, even a multivitamin, to your physician.

Finally, pay attention to the doses of any vitamins and minerals you're taking. Many researchers and doctors feel that the Daily Values for certain nutrients—vitamin C, for example—should be set much higher. They've also found that the body's need for nutrients goes way, way up when it's fighting disease. That's why you'll find the recommendations in this book often go way beyond the Daily Values for many nutrients.

Here's wishing you all of the healing that nature's nutrients can supply.

PART ONE
VITAMINS AND MINERALS FOR HEALTH

BETA-CAROTENE

Daily Value: None established

Good Food Sources: Sweet potatoes, carrots, cantaloupe, spinach and other dark green leafy vegetables

The evidence is overwhelming! People who eat three or more servings a day of beta-carotene-rich fruits and vegetables have a lower risk of heart disease and many types of cancer. However, the scientific community isn't as enthusiastic about the effects of beta-carotene supplements.

During the early 1990s, studies sang the praises of beta-carotene-rich foods and their ability to lower the risk of cancer and other diseases. In response to those promising findings, many doctors recommended beta-carotene supplements to their patients. But in 1994, a study of 29,000 male Finnish smokers found that men who took 20 milligrams (about 33,000 IU) of beta-carotene a day actually had an increased incidence of both lung cancer and heart disease. The result was unexpected, and accolades for beta-carotene supplements died down.

Some scientists speculated that the devastating effects of alcohol and 3 decades' worth of smoking were well under way before the study began. A poor diet and heavy drinking and smoking put these men at a higher risk of heart disease and cancer before beta-carotene supplements were handed out.

Six years later, another study called the Carotene and Retinol Efficacy Trial, or CARET, was halted when researchers discovered that patients receiving just 30 milligrams of beta-carotene supplements a day had a 46 percent higher risk of dying from lung cancer. Since then a review of over 60 randomized trials, conducted by the respected Cochrane Collaboration, concluded that beta-carotene supplements significantly increased the risk of mortality.

In light of recent findings, the Institute of Medicine doesn't believe that beta-carotene supplements are advisable for the general public (but does concede that supplements may be beneficial for people with vitamin A deficiencies). Today doctors are understandably cautious about recommending beta-carotene supplements, especially for people who smoke and who have had high levels of asbestos exposure.

Contributing to their reluctance and caution in recommending supplements is the growing body of research showing that most foods containing beta-carotene also contain other powerful disease-fighting members of the carotenoid family such as alpha-carotene, lycopene, zeaxanthin, and lutein. In fact, some experts suspect that it may be these substances that have been doing most of the disease-preventive work while beta-carotene has been garnering all of the credit.

Using Beta-Carotene Safely

Most experts agree that people should be reaching for carotenoid-rich foods rather than supplements. Beta-carotene is plentiful in vegetables and fruits, and population studies have strongly suggested that eating three or more servings can significantly reduce the risk of heart disease and many forms of cancer.

Too much beta-carotene in the body can turn the skin orange. The discoloration fades as levels of the nutrient return to normal.

BIOTIN

Daily Value: 300 micrograms

Good Food Sources: Brewer's yeast, barley, oat bran, soybeans, filberts, walnuts, peanuts, bananas, cauliflower, milk, egg yolks, salmon

Your nails are a disaster. They've been clipped, filed, and buffed, then coated with polish. And they still look thin, brittle, and pathetic.

They will never appear in *Vogue*. But they do happen to be just about the first thing folks notice when you shake hands or pet their dogs. So what are you going to do?

Well, you may want to try your luck with biotin, a B-complex vitamin that your body needs to process carbohydrates, fats, and amino acids (the building blocks of protein). Years ago researchers discovered that hoof abnormalities in horses could be successfully treated with biotin supplements. Since then biotin has been touted as a nail and hair strengthener. Some research has shown that biotin supplements can improve the condition of brittle nails. However, those studies were small and/or inconclusive. Larger placebo-controlled studies are needed before any positive conclusions can be made.

Biotin deficiency is uncommon and is usually limited to those who are being fed intravenously over a long period of time or have a genetic inability to absorb biotin. Most people really don't need to worry about whether or not they're getting enough. That's because unless you have a genetic defect that alters the way your body uses this nutrient, either you get enough of it through the eggs, milk, and cereals in your diet or your body will manufacture what you need.

People with type 2 (non-insulin-dependent) diabetes may prove to be a different story. They often have lower levels of biotin than people without the disease. Fortunately, researchers are finding that biotin supplements may help those with type 2 diabetes manage their glucose levels. When researchers at Yale University School of Medicine gave 43 patients with poorly controlled type 2 diabetes a biotin/chromium supplement, their glucose and lipid levels were significantly improved after just 4 weeks.

Research is also showing that biotin can decrease symptoms associated with peripheral neuropathy, a complication of long-term diabetes that causes numbness, tingling, pain, and weakness in the extremities due to nerve damage. People with peripheral neuropathy have reported an improvement of symptoms after 1 month of taking biotin supplements. (For the full details on using nutrients to treat diabetes, see page 213.)

Using Biotin Safely

Biotin may be one of the safest of all vitamins. There are no reports of toxicity, even when it's taken in high doses up to 600 micrograms.

Biotin is destroyed by certain food-processing techniques such as canning and heat curing. So it's always better to choose fresh fruits, vegetables, and meats over canned or cured foods.

CALCIUM

Daily Value: 1,000 milligrams

Good Food Sources: Skim milk, nonfat yogurt, cheeses, collard greens, mustard greens, kale, broccoli, canned salmon with bones, sardines with bones, corn tortillas processed with lime, calcium-fortified orange juice

By now, just about everyone knows that getting enough calcium helps prevent diseases such as osteoporosis. Less well known is just how calcium goes about doing this.

When you eat cheese or drink milk, the calcium in these foods is absorbed through your small intestine and into your blood. The amount of calcium in your blood is regulated by a substance called parathyroid hormone. When calcium intake is low, parathyroid hormone signals for bone to be broken down, releasing calcium into the bloodstream. "Diets with adequate calcium intake produce less parathyroid hormone, so that we conserve more calcium and more bone," says John Anderson, PhD, professor of nutrition in the Schools of Public Health and Medicine at the University of North Carolina at Chapel Hill.

Calcium then combines with phosphorus to help form hard, crystal-like substances that create the latticework that undergirds strong bones and teeth. In fact, 99 percent of the calcium in your body is stored in your skeleton. Researchers call this ongoing process of removing old bone and forming new bone remodeling.

You also need a stable level of blood calcium for a normal heartbeat, nerve and muscle function, and blood clotting. Living cells require calcium to act as a messenger and to help respond to hormones and neurotransmitters.

Even though calcium is vital for bone growth and maintenance in everyone, experts don't advise a one-size-fits-all intake. Here are the Adequate Intakes (AIs) of calcium as set by the Institute of Medicine.

- Infants, birth through age 6 months: 210 milligrams
- Infants, ages 7 to 12 months: 270 milligrams
- Children, ages 1 to 3 years: 500 milligrams
- Children, ages 4 to 8 years: 800 milligrams
- Children, adolescents, and young adults, ages 9 to 18: 1,300 milligrams
- Pregnant and nursing women, ages 14 to 18: 1,300 milligrams
- Pregnant and nursing women, ages 19 to 50: 1,000 milligrams
- Adults, ages 19 to 50: 1,000 milligrams
- Adults, ages 51 and older: 1,200 milligrams

Using Calcium Safely

Not all calcium supplements are created equal. The actual amount of calcium contained in a supplement, called elemental calcium, varies from one form of calcium to the next. Calcium citrate, which contains about 21 percent of elemental calcium, is the most easily absorbed and digested by the body. Calcium carbonate has a higher concentration of elemental calcium (40 percent), but it's slightly more difficult to absorb, especially for people with decreased stomach acid, so it should always be taken with food.

A newer form of calcium called calcium formate has more absorbable calcium than calcium citrate, but it's not widely available. There are several other forms of calcium to consider, but most of them have lower concentrations of elemental calcium or they aren't nearly as digestible as calcium citrate. Calcium lactate and calcium gluconate contain only 13 percent and 9 percent elemental calcium, respectively. Calcium phosphate has a much higher percentage of calcium, but it's difficult to absorb.

Another consideration when choosing a supplement is how the calcium was obtained. Supplements that are products of oyster shells, dolomite, and bone meal may contain traces of lead, mercury, or arsenic. Many manufacturers have taken steps to reduce these traces, and some labels indicate that the supplements are "lead-free."

Calcium is best absorbed when it's taken with food and at a dose not exceeding 500 milligrams. This means that if you're taking supplements exceeding that amount, you should take them in divided doses throughout the day.

High calcium intake (more than 2,000 milligrams a day) may cause constipation and kidney stones and inhibit the absorption of minerals, like zinc and iron.

FOLIC ACID

Daily Value: 400 micrograms

Good Food Sources: Fortified cereals, pinto beans, navy beans, asparagus, spinach, broccoli, okra, brussels sprouts

Folic acid is a nutritional powerhouse that makes things happen within the body. It works with approximately 20 different enzymes to build DNA, the material that contains the genetic code for your body, and is essential for normal nerve function.

It also seems to prevent heart disease and stroke by reducing the body's levels of homocysteine, an artery-attacking chemical that accumulates in the blood of people who eat meats.

What's more, folic acid may help protect against cancer of the ovaries, colon, and cervix. In a study at the University of Alabama at Birmingham, researchers found that women with high levels of folate (the naturally occurring form of folic acid) were two to five times less likely than women with low folate levels to develop cervical dysplasia in conjunction with various risk factors such as cigarette smoke, human papillomavirus, contraceptives, and childbirth. (Cervical dysplasia is a condition involving the development of abnormal cells in the cervix. This condition can progress to cancer in some women.)

Folic acid also protects a woman's fetus from life-threatening birth defects of the brain and spine. Studies show that 50 to 70 percent of neural tube defects, like spina bifida, could have been prevented if mothers had taken folic acid supplements before and during their pregnancies. Because of the strong link between birth defects and folate deficiency, in 1998 the U.S. government mandated that folic acid be added to all grain and cereal products. Unfortunately, a survey by the March of Dimes has found that two-thirds of women of reproductive age still aren't getting the recommended 400 micrograms of folic acid they need to prevent birth defects, and only 7 percent knew that folic acid should be taken before pregnancy.

Using Folic Acid Safely

Folic acid has virtually no side effects, even when taken in high amounts. For most people, taking more than 1,000 micrograms has no benefit. Unless a doctor prescribes high doses of folic acid, supplements shouldn't exceed 1 milligram (1,000 micrograms) a day. Doses of more than 400 micrograms a day can mask symptoms of pernicious anemia, a potentially fatal disease due to vitamin B_{12} deficiency.

"In general, 0.4 milligram (400 micrograms) of folate is a good amount to get in a day, and with careful planning that can be achieved," says Meir Stampfer, MD, DrPH, professor of nutrition and epidemiology at Harvard School of Public Health. A day's worth of folate could look like this: 1 cup of orange juice (110 micrograms) and 1 cup of folate-fortified cereal (160 micrograms) plus a cup of raw spinach in a lunch or dinner salad (130 micrograms).

Although folate is available in these and many other foods, be aware that as much as 50 percent of the nutrient is destroyed during food processing, storage, and household preparation. In general, much of the folate in foods is killed by heat and light.

Several substances can increase your need for the vitamin, including alcohol, tobacco, aspirin and other nonsteroidal anti-inflammatory drugs, oral contraceptives, pancreatic extracts, estrogen, antacids, arthritis drugs such as methotrexate, and medications prescribed for convulsions, malaria, and bacterial infections.

IRON

Daily Value: 18 milligrams

Good Food Sources: Beef, Cream of Wheat cereal, baked potatoes, soybeans, pumpkin seeds, clams

There's no doubt that many of us can use more iron than we're getting. Roughly 20 percent of Americans are deficient in this mineral. The group most likely to be coming up short: women in their reproductive years.

"I would say that women need to be a little more thoughtful than men about iron, probably in the same way that women should be a little more cautious about calcium intake because of osteoporosis," says Adria Sherman, PhD, professor of nutritional sciences at Rutgers University in New Brunswick, New Jersey.

Iron, which is absorbed in the intestines, comes in two forms: heme and nonheme. Found in meats, the heme form is well absorbed. Men get about two-thirds of their iron needs met by heme iron; the amount varies for women. Nonheme iron is found in vegetables and isn't as well absorbed.

Most of the iron you consume goes to form hemoglobin, the substance that helps your red blood cells transport oxygen from your lungs to the rest of your body. The remainder is stored in the bone marrow, liver, spleen, and other organs.

Because iron also plays a key role in helping to prepare your immune system's infection fighters for battle, a deficiency may lead to colds. Low iron levels can also cause fatigue, pallor, and listlessness—hallmarks of anemia, says Dr. Sherman. In children, low iron levels can cause stunted growth and impaired learning. Other symptoms of iron deficiency include split nails, a sore tongue, and cold hands and feet. An annoying condition called restless legs has also been linked to low iron.

Some experts even believe that vague gastrointestinal problems such as gas, belching, constipation, and diarrhea may be rooted in iron deficiency. If you suspect that you may be deficient in iron, ask your family doctor or your gynecologist to test your blood at your yearly exam.

Using Iron Safely

Here's a fact about iron supplements that should encourage healthy respect: The leading cause of fatal poisoning in children under 6 years old is accidental overdosing on products with iron. So make sure your iron supplements are tightly capped and kept out of their reach.

Although accidental iron poisonings occur most often in children who ingest supplements containing iron that are formulated for adults, high levels of iron can also be toxic to adults. Therefore, most experts recommend that you don't take iron supplements unless your doctor confirms the need with a blood test.

A daily intake of 25 milligrams or more for an extended period of time may cause undesirable side effects. Symptoms of acute iron poisoning include pain, vomiting, diarrhea, and shock. Still, doctors normally recommend iron supplementation for pregnant women and for infants.

Among the variety of iron supplements, experts say those made with ferrous salts are better absorbed. Among them, ferrous sulfate is considered best. Slow-release and coated iron tablets may cause less diarrhea, nausea, and abdominal pain, but since the site of maximum absorption is the beginning of the small intestine, delaying the time of release decreases the overall amount of iron absorbed by your body. Taking the tablets with a meal could go a long way in helping to reduce stomach upset, but then again, the food may interfere with the iron absorption. Therefore, since it is advantageous for absorption, experts recommend taking iron supplements between meals if you do not experience side effects or you can tolerate iron taken in this manner.

MAGNESIUM

Daily Value: 400 milligrams

Good Food Sources: Brown rice, avocados, spinach, halibut, almonds, oatmeal, baked potatoes with skin, kidney beans, pinto beans, broccoli, bananas, raisins

Imagine a product that not only may help prevent a heart attack but also may successfully ease premenstrual syndrome, high blood pressure, heart arrhythmia, asthma, and kidney stones.

This single-source solution to some of our most vexing health problems doesn't come from the high-tech laboratory of some pharmaceutical company. It's magnesium, an essential mineral that's often missing from our diets. And the more studies researchers conduct, the more impressive this mineral looks.

"Magnesium is an important element for health and disease," says Herbert C. Mansmann Jr., MD, honorary professor of pediatrics and director of the Magnesium Research Laboratory at Jefferson Medical College of Thomas Jefferson University in Philadelphia. "The research papers on this topic are increasing exponentially."

Investigators have been breaking new ground, but magnesium has a long healing history. Epsom salts—first discovered in Epsom, England, in 1808, and essentially made of magnesium sulfate—have long been the key ingredient of soothing hot foot soaks. Inside your body, magnesium serves several crucial roles, especially as an assistant to 350 enzymes. This includes helping to turn food into energy and helping to transmit electrical impulses across nerves and muscles. These impulses generate what's called neuromuscular contraction, literally enabling your muscles to flex. Take away magnesium, and muscles—even the smooth muscles that routinely squeeze blood vessels—will cramp.

Magnesium is also vital for making sure that calcium is used properly by keeping calcium out of the cells. Too much calcium, however, can cause you to lose magnesium in your urine.

Healthy kidneys will limit the amount of magnesium excreted in the urine when the body has a low intake of magnesium. However, some asthma and cardiovascular medications, diuretics, antibiotics, and fiber laxatives (except for ones that contain polycarbophil) can cause the kidney to release too much magnesium. Alcohol is notorious for removing magnesium from your body. Between 30 and 60 percent of alcoholics have low levels of magnesium, and in patients going through withdrawal it's nearly 90 percent. People with diabetes who have high blood sugar lose a lot of magnesium in the urine.

"It's very easy to not get enough into the system or to lose what's in there. And that's rarely recognized until someone has advanced magnesium deficiency, with a low blood level of magnesium," says Dr. Mansmann. But this much is known: Up to 40 percent of the American population gets less than 75 percent of the Daily Value of magnesium, says Dr. Mansmann. Just how many suffer needlessly from health problems related to magnesium deficiency is anyone's guess, but it could help explain why many of us suffer, or know someone who suffers, with the common symptoms of low magnesium levels. They include constipation, hypertension, migraine, muscle cramps, osteoporosis, and premenstrual syndrome. Prolonged symptoms of magnesium deficiency lead to muscle weakness, tremors, seizures, and heart arrhythmias.

Using Magnesium Safely

Picking a magnesium supplement may not seem like a decision worthy of intense study, but select the wrong one and the wrong dose, and you may not get the appropriate benefit.

Magnesium is usually mixed with compounds, the most common one being salt. The weight of magnesium salt is heavy, and labels typically provide that number rather than the actual weight of the magnesium. Always look at how much *elemental* magnesium supplements have, which is a truer representation of the magnesium amount.

There are several forms of magnesium, and the absorption of each type determines how it should be used. For example, supplements with magnesium L-lactate dehydrate (Mag-Tab SR by Niche Pharmaceuticals, Inc. is one) are best for long-term use, according to Dr. Mansmann. Magnesium gluconate is excellent for cardiac arrhythmias and migraines because most of it is absorbed quickly in the stomach.

Dose for dose, magnesium gluconate causes less diarrhea than magnesium oxide or magnesium chloride. It can be taken on an empty stomach, while some of the other salts can cause stomach upset in some people. As a general rule, you need about 6 milligrams of elemental magnesium for every kilogram (2.2 pounds) of body weight. That means that if you weigh 150 pounds, you should be getting about 400 milligrams a day. If you develop diarrhea, simply take your magnesium in divided doses throughout the day, or reduce the dose by 20 to 25 percent until normal soft bowel movements return, says Dr. Mansmann.

If you have kidney or heart problems, always check with your doctor before taking supplemental magnesium.

NIACIN

Daily Value: 20 milligrams

Good Food Sources: Chicken breast, tuna, veal, fortified breads and cereals

The niacin story is one of triumph and potential tragedy. The triumph: One form of niacin, nicotinic acid, lowers the risk of heart disease at a fraction of the cost of prescription drugs. The tragedy: Used improperly, slow-release niacin can cause severe side effects, including liver damage.

"In the right hands, it's a very useful medication. It lowers harmful cholesterol and raises good cholesterol better than any drug we have," says James McKenney, PharmD, professor emeritus in the School of Pharmacy at Virginia Commonwealth University in Richmond. "But taken indiscriminately by an uninformed person without a professional monitoring his condition, it can be dangerous."

When taken in doses over 1,500 milligrams daily, the slow-release or long-acting forms of niacin that are available without a prescription can result in an accumulation of a niacin by-product that is toxic to the liver. This problem doesn't occur with the short-acting nonprescription forms of niacin.

A less controversial use of niacin has positive results. Niacin prevents pellagra, a now rare condition that often starts with skin inflammation, includes diarrhea and depression, and ends in death. In the Deep South at the turn of the 20th century, this ailment afflicted over 100,000 people, largely because their diets consisted mainly of cornmeal. Not only does corn contain a form of niacin that the body cannot readily use, but a diet consisting of nothing but corn can also create an amino acid imbalance. Thanks to the fortification of flours and cereals with niacin, pellagra is rare in all but alcoholics and people suffering from severe gastrointestinal problems.

Niacin may also reduce the risk of Alzheimer's disease. Researchers at the Rush Institute for Healthy Aging in Chicago followed the diets of over 3,500 people 65 years of age and older for 5½ years. They found that those who got the least amount of niacin were 70 percent more likely to have Alzheimer's disease. The participants who took niacin supplements and ate niacin-rich foods, such as fish, beans, and fortified grains, showed less cognitive decline.

Using Niacin Safely

It's virtually impossible to get too much niacin in your diet. But when you take niacin supplements in the doses needed to improve your cholesterol levels (1,000 to 2,000 milligrams), you are likely to experience side effects, especially flushing and itching with the immediate-release form (a bothersome but not dangerous side effect) and liver damage with the slow-release form (a dangerous side effect). That's why this kind of therapy needs to be taken under medical supervision.

Niacinamide, a form of niacin that is included in multivitamin/mineral supplements, does not produce the side effects associated with niacin itself. It also does not reduce blood cholesterol levels.

PANTOTHENIC ACID

Daily Value: 10 milligrams

Good Food Sources: Eggs, fish, milk and milk products, whole grains, legumes, white and sweet potatoes, yeast, lean beef

In a world that pops painkillers for hangnails and spreads toxic chemicals on lawns to produce greener grass, pantothenic acid may mean the difference between life and death.

In a study at the University of Windsor in Canada, researchers have found that tissue cells treated with water-soluble coenzyme Q10, a substance containing pantothenic acid, can detoxify many of the harmful synthetic compounds found in herbicides, insecticides, and drugs.

Recognition of the protective benefits of pantothenic acid—one of the B vitamins—is long overdue. For years it was taken for granted, but word of its life-sustaining abilities is spreading. Pantothenic acid, also known as vitamin B_5, is involved in so many different metabolic pathways, including the conversion of food to energy, the synthesis of important hormones, and the body's utilization of body fat and cholesterol.

Those most likely to be deficient in pantothenic acid are people who are at high risk of malnutrition, such as older folks, people with serious drinking problems, and people who aren't able to eat on their own.

Signs of deficiency rarely occur except with severe life-threatening malnutrition. In fact, pantothenic deficiency is so rare that the only proven effects are those seen in animal experiments. Most people take in sufficient levels of pantothenic acid through their diets.

Using Pantothenic Acid Safely

Pantothenic acid is not known to be toxic in high doses. Supplements up to 1,200 milligrams a day have been taken with no ill effects reported except an occasional case of gastrointestinal problems, like nausea, heartburn, and diarrhea. The amount of pantothenic acid required to detoxify all of the synthetic chemicals to which people are exposed is unknown.

Up to 75 percent of pantothenic acid is destroyed by processing, canning, or freezing. That's why the best sources are unprocessed whole grains, fortified or enriched cereals to which the nutrient has been added, and multivitamin/mineral supplements.

PHOSPHORUS

Daily Value: 1,000 milligrams

Good Food Sources: Halibut, nonfat yogurt, salmon, skim milk, chicken breast, oatmeal, extra-lean ground beef, broccoli, lima beans

What do a Bengal tiger and a teenager have in common? Depending on their chow, they may both be getting too much phosphorus.

Years ago, after noticing that the big cats in some zoos simply lay in their cages all day, researchers found that the animals' feed was high in phosphorus and dangerously low in calcium. Of course, a calcium-phosphorus imbalance has yet to be linked to teenage couch-potato syndrome. But some experts believe teens who drink too much soda may have a phosphorus imbalance that could lead to osteoporosis later in life.

The mineral phosphorus is needed for many of the chemical reactions in the body. Phosphorus compounds help regulate the release of energy that fuels us. By combining with calcium, phosphorus also helps form hard, crystal-like substances that create the latticework that undergirds strong bones and teeth. In fact, 85 percent of the body's phosphorus is located in bone.

That may be part of the problem. The mechanism regulating the body's balance of calcium and phosphorus is so finely calibrated that getting too much phosphorus actually causes calcium to be removed from your skeleton and sent to your blood. Long-term calcium loss has been found to cause osteoporosis, a weakening of the bones that can lead to tooth loss and fractures.

Eating natural forms of phosphorus, which is found in everything from chicken and broccoli to milk and fruits, isn't likely to give you too much of this mineral. But some experts are worried that drinking too much soda—such as cola, root beer, and even clear drinks—can tip your delicate calcium-phosphorus balance in the wrong direction. Moreover, by forsaking milk for soda, you're further reducing your calcium intake, says John Anderson, PhD, professor of nutrition in the Schools of Public Health and Medicine at the University of North Carolina at Chapel Hill.

"That's where you get hurt the worst. You are compounding the problem. You are getting low calcium and high phosphorus," says Dr. Anderson.

It seems soda and many processed foods contain either phosphoric acid or some form of phosphate, both of which are hefty sources of phosphorus.

"Phosphoric acid is used in cola soft drinks to give them an acid taste," says Dr. Anderson. "Added to foods, phosphates may act as preservatives or perhaps even help alter the physical quality."

In rare cases, people who use antacids containing aluminum hydroxide for long periods of time might suffer from weakness, loss of appetite, malaise, and bone loss. This chemical apparently prevents phosphorus from being absorbed.

Using Phosphorus Safely

Experts say there's virtually no reason to ever take a phosphorus supplement. It's easy to get enough phosphorus from your diet.

POTASSIUM

Daily Value: 3,500 milligrams

Good Food Sources: Dried apricots, baked potatoes, dried prunes, cantaloupe, bananas, spinach, salmon, carrots, mushrooms, pears, apples, citrus fruits

When combined with water in a laboratory, pure potassium will actually burst into flames.

Luckily for us, it reacts quite differently in the body. When derived from food and supplements, potassium can take on a number of important roles, from maintaining normal fluid balances to promoting cell and muscle growth.

One of potassium's most well-known roles, however, is its ability to regulate blood pressure. Scientists believe this may have something to do with potassium's ability to pump sodium out of the body's cells and reduce body fluid. Potassium may also affect blood vessel tone, or resistance. Or it may be that potassium modifies the way blood vessels react to circulating hormones that affect blood pressure, such as vasopressin and norepinephrine.

In any case, potassium's ability to lower blood pressure is such that some scientists suspect low dietary levels of the mineral may actually trigger high blood pressure in certain people.

Aside from its miraculous effect on blood pressure, potassium appears to have other heart-healthy benefits. Specifically, it might help prevent stroke, death caused by stroke, and cardiovascular disease. And other recent studies point to a connection between high potassium intake and a reduced risk of developing kidney stones.

Potassium is also necessary for good muscle contraction, healthy electrical activity in the heart, and rapid transmission of nerve impulses throughout the body. This is why heartbeat irregularities are considered a classic sign of potassium deficiency. Other symptoms of deficiency can include muscle weakness, numbness and tingling in the lower extremities, nausea, vomiting, confusion, and irritability.

Using Potassium Safely

Most of us get around 2,650 milligrams of potassium every day, reports the National Center for Health Statistics. And while that may be enough for some people, it's best to shoot for the FDA's recommended Daily Value of 3,500 milligrams. To get this, you probably need to add at least three more servings of potassium-rich fruits and vegetables to your diet every day. And there are a number of good reasons for doing this: Studies suggest that even adding just one more serving of potassium-rich fruits and vegetables every day can reduce your risk of stroke by 40 percent.

A well-balanced diet should provide all the potassium that most people need. But potassium supplements—available over the counter or, in larger doses, by prescription—may be necessary for those who take diuretic medications. Diuretics help the body lose excess water but also deplete its potassium supply. (Digitalis, a heart medicine, can also cause you to excrete potassium.) If you use over-the-counter supplements, it is usually best to keep your total daily potassium intake from diet and supplements to 3,500 milligrams.

When a potassium supplement is required, talk to your doctor or pharmacist about which kind is best for you. Supplements containing more than 99 milligrams of potassium are available only by prescription.

Too much potassium (more than 5,000 milligrams a day) can upset the balance of minerals in your body and cause heart and kidney problems. Other potential side effects include muscle weakness; tingling in the hands, feet, or tongue; and a slow or irregular pulse.

People with diabetes or kidney disease should consult their doctor before taking potassium supplements, as should people on certain medications, including nonsteroidal anti-inflammatory drugs, potassium-sparing diuretics, ACE inhibitors, and heart medicines such as heparin.

RIBOFLAVIN

Daily Value: 1.7 milligrams

Good Food Sources: Almonds, brewer's yeast, liver, eggs, milk, mushrooms, seafood, leafy green vegetables, wheat germ, wild rice, fortified grains and cereals

Riboflavin will probably never bathe in the nutritional spotlight like vitamin C, magnesium, and vitamin E. But a smattering of experts say that it's about time we give this nutrient, also known as vitamin B_2, its due.

Emerging research shows that riboflavin can act as an antioxidant, potentially helping to prevent cancer and control cholesterol buildup by helping to tame harmful free radicals. Free radicals are naturally occurring renegade molecules that damage your body's healthy molecules by stealing electrons to balance themselves. Antioxidants neutralize free radicals by offering their own electrons and thus protect the healthy molecules from harm.

Some research suggests that riboflavin's antioxidant action is particularly helpful in the lungs, brain, and heart. In the brain, riboflavin appears to help correct small deficiencies in brain cells, thus preventing the occurrence of migraine headaches. In the heart, it appears to help break down the amino acid homocysteine. High levels of homocysteine have been linked to increased odds of heart disease, as well as stroke. Interestingly enough, riboflavin also appears to play a role in preventing esophageal cancer, as well as the formation of cataracts.

Riboflavin also assists a number of important chemical processes in the body. Folate and vitamin B_6, for example, need riboflavin to undergo the chemical changes that make them useful. Amino acids are transformed by riboflavin into what are called neurotransmitters, chemicals crucial for thinking and memory. A shortage of red blood cells, which causes symptoms such as anemia, has been linked in some cases to a lack of riboflavin. The vitamin is also involved with muscle energy metabolism, which is why some research suggests that riboflavin may boost performance in athletes.

Riboflavin deficiency can affect your vision, causing your eyes to become light-sensitive and easily fatigued. Other symptoms of deficiency include blurred vision and itching, watering, sore, or bloodshot eyes. Severe dermatitis, particularly itching, peeling skin on the nose or scrotum, is another hallmark of riboflavin deficiency.

During World War II, manufacturers began fortifying cereals and flours with riboflavin. But research suggests that you may need other sources of the vitamin as well. It appears that people who choose to limit their dairy and meat consumption may still be at risk for deficiency.

People who exercise regularly may not be getting enough riboflavin, either, since activity seems to help speed the vitamin's removal from the body.

Using Riboflavin Safely

There's no need to worry about a riboflavin overdose. Any excess of this particular vitamin is excreted from your system. And unlike most other vitamins, this one quickly lets you know that you've reached your saturation point. Two hours after taking a supplement containing riboflavin, your urine will turn bright yellow.

Huge amounts of riboflavin, 2,000 times the Daily Value, have been known to cause kidney stones, but there is no reason to take this much. Also, both oral contraceptives and alcohol seem to reduce your body's ability to absorb riboflavin.

With all this in mind, you may want to consider taking a multivitamin or B-complex vitamin supplement to get your daily intake of riboflavin. Most people, particularly alcoholics, infants, and the elderly, don't get enough of the vitamin from food alone.

SODIUM

Daily Value: 2,400 milligrams

Good Food Sources: Cheeses, including cottage cheese; most meats, especially ham and bacon; canned soups; canned vegetables; processed lunchmeats; shellfish; canned tuna; cereals; breads; baked goods; salad dressings; potato chips; pickles; sauces. *Note:* Although we all need a certain amount of sodium to survive, most people get too much rather than too little.

You probably don't think about the amount of sodium you eat every day. But pair that little element up with chlorine to make the chemical compound sodium chloride, and you get salt—a food additive you are no doubt more than familiar with.

In the form of salt, sodium gets a bad rap for its role in raising blood pressure. But despite this, sodium is a mineral that your body needs as much as any other. It regulates the amount of fluid that your body contains; it facilitates nerve and muscle impulses; and together with potassium, it maintains the permeability of your cells' walls. This is a vital job if nutrients and other substances involved in cell maintenance are to be able to come and go as they're needed.

Clearly, your body needs sodium to function properly. The problem is that the modern American diet gives us all the sodium we need—and then some. Though the Daily Value of sodium is just 2,400 milligrams—and some research suggests that as little as 1,500 milligrams may help lower blood pressure—most Americans get over 4,000 milligrams a day. A number of factors are to blame for this overabundance of salt in the American diet. But perhaps the biggest factor is the high level of salt found in prepackaged "convenience" foods that have become staples in most American homes.

Over the past decade, two facts about our sodium intake have become abundantly clear. Fact one is that Americans are consuming almost twice as much as they should. Fact two is that high sodium intake and high blood pressure are pretty clearly linked. "A number of recent studies have essentially ended the sodium debate," says David L. Katz, MD, MPH, director of the Yale-Griffin Prevention Research Center in Derby, Connecticut, and author of *The Way to Eat*. "The connection between sodium and high blood pressure is fairly evident."

Perhaps the best evidence comes from the DASH (Dietary Approaches to Stop Hypertension) studies conducted by the National Heart, Lung, and Blood Institute. One of the studies, called DASH-Sodium, showed on a large scale that a diet with the lowest level of sodium (around 1,500 milligrams a day) had the greatest blood-pressure lowering effects. In addition, INTERSALT, a massive epidemiological study that included over 10,000 men and women in 32 countries, also affirmed that lower sodium intake equals lower blood pressure.

Using Sodium Safely

Considering the most recent research, it's apparent that limiting sodium intake will be helpful for most. Though the Daily Value is 2,400 milligrams, research indicates that even less—like 1,500 milligrams—may be better.

The problem is that it doesn't take much salt to reach that Daily Value: 2,400 milligrams of sodium equals just 1 teaspoon of table salt. Couple this with the fact that salt is almost everywhere in the modern American diet, and the challenge can seem overwhelming.

Luckily, the National Heart, Lung, and Blood Institute has a number of tips that can help you limit your sodium intake. Some of these include using fresh fruits, vegetables, and meats instead of canned choices whenever possible. And when you have to use canned products, choose low-sodium versions when available. Also, rinsing canned items in water can help remove some of the salt. Finally, choose herbs and spices rather than salt to add more flavor to meals.

For even more tips on lowering sodium in your diet, refer to the National Heart, Lung, and Blood Institute's Web site at www.nhlbi.nih.gov/hbp/prevent/sodium/sodium.htm.

SULFUR

Daily Value: None established

Good Food Sources: Meats, poultry, fish, eggs, legumes, garlic, onions, brussels sprouts, asparagus, kale, wheat germ

When most of us think of sulfur, the first thing that comes to mind is that "rotten egg" smell produced by sulfur dioxide gas. You'll usually notice this around natural hot springs or volcanic craters.

Within the body, however, sulfur can play a role that will make you forget all about that awful smell. Absorbed from protein-based foods, drinking water, and even noxious air, the sulfur taken into our bodies combines with toxins to form harmless compounds that can then be escorted to the nearest exit. Sulfur is also combined with the proteins that structure cartilage, tendons, and bone in the body, as well as with the proteins in our hair and nails.

Sulfur is available in two supplement forms—dimethyl sulfoxide (DMSO) and methylsulfonylmethane (MSM)—that have been shown to be quite useful in treating pain. And sulfur baths have proven their worth as remedies for numerous skin conditions, as well as the pain related to arthritis.

Sulfur is not related to sulfa drugs or sulfites, which are sometimes added to foods.

Using Sulfur Safely

Sulfur is so widely available from foods, water, and air that the Food and Drug Administration Research Council has established no Daily Value. It also seems to be impossible to get the wrong amount of sulfur—either too much or too little.

THIAMIN

Daily Value: 1.5 milligrams

Good Food Sources: Black beans, navy beans, brewer's yeast, cashews, peas, pork, potatoes, soy nuts, sunflower seeds, whole grains, whole-grain pasta, oatmeal and other cereals

Thiamin, also known as vitamin B_1, has the interesting distinction of being the first B vitamin to be discovered. In fact, when German chemist Casimir Funk first isolated the nutrient in 1911, he actually created the term *vitamin* to explain the "vital" role of the nutrient.

Time and research have shown that Casimir knew what he was talking about. Though its Daily Value is only 1.5 milligrams, thiamin is critical to the function of many organs. It plays a key role in breaking down carbohydrates, which makes it one of the most important nutrients required for producing energy for the body.

Perhaps thiamin's greatest role is in the health of the heart, where it has been shown to ease the symptoms of congestive heart failure. Thiamin also may delay the onset of heart disease in people with diabetes, and it may even slow the progression of HIV.

Because many cereals, pastas, and other foods in the United States are fortified with thiamin, deficiency is usually not a problem here. But many parts of the world still don't fortify food with thiamin.

Although rice and whole grains—dietary staples throughout the world—naturally contain thiamin, the process of refining them for consumption removes the nutrient. Folks living on little but devitalized rice and grains soon become thiamin-deficient and develop a disease called beriberi, with symptoms such as weakness, heart enlargement, and limb swelling that make even walking difficult.

Thiamin deficiencies have also been found to cause mood changes, vague feelings of uneasiness, fear, disorderly thinking, and other signs of mental depression—symptoms that researchers say often affect memory.

Using Thiamin Safely

Although thiamin toxicity—its symptoms include itching, tingling, and pain—has been caused by massive doses administered by injection, there has been no evidence of toxicity from oral thiamin, even when doses as high as 500 milligrams (333 times the Daily Value of 1.5 milligrams) were taken daily for a month. Experts say that excess thiamin is easily cleared by the kidneys.

TRACE MINERALS

Many of the nutrients we ingest every day—such as copper, chromium, manganese, and others—are known as trace minerals. But don't let the word *trace* mislead you. Though you need less of these minerals than some of the biggies like calcium or magnesium, they are no less important to your general health and well-being.

Several trace minerals—copper, chromium, cobalt, manganese, and molybdenum—are firmly established as essential to humans. And even though you only need a few micrograms (one thousandth of a milligram) of them instead of milligrams, you still can't live without them, at least not for very long. These minerals are necessary for certain vital chemical reactions in the body to occur, and no other elements can take their places. That's why the National Research Council has developed daily intake guidelines to help you make sure that you are getting enough.

The Estimated Safe and Adequate Daily Dietary Intakes were established for essential nutrients (including many trace minerals) that have some research to support an estimated range of requirements, but not enough to establish a Recommended Dietary Allowance or a Daily Value.

Luckily, trace minerals are found in a variety of foods and in water, so we usually get enough of every one of them to function normally, though we may not always get optimum amounts.

Several additional trace minerals, including boron, silicon, and vanadium, have been proven essential to assorted bacteria, fungi, and other microbes. And all plants need boron in order to grow. As technology improves and research deepens, these minerals may one day be shown to be essential to humans as well.

Many trace minerals act as coenzymes, so-called catalysts in chemical reactions. That means they function as spark plugs, getting chemical reactions going without actually being changed in the process. That's important, because our bodies are giant laboratories, where billions of chemical reactions are taking place all the time.

Trace minerals play roles in your body's production of neurotransmitters, biochemicals that send messages through your nervous system; in the production of major hormones secreted by your thyroid and adrenal glands; and in your body's ability to burn carbohydrates and fat for energy and to weave molecules into the tissues that become your bones, blood vessels, skin, and teeth. Along with other food components, trace minerals help you grow, reproduce, and maintain your body over the years.

Getting enough trace minerals is a perfect reason to abide by one important bit of nutritional advice: Eat a varied diet that contains whole foods. Whole grains, nuts, seeds, beans, fresh fruits and vegetables, mushrooms, shellfish, herbs, and spices are the richest sources of trace minerals. A few processed foods also contain high amounts: ham, canned pineapple juice, cocoa, and beer, which contains trace minerals from the brewer's yeast used to concoct the stuff. Yes, chocolate and beer fit into a healthy diet—in moderation, of course. And you heard it here first!

Aside from these foods, one of the best ways to get adequate doses of trace minerals in your diet is to pick a good multivitamin/mineral supplement that supplies an array of trace minerals in the ranges recommended on the following pages. With very few exceptions, there's no reason to take supplements of individual trace minerals. That's because most trace minerals are toxic in high amounts. Until more is known about these elements, especially how they interact with other nutrients, it's prudent to stick to amounts that researchers know are safe. And if you have health problems, get your doctor's okay before you begin taking any supplement.

Boron

Daily Value: None established

Good Food Sources: Cooked dried beans and peas; nuts; dark green leafy vegetables; grape juice; legumes; noncitrus fruits like blueberries, peaches, and plums

Though it's just a trace mineral, boron has been cropping up recently in a number of new supplements. Some suggest that boron can enhance memory, cognitive function, and hand-eye coordination. It's also become big in the bodybuilding world, where it is believed that boron can increase strength and muscle mass, as well as testosterone levels.

However, most experts advise steering clear of boron as a supplement. Hard scientific evidence is lacking, and doses of boron greater than 50 milligrams a day can be toxic (see "Using Boron Safely" below).

What seems more certain is that boron plays a role in bone health. It is found in high concentrations in bone. And though it's not known if boron affects bone health directly, it does enhance the absorption of calcium, magnesium, copper, and vitamin D, all of which improve bone density.

As long as you're getting enough plants in your diet, you should be getting enough boron (see "Good Food Sources" above). Meat eaters may want to add a plant every now and then to up their intake, though.

Using Boron Safely

There is no Daily Value for boron. So how much should you get? Probably about the amount you're getting now, if you're eating a well-balanced diet that contains at least five servings of fruits and vegetables a day. That's 1.5 to 3 milligrams of boron a day.

However, consumers should be leery of the number of new boron supplements on the market. Doses of boron greater than 50 milligrams a day can be toxic and cause lethargy, diarrhea, skin rashes, loss of appetite, or vomiting. Children or women who are pregnant or nursing should avoid boron supplements.

Chromium

Daily Value: 120 micrograms

Good Food Sources: Beer, black pepper, bran, cheese, coffee, lean meat, molasses, whole-grain breads and cereals

Sure, this element is essential for making the shiny stuff on cars and motorcycles. But it might be even more essential in the body. This trace mineral is important to the body for a number of reasons, but it might show the greatest promise as a treatment for diabetes. And since almost 90 percent of the population doesn't get enough chromium, it may be more important than we realize.

Think of chromium as the shovel that gets the fuel into the furnace. This trace mineral hooks up with insulin to help transport glucose (blood sugar) across cell membranes and into cells, where it can be burned for energy. People who don't get enough chromium may develop a condition called glucose intolerance; they have high blood sugar levels and often high insulin levels. The high blood sugar levels do not drop much when additional insulin is given, but they do go down when people get the chromium they need. Glucose intolerance can set the stage for type 2 (non-insulin-dependent) diabetes.

Signs of chromium deficiency include diabetes-like symptoms of high blood cholesterol and problems with insulin levels.

Since chromium helps insulin work better, it may also raise blood sugar levels in people with low blood sugar, as shown in studies by researchers with the U.S. Department of Agriculture. Chromium has also lowered the amount of insulin needed by diabetes patients in some recent studies.

Other research seems to indicate that chromium has a positive role in your heart health as well. One study found that chromium supplements helped raise HDL cholesterol, the good kind that helps escort bad cholesterol out of your body, in men taking beta-blocker drugs. Another study showed that chromium lowered triglyceride levels by as much as 20 percent in people with obesity and diabetes.

Though chromium is deficient in a number of people, the biggest problems seem to be in the elderly, people who exercise a lot, people with a lot of stress, or those who eat poor diets and a lot of sugar.

Using Chromium Safely

Even balanced diets designed by dietitians contain less than 50 micrograms of chromium and average about 15 micrograms per 1,000 calories, far less than the 120 micrograms that's recommended.

Trivalent chromium, the kind found in foods and supplements, is considered to be quite safe. Still, it's best to get no more than 200 micrograms a day from supplements without medical supervision.

On the other hand, if you work around chromium-containing compounds, you'll want to steer clear of fumes and dust. Industrial chromium, a completely different form than that found in foods, is toxic.

People with diabetes who take chromium should be under medical supervision, since their insulin dosage may need to be reduced as blood sugar drops.

Many studies detailing chromium's benefits have used chromium picolinate, an easily absorbed form. Chromium nicotinate and amino acid forms of chromium are less easily absorbed than chromium picolinate but can supply adequate amounts of the mineral. The least absorbable form is chromium chloride, which is found in some multivitamin/mineral supplements. This type binds with other components in foods and becomes mostly unabsorbable.

Chromium is sometimes sold as glucose tolerance factor (GTF), a combination of chromium, nicotinic acid (a form of niacin), and amino acids. GTF may vary so much in composition that it is not a reliable source of chromium.

Cobalt

Daily Value: None established

Good Food Sources: Dairy and other animal products

Cobalt is at the core of every molecule of vitamin B_{12}, a nutrient that's essential for the body's formation of red blood cells. That function is vital, and it's the only known function of cobalt in humans.

Using Cobalt Safely

No Daily Value has been set for cobalt; you get the amount you need from preformed vitamin B_{12}. Although B_{12} deficiency is not uncommon (some true vegetarians may develop B_{12} deficiency), cobalt deficiency has never been seen in people.

Copper

Daily Value: 2 milligrams

Good Food Sources: Beef, black pepper, cashews, clams, crab, green leafy vegetables, lentils, liver, lobster, mussels, nuts, oysters, pistachios, shellfish, soybeans, squid, unsweetened baker's chocolate, whole grains

It's hard to think of copper without imagining electrical wire, pipes, and, of course, shiny new pennies. But this bright orange metal does a lot more than keep our houses and the economy going strong. It does the same for our bodies, as well. Anyone who is concerned about heart disease or osteoporosis, and that's just about everyone, should be paying attention to copper.

Deficiencies of copper seem to help cause the onset of both of these conditions. And though more research is needed, copper supplementation might help prevent them. Copper also seems to be critical in the development of immunity, brain function, bone strength, iron transport, and the health of developing infants.

Copper plays a role in the body's formation of strong, flexible connective tissue, in the production of neurochemicals in the brain, and in the functioning of muscles, nerves, and the immune system.

"One of copper's best-understood roles so far is its function in the cross-linkage of collagen and elastin," explains Leslie Klevay, MD, ScD, professor of internal medicine at the University of North Dakota School of Medicine and Health Sciences in Grand Forks. "Copper helps knit together these two very important connective tissues, which are used throughout the body to build other tissues."

Copper-deficient animals have weakened hearts and blood vessels and may die from heart failure or a ruptured aorta, the main artery from the heart. They also have bone defects that are identical to osteoporosis. "Copper is essential for the network of connective tissue in bone on which minerals such as calcium are deposited," Dr. Klevay explains.

Copper also interacts with iron, so copper deficiency eventually leads to anemia.

Copper deficiency may be more prevalent than we know. It may be more of a marginal condition than a true deficiency in people eating normal diets, Dr. Klevay says. Still, some experts suspect that many people are getting less than optimum amounts and may suffer from chronic illnesses such as heart disease and osteoporosis as a result.

Using Copper Safely

Copper is often found in multivitamin/mineral supplements. If you want to get additional copper that way, look for a supplement that offers 1.5 to 3 milligrams of copper gluconate, Dr. Klevay says. "I prefer that people get their copper from foods," he adds.

Few people get more than 2 milligrams of copper a day from diet alone, and a fair number of people consume less than 1.5 milligrams a day, an amount that Dr. Klevay considers the bare minimum.

Copper is toxic in large amounts (it's most likely to cause vomiting), so there's simply no good reason to take more than 3 milligrams a day, Dr. Klevay says.

Zinc interferes with the body's ability to absorb copper, which is why experts who recommend zinc supplements often suggest extra copper as well, generally in a ratio of 1 milligram of copper to 10 milligrams of zinc. So if you're taking 15 milligrams of zinc (the Daily Value), you should be getting 1.5 milligrams of copper a day. And copper supplements are definitely off-limits to people with Wilson's disease, an inherited disorder that makes copper accumulate in the liver.

In addition, people who are taking large doses of vitamin C, iron, or zinc should wait at least 2 hours before taking copper supplements.

Fluoride

Estimated Safe and Adequate Daily Dietary Intake: Adults, 1.5 to 4 milligrams. Children up to age 6 months, 0.1 to 0.5 milligram; ages 6 to 11 months, 0.2 to 1 milligram; ages 1 to 3 years, 0.5 to 1.5 milligrams; ages 4 to 6 years, 1 to 2.5 milligrams; ages 7 to 18 years, 1.5 to 2.5 milligrams.

Good Food Sources: Fluoridated water; tea; marine fish with bones, such as canned salmon and mackerel

You might think that because fluoride is added to water and toothpaste, it's one of those nutrients that you just can't live without. That's not the case, although its potential for making visits to the dentist more pleasant is undisputed.

Both oral and topically applied fluoride are incorporated into tooth enamel. Fluoride protects the enamel, so it is less likely to dissolve under assault from the acid-producing bacteria that thrive in your mouth. Even adults can benefit from fluoride's tooth-toughening talents.

Fluoride is also taken up by bone tissue, making the tissue stronger, too. But studies using fluoride to strengthen bones weakened by osteoporosis have had mixed results. (For the full story on using nutrients to prevent and treat osteoporosis, see page 427.)

Using Fluoride Safely

People who drink fluoridated water get about 1 milligram per liter of water. People who don't drink fluoridated water may get very little fluoride in their diets, unless they're big tea drinkers. One cup of tea offers 1 to 3 milligrams of fluoride.

Up to 10 milligrams of fluoride a day from foods and water is considered safe for adults. You should not take more than 4 milligrams a day of supplements of rapid-release sodium fluoride.

Although fluoride supplements are available only by prescription, rapid-release forms are not safe to take in large amounts. Large amounts can cause bone pain and, in children, mottled, brown teeth.

Iodine

Daily Value: 150 micrograms

Good Food Sources: Iodized salt, lobster, shrimp, cooked oysters, marine fish, seaweed, breads, milk

Iodine is used by the thyroid gland to produce an important hormone called thyroxine. This hormone helps regulate energy production, body temperature, breathing, muscle tone, and the manufacture and breakdown of tissues. Iodine deficiency usually results in an enlargement of the thyroid gland known as goiter, visible as swelling on the front of the throat.

Recently, iodine has gained interest as a treatment for fibrocystic breast disease and even breast cancer. The trace mineral seems to be remarkably effective in breaking down the growths of tissue associated with the conditions.

"Iodine research has become a scientifically impressive area in breast disease," says Bernard A. Eskin, MD, MS, a professor at Drexel University College of Medicine in Philadelphia. "Studies on human cancer cultures show a positive or improved effect with iodine. This is indicated by a reduction of the cancerous tissue and protection from further growth as long as it is used."

The only iodine supplement currently on the market is Iodoral, a formulation that contains 5 milligrams of iodine and 7.5 milligrams of potassium iodide per tablet. The recommended dosage is one to four tablets daily, though you should work closely with a physician in establishing this dosage.

Using Iodine Safely

Thanks to iodine-fortified salt, there's no need to worry about getting enough iodine. Most people get several times the Daily Value with no ill effects. The iodine in your medicine cabinet should never be consumed, however.

Manganese

Daily Value: 2 milligrams

Good Food Sources: Canned pineapple juice, wheat bran, wheat germ, whole grains, seeds, nuts, cocoa, shellfish, tea

At first glance, manganese might easily be confused with magnesium. But though you need much less of this trace mineral, it's of equal important to your health. The word *manganese* is derived from the Greek word for *magic*. And this little-known trace mineral can apparently work its own magic in the body.

Manganese is an essential part of biochemical reactions that affect bone, cartilage, brain function, and energy supply. Manganese helps your body build and maintain strong bones. It makes up a part of molecules known as mucopolysaccharides. These molecules are used to form collagen, the strong, fibrous connective material that builds tissues throughout the body, including bone and cartilage, the rubbery cushioning found where bones meet.

In bone, a mesh of collagen provides the framework on which calcium, magnesium, and other bone-hardening minerals are deposited. Animals deficient in manganese have bone problems similar to those that develop in people with osteoporosis. Under a microscope, these animals' bones actually appear riddled with holes. Other animals that are manganese-deficient develop tendon problems.

In one study, women with osteoporosis had lower blood levels of manganese than women without osteoporosis. Another study found that supplements of calcium, manganese, zinc, and copper helped stop bone loss, but the effect of manganese alone was not tested.

Manganese is also necessary for proper brain function. Low levels have been associated with seizure disorders such as epilepsy. Manganese also helps your body break down carbohydrates and fat for energy.

Manganese deficiency has never been detected in people eating normal diets. Whether that's because people are getting enough of the mineral through foods or because deficiency symptoms go unrecognized has yet to be determined. What's interesting is that people used to get around 8 milligrams of manganese a day back in the early 20th century, thanks mostly to a diet based around whole grains, nuts, and seeds. Nowadays, changes to our diet have cut that number back to 2 to 3 milligrams.

Though the Daily Value of manganese is only 2 milligrams, some experts believe that between 3 and 5 milligrams is even more helpful. So it's best to try to eat more of the foods mentioned on page 31 to achieve that level.

Using Manganese Safely

Research indicates that amounts of up to 10 milligrams of manganese a day are safe, but there's no need to get more than 3.5 to 5 milligrams daily. To get your manganese, stick to foods that can provide you with enough of this and other trace minerals. One of the best sources of manganese is canned pineapple juice.

Some multivitamin/mineral supplements contain manganese. If you decide to take a supplement that includes this mineral, look for one that offers no more than 2 milligrams of manganese chloride, a very absorbable form. Single supplements of manganese are not available, nor are they desirable, since taking too much of this trace mineral can be toxic.

Calcium supplements may interfere with your body's ability to absorb manganese. In one study, a dose of 800 milligrams of calcium inhibited the absorption of manganese. So if you're taking calcium supplements, you might consider eating manganese-rich foods at other times of the day. You also may want to take calcium separately from a multivitamin/mineral supplement containing manganese.

Manganese toxicity has been seen in industrial exposure to the mineral and in people drinking contaminated well water. High amounts can cause symptoms similar to those of Parkinson's disease, including trembling, shuffling, and slow movement.

Molybdenum

Daily Value: 75 micrograms

Good Food Sources: Beans, whole grains, cereals, milk and milk products, dark green leafy vegetables

Come on, you can spit it out: *mo-LIB-duh-num*. This fabulous trace mineral with the funny name is a component of three enzymes, which act in the body to get important chemical reactions going.

Molybdenum is part of sulfite oxidase, an enzyme that helps the body detoxify sulfites, compounds found in proteins and used as chemical preservatives in some foods and drugs. People who can't break down sulfites have toxic buildups of this chemical in their bodies, explains Judith Turnlund, RD, PhD, of the U.S. Department of Agriculture/Agricultural Research Service Western Human Nutrition Research Center at the University of California, Davis. "Infants born with this disorder are very sick and usually don't live long," she says. These infants have a rare genetic disorder that inhibits molybdenum-containing enzymes in their bodies, and giving them extra molybdenum doesn't usually help, she says.

Some people are supersensitive to the sulfites used as additives, developing asthma and other life-threatening breathing problems. "Unfortunately, supplemental molybdenum would not be particularly helpful in reducing sulfite sensitivity in people with asthma," says Dr. Turnlund.

Molybdenum is also part of two other enzymes, xanthine oxidase and aldehyde oxidase. Both are involved in the body's production of genetic material and proteins. Xanthine oxidase also helps the body produce uric acid, an important waste product.

Physical signs of molybdenum deficiency are considered extremely rare, Dr. Turnlund says. Only one case, a man on long-term tube feeding, has ever been confirmed. Molybdenum deficiency is difficult to induce even in animals. "People eating fairly normal diets simply don't become deficient in this nutrient," Dr. Turnlund says. Most people get about 180 micrograms daily from foods.

Using Molybdenum Safely

Up to 500 micrograms of molybdenum a day has been found to be safe in research studies, but there's no reason to take that much, Dr. Turnlund says. Amounts higher than 500 micrograms may interfere with your body's metabolism of copper, another essential trace mineral.

There's also no need to get this trace mineral in supplement form, Dr. Turnlund says. Some multivitamin/mineral supplements do supply molybdenum. Stick to one that provides no more than 75 to 250 micrograms, Dr. Turnlund advises.

People with gout or high blood levels of uric acid should consult their doctor before taking supplements that contain molybdenum.

Selenium

Daily Value: 70 micrograms

Good Food Sources: Brazil nuts, seafood, meat, dairy foods, wheat germ, nuts, oats, whole-grain bread, bran, brown rice, garlic, orange juice

Call selenium the "little nutrient that could."

Though it's just a trace mineral—and rarely even listed on food nutrition labels—recent studies have shown that selenium has powerful antioxidant properties that positively affect the body in a number of ways.

Researchers used to think that industrial forms of selenium were actually carcinogenic. The reason this seems so ironic today is that recent research suggests that selenium actually helps fight certain forms of cancer, including lung, prostate, and colorectal cancer. The National Cancer Institute is in the process of conducting a large study right now to determine selenium's role in fighting cancer.

Other research has shown that selenium seems helpful in fighting viruses, most notably hepatitis and HIV. The mineral has other important roles in the body as well. It activates substances that protect the eyes from cataracts and the heart from muscle damage. It binds with toxic substances such as arsenic, cadmium, and mercury to make them less harmful. And it boosts several infection-fighting elements of your immune system.

While the research initially looked promising, recent studies have not shown supplemental selenium to have a beneficial effect on cardiovascular disease. Nonetheless, getting a daily dose of selenium from food may still provide heart-protective properties.

As an antioxidant (it's actually part of an antioxidant enzyme called glutathione peroxidase), selenium's effect seems comparable to vitamin E. In fact, selenium and vitamin E work so well together against free radicals that they frequently substitute for one another. That's why a deficiency of one of these nutrients can frequently lead to a deficiency of the other.

Using Selenium Safely

As far back as the 13th century, the famous explorer Marco Polo noted that certain forages on which his animals grazed in western China caused the animals' hooves to drop off.

In subsequent centuries, scientists found that the cause was a toxic level of selenium in the plants that animals ate and that high levels of selenium in the diet could affect humans as well as horses. The only difference seems to be that humans lose hair and nails as opposed to hooves. Other side effects of excessive selenium intake include a persistent garlic odor on your breath and skin, a metallic taste in your mouth, dizziness, and nausea for no apparent reason.

Today we know that the recommended Daily Value is 70 micrograms. Some experts suggest that you look for a selenium supplement labeled "l-selenomethionine" and avoid those marked "sodium selenite" because l-selenomethionine is less likely to cause side effects and won't react with vitamin C to block selenium absorption. Scientists caution that selenium supplements in excess of 400 micrograms per day should be taken only under medical supervision. According to one study that appeared in the August 21, 2007, issue of *Annals of Internal Medicine*, long-term supplementation may increase a person's risk of type 2 diabetes. Further research is necessary to confirm this link.

There is some debate over whether we need to take selenium supplements. Acid rain and the use of fossil fuels may be depleting the amount of selenium in the food chain. A further reduction in selenium intake can be linked to the many processed foods we eat. For these reasons, some experts have argued that the optimum amount of selenium may be much higher than the Daily Value suggests. The Brazil nut seems to be the richest source of selenium available. One ounce of the nuts, dried and unblanched, contains a whopping 550 micrograms.

If you are counting on the foods you eat as your primary source of selenium, here's something for you to think about. Plants get their selenium contents directly from the soil in which they grow. Generally, the soil in those states east of the Mississippi and west of the Rockies has a low selenium content. Crops that are grown in these areas will also have low selenium contents. Livestock is also affected, because the animals graze on plants grown in the same soil as our crops. Compounding this problem are the ions produced when we burn fossil fuels such as coal and oil. These ions acidify the soil, which hinders selenium uptake and reduces the amount of selenium found in the crops even more.

For these reasons, as well as the myriad health benefits that selenium seems to provide, you may want to make sure your daily multivitamin/mineral supplement contains selenium.

VITAMIN A

Daily Value: 5,000 IU, with a minimum of 2,331 IU for women and about 3,000 IU for men

Good Food Sources: Carrot juice, pumpkin, sweet potatoes, carrots, spinach, butternut squash, tuna, dandelion greens, cantaloupe, mangoes, turnip greens, beet greens

Give 200,000 IU of vitamin A to a malnourished child in Indonesia, Nepal, India, or Ghana, and it could save his or her life. Give 25,000 IU of beta-carotene, a vitamin A precursor, to an adult every day, and it could help prevent macular degeneration, which, after cataracts, is the leading cause of blindness in people age 50 and older.

"There was a famous physician by the name of Paracelsus who said, 'All substances are poisons. There is none which is not a poison. The right dose differentiates a poison and a remedy.' And vitamin A is a perfect example," says Narinder Duggal, MD, clinical pharmacy specialist, internist, and medical director of Liberty Bay Internal Medicine in Poulsbo, Washington. "From our understanding now, vitamin A is protective to a certain level and then becomes counterproductive; at low levels, it's an antioxidant, but at high levels, the body becomes saturated and it acts as an oxidizer, especially in people who smoke and are therefore already under oxidative stress," he says.

What is this powerful substance that can do both good and bad things in the body? Actually, vitamin A is the generic name given to a group of naturally occurring molecules called retinoids. Study after study shows that your body uses these retinoids, which are powerful compounds drawn from plant and animal sources, to build or maintain an effective immune system. Vitamin A also helps the body reproduce cells, which helps prevent cancer, and it appears to help maintain the health and function of ovaries, egg cells, sperm cells, and the placenta.

Without an adequate amount of vitamin A, your body is vulnerable to a whole host of infectious creatures that can cause anything from measles to AIDS. Those who lack vitamin A on their defense teams also face increased risk of skin problems, cancer, and blindness.

Symptoms of a vitamin A deficiency include night blindness, difficulty recovering vision (after looking into the headlights of an oncoming car, for example), distorted color vision, dry eyes, loss of appetite, poor sense of taste and smell, and difficulty keeping your balance.

Fortunately, most people in the United States get enough vitamin A from their diets. Those most at risk are people who have cancer, tuberculosis, pneumonia, chronic nephritis, urinary tract infections, or prostate disease, all of which may increase the body's demands for vitamin A. People who have digestive conditions that impair fat absorption—celiac disease and cystic fibrosis are two examples—are also at risk.

Vitamin A is a fat-soluble substance. "For vitamin A and most other vitamins, the recommendation is still that you get the bulk of them through dietary means rather than supplements," says Boyd Lyles, MD, director of the HeartHealth and Wellness Center in Dallas and medical director of L A Weight Loss. There are two reasons doctors recommend getting vitamin A from foods versus supplements: (1) foods contain hundreds of other substances that may have healthful benefits, and (2) although excessive amounts of vitamin A are usually toxic, large amounts of beta-carotene—the form that is often found in foods—usually are not. And your body will turn beta-carotene from yellow and orange vegetables into the vitamin A it needs. There is one exception: Both vitamin A and beta-carotene can damage the liver in someone who drinks heavily.

Although vitamin A deficiency is rare in the United States, there are some people in this country who do not get the vitamin A they need. "In people who are not consuming enough vitamin A–rich foods like liver, fish, egg yolks, carrots, and yellow vegetables, there may be some benefit in taking vitamin A supplements," Dr. Lyles says. If you do decide to take supplements, taking beta-carotene can be safer than taking vitamin A because beta-carotene doesn't build up in the body the way vitamin A does. And children, people with kidney or liver disease, and pregnant women should *always* take beta-carotene instead of supplemental vitamin A.

Using Vitamin A Safely

For centuries, Arctic adventurers, Eskimos, and even sled dogs have known that eating polar bear liver can make them sick. The reason? It's loaded with enough vitamin A to poison a full-grown adult. A single meal consisting of a half-pound to 1 pound of polar bear liver contains a whopping 3 million to 13 million IU of vitamin A, which is 6 to 26 times the amount needed to cause acute vitamin A poisoning.

Only 500,000 IU of vitamin A, taken over a short period of time, can cause irritability, headaches, vomiting, bone pain, weakness, and blurred vision. Regular use of even 50,000 IU a day can cause hair loss, weakness, headaches, enlarged liver and spleen, anemia, stiffness, and joint pain. And at least one death has been reported from the regular use of 25,000 IU every day. "These days, we tend to think that more than 2,500 IU on a chronic basis, or more than 25,000 IU on an acute basis, is too much," Dr. Duggal says. As a result, the safe upper limit for vitamin A has been set at 10,000 IU.

Women of childbearing age need to be particularly careful when supplementing vitamin A. Daily doses of 10,000 IU during the first 3 months of pregnancy have been linked to a high risk of birth defects. And 25,000 IU daily is known to cause spontaneous abortions when taken early in pregnancy. For these reasons, women of childbearing age should take beta-carotene instead of supplemental vitamin A and check with their doctor before they do so. They should also check their multivitamin/mineral supplements to make sure they are not getting more than the safe upper limit of 10,000 IU.

The bottom line? In different amounts and situations, vitamin A can be either a miraculous healing agent or it can be a malicious, toxic compound. It's a good idea to try to get it from foods and to consult your doctor before supplementing.

VITAMIN B$_6$

Daily Value: 2 milligrams

Good Food Sources: Bananas, potatoes with skin, avocados, chicken, beef, brewer's yeast, eggs, brown rice, soybeans, oats, whole wheat, peanuts, lentils, walnuts

From migraines and memory loss to diabetes and PMS, the list of conditions for which vitamin B$_6$, also called pyridoxine, is gaining acceptance as a possible treatment is long.

Vitamin B$_6$ serves the important purpose of ensuring that biological processes, including immune function and fat and protein metabolism, take place in the body. "And there is evidence that B$_6$ helps with blood sugar regulation," says Boyd Lyles, director of the HeartHealth and Wellness Center in Dallas and medical director of L A Weight Loss. Specifically, B$_6$ helps ensure that you have an adequate supply of glucose in your blood. When you're not using glucose, it is stored in your muscles. B$_6$ helps release it into your blood so you can use it. When it comes to diabetes, a shortage of vitamin B$_6$ has been linked to something called glucose intolerance, which is an abnormally high rise in blood sugar after eating. Lack of vitamin B$_6$ may also impair the secretion of insulin and glucagon, the hormone that tells your pancreas when to stop producing insulin.

Vitamin B$_6$ is also important in brain function. This nutrient is vital in helping to create neurotransmitters, the chemicals that allow brain cells to communicate with one another. As a result, a lack of B$_6$ impairs your memory, causing trouble with your ability to register, retain, and retrieve information.

Because of their positive effects on the immune system, shortages of the B vitamins can also lead to nerve damage in the hands and feet. Some studies indicate that people with diabetes experience less of the numbness and tingling of diabetes-caused nerve damage if they get supplemental amounts of B vitamins such as B$_6$ and B$_{12}$.

In addition, there are some good data showing that women with PMS experience a reduction in symptoms with vitamin B$_6$, says Narinder Duggal, MD, clinical pharmacy specialist, internist, and medical director of Liberty Bay Internal Medicine in Poulsbo, Washington. "The thinking is that B$_6$ may ease PMS symptoms because it helps in the clearing of excess estrogen from the body, and it can also help ease depression. Individuals with PMS suffer from both mood instability and a hormonal imbalance, and B$_6$ seems to help with both," he says. There is also some evidence that vitamin B$_6$ is useful in preventing migraines, both general migraines and menstrual migraines associated with PMS, he adds.

Another potential use of vitamin B$_6$ is on the horizon. Several studies show that people with cardiovascular disease tend to have lower levels of B$_6$, which may have something to do with the relationship between B$_6$ and homocysteine, a substance that has been linked with a higher risk of cardiovascular disease. B$_6$ is one of the vitamins that can help decrease the amount of homocysteine in the blood, thus potentially lowering heart disease risk, she says.

Using Vitamin B$_6$ Safely

Even the foods richest in vitamin B$_6$—such as bananas, avocados, brewer's yeast, and beef—provide barely a single milligram. But that doesn't necessarily mean you'll need to reach for a supplement, since the Daily Value is only 2 milligrams.

And if you do opt for a supplement, you should use caution. Too much vitamin B$_6$ has been linked to serious nerve disorders as well as to oversensitivity to sunlight, which produces a skin rash and numbness.

Experts recommend you consult with your health care professional before taking more than 100 milligrams of vitamin B$_6$ a day. It's also a good idea to get vitamin B$_6$ as part of a B-complex tablet that provides the Daily Value of all the B vitamins. People who are undergoing levodopa therapy for Parkinson's disease should avoid vitamin B$_6$ supplements altogether, because B$_6$ has been found to reduce the drug's effectiveness.

Vitamin B$_6$ has also been shown to reduce the levels of isoniazid, for tuberculosis; monoamine oxidase (MAO) inhibitors; and penicillamine, for Wilson's disease. And some antibiotics, cardiac medications, estrogen, and diuretics may cause depleted levels of B$_6$ in the blood. If you are taking any of these drugs, you might want to talk to your doctor before taking a B$_6$ supplement.

VITAMIN B$_{12}$

Daily Value: 6 micrograms

Good Food Sources: Clams, ham, cooked oysters, king crab, herring, salmon, tuna, cheese, organ meats

Short of an accident, there are few faster ways to short-circuit your body than bypassing vitamin B$_{12}$. That's because B$_{12}$, also called cobalamin, is vital to the production of myelin, the fatty sheath that insulates nerve fibers, keeping electrical impulses moving through your body.

Because of the nutrient's important nerve-protecting function, a whole host of problems have been linked to low levels of vitamin B$_{12}$, including memory loss, confusion, delusion, fatigue, loss of balance, decreased reflexes, impaired touch or pain perception, numbness and tingling in the arms and legs, tinnitus, and noise-induced hearing loss. Deficiencies of B$_{12}$ have also been linked to multiple sclerosis–like symptoms and dementia. When someone is deficient in B$_{12}$, the lack of healthy myelin will lead to disrupted nerve transmission, which, in turn, leads to tingling in the fingers and the bottoms of the feet.

But healthy myelin is only the beginning of vitamin B$_{12}$'s importance. Researchers have discovered that a deficiency raises blood levels of a substance known as homocysteine. Vitamin B$_{12}$ helps convert homocysteine into methionine, which brings down homocysteine levels. In addition to being toxic to brain cells in high doses, raising serious questions about its possible role in Alzheimer's disease, homocysteine may be one of the primary causes of heart disease. So the lower your homocysteine level, the lower your risk for heart disease. There's evidence that in some people, the accumulation of homocysteine may be caused by a genetic defect, while in others, it's simply the result of a vitamin B$_{12}$ deficiency. Such homocysteine buildup also seems to occur with folate and B$_6$ deficiencies.

Because vitamin B$_{12}$ is also important for the production of red blood cells, a severe deficiency, called pernicious anemia, can lower energy levels. "There is a type of anemia called macrocytic anemia, and the most common cause of macrocytic anemia is folate and B$_{12}$ deficiency," says Narinder Duggal, MD, clinical pharmacy specialist, internist, and medical director of Liberty Bay Internal Medicine in Poulsbo, Washington. "What happens with macrocytic anemia is that your blood cells are larger than they should be because they are not dividing properly," he says.

Because vitamin B$_{12}$ is found in animal products, vegans—strict vegetarians who avoid dairy products and eggs as well as meats—are at risk for becoming B$_{12}$-deficient. If someone is consuming animal products and then becomes a vegetarian or a vegan, he or she will generally have stored up enough B$_{12}$ to last a few years. The vitamin gets circulated throughout the body and reabsorbed in the intestinal tract. So a person may not have symptoms for a while and then start to show signs of B$_{12}$ deficiency after a few years of not eating meat. In fact, one study documented cases of children of vegans whose growth was stunted because they did not get adequate B$_{12}$.

Even some people who do eat meats and dairy products can have what's known as food-bound malabsorption. People with food-bound malabsorption can't absorb B$_{12}$ from food because the B$_{12}$ is attached to protein, and the body needs to be able to remove the B$_{12}$ from that protein in order to absorb it. So even when they eat enough vitamin B$_{12}$ foods, people with food-bound malabsorption may be B$_{12}$-deficient. These people *can* absorb B$_{12}$ from supplements, however.

In addition, there are a lot of people in this country who have had bariatric or weight loss surgery. The surgery changes the size of the stomach and, therefore, the amount of stomach acid produced, so less B_{12} gets absorbed. Plus, the surgery often bypasses part of the small intestine where nutrient absorption—B_{12} included—takes place.

Using Vitamin B₁₂ Safely

It's easy to get adequate amounts of vitamin B_{12} from food sources, because you need so little of it. So there's really no need to take a supplement unless you fit into one of the previously mentioned categories or your doctor tells you to do so.

Doctors often prescribe shots for those who have trouble absorbing vitamin B_{12}, however. It's becoming more common for people with B_{12} deficiencies to get monthly intramuscular injections. If you have absorption problems, doctors recommend using sublingual B_{12} tablets, normally placed under the tongue, or a B_{12} nasal gel. Both are available in health food stores. For those without absorption problems, oral tablets are available, but doctors recommend both sublingual tablets and nasal gel as alternatives.

Vitamin B_{12} supplements are considered extremely safe; even huge excess doses are harmlessly excreted in your urine. If you get injections, there may be some discomfort at the injection site, and in rare cases, sensitive people could have allergic reactions to B_{12}. If you have any of the following conditions, you should check with your doctor before using B_{12}: folate deficiency, iron deficiency, any kind of infection, Leber's disease, polycythemia vera, or uremia.

VITAMIN C

Daily Value: 60 milligrams

Good Food Sources: Pineapple, broccoli, peppers, cantaloupe, strawberries, oranges, kiwifruit, pink grapefruit, papaya, cauliflower, chili peppers

Linus Pauling is gone, dead at the age of 93 from cancer. But at the Linus Pauling Institute at Oregon State University in Corvallis, and in research labs across the country, his scientific legacy lives on. Experts continue to investigate the healing potential of vitamin C, also called ascorbic acid.

"We're conducting research projects that explore the role of vitamin C in cardiovascular disease, cancer, immunity, cataracts, skin health, and other physiological and pathological conditions," says Stephen Lawson, MD, administrative officer of the Institute.

There's good reason to believe that further research will bear even more fruit. While skeptics continue to carp, already dozens of studies strongly suggest that vitamin C plays a role in preventing a variety of diseases. And there are a growing number of doctors who are using the nutrient to treat disease as well.

Vitamin C is thought to help protect the esophagus, oral cavity, stomach, and pancreas—and possibly the cervix, rectum, and breasts—from cancer. How does it do all of that?

Some forms of cancer are thought to be caused by what are called free radicals, naturally occurring renegade molecules that damage the body's healthy molecules (such as DNA, in the case of cancer) by stealing electrons to balance themselves. Vitamin C and other substances known as antioxidants neutralize free radicals by offering their own electrons, minimizing oxidative damage to DNA and other molecules. "The best way to describe it is this: If you cut an apple in half and let it sit on a shelf for a few hours, it will turn brown," says Narinder Duggal, MD, clinical pharmacy specialist, internist, and medical director of Liberty Bay Internal Medicine in Poulsbo, Washington. "But if you put lemon juice on the apple, it will last forever on the shelf because the vitamin C in the juice acts as an antioxidant," he says. Nitrites, potentially cancer-causing preservatives found in foods such as hot dogs and lunchmeats, and nitrates—found naturally in vegetables and drinking water—are also neutralized by vitamin C.

The long arm of vitamin C's antioxidant protection may also extend to heart health. In the National Health and Nutrition Examination Survey (NHANES I), participants who consumed more than 50 milligrams of vitamin C per day from foods together with vitamin C supplements (for a total daily intake of 300 milligrams of vitamin C) had a lowered risk of cardiovascular disease. Specifically, the study found that the risk of death from cardiovascular disease was 42 percent lower in men and 25 percent lower in women. In addition, a recent analysis of several large-scale studies in adults found that taking more than 700 milligrams per day of vitamin C for 10 years reduced the risk of heart disease by 25 percent, Dr. Lawson says.

Vitamin C also appears to help prevent stroke. A community of Japanese women who took vitamin C were followed for about 20 years and found to have a lower risk of stroke. However, these women also had a very high intake of fruits and vegetables, so it's not fully understood whether it was the vitamin C by itself or the combination of vitamin C and the fruits and vegetables that lowered the risk of stroke.

There have also been some studies showing that vitamin C can help with blood vessel dilation in doses of 500 milligrams per day. Vitamin C also helps make and stabilize nitric oxide, a signaling molecule that helps relax arteries. "And many studies have shown that doses of 500 milligrams to 2,000 milligrams of vitamin C lowered blood pressure in people with hypertension," Dr. Lawson says.

Vitamin C's role as an antioxidant may even help delay or prevent cataract formation. The nutrient may be beneficial because ultraviolet light and oxidative stress in the lens of the eye are thought to be leading causes of cataract formation. Vitamin C can help prevent the damage caused by oxidative stress.

"Higher intakes than a few hundred milligrams per day may be necessary to help prevent cataracts," Dr. Lawson says.

Cold sufferers have raved for years about vitamin C's effect on what ails them. Research shows that high intake of this water-soluble vitamin actually supercharges some of the immune system's most important defense cells, helping them move faster while tracking down potential pathogens such as bacteria and viruses. That means you may not be able to prevent a cold by taking vitamin C, but you can probably make it shorter and less severe. Not only that, but vitamin C has also been found to reduce levels of histamine, a chemical released by the body that can dampen immune response, says Carol S. Johnston, PhD, RD, professor and chair of the department of nutrition at Arizona State University in Mesa.

This antihistamine benefit may also be good news for folks suffering from asthma or allergies. Researchers at Harvard Medical School found that people who got at least 200 milligrams of vitamin C a day had a 30 percent reduced risk of bronchitis or wheezing compared with people who got about 100 milligrams of vitamin C a day.

Researchers at the Linus Pauling Institute have found that vitamin C inhibits replication of HIV, at least in infected cells in the laboratory. And some studies show that vitamin C may also be beneficial for people with diabetes, specifically because it may help minimize the effects of the disease on the kidneys, eyes, and nerves. As if all of that weren't enough, vitamin C has long been known to protect gums, joints, ligaments, artery walls, and skin. It also improves wound healing by aiding the production of collagen, the building block of tissues. "About one-third of your body's protein is collagen, which means you're in pretty bad shape without vitamin C," says Dr. Johnston.

Although most people have heard of vitamin C's healing benefits, many may be depleted of this important nutrient. In a study conducted at Arizona State University, Dr. Johnston found that 60 percent of the participants got about 125 milligrams of vitamin C a day, more than twice the Daily Value. Between 18 and 20 percent, however, were depleted, and roughly 3 percent had blood vitamin C levels that indicated they should be suffering from scurvy, a potentially fatal deficiency disease once common among sailors. "We saw in our population that the ones who were deficient ate less than one serving of fruits and vegetables a day, when it is recommended that you eat five to nine servings," says Dr. Johnston.

Early signs of vitamin C depletion include weakness and lethargy, followed by delayed wound healing. If stores of vitamin C are completely exhausted, a rare occurrence today, scurvy appears. Its symptoms include dementia, bleeding gums, tooth loss, hemorrhages, and pain in muscles, bones, and joints.

Using Vitamin C Safely

Scan the shelves in your local health food store, and you may see more forms and brands of vitamin C than new cars at a dealership.

But don't worry about which one to buy. All of the forms are good sources of vitamin C. Whether the vitamin C is top-of-the-line or bargain-basement, the amount that your body uses is the same. "I compared ones that are expensive with those that are dirt cheap—two bucks a bottle—and there was no difference," says Dr. Johnston. "In other words, additives like rose hips, manipulation like buffering, and cost didn't have any impact on bioavailability." There may be one small difference, however: Buffered vitamin C could cause slightly less diarrhea in high doses than other forms.

And high doses do seem to be safe. Megadoses of vitamin C, between 500 and 2,000 milligrams every 4 hours, have been used to acidify urine, which affects the way some medications are absorbed. In no fewer than five clinical studies, folks who took 5,000 milligrams a day for more than 3 years reported no side effects. However, you may be wasting your money. "Except in the case of an acute cold, which may be shortened by taking 1,000 milligrams of vitamin C two to three times a day, all you really need on a chronic basis is 250 to 500 milligrams two to three times a day," Dr. Duggal says. Large doses of vitamin C may inhibit the absorption of tricyclic antidepressants and may interfere with the results of some diagnostic urine and blood tests. Therefore, if you are taking antidepressants or undergoing any tests, be sure to tell your doctor that you are also taking large doses of vitamin C. And do not exceed 1,000 milligrams of vitamin C a day if you are taking statins, because the vitamin can dramatically reduce the benefits of statin drugs. And as mentioned, high doses of vitamin C—usually more than 2,000 milligrams—can cause diarrhea. (If you experience this reaction, experts recommend taking the vitamin in divided doses with meals throughout the day.)

People who have deficiencies in a red blood cell enzyme called glucose-6-phosphate dehydrogenase should not take large doses of vitamin C because it can damage their red blood cells and cause anemia. This deficiency is most common among people of African, Mediterranean, or Asian descent. Some experts recommend limiting the use of chewable vitamin C tablets because they can cause enamel loss from the surface of the teeth and other dental problems.

VITAMIN D

Daily Value: 400 IU

Good Food Sources: Herring, sardines, salmon, fortified milk, eggs, fortified cereals, veal, beef, egg yolks

The *D* in vitamin D could very well stand for *different*. How else to describe the only nutrient that's both made by your body (vitamin D is synthesized through your skin by the action of ultraviolet light that's present in sunlight) and required in your diet?

Without it, another *D* word comes to mind: *devastating*. Children who don't get adequate vitamin D develop rickets, a condition characterized by flaring ankles and wrists that have noticeable knobby bumps and by weak, soft leg bones that bow under the child's own weight. Similarly, adults risk developing osteomalacia, a condition similar to rickets but occurring in developed bones. Some experts believe that not getting enough vitamin D can make osteoporosis worse. Osteoporosis is a bone-weakening disease that leads to fractures and tooth loss.

Vitamin D is responsible for getting the important bone builders calcium and phosphorus to the places in the body that they need to go to help bone grow in children and remineralize in adults. It does this first by making certain these minerals are absorbed in the intestines, second by bringing calcium from bones into the blood, and third by helping the kidneys reabsorb the two minerals. In the case of rickets, the body is desperately trying to make bone, but adequate calcium and phosphorus aren't available. It's a poor effort. The result is a mass of unmineralized bone accumulation.

"Vitamin D is a huge player in osteoporosis right now," says Narinder Duggal, MD, clinical pharmacy specialist, internist, and medical director of Liberty Bay Internal Medicine in Poulsbo, Washington. Calcium is important for the density of bone, but vitamin D appears to be equally important for the *quality* of bone, meaning the strength of the bone, as well as the strength of the tendons and ligaments that help support it, Dr. Duggal says.

In addition to its role in bones, more extensive roles for vitamin D have recently been suggested by the discovery of the vitamin D receptor (VDR) in tissues that are not involved in calcium and phosphate metabolism, including immune system regulation and cancer prevention, says Gerard Mullin, MD, director of integrative GI nutrition services and capsule endoscopy in the division of gastroenterology and liver diseases at Johns Hopkins Hospital in Baltimore. Vitamin D deficiency has also been linked to type 1 and type 2 diabetes. Fortified milk is one ready source of vitamin D, although it takes a quart to provide the Daily Value. But you shouldn't rely on diet alone to give you the vitamin D you need. Most experts recommend at least 15 minutes of bright sunlight a day—without sunblock—to help your body make what it needs.

"It depends on where you are in relation to the equator, but in northern climates during the winter, the sun is at such an angle that the light rays don't penetrate the skin to make vitamin D," says H. F. DeLuca, PhD, chairman of the department of biochemistry at the University of Wisconsin-Madison. "During the summer, you can store up quite a bit of vitamin D in your fat cells. If your diet is good, it will probably last you through the winter." Sitting next to a sun-filled picture window or driving in a car doesn't count; the glass filters out the rays you need.

Fortunately, kids are born with enough vitamin D to last them 9 months. Adults aren't as lucky, however. Many Americans have indoor jobs, so getting 10 to 15 minutes per day is hard for a lot of people, says Carol Wagner, MD, a professor in the department of pediatrics at the Medical University of South Carolina in Charleston who has done extensive research on vitamin D.

In addition, "there is mounting evidence that vitamin D deficiency in elderly people is a silent epidemic that results in bone loss and fractures," reports Michael F. Holick, MD, PhD, professor in the section of endocrinology, diabetes, nutrition, and weight management and director of the General Clinical Research Center at Boston University Medical Center. A study published in the *American Journal of Clinical Nutrition* showed that 10 percent of older people were deficient in vitamin D, and 37 percent had insufficient levels.

Vitamin D also plays a role in immune function. "Vitamin D regulates the balance of pro- and anti-inflammatory molecules that are produced by the cells in the immune system, so it acts kind of like a master regulator of immunity," says Dr. Mullin. Vitamin D also appears to help prevent cancer "by acting as a DNA editor," says Narinder Duggal, MD, clinical pharmacy specialist, internist, and medical director of Liberty Bay Internal Medicine in Poulsbo, Washington. "Vitamin D works to clean up the mistakes in DNA that can lead to cancer," he says.

Using Vitamin D Safely

When eight people in Massachusetts developed symptoms such as nausea, weakness, constipation, and irritability just from drinking fresh vitamin D-fortified milk, doctors scratched their heads—that is, until they discovered that the milk had accidentally been fortified with more than 580 times the proper amount of vitamin D.

Such massive overfortifications are rare. But they're a good example of what can happen when you get too much vitamin D. Because the nutrient is stored in fat cells, long-term high doses can cause calcium to be deposited in the soft tissues of the body and can result in irreversible damage to the kidneys and cardiovascular system. High intake of vitamin D can even lead to coma.

Because vitamin D can be so toxic, you should never take doses exceeding 2,000 IU unless prescribed by your doctor. "Vitamin D is different from vitamins such as A, where you have to get nervous about toxicity at a particular level," Dr. Mullin says. "Everyone has a different response to it in terms of toxicity," he says. To make sure you are getting—and making—an appropriate amount of vitamin D, experts recommend asking your doctor to have your levels tested periodically.

VITAMIN E

Daily Value: 30 IU

Good Food Sources: Vegetable and nut oils, including soybean, safflower, and corn; sunflower seeds; whole grains; wheat germ; spinach

Vitamin E may well prove to be one of the most powerful antioxidants around.

Studies indicate that it fights heart disease, specifically by lowering LDL cholesterol; prevents cancer; alleviates respiratory problems; and boosts your immune system's ability to fight off infectious disease. It may also prevent some of the damage that diabetes does to the body, particularly to the eyes.

How does a simple vitamin achieve such complex results? Vitamin E works in a variety of ways, but a key mechanism seen in the laboratory is its ability to neutralize free radicals, naturally occurring unstable molecules that can damage your body's healthy molecules by stealing electrons to balance themselves.

The main function of vitamin E is as an antioxidant. It helps defend against free radicals formed during normal metabolism or through exposure to environmental toxins such as cigarettes or pollution. Free radicals can damage the fats found in cell membranes, which leaves cells vulnerable to destruction.

"Vitamin E appears to help with bloodflow and, therefore, healing," says Boyd Lyles, MD, director of the HeartHealth and Wellness Center in Dallas and medical director for L A Weight Loss.

What happens in the laboratory seems to translate into what happens in real life…at lower doses, that is. Although some past animal and observational studies have shown that high doses of vitamin E could help prevent both cardiovascular disease and cancer, the latest research is contradictory. A study published in the *Annals of Internal Medicine* looked at death rates in 14 published clinical trials on vitamin E supplementation (average supplementation was 400 IU per day) that took place from 1993 to 2004. They found that 200 IU of vitamin E or less per day was safe—and even potentially beneficial—for preventing and treating heart disease. But the study found that individuals who take more than 400 IU per day were 10 percent more likely to die than those who did not.

"When vitamin E was tested in individuals with heart disease, it was shown to have a benefit for those individuals, but for normal healthy people, the question remains open," says Meir Stampfer, MD, DrPH, professor of nutrition and epidemiology at Harvard School of Public Health.

Vitamin E seems to benefit people with heart disease in two ways. First, it seems to be especially effective in lowering bad LDL cholesterol, thus preventing the buildup of plaques in the arteries. And second, it acts as a blood thinner, which allows blood to flow more easily through the arteries.

Yet despite this vitamin's potential ability to prevent disease, research shows that many older adults do not get even the Daily Value of 30 IU of vitamin E. It's always a good idea to try to get vitamin E from food first. But if you can't seem to get enough nuts and/or oils to get enough, you will have to take supplements.

There are eight different forms of the vitamin. But the supplement labeled "d-alpha-tocopherol" is the one that will give you the biggest bang for your buck. It makes more vitamin E available to your body than any other form.

D-alpha-tocopherol loses its potency when exposed to air, heat, and light, so make sure it's stored in a cool, dark place. It should be taken with a meal that contains fat; otherwise your body cannot absorb it adequately. It should not be taken at the same time as an iron supplement, since iron seems to destroy vitamin E before it can get down to business.

Using Vitamin E Safely

People who are taking anticoagulants (sometimes called blood thinners or heart medicine) should not take vitamin E supplements because they can be harmful. Some experts think it's also a good idea for people who have had strokes or bleeding problems to consult their doctors before taking supplements. Vitamin E can also interfere with the absorption and action of vitamin K, which is involved in blood coagulation.

Also, researchers at the Linus Pauling Institute in Corvallis, Oregon, have discovered that vitamin C recycles vitamin E in people. In other words, vitamin E is more effective when taken along with vitamin C.

On the other hand, those who are taking anticonvulsants, cholesterol-lowering drugs, tuberculosis drugs, ulcer medication, or the antibiotic neomycin should probably talk to their doctor about increasing the amount of vitamin E they take. All of these medications can increase the body's need for the nutrient.

VITAMIN K

Daily Value: 80 micrograms

Good Food Sources: Cauliflower; broccoli; green leafy vegetables such as spinach and kale; some vegetable oils such as canola, olive, soybean, and cottonseed

Unless you were born within the past couple of minutes, your chances of having a vitamin K deficiency are pretty slim. Your body needs such tiny amounts of this nutrient to help blood clot when you're injured—this is vitamin K's primary job—that you most likely get more than enough without making any effort at all. You can even manufacture your own vitamin K. About half of the vitamin K your body needs is normally produced by your own intestinal bacteria.

Babies are the big exception. They lack the bacteria necessary to produce vitamin K, and they're usually not up to a diet of green leafy vegetables for quite a while. And although breast milk has a small amount of the nutrient, it's one of the few instances in which breast milk is simply not enough. So babies are generally given a shot of vitamin K at birth.

The only other folks who need an extra boost of supplemental vitamin K are people with diseases that can affect vitamin K absorption, such as cystic fibrosis, celiac disease, Crohn's disease, and gallbladder disease.

But there are some folks who are afraid that they get too much vitamin K. Many people who are taking anticoagulants, or blood thinners, to prevent heart attack and stroke actually cut down on the amounts of green leafy vegetables they eat for fear of triggering the same events that their medications are trying to prevent. But reducing intake of vitamin K may increase the effect of anticoagulants, in turn raising the risk of bleeding.

The better thing to do is to keep your consumption of leafy green vegetables about the same when you're taking a blood-thinning drug, says Arthur I. Jacknowitz, PharmD, distinguished chair and professor of clinical pharmacy at West Virginia University in Morgantown. The reason? Every individual's anticoagulant dose is custom-tailored to his or her particular needs. Those needs are identified through a series of blood tests when the anticoagulants are started. The amount of anticoagulant then prescribed is intended to strike a very delicate balance, giving your body enough vitamin K to clot and heal wounds but not enough to clot and cause a heart attack.

Therefore, it's important to get about the same amount of vitamin K as you normally do in your diet when you're taking an anticoagulant rather than cutting back on the nutrient.

You'll also find vitamin K in supplements that help strengthen bones. That's because vitamin K helps usher calcium into bones and keep calcium from escaping in urine. Researchers have found that people with osteoporosis tend to have low levels of vitamin K.

After following more than 72,000 women for 10 years, investigators for the Nurses' Health Study found that women with the lowest intake of vitamin

K were at 30 percent higher risk for suffering a bone fracture than women with the highest intake. Meanwhile, the Framingham Heart Study found that getting 250 micrograms of vitamin K a day, which is approximately the amount in a half-cup of broccoli or mixed greens, lowered the risk of hip fractures in elderly men and women.

In general, a multivitamin will include 10 to 25 micrograms of vitamin K, according to the Linus Pauling Institute at Oregon State University in Corvallis. Supplements to strengthen bones may contain 100 to 120 micrograms of the vitamin.

Using Vitamin K Safely

Since your body can absorb vitamin K only when it's accompanied by dietary fat, it's best to eat your leafy greens with a food that contains at least some fat. A dollop of oil-based salad dressing on a bed of greens or even a serving of lettuce on a lean burger will make sure your vitamin K is there when you need it.

ZINC

Daily Value: 15 milligrams

Good Food Sources: Cooked oysters, beef, lamb, eggs, whole grains, nuts, yogurt

When you think zinc, think productivity. From helping to create new skin and sperm cells to boosting the immune system, this mineral works overtime to produce the cells you need to keep healthy.

"Healing, growth, pregnancy, and lactation are all situations where there is an increased need for zinc because of the need for more cells," says Adria Sherman, PhD, professor of nutritional sciences at Rutgers University in New Brunswick, New Jersey.

A classic example is immune defense. Before your body can battle a foreign invader, zinc and chemicals called zinc-dependent enzymes work together to help build new immune system cells and whip them into fighting trim. That's why zinc is helpful in fending off viral infections.

Zinc's effect on your immune system may even help you get through busy, stressful times when you're not eating right or avoiding the gym.

By the same token, too much zinc—just 25 milligrams a day in one study—has been found to decrease immunity.

Zinc's quick cell replication skills come in handy when you have cuts or wounds. It's vital for the production of collagen, the connective tissue that helps wounds heal. Without zinc, wounds don't heal as quickly.

Although research is preliminary, some doctors recommend zinc to treat an enlarged prostate. The high levels of zinc in pumpkin seeds have been shown to help shrink an enlarged prostate in studies. In addition to eating a handful of pumpkin seeds every day, drizzling pumpkin seed oil over salads, meat, or chicken may help.

Even several key enzymes that protect and preserve your vision can't be formed without zinc. A large national trial found that people who took a combination of antioxidants and zinc lowered their risk of developing age-related macular degeneration by 25 percent, even though they are at high risk for the disease.

The benefits of zinc aside, it's likely that most Americans simply don't get enough of this mineral. In fact, one study found that 30 percent of healthy elderly people are zinc deficient.

Another potential problem: Increased calcium intake, recommended to prevent osteoporosis, removes some zinc from the body. In a study of post-menopausal women, giving them 890 additional milligrams of calcium a day reduced their absorption of zinc.

Signs of possible deficiency include impaired immunity, weight loss, bloating, loss of appetite, rashes and other skin changes, bedsores, hair loss, diminished sense of taste or smell, absence of menstrual periods, and depression.

Using Zinc Safely

While it's best to get zinc from foods, you can choose from several zinc supplements. But be careful not to take too much. More is not necessarily better. Excessive amounts can cause nausea, headaches, lethargy, and irritability. In fact, taking more than 2,000 milligrams of zinc sulfate has been known to cause stomach irritation and vomiting.

Even taking between 30 and 150 milligrams of zinc daily for several weeks interferes with copper absorption and can cause copper deficiency. (For this reason, doctors often recommend that those using zinc supplements take additional copper, in a ratio of 1 milligram of copper to 10 milligrams of zinc.) More than 30 milligrams of zinc a day can increase your risk of developing anemia. Such high doses have also been found to lower levels of HDL, the "good" cholesterol, while raising levels of LDL, the "bad" cholesterol. (A doctor may, however, recommend amounts this high to treat Wilson's disease, a condition involving excess copper in the body.) And increased dietary zinc has been shown to markedly decrease mental functioning in people with Alzheimer's disease.

Although small amounts of zinc may help the prostate, researchers are finding that more than 100 milligrams of zinc a day can lead to prostate cancer. In a study of 47,000 men, the National Cancer Institute found that those taking more than 100 milligrams of zinc a day had double the risk of develop-

Drugs Can Sabotage Your Nutrition

You're doing everything you can to eat right. You pay careful attention to getting all of the right nutrients, and that means you're probably taking vitamin and mineral supplements. And you're sure that you have all your nutritional bases covered. But do you really?

If you regularly take medication, either prescription or over-the-counter, you should be aware that some drugs are potential nutrition robbers. Nutrition researchers now know that drug-nutrient interaction is a potentially serious problem. Some drugs can remove nutrients from the body, prevent absorption of nutrients, or affect the body's ability to convert nutrients into usable forms.

For instance, proton-pump inhibitors, which include over-the-counter and prescription medications such as omeprazole (Prilosec) to treat gastroesophageal reflux disease, alter the pH of the stomach and by doing so may inhibit the absorption of calcium, says Arthur I. Jacknowitz, PharmD, distinguished chair and professor in the department of clinical pharmacy at West Virginia University in Morgantown. As a result, you're at a higher risk of developing osteoporosis when you take these drugs for a long period of time, especially if you're elderly or are at risk for developing the disease.

Also, diuretics and antihypertensive agents may deplete minerals and electrolytes in your body, such as calcium, potassium, and magnesium. Diuretics are used to treat hypertension and work to reduce salt in the body, Dr. Jacknowitz says. A depletion of minerals and electrolytes can result in feelings of tiredness and sleepiness, which, if not recognized, can proceed to coma, seizures, and even death, he says.

In fact, medical experts have determined that of the top 25 drugs prescribed most often, 19 have the potential for causing serious nutrient deficiencies.

Pregnant and nursing women, infants, and the elderly may be even more at risk. They may be more deficient in essential nutrients to begin with.

See the table on pages 56–57 for a list of some common prescription drugs and their nutrient interactions. If you're taking any of these

ing advanced prostate cancer, compared with men who didn't take zinc.

Because of these risks, doctors recommend that zinc supplements in excess of 15 milligrams a day be taken only under medical supervision.

Because zinc can cause stomach upset, it may be taken with food. Dairy products, bran products, and foods high in calcium and phosphorus, such as milk, may decrease zinc absorption. Protein-rich foods such as lamb, beef, and eggs enhance absorption.

---

drugs, you may want to check with your doctor to see if you should increase your intake of the nutrients that the medication affects.

How can you prevent nutrient deficiencies caused by medication and other drug-nutrient interactions? Here are several suggestions from Dr. Jacknowitz.

- Take your medications with water. Over the past 10 years, researchers have learned that grapefruit juice can increase or decrease the effect of many drugs, including the blood pressure medication felodipine (Plendil), the cholesterol drugs atorvastatin calcium (Lipitor) and simvastatin (Zocor), and the antidepressant sertraline hydrochloride (Zoloft). Orange juice may also have an effect. The best beverage to choose to wash down your pills is water.

- Your vitamin and mineral supplements are considered medications, so you should always tell your doctor about everything you're taking.

- Make sure you understand the patient information provided to you with your prescription drug. If you have any questions, ask the advice of your doctor or pharmacist.

- When you buy an over-the-counter product, read the label carefully. If you're confused about ingredients, don't hesitate to ask the pharmacist.

- Follow your doctor's instructions about when to take a medication.

- The actions of some drugs may be enhanced or lessened by certain foods and beverages. Don't be afraid to ask your doctor or pharmacist how drugs may interact with your favorite foods, especially if you eat large amounts of them.

- Eat a nutritionally well-balanced diet with a wide variety of foods. Caffeine, alcohol, and even high-fat foods can affect the efficacy of your drugs. For instance, eating a fatty meal with the insomnia drug zaleplon (Sonata) can decrease the effectiveness of the medication. If you're taking a blood-thinning drug such as warfarin, don't increase your intake of green leafy vegetables, as they may affect the action of the drug.

(continued)

Drugs Can Sabotage Your Nutrition (*cont.*)

Drug Class	Treatment for . . .
Antacids	Indigestion
Antibacterial agents	Chronic bronchitis, tuberculosis, urinary tract infections
Antibiotics	Bacterial infections
Anti-cancer drugs	Tumors
Anticoagulants	Blood clots
Anticonvulsants	Epilepsy, seizures
Antihypertensive agents	High blood pressure
Anti-inflammatory agents	Inflammation, swelling
Antimalarials	Malaria
Diuretics	High blood pressure, water retention
H_2 receptor antagonists	Peptic ulcers
Hypocholesterolemic agents	High blood cholesterol
Laxatives	Constipation
Proton-pump inhibitors	Gastroesophageal reflux disease
Tranquilizers	Depression, sleeping problems

Generic Name	May Interfere with . . .
Aluminum hydroxide, sodium bicarbonate	Calcium, copper, folate
Boric acid	Riboflavin
Isoniazid	Niacin, vitamin B_6, vitamin D
Trimethoprim	Folate
Gentamicin	Magnesium, potassium
Tetracycline	Calcium
Cisplatin	Magnesium
Methotrexate	Calcium, folate
Warfarin	Vitamin K
Phenobarbital, phenytoin, primidone	Vitamin D, vitamin K
Hydralazine	Vitamin B_6
Aspirin	Folate, iron, vitamin C
Colchicine	Vitamin B_{12}
Prednisone	Calcium
Sulfasalazine	Folate
Pyrimethamine	Folate
Furosemide	Calcium, magnesium, potassium
Thiazides	Potassium
Triamterene	Folate
Cimetidine, ranitidine	Vitamin B_{12}
Colestipol	Folate, vitamin A, vitamin B_{12}, vitamin K
Mineral oil	Vitamin D, vitamin K
Senna	Calcium
Lansoprazole	Calcium
Chlorpromazine	Riboflavin

PART TWO

THERAPEUTIC PRESCRIPTIONS FOR HEALING

AGE SPOTS

GOING, GOING, GONE

Ours is a culture with little appreciation for spots. None of us like getting a spot on our record, on our reputation, or on our shirt. And we certainly don't like seeing spots when we're looking into a mirror!

But as we age, many of us do begin to see spots, especially on our hands, feet, and face.

And whether we call them liver spots, age spots, or sun spots, the reaction is likely the same: We want a spot remover.

Technically known as lentigines, age spots are the result of excess pigment being deposited in the skin during years of sun exposure. So along with treatment, dermatologists also recommend avoiding exposure to the sun.

Note: Though the majority of age spots are harmless blemishes that require no more than a trip to the dermatologist, early stages of skin cancer can masquerade as innocent-looking age spots. If any spot enlarges, thickens, changes color, has an uneven rather than a round edge, bleeds, or itches, have it checked by a doctor. For extra protection, also include a skin examination in your annual checkup.

The good news is, if your spots really are just age spots, dermatologists today have an assortment of treatments at their disposal that can fade them, if not remove them completely. These include topical application of a vitamin A acid called retinoic acid.

Fade 'Em Away with Retin-A

Originally developed as an acne medication to unplug clogged pores, retinoic acid, the active ingredient found in products like Retin-A and Differin, has found resounding success as an anti-aging ointment. Though not a fountain of youth, retinoic acid works to eliminate fine wrinkles, blemishes, and age spots by stimulating cell turnover in a metabolic process that still is not entirely understood, says Retin-A creator Albert Kligman, MD, PhD, professor emeritus of dermatology at the University of Pennsylvania School of Medicine in Philadelphia.

To remove an age spot, dermatologists often recommend applying the strongest dosage of retinoic acid that you can tolerate directly on the spot. The area will proceed to peel, and after a few months, the spot should diminish and possibly even disappear.

If you're like the people who were in a research group at the University of Michigan School of Medicine in Ann Arbor, you may even see results after just 1 month. In a 9-month study of 83 people with age spots, researchers found that people treated with a retinoic acid gel experienced lightening of these spots after 1 month. After 9 months, 57 percent of those treated with the gel showed significant lightening of their age spots.

Retinoic acid can be even more effective when used in combination with other treatments, says John F. Romano, MD, clinical assistant professor of dermatology at New York Hospital–Cornell Medical Center and St. Vincent's Hospital, both in New York City.

"I often have people apply glycolic acid in the morning and retinoic acid at night. Or I may combine it with a bleaching cream," says Dr. Romano.

Retinoic acid cream comes in a variety of concentrations, but it's available only by prescription, so you'll need to work with your dermatologist to find the dosage that's right for you.

And because retinoic acid continually sloughs off the outermost, dead layer of skin, it can not only eliminate existing spots but also nip new spots in the bud. The downside of this process is that an area of skin previously

Food Factors

Unfortunately, there are no magical foods that, if eaten, will fade age spots. There are, however, a few that can increase your sensitivity to the mother of age spots, the sun. Here's what you might want to avoid before playing in the sunshine.

Hold the lime. Certain fruits and vegetables—particularly celery, parsnips, carrots, and limes—contain psoralens, chemicals that can increase your sensitivity to the sun. Unless you're sensitive to psoralens, eating these foods before going out in the sun is not likely to be a problem, says Douglas Darr, PhD, a biotechnology industry consultant in Research Triangle Park, North Carolina. You'd best wash your hands—which are already susceptible to sun exposure and age spots—after handling these foods, however. Anyone's skin can be more susceptible to burning after direct contact with psoralens.

sheltered from evaporation and the elements is exposed. That's why a common side effect of retinoic acid is dry, sun-sensitive skin that can be irritated and scaly. Though this effect typically diminishes with time, if you're using retinoic acid, you'll likely need a moisturizer. Sunscreen is also a must once you start using retinoic acid.

Protect Your Skin with Vitamin C

If vitamin D is the sunshine vitamin, then vitamin C is the sunblock vitamin, say some researchers—many of whom also proclaim it the healthy skin vitamin.

"In general, vitamin C is important for keeping the skin younger looking," says Lorraine Meisner, PhD, professor of population health sciences at the University of Wisconsin School of Medicine and Public Health in Madison. She recommends a safe daily vitamin C intake of about 300 to 500 milligrams to maintain skin quality.

Studies have shown that just a minimal amount of ultraviolet rays can deplete exposed skin of vitamin C by 30 percent. Exposure to the ozone in a polluted city can decrease levels of vitamin C by as much as 55 percent. Medical researchers have also found vitamin C to be of some help when applied topically. It has been shown to significantly reduce the amount of so-called free radical damage that occurs from sun exposure. Free radicals are naturally occurring unstable molecules that steal electrons from the body's healthy molecules to balance themselves. Unchecked, they can cause significant tissue damage. Antioxidants—vitamin C is one—neutralize free radicals by offering their own electrons and so protect healthy molecules from harm.

"Since vitamin C prevents skin damage from sun exposure, it's reasonable to suspect that it can also prevent the consequences of that damage, including wrinkling and age spots," says Douglas Darr, PhD, a biotechnology industry consultant in Research Triangle Park, North Carolina. Dr. Darr advocates using topical vitamin C as an adjunct to sunscreen.

One such topical vitamin C product is Cellex-C, which is available in a 10 or 17 percent vitamin C lotion or cream. It can be purchased without a prescription from dermatologists, plastic surgeons, and licensed aestheticians (full-service beauty salon operators) and by mail order from Cellex-C International (www.cellex-c.com). For optimum sun protection, the product should be applied once a day along with a sunscreen, according to Dr. Meisner, whose patented technology led to the development of Cellex-C.

Damage Control with Vitamin E

Vitamin E, an antioxidant vitamin added to everything from nail polish remover to shampoo, is also helpful in preventing sun damage.

Researchers have shown that d-alpha-tocopherol, natural vitamin E oil, can prevent inflammation and skin damage if applied before sun exposure.

Prescriptions for Healing

The only vitamin approved by the FDA as safe and effective in reducing some of the effects of the sun is vitamin A, applied topically as retinoic acid. But there are several promising nutrients that may prevent the harmful effects of the sun that lead to age spots. Here's what some experts recommend as the best dosages.

Nutrient	Daily Amount/Application
Oral	
Selenium	50–200 micrograms (l-selenomethionine)
Vitamin C	300–500 milligrams
Vitamin E	400 IU (d-alpha-tocopherol)
Topical	
Vitamin A	0.025% or higher cream (retinoic acid), depending on skin type
Vitamin C	10% or 17% lotion (Cellex-C), depending on skin type
Vitamin E	At least 5% cream or oil, applied after sun exposure

MEDICAL ALERT: Selenium can be toxic in daily doses exceeding 400 micrograms, so if you'd like to try this therapy to protect your skin, you should discuss it with your doctor.

If you are taking anticoagulant drugs, you should not take oral vitamin E supplements. (Though generally a dose of up to 1,500 IU of vitamin E a day is considered safe, some recent reports suggest that taking more than 400 IU a day could be harmful to people with cardiovascular or circulatory disease or with cancer. If you have such a condition, be sure to consult your doctor before you begin supplementation.)

Vitamin E oil can be bought over the counter in drugstores, as can vitamin E-fortified creams. Research has shown that if the cream or oil contains at least 5 percent vitamin E, it can also be effective in reducing post–sun damage.

You can also reap some of vitamin E's sun-protective properties by taking supplements, adds Karen E. Burke, MD, PhD, a dermatologic surgeon and dermatologist in private practice in New York City. "It's highly effective as an anti-inflammatory agent, and it reduces sun damage to the skin," she says. Dr. Burke recommends that people take 400 IU of vitamin E daily in the natural form of d-alpha-tocopherol.

Good dietary sources of vitamin E include polyunsaturated vegetable oil, wheat germ, spinach, and sunflower seeds.

Try Some Selenium Sun Protection

You might want to boost your dietary intake of the antioxidant mineral selenium as well, says Dr. Burke.

"Selenium can prevent solar damage, pigmentation, and dark spots, but because the selenium content of water varies across the country, not everyone is getting enough to be beneficial," says Dr. Burke, citing the Southeast in particular as an area deficient in selenium.

To quench the free radicals caused by sun exposure and to prevent skin damage, Dr. Burke recommends daily supplements of 50 to 200 micrograms of selenium in the form of l-selenomethionine. Your dosage depends on where you live and whether you have a family history of cancer. Selenium can be toxic in very high doses, so if you'd like to try this therapy to protect your skin, you should discuss it with your doctor before taking any more than 400 micrograms a day. Children should not take extra selenium until they have their adult teeth.

To get more selenium in your diet, try tuna; a 3-ounce can serves up a full 99 micrograms. Or treat yourself to an ounce of baked tortilla chips for a whopping 284 micrograms.

AGING

A RADICAL SOLUTION

At age 38, Elizabeth lies on Litchfield Beach in South Carolina, sunscreen carefully smoothed over her wrinkle-free skin, her naturally dark hair tucked under a scarf and a pair of dense wraparound sunglasses shielding her lovely blue eyes from the morning sun.

Beside her is a cooler containing several bottles of springwater and a fresh fruit salad of watermelon, cantaloupe, and honeydew for lunch. Next to her on the sand is a pair of well-used sneakers for the 2-mile walk she takes along the water's edge every day.

Elizabeth knows that she's gorgeous. There are no wrinkles or stretch marks marring her perfect body. And she's determined that there never will be. She'll do whatever it takes to defy aging until the day she dies.

What are the odds that she'll make it? Better than they were a decade ago. Back then scientists had already found the reasons that we deteriorate into wrinkles, bags, age spots, flab, and life-threatening conditions. The reasons were, and still are, genetics, disease, environmental factors such as smoking and diet, and the aging process itself. Today these scientists also know that every single one of these factors may be directly influenced and perhaps even altered by getting enough of the right kinds of vitamins and minerals.

A Chemical Blitzkrieg

Both the diseases that contribute to aging and the physical and mental "damage" that we associate with old age seem to be triggered by a lifelong blitzkrieg of damaging molecules that affect us on many levels.

These molecules, sometimes called free radicals by scientists, are sent zinging through our bodies by cigarette smoke and chronic infection as well as by the normal cell metabolism that converts the carbohydrates and fat we eat into the energy required to power our cells. Yes, just eating your daily breakfast normally produces untold numbers of these harmful molecules. There's no way to avoid them completely.

Unfortunately, free radicals have the nasty habit of stealing electrons from your body's healthy molecules to balance themselves. In the process, they damage cells and their DNA, the genetic blueprint that tells a cell how to do its job. And without a perfect copy of that DNA blueprint, a cell doesn't know what it's supposed to do. Yet biochemists estimate that every cell in the body is hit 10,000 times every day by free radicals.

The result? Depending on how badly they're hit and how quickly they're returned to service by cellular repair squads, the cells may mutate or die. And when either of these events happens, it may initiate the underlying biochemical processes that cause many of the diseases that accelerate aging: heart disease, high blood pressure, Parkinson's disease, cancer, cataracts, diabetes, and even Alzheimer's disease.

Some scientists also believe that free radicals affect the aging process even more directly. In fact, there's a growing consensus that aging itself is due to free radical reactions.

The idea is that there may be an accumulation of damage from the constant cellular bombardment by free radicals. A cell gets hit once, the cellular repair squads come to the rescue and cut out the damage to the cell's DNA blueprint, and the cell bounces back into action. But when the cell gets hit over and over again, there may come a point at which the repair squads can't patch everything back together the way it was. So the cell continues to do its job, but not as well as it had been.

If it's a skin cell, for example, you might end up with wrinkled skin rather than smooth, polished skin. If it's an eye cell, maybe you just can't see as clearly as you used to.

In any event, scientists have found that up to 40 percent of all of the proteins in an older person may be damaged by free radicals. Proteins are involved in myriad functions in the body, from guiding chemical reactions to supplying energy to maintaining the body's structures.

And that, plus the fact that studies indicate that damaged proteins shorten the life span of laboratory animals, has led some scientists to suspect that free radicals may directly cause aging.

Natural Antioxidants

Although millions of free radicals bombard your cells on a daily basis, the fact that it takes as long as it does for them to cause damage or disease is a tribute to the natural free radical–fighting systems with which you were born. These systems are fighting free radicals every moment of every day.

Each system is ingeniously designed to produce an antioxidant, a naturally occurring chemical that binds to the free radical (or the oxidant, as it is sometimes called) before it reaches the cells. In doing so, the antioxidant helps preserve your body's healthy molecules.

Each antioxidant is designed to work in a different way in a different part of the cell. Its marching orders come from the genetic instructions on your chromosomes, and its power comes from a ready supply of specific nutrients in your diet. One natural antioxidant is dependent upon the availability of copper, zinc, and manganese. Another is dependent on iron, and a third is dependent on selenium.

Food Factors

Although a rich supply of vitamins and minerals is clearly a priority in any anti-aging program, here are four other factors to consider.

Serve up gazpacho. This cold soup staple of Spain increases your army of antioxidants and guards cells against the damage of free radicals. A study by the Jean Mayer USDA Human Nutrition Research Center on Aging at Tufts University in Boston found that volunteers who had two servings of gazpacho every day raised their levels of vitamin C and lowered their levels of oxidative stress. In another study of the benefits of a Mediterranean diet on over 900 men and women with an average age of 66, researchers at the Stanford University School of Medicine found that gazpacho lowered levels of inflammation, which is linked to heart disease. This chilled soup, usually made with tomatoes, garlic, peppers, onions, and olive oil, is easy to make and a zesty way to build up your defenses.

Feel blue. There's more to blueberries than their natural deliciousness and beautiful hue—they may actually have anti-aging properties. Aged animals fed wild blueberries, native to North America, for 8 weeks showed improvements in muscle strength, coordination, balance, stamina, and short-term memory. Scientists at the Human Nutrition Research Center on Aging say it may be that polyphenol, a compound found in blueberries that has antioxidant and anti-inflammatory abilities, is responsible for these exciting results. So mix some of these plump berries into your breakfast cereal or eat them au natural to put a spring back in your step.

How much do you need? That all depends on what it takes to maintain an ideal balance of antioxidants. But since scientists are just beginning to understand what's necessary, the best that we can do right now is eat a variety of antioxidant-rich fruits and vegetables.

Supplementing the Body's Natural Antioxidants

Although the body produces natural antioxidants to neutralize free radical damage, it doesn't produce enough to handle the free radical bombardment generated by the modern world. Your body's natural antioxidant systems were simply not designed to handle rooms full of cigarette smoke, a

Eat protein. For years researchers believed that high-protein diets promoted calcium loss, which can lead to a weakening of the bones. However, a study from the Human Nutrition Research Center on Aging and the New England Research Institutes (located in Watertown, Massachusetts) found that protein doesn't cause the body to excrete excess calcium, and may actually help strengthen bones. Researchers increased the dietary protein of one group of healthy men and women over the age of 50 by 58 grams a day. The other group was assigned a low-protein diet. All of the participants were already meeting their daily requirements of 800 milligrams of calcium. The participants on the high-protein diet had 25 percent higher levels of bone regrowth.

Older people may sometimes have birdlike appetites, but the amount of protein that they need to stay active is elephantine. According to the Alliance for Aging Research, nearly 50 percent of all seniors don't consume enough high-protein foods. Two great sources of protein are chicken and fish. A 3-ounce portion of chicken breast and a 3-ounce portion of tuna contain 27 and 25 grams of protein, respectively. Add a cup of skim milk to that, and you'll be consuming another 10 grams of protein.

Forgo fat. Medical research has shown that dietary fat is a prime generator of free radicals, the naturally occurring unstable molecules that damage your body's healthy molecules by stealing their electrons and, in the process, contribute to aging. Here's yet another reason to stick to a low-fat diet.

diet loaded with fat, and constant exposure to new and more virulent viruses.

This may change once scientists learn how to alter our genes so that we produce more natural antioxidants. But in the meantime, we do have another option: enhancing our natural antioxidants with synthetic antioxidants—in a word, supplements.

Laboratory studies indicate that antioxidant supplements, predominantly vitamins C and E plus beta-carotene and selenium, seem to be able to neutralize free radicals caused by exposure to environmental pollutants.

Does that mean that supplements can actually slow the aging process? Nobody knows yet, but scientists are actively trying to figure that out.

Prescriptions for Healing

The exact amount of vitamins and minerals required to slow aging and to prevent many of the diseases that accelerate aging is a hot topic of debate among scientists. Until more research provides further information, experts conducting the research suggest getting the Recommended Dietary Allowance of antioxidants.

Nutrient	Daily Amount
Selenium	55 micrograms
Vitamin A	5,000 IU
Vitamin C	60 milligrams
Vitamin E	30 IU

Plus a multivitamin/mineral supplement containing the Daily Values of all essential vitamins and minerals.

MEDICAL ALERT: *Selenium in doses exceeding 400 micrograms daily should be taken only under medical supervision.*

If you are taking anticoagulant drugs, you should not take vitamin E supplements. (Though generally a dose of up to 1,500 IU of vitamin E a day is considered safe, some recent reports suggest that taking more than 400 IU a day could be harmful to people with cardiovascular or circulatory disease or with cancer. If you have such a condition, be sure to consult your doctor before you begin supplementation.)

Although antioxidant supplements perform well on laboratory animals, it may be some time before science can answer that question for humans.

Yet while we're waiting to find out, one thing seems absolutely clear: Those folks who take supplemental antioxidants or who enrich their diets with antioxidant-rich fruits and vegetables certainly seem to be preventing development of the diseases that can accelerate the aging process. A long-term study conducted by French researchers called the SUpplémentation en VItamines et Minéraux AntioXydants (SU.VI.MAX) set out to assess the effects of vitamin and minerals supplements on chronic diseases, such as cancer and heart disease. They looked at whether a cocktail of antioxidants at doses that are available through a healthy balanced diet could reduce the risk of disease over a period of 7½ years. Over 13,000 adults between the ages of 45 and 60 were given either a placebo or a supplement containing 120 milligrams of vitamin C, 30 milligrams of vitamin E, 6 milligrams of beta-carotene, 100 micrograms of selenium, and 20 milligrams of zinc. After 7½ years, the researchers found that the men in the group taking the supplements had a lower incidence of cancer.

Hundreds of population-based studies like this one conducted over the past 2 decades have demonstrated that high intake of antioxidants, through food or supplements, reduces the risk of diseases that accelerate us into old age and helps us maintain a high quality of life. However, clinical studies of antioxidant supplements taken singly or at high doses over an extended period of time aren't as consistently positive.

Getting people to eat a more nutrient-dense diet as they age is important, says Jeffrey Blumberg, PhD, director of the antioxidants research laboratory at the Jean Mayer USDA Human Nutrition Research Center on Aging at Tufts University in Boston. But what you eat is also important, he adds.

"In essence, eating a super high-quality diet is crucial if you want to do all that you can to stay young longer," says Dr. Blumberg. "It's especially important to key in on good food sources of vitamins C and E and carotenoids like beta-carotene." Good sources include orange and yellow vegetables, fruits, and whole grains.

"In addition, I'd go so far as to advise people who want to take steps to slow down the aging process to take a daily multivitamin/mineral supplement," he says. "The idea behind this is that you can die 'young' as late as possible."

ALCOHOLISM

REPAIRING NUTRITIONAL DAMAGE

You probably know someone with a drinking problem. In fact, maybe that person is you.

Problems with alcohol are fairly common in the United States. "Two-thirds of all Americans drink," says Charles H. Halsted, MD, professor emeritus of internal medicine at the University of California, Davis. "Sixty percent are light to moderate drinkers, but up to 10 percent drink excessively."

The light to moderate drinkers are probably in pretty good health, according to Dr. Halsted. "Moderate drinking is safe and may be beneficial, since it lowers the risk of cardiovascular disease," he says.

But excessive alcohol consumption is another story. Excessive drinking on a daily basis—more than three drinks for a woman and more than six for a man—increases your risk of cancer and can damage the liver, pancreas, heart, and brain, and also increases the risk of breast cancer in women, says Dr. Halsted. It can cause vitamin deficiencies resulting in anemia, memory loss, osteoporosis, and night blindness. Although rare in this country, when scurvy due to vitamin C deficiency and pellagra due to niacin deficiency do occur, it's usually in alcoholics.

The Liquid Saboteur

How does alcohol damage your health? It hinders your body's ability to absorb, process, use, and store the nutrients found in food—plus it tends to edge out food in your diet.

Alcoholic beverages are essentially made up of water, pure alcohol, and sugars, so they offer virtually no nutritional value, says Charles S. Lieber, MD, professor of medicine and pathology at Mount Sinai School of Medicine in New York City and chief of the Alcohol Research and Treatment Center at the James J. Peters Veterans Affairs Medical Center in New York. "Alcoholic beverages are full of empty calories. If you're a heavy drinker, those empty calories replace other nutrients in the diet. In addition, alcohol has a direct, toxic effect on the gastrointestinal tract."

The result is that many, if not most, of the vitamins, minerals, and other nutrients extracted from food during digestion cannot be absorbed through the gastrointestinal tract and into the bloodstream. Compounding the problem is the fact that alcohol is toxic to the liver, the organ that processes nutrients. Normally the liver stores the nutrients it receives and turns food into the energy your body needs.

But once the liver is damaged, your body's ability to properly use many vitamins and minerals such as thiamin, B_6, and folate (the naturally occurring form of folic acid) is significantly reduced. And since a damaged liver produces less bile, a substance the body uses to prepare fat-soluble vitamins for absorption by the intestines, your body's ability to absorb vitamins A, D, and E is also impaired.

Antioxidant Protection

Although alcohol devastates the body both directly as a toxin and indirectly through nutrient loss, scientists suspect that it may also affect the body's natural antioxidant defenses. Antioxidants are substances that protect your body's healthy molecules against damage by unstable molecules called free radicals. Heavy alcohol use not only increases the production of free radicals, but it also depletes stores of antioxidants, like vitamins C and E. That means that while those nasty rogue molecules are increasing exponentially, the natural warriors needed to fight them off are decreasing rapidly. This imbalance is called "oxidative stress."

There is some experimental evidence that when combined with abstaining from alcohol, supplemental antioxidants like vitamin C, vitamin E, and selenium may prevent the progression of liver damage. Many doctors who treat alcoholism put patients on a supplemental program designed around their own antioxidant deficiencies. However, everyone, from teetotalers to problem drinkers, will benefit by getting the Daily Values of antioxidants.

The recommended daily intake is 30 IU for vitamin E and 60 milligrams for vitamin C, and the Daily Value is 70 micrograms for selenium.

Vitamin A: Finding the Right Balance

Research suggests that long-term alcohol use causes the liver to excrete vitamin A and impairs the body's ability to convert beta-carotene to vitamin A.

So it should come as no surprise that people with cirrhosis of the liver, a disease commonly caused by chronic alcohol use, are frequently deficient in vitamin A. Vitamin A plays an important part in helping you to reproduce, to grow new cells, to fight infection, and, because of its important role in the retina, to see at night.

Although it seems like common sense that the answer to a vitamin A deficiency is to simply pop a couple of pills, giving supplemental vitamin A to people with alcohol problems is tricky, cautions Dr. Lieber.

Vitamin A is not only toxic to the liver if taken in large amounts, but alcohol intensifies that toxicity. "So if you supplement vitamin A in an alcoholic, you have to be careful not to add insult to injury and enhance the toxic effects of alcohol," Dr. Lieber says. "It's important to correct the deficiency. But at the same time, it's important to avoid any excess. There's a very small therapeutic window." Even the usual doses of vitamin A can be harmful to alcoholics, so vitamin A supplements should only be taken under the supervision of a doctor. "It's a short hop from helping to hurting with vitamin A," says Dr. Lieber.

For a while, researchers wondered if they could avoid the toxic effects of supplementation and still prevent a vitamin A deficiency by prescribing beta-carotene, a nontoxic precursor of vitamin A that occurs naturally in dark green leafy vegetables and in orange and yellow vegetables. But for a drinker,

---

Food Factors

When alcohol replaces food in the diet, as it frequently does in people who have drinking problems, it speeds up the body's metabolism and can cause muscle breakdown and a protein deficiency that sabotages the body's ability to repair normal wear and tear.

That's why people with chronic drinking problems tend to lose weight, says Charles H. Halsted, MD, professor emeritus of internal medicine at the University of California, Davis. Here's what you can do to help correct the problem.

First, abstain. Not drinking is a prerequisite to correcting or restoring nutritional health.

Eat hearty. To counteract weight loss and protein deficiency, Dr. Halsted suggests that people with drinking problems eat at least 2,000 calories a day. Most of those calories—about 60 percent—should be in the form of fruits and vegetables, as well as breads, pastas, and other grains, with at least one meal a day containing animal protein.

beta-carotene has the same problem as vitamin A itself, says Dr. Lieber. Although it's seemingly nontoxic to everyone else in the world, too much beta-carotene can damage an alcoholic's liver just as easily as vitamin A.

Think Thiamin for the Brain

The unsteady gait, confusion, and poor memory that many of us associate with someone who drinks excessively are also symptoms of brain damage caused by long-term alcohol abuse. Alcohol not only affects the brain indirectly by impairing absorption of vital nutrients, but it's directly toxic to the brain as well. Studies using brain imaging have consistently found that alcoholic men and women have greater brain shrinkage than nonalcoholics. The cerebellum, the part of the brain responsible for coordination and some forms of learning, seems to be especially vulnerable to alcohol. The cerebellum is also affected by the body's stores of thiamin, which regulates the metabolism of brain cells.

"Thiamin is an important player in the way the brain works," explains Dr. Halsted.

And although the brain requires a continuous supply of thiamin, the body does not store it in any appreciable amount. Up to 80 percent of alcoholics have a thiamin deficiency. Laboratory studies indicate that a thiamin deficiency from alcohol abuse disrupts the ability of brain cells to do their job, resulting in impaired function and cell death. This may eventually lead to Wernicke-Korsakoff syndrome, a brain disorder characterized by an unsteady gait, confusion, and memory loss.

Some doctors prescribe 50 milligrams of thiamin a day to temporarily supplement the diets of alcoholics, but brain damage caused by a thiamin deficiency cannot be reversed, says Dr. Halsted.

Building with Bs

Aside from a thiamin deficiency, excessive drinking can also cause a deficiency of vitamin B_6, a nutrient needed for formation of red blood cells as well as reactions involved in normal cell functions. "Pyridoxine, or vitamin B_6, is more rapidly eliminated from the body during heavy drinking," says Dr. Halsted. Over 50 percent of those who drink excessively seem to have deficiencies. Eating a well-balanced diet that includes 1.3 milligrams of vitamin B_6 can correct the problem, says Dr. Halsted, but only if no further alcohol is ever consumed. Good food sources of pyridoxine include meat, fish, poultry, or fortified cereals.

Folate, another B vitamin, is also in low supply when people drink excessively, says Dr. Halsted. Since folic acid is one vitamin that does not significantly alter the taste of any beverage in which it's dissolved, some scientists have recommended that manufacturers add folic acid to alcoholic beverages as they are bottled or canned, but this hasn't occurred and beverages except beer are completely devoid of folate.

A well-balanced diet may prevent folate deficiency in nondrinkers, but folate is lost from the body more rapidly in heavy drinkers. A folic acid supplement of 400 micrograms a day may prevent folate deficiency in drinkers, says Dr. Halsted.

Reversing a Mineral Deficiency

Because alcohol can derail the transportation system that escorts minerals such as zinc and magnesium out of the liver and into your bloodstream, researchers agree that anyone with a drinking problem also runs the risk of zinc and magnesium deficiencies.

Both zinc and magnesium are excreted in relatively large amounts when people are drinking excessively, says Dr. Halsted. They can be replaced by eating a well-balanced diet, he adds. Shellfish, pot roast, and eggs are all good sources of zinc, while nuts, whole grains, vegetables, and tofu are pretty decent sources of magnesium.

If you have heart or kidney problems, it's important that you talk to your doctor before taking magnesium supplements.

Preventing Bone Loss

Research shows that long-term alcohol consumption can decrease the density of bones, making them more susceptible to fractures. For menopausal women who are especially vulnerable to osteoporosis, long-term alcohol use is particularly damaging. In the Framingham Osteoporosis Study, researchers found that women between the ages of 67 and 90 who consumed more than 3 ounces of alcohol a day had more significant bone loss than women who drank moderate amounts of alcohol.

Calcium is one of the many nutrients that bones need to remain strong. Therefore, it is a good idea to take over-the-counter calcium and vitamin D,

Prescriptions for Healing

Alcohol abuse causes damage to the liver, pancreas, intestines, and brain. The process of reversing that damage begins when you stop drinking and start eating a balanced diet that provides at least the Daily Values of certain vitamins and minerals. Here's what doctors say that you need. If you find that you can't get these amounts from your diet, taking a general multivitamin/mineral supplement may help.

Nutrient	Daily Amount
Calcium	600 milligrams 3 times a day
Folic acid	400 micrograms
Magnesium	400 milligrams, with a doctor's supervision
Selenium	55 micrograms
Thiamin	50 milligrams
Vitamin A	5,000 IU, with a doctor's supervision
Vitamin B$_6$	1.3 milligrams
Vitamin C	60 milligrams
Vitamin D	200 milligrams, 3 times a day, plus 400 milligrams twice a day
Vitamin E	30 IU
Zinc	15 milligrams, with a doctor's supervision

Or a multivitamin/mineral supplement containing the recommended amounts of these vitamins and minerals

MEDICAL ALERT: *If you have a drinking problem, you should seek professional care.*

If you have heart or kidney problems, you should consult your doctor before taking magnesium supplements.

Selenium in doses exceeding 400 micrograms daily should be taken only under medical supervision.

If you are taking anticoagulant drugs, you should not take vitamin E supplements. (Though generally a dose of up to 1,500 IU of vitamin E a day is considered safe, some recent reports suggest that taking more than 400 IU a day could be harmful to people with cardiovascular or circulatory disease or with cancer. If you have such a condition, be sure to consult your doctor before you begin supplementation.)

says Dr. Halsted. These usually come together with 600 milligrams of calcium and 200 milligrams of vitamin D, which should be taken three times a day. However, this is insufficient for vitamin D, so another two capsules at 400 milligrams each should be taken each day.

Vitamins Won't Correct the Addiction

There are three things you should remember about alcohol and nutrition, says Dr. Halsted.

First, there is no nutrient that will reduce the craving for alcohol, as some early scientific reports may have led people to believe. "The sum total of evidence seems to point more toward an addictive gene that causes the craving and results in excessive alcohol consumption," says Dr. Halsted. "So there's no way that nutrition will affect it."

Second, since nutrient levels can vary so widely from person to person, anyone who has a problem with alcohol should have his or her nutritional status individually evaluated by a doctor. If your doctor doesn't seem to know much about nutrition, you can contact the American Board of Physician Nutrition Specialists for a referral to a doctor in your area who does. Write to the American Board of Physician Nutrition Specialists, University of Alabama at Birmingham, 439 Susan Mott Webb Nutrition Sciences Building, 1675 University Boulevard, Birmingham, AL 35294-3360, or go to the Web site at www.ipnec.org.

The third thing you should remember is this: "For the alcoholic, the only cure is abstinence," says Dr. Halsted. "There's no point in popping a vitamin pill or eating a balanced diet while you're still drinking. You can eat a balanced diet and take vitamins, but if you still drink in excess for 5 to 10 years, you run the risk of getting liver disease."

After you've stopped drinking, there is some good nutritional news, however. "If it has not progressed too far, alcoholic liver disease may be reversible once you're on a regular, balanced diet that meets the Recommended Dietary Allowances for vitamins and minerals," says Dr. Halsted.

ALLERGIES

NUTRIENTS THAT EASE
THE SNEEZE

Allergies are versatile. They can show up just about anywhere in your body and create an incredible variety of symptoms. They can affect your nose, eyes, throat, lungs, stomach, skin, and nervous system. They can make you itch, wheeze, and sneeze, make your nose run and your eyes weep, give you a headache or a bellyache, and even bring on fatigue and depression.

So with all of these possible symptoms, what is it that makes an allergy an allergy? To put it another way, what exactly is going on in your body when you have an allergy?

Allergy symptoms occur when your body's immune system overreacts to substances in your environment. Most people can live with a little cat dander, dust, or pollen, for example. (Some folks can live with a lot!) But people with allergies have immune systems that can react to just about anything that comes along. "It fights these foreign substances just as it would bacteria or viruses," explains Jeremy Kaslow, MD, an Orange County, California, allergy specialist and past associate professor of medicine at the University of California, Irvine.

The main causes of run-of-the-mill allergy symptoms are histamine and leukotrienes, biochemicals that your immune system releases. Your immune system is an incredibly complex system of several different kinds of cells working in tandem. The overly sensitive cells involved in allergies are mainly mast cells and basophils. Mast cells are found in tissues such as your skin, lungs, throat, stomach, and intestines, while basophils hang out in your blood vessels. As you can see, these cells monitor nearly every part of the body.

Why Your Nose Runs

Histamine is usually stored in granules inside mast cells. When a mast cell is exposed to a substance that triggers an allergic reaction, however, the cell releases its histamine into surrounding tissues.

"Histamine plays an important role in certain types of allergic reactions,"

Dr. Kaslow explains. "It causes small blood vessels to widen and become more permeable to fluid, allowing fluid to pass from the bloodstream into surrounding tissues, causing nasal congestion, runny eyes and nose, and sometimes hives."

Histamine makes the smooth muscles in the walls of the lungs, blood vessels, stomach, intestines, and bladder contract. That contraction brings on a wide range of symptoms. In the lungs, for example, histamine may cause wheezing. Histamine release also indirectly stimulates the production of thick, sticky mucus.

You can blame Mom and Dad for the fact that you're allergic; the tendency is inherited. But some doctors believe a healthy diet and certain nutritional supplements can balance your immune system, keeping it strong but not overreactive.

"To crack the underlying problem, you really need a healthy nutritional foundation that's based on diet," says Dr. Kaslow. "If you continue to eat poorly and simply take a few supplements, you aren't likely to see much of a benefit."

With that in mind, here are particulars on the nutrients that may be helpful in fighting allergies.

Antioxidants May Stifle the Sneeze

There's no doubt that antioxidants play an important role in almost every function of the body, but scientists have been zeroing in on antioxidants' ability to defend against respiratory illnesses, such as allergies and asthma. Researchers from the Royal Brompton Hospital and National Heart and Lung Institute in London studied the diets of people on the Greek island of Crete, where very few children suffer with allergies. They surveyed 690 children between the ages of 7 and 18 and gathered data from questionnaires that were completed by their parents. The researchers discovered that those who ate fresh foods high in antioxidants, such as grapes, oranges, tomatoes, and nuts, were less likely to have wheezing and other respiratory symptoms. In yet another British study of over 2,500 middle-aged men, those who ate five apples a week had greater lung functioning than those who ate no apples. The researchers believed that healthy compounds found in apples, like antioxidants, have allergy-fighting effects.

It's not clear if antioxidant supplements, particularly vitamins C and E, have the same effect. When inflammatory cells located in the airways and

Food Factors

Some of the most serious allergic reactions—including deadly shock—can involve food. People with serious allergies usually find out through tests which foods they need to avoid. Components of certain foods may also help trigger allergies. Here's what you need to know.

Pinpoint your problem foods. If you suspect food is the culprit, see a specialist who can help you determine which foods are aggravating your symptoms, experts suggest. Peanuts, nuts, eggs, milk, soy, and fish and other seafood have all been implicated in allergic reactions. And gluten, a protein found in wheat, rye, barley, and oats, can cause allergy-related intestinal problems in some people.

Watch out for cross-reactions. Some people with inhalant allergies develop allergies to foods that contain similar substances.

"Someone who reacts to birch pollen, for instance, may get itching or swelling of the lips, tongue, throat, or roof of the mouth if he eats apples," reports John W. Yunginger, MD, professor of pediatrics at Mayo Medical School in Rochester, Minnesota. People allergic to ragweed, on the other hand, may react to melons, he says.

The foods most likely to cause reactions confined to the mouth: uncooked fruits, nuts, and vegetables.

---

lungs, called eosinophils and neutrophils, are activated, they create oxidants, which irritate the lungs and cause mucus. Several studies have shown that vitamins E and C can help tame that reaction when it's caused by smog and other air pollutants. Vitamin C is believed to be a natural antihistamine, and vitamin E is said to enhance the function of immune cells to better ward off free radicals. A long-term study sponsored by the National Center for Complementary and Alternative Medicine is taking a closer look at how these antioxidants function in the lungs and whether supplemental therapy will decrease inflammation produced by allergens. Until the results of that study are in, alternative medicine experts believe the best reason to take antioxidant supplements is to accomplish what allergy drugs cannot: addressing the underlying problem of allergies by strengthening the immune system. Doctors recommend taking 500 milligrams of vitamin C and 400 IU of vitamin E to balance and strengthen the immune system naturally.

Although the Daily Value for vitamin C is only 60 milligrams, these higher doses are considered safe for most people. Extremely high doses can cause stomach upset, nausea, and diarrhea in some people. If you experience any discomfort, you might want to cut back. Recent reports suggest that a daily dose of vitamin E greater than 400 IU can be harmful, so it's best not to exceed this dosage.

Extra Help from Bioflavonoids

Food-based vitamin C supplements contain bioflavonoids. These colorful chemical compounds are intimately related to the ascorbic acid compound of vitamin C. The chemical structure of bioflavonoids is similar to that of a drug called cromolyn, used in inhalers to reduce asthma-related inflammation.

Bioflavonoids reportedly help reduce the release of symptom-producing histamine, reduce inflammation, and promote healthy connective tissue, explains Dr. Kaslow.

Prescriptions for Healing

For the best allergy-alleviating action, some doctors suggest adding these nutrients to a healthy, balanced diet.

Nutrient	Daily Amount
Magnesium	400 milligrams
Vitamin C	500 milligrams
Vitamin E	400 IU

Plus a multivitamin/mineral supplement

MEDICAL ALERT: *If you have heart disease or kidney problems, check with your doctor before taking magnesium supplements.*

Some people may experience diarrhea when taking excessive amounts of vitamin C.

If you are taking anticoagulant drugs, you should not take oral vitamin E supplements. (Though generally a dose of up to 1,500 IU a day is considered safe, some recent reports suggest that taking more than 400 IU a day could be harmful to people with cardiovascular or circulatory disease or with cancer. If you have such a condition, be sure to consult your doctor before you begin supplementation.)

Unfortunately, experience with one of the common bioflavonoids, quercetin, suggests that it isn't readily absorbed, so the effectiveness in influencing allergic reaction doesn't always match the research done in the laboratory, Dr. Kaslow says.

Researchers are still investigating the role of bioflavonoids in allergy relief. For now, Dr. Kaslow says, don't rely on supplements alone; instead, emphasize better food choices, including bioflavonoid-rich foods such as citrus fruits, cherries, dark grapes, broccoli, red and green peppers, and herb teas (stinging nettle is specifically recommended for allergies). You'll be getting a host of other helpful nutrients as well.

Magnesium May Ease Breathing

Some doctors who treat people with allergies recommend that their patients get the Daily Value of magnesium, which is 400 milligrams. That's because population-based studies have suggested that low levels of dietary magnesium are associated with an increased risk of airway reactivity and respiratory symptoms. Research also indicates that high intake of this essential mineral can improve lung function and reduce the risk of wheezing. In a 2-month study of 37 children and adolescents, Brazilian researchers found that those taking 300 milligrams of magnesium a day had on average 28 percent fewer days of severe asthma reactions. The participants taking the supplements also used their inhaled medication 40 percent less.

It's possible that magnesium's ability to relax body and blood vessels is what's at work here, but more large-scale studies are still needed to fully understand the respiratory effects of magnesium.

Studies show that most men and women don't get adequate amounts of magnesium in their diets. Adults over the age of 70 usually take in far less magnesium than younger adults. The very best sources of magnesium are nuts, beans, and whole grains. Green vegetables are another good source, as are bananas. Most processed foods contain very little of this essential mineral.

Fortunately, you don't need to load up on magnesium to get healthful benefits. If you do, you'll soon find your maximum tolerable dose: You'll end up with diarrhea. (That's why milk of magnesia is such a good laxative!) People with kidney disease, kidney failure, or heart block and those who have had an ileostomy should not take magnesium.

Nutrients to Protect Mucous Membranes

Dr. Kaslow also recommends other nutrients: vitamin A, selenium, and zinc. These nutrients play important roles in the health of mucous membranes, your body's internal skin.

"If you have healthy mucous membranes, your chances of having significant allergy problems will be less," Dr. Kaslow says. The mucous membrane is a layer of cells that secrete the slimy substance we all know and should love, because it contains an array of infection-fighting biochemicals. Mucus also shields cells from direct contact with pollen and other allergens, substances that trigger allergies.

"This mucus layer protects cells from the damaging effects of air pollution," Dr. Kaslow says. "Studies show that people who are exposed to both air pollution and allergens are more likely to have severe allergic reactions than those exposed only to allergens."

The allergic reaction itself also leads to the generation of unstable molecules called free radicals, which injure your body's healthy molecules by stealing electrons to balance themselves. In the process, free radicals injure mast cells and may make them even more twitchy and prone to histamine release, Dr. Kaslow adds.

Dr. Kaslow suggests nixing junk foods and eating more unprocessed foods to get an adequate supply of all of these nutrients. Some doctors recommend taking a multivitamin/mineral supplement that covers all the bases. For some people with allergies, avoiding certain foods can be dramatically helpful for all of their symptoms.

ALZHEIMER'S DISEASE

FIGHTING THE MEMORY THIEF

Few health problems are as feared as Alzheimer's disease. The fourth leading cause of death in older adults (after heart disease, cancer, and stroke), Alzheimer's affects approximately five million Americans. And this figure is expected to more than triple by the middle of the century.

Alzheimer's is a disease that sneaks up slowly, ever so quietly stealing away elderly people's memory and personality, eventually eroding their ability to take care of themselves. Elderly people with Alzheimer's are then forced to rely on family or health care professionals for survival. Is there no hope?

Actually, yes, there is. A cure is still probably years away. But even in the high-tech world of brain research, some of the most promising treatments on the horizon may include the use of a few simple vitamins.

Investigating an Elusive Enemy

A look at what's going on in the brain of someone with Alzheimer's disease makes the memory loss and other personality problems at least understandable. Once-healthy brain cells begin to die off.

"We are just beginning to understand what is happening to brain cells," says James E. Galvin, MD, MPH, a neurologist and researcher at the Alzheimer's Disease Research Center at Washington University in St. Louis. Research has focused on the presence of microscopic plaques, made of a substance called beta-amyloid, as the most likely cause of Alzheimer's disease. As amyloid accumulates in the brain area responsible for memory, personality, and mental functioning, the symptoms of the disease become detectable.

As it turns out, amyloid probably has quite a few partners in crime—and at least one could be hiding in your family tree. Some forms of a blood protein called apolipoprotein E (apoE) that normally ferry cholesterol through the blood also appear to be associated with an increased risk of amyloid deposition in the brain, says Dr. Galvin. And the evidence implicating one form, apoE-4, as a risk factor for this disease is convincing. Whites and African Americans with two apoE-4 genes are 15 times and six times more likely to develop Alzheimer's, respectively, as those who inherit only apoE-2 or apoE-3 genes. Even the presence of one apoE-4 gene increases the risk by three times over people without apoE-4 genes.

However, people shouldn't go out and be tested for these genes, since they are only risk factors and are not predictive of who will get the disease, says Dr. Galvin. Other risk factors include high cholesterol levels, uncontrolled diabetes, and head injuries.

Other researchers think zinc and copper can potentially increase the amount of toxic amyloid deposited in the brain. In laboratory experiments, investigators at Massachusetts General Hospital in Boston found that a slight increase in zinc caused beta-amyloid protein "to curdle into gluelike clumps" within just 2 minutes. These clumps have been shown to interfere with synaptic activity and neurotransmission. More information is needed on the role of dietary zinc in Alzheimer's, according to the study's lead researcher, Rudolph Tanzi, PhD, director of the Genetics and Aging Unit at Massachusetts General Hospital and Harvard Medical School. But now there is enough evidence to warn against megadoses of elemental zinc or copper. Because increased dietary zinc has been shown to markedly decrease mental functioning in people with Alzheimer's, Dr. Tanzi suggests that they get no more than the Daily Value of 15 milligrams. In 1997, Dr. Tanzi started a company called Prana Biotechnology, Ltd., which has begun clinical trials aimed at treating Alzheimer' disease by blocking the interaction between zinc and copper and the beta-amyloid protein in the brain.

Brain Rust Sets In

No matter what the cause of Alzheimer's may ultimately be, some researchers are convinced that the oxidative damage your brain suffers over a lifetime may play an important role in the development of this disease. When the body burns oxygen to produce energy, the process also produces chemically unstable molecules, known as free radicals, as by-products. These molecules steal electrons from your body's healthy molecules to balance themselves, damaging all kinds of cells, including brain cells, in the process.

A number of things contribute to the production of free radicals: pollution, cigarette smoke, alcohol—in other words, living in the 21st century. "What makes me think oxidative damage is important is that one of the main risk factors for Alzheimer's is getting old," says Dr. Galvin. "Oxidative damage accumulates during aging just from normal metabolism of brain cells."

In fact, 10 percent of people ages 65 and older have Alzheimer's, while 50 percent of those over age 85 have it.

One theory suggests that the oxidation process might make amyloid even more damaging—and might kill some brain cells on its own. In addition, the formation of amyloid may increase the production of free radicals, leading to a vicious cycle.

Further complicating the search for an Alzheimer's cure is that multiple factors such as apoE-4, oxidative damage, and even inflammation may each play some small role in the cause and the progression of the disease. "There probably won't be a single solution," says Dr. Galvin. "The same symptoms and the same plaques and tangles come about from multiple different causes. Only now are we beginning to understand the role vitamins, minerals, and other

Food Factors

Just like every other organ in the body, the brain relies on the right balance of nutrients in order to function properly. However, there's still much to learn about the impact of nutrition on Alzheimer's disease. Alzheimer's research is growing by leaps and bounds as the aging population continues to grow. Here's some food for thought.

Cruise the Mediterranean diet. In a study of over 2,000 elderly adults over the course of 4 years, researchers found that those who followed the "Mediterranean diet," which is rich in fruits, vegetables, fish, legumes, and olive oil, were less likely to develop Alzheimer's than the people who didn't follow the diet. While more research needs to be done on the effects of diet on Alzheimer's, it makes sense that foods high in nutrients, fiber, and omega-3 fatty acids would reduce the risk of heart disease and diabetes and therefore encourage good blood flow to the brain.

Add some spice. Curcumin, an Indian curry spice derived from turmeric, may do more than add kick to your dish. Researchers at UCLA discovered that curcumin reduces inflammation, oxidative damage, and plaque by 43 to 50 percent in the brains of Alzheimer-prone mice. The study authors note that India, where curcumin is a staple, has a very low incidence of Alzheimer's disease.

Go fish. Maybe Grandma was right—fish might really be "brain food." A study at the Department of Veterans Affairs and UCLA showed that a diet high in an omega-3 fatty acid called docosahexaenoic acid (DHA) dramatically slowed the progression of Alzheimer's in mice. Rodents that were fed DHA-fortified chow had 70 percent less amyloid protein than those who weren't given DHA food. Scientists believe that boosting intake of DHA, found in cold-water fish like salmon, halibut, and mackerel, may even delay the disease in people who are predisposed to it.

antioxidants such as omega-3 fatty acids may play in preserving a healthy brain and reducing the risk of Alzheimer's disease and other brain disorders."

Vitamin E Might Provide Some Protection

While researchers explore different approaches for conquering Alzheimer's, at least one research team has turned to a vitamin breakthrough in stroke treatment for answers.

During a stroke, damaged brain cells release a neurotransmitter called glutamic acid. This chemical causes a chain reaction that destroys more brain cells, releasing even more dangerous glutamic acid.

Exposing brain cells to vitamin E in the laboratory seems to shield them from the effects of a stroke, says David Schubert, PhD, professor of neurobiology at the Salk Institute for Biological Studies in San Diego. "Vitamin E actually has a protective effect on brain cells, limiting the number killed by the glutamic acid," he explains.

In another study, Dr. Schubert's laboratory showed that bathing brain cells in vitamin E protects them from a toxic protein found in amyloid plaques.

How? Just as soaking a peeled apple in lemon juice prevents oxidation from turning it brown, antioxidants such as vitamin E protect brain cells by neutralizing free radicals.

There's a hitch, however, in using vitamin E to prevent and treat Alzheimer's. In animal studies of stroke and in a clinical trial in human

Prescriptions for Healing

Doctors are studying several nutrients as potential treatments for Alzheimer's disease. Here's what they recommend, based on very preliminary research.

Nutrient	Daily Amount
Folic acid	400 micrograms
Thiamin	5,000 milligrams
Vitamin E	400 IU

MEDICAL ALERT: *Anyone with Alzheimer's disease should be under a doctor's care.*

This amount of thiamin is thousands of times beyond the Daily Value and caused nausea in some people when it was tested. Make sure you get your physician's approval before trying this therapy.

If you are taking anticoagulants, you should not take vitamin E supplements. (Though generally a dose of up to 1,500 IU a day is considered safe, some recent reports suggest that taking more than 400 IU a day could be harmful to people with cardiovascular or circulatory disease or with cancer. If you have such a condition, be sure to consult your doctor before you begin supplementation.)

Alzheimer's, "vitamin E is not as effective as laboratory experiments would suggest, although it had some positive effect in the Alzheimer's trial and is still used in conjunction with other medications in the clinical treatment of Alzheimer's," says Dr. Schubert.

In the quest for a cure, however, researchers are attempting to fuse vitamin E with something like a steroid to make a drug that's more potent, says Dr. Schubert.

It's too early to tell whether vitamin E supplements alone can help ward off Alzheimer's disease. But Dr. Schubert says there's enough potential to warrant taking supplements. "Vitamin E is pretty hard to get in your normal diet, because it's primarily in vegetable oils," he says. "And if you don't eat enough, the vitamin E in your blood and brain actually decreases as you get older. That can be elevated somewhat by vitamin E supplements."

Although you should see your doctor first, about 400 IU of vitamin E a day should be enough for most people, he says. The Daily Value for vitamin E is 30 IU.

Folic Acid May Preserve Memory

Folic acid, or vitamin B_9, is earning scientific attention when it comes to maintaining cognitive function in the aging brain. Research has shown that folic acid may reduce levels of homocysteine, a protein that's suspected of increasing the risk of Alzheimer's. A study reported at the Alzheimer's Association International Conference on the Prevention of Dementia found that daily doses of 800 micrograms of folic acid helped older adults perform better on tests of memory, reaction time, and thinking speed. While folic acid appeared to benefit mental functioning, this study didn't focus on whether it has the ability to prevent Alzheimer's.

However, a larger, long-term study did take a closer look at how folic acid may affect Alzheimer's. Researchers for the Baltimore Longitudinal Study of Aging, funded by the National Institutes of Health, analyzed the diet and supplement use of 579 participants over the course of 9 years. They found that older adults who consumed 400 micrograms of folic acid every day reduced their risk of Alzheimer's by more than 50 percent. Researchers didn't find any added benefit to taking more than 400 micrograms, the Recommended Dietary Allowance. Participants maintained their folic acid intake through a combination of folate-rich foods and folic acid supplements.

The Thiamin Connection

While vitamin E researchers try to protect the brain against the ravages of amyloid plaques, those studying thiamin have taken a different approach: improving the memory of people with Alzheimer's.

In a study at the Medical College of Georgia in Augusta, researchers treated 18 Alzheimer's patients for 5 months with megadoses of thiamin ranging from 3,000 to 8,000 milligrams a day, with the dose changing from month to month.

At the end of each month, the participants were given a brief bedside exam that included questions about the date, the name of the hospital, and the city, county, and state, says Kimford Meador, MD, former head of the section of behavioral neurology at the college. When the results were analyzed, Dr. Meador says, the research team discovered that some participants improved slightly the month they took 5,000 milligrams of thiamin a day.

"Overall, even in those whose scores dropped, they didn't drop as fast as they 'should have,'" says Dr. Meador, who is now the Melvin Greer professor of neurology and director of the clinical Alzheimer program at the University of Florida in Gainesville. In other words, he would have expected people in the later stages of the disease to perform poorly, but while taking the vitamin, they were doing better than expected.

"In particular, on the bedside exam you can expect a three-point drop almost every 4 to 6 months. We didn't see that in these people," he explains. "Our people either maintained where they were or dropped a point or two—not as far as they should have. At this stage of the research, this is pretty much the best you can hope for."

Why might something like thiamin help protect memory? It's possible that thiamin helps make an important neurotransmitter called acetylcholine, which helps the nerve impulses that carry thought leap across the gaps between brain cells, more available in the brain, explains Dr. Meador. And acetylcholine levels are lower in people with Alzheimer's. Interestingly, research shows that thiamin deficiency in older folks may run as high as 37 percent, Dr. Meador says.

Does this mean that people with Alzheimer's could benefit from taking large doses of thiamin? Much more research needs to be done before answering that question for sure, says Dr. Meador. "The effect of the treatment is not tremendous in and of itself, but it looks like it's an innocuous treatment and of mild benefit," he says. "I'd like to stress that it's not a final answer and that we studied small numbers. But until something better comes along, why not?" Taking 5,000 milligrams of thiamin a day caused only mild nausea in some people, says Dr. Meador. If you or a family member would like to try this therapy, make sure you discuss it with your doctor.

ANEMIA

GETTING BACK IN THE PINK

The old doctors' joke—that the first order of business is to find the pale patient against the white sheet—makes one good point about anemia: It tends to drain the color out of you, as surely as it pulls the plug on your energy supply.

Anemia is a blood disorder that results from a shortage of hemoglobin in the red blood cells, the disk-shaped cells that carry oxygen to all parts of the body. No matter what kind of anemia you have—and there are several varieties—the symptoms tend to be the same. Along with being pale and fatigued, you can feel weak and short of breath, your heart rate may climb, and you may find it hard to concentrate.

These symptoms occur because without sufficient hemoglobin in the red blood cells, all parts of the body, including the brain, are starved for oxygen. Thus, the heart tries to compensate by pumping more blood more often, explains Christine Gerbstadt, MD, RD, national spokesperson for the American Dietetic Association and nutritionist at Drexel University in Philadelphia.

Doctors can usually diagnose anemia by examining red blood cells under a microscope to determine their shape, size, and number and by doing tests that measure levels of different blood components.

"Even after we've determined the type of anemia, it's important to figure out what's causing it," Dr. Gerbstadt says. Everything from excessive bongo playing (the constant impact on the hands damages blood cells) to arctic temperatures and toxic drugs can cause the disease.

"Nutritional deficiencies are a fairly common cause of anemia, too," Dr. Gerbstadt says. In addition to iron deficiency, a shortage of folate (the naturally occurring form of folic acid) or vitamin B_{12} can be a culprit. Rarely, the problem turns out to be an inadequate supply of copper, riboflavin, or vitamins A, B_6, C, or E.

Here's what studies show.

Iron Out an Oxygen Shortage

We've all heard about iron-poor blood, and for good reason. Iron deficiency is by far the most common cause of anemia. Up to 58 percent of healthy young women may be short on iron, although not always to the point of anemia.

The problem is that many women don't consume enough iron each day to make up for the 2.5 milligrams or so they lose each month during menstruation. Pregnant women need even more iron. Teens and women nearing menopause also often come up short.

Studies show that women ages 18 to 24 get about 10.7 milligrams a day, which is nowhere near the Daily Value of 18 milligrams.

An iron shortage leads to a reduction in hemoglobin, the iron-based protein in red blood cells that lets these cells pick up oxygen in the lungs and release it in tissues where oxygen is low. "It's simple enough," Dr. Gerbstadt says. "These cells simply can't transport the oxygen you need." The cells even look pale under a microscope.

If you do have iron-deficiency anemia, your doctor will initially prescribe large amounts of iron—often 200 to 240 milligrams a day, usually in a form called ferrous sulfate. (Experts caution against taking this much iron without medical supervision.) Avoid using over-the-counter preparations such as enteric-coated iron tablets or capsules containing slow-release granules, experts say. Both can interfere with the body's ability to absorb the iron. And make sure your doctor continues your treatment for a sufficient amount of time. Although your anemia will be corrected in 3 to 4 months, it takes an additional 6 to 12 months of therapy for your body's iron stores to be replenished.

The large amount of iron used to correct anemia is not available through food, says Lona Sandon, RD, MEd, assistant professor of nutrition at the University of Texas Southwestern Medical Center at Dallas and American Dietetic Association spokesperson. "We still encourage women to eat more iron-containing foods, however," she says. Even beef, a food often avoided since cholesterol became a bad word, is recommended to anemic women, she says. "It's an unbeatable source of easily digested iron," she notes.

Getting Enough Copper

While you're stocking up on iron, you'll also want to make sure you're getting 2 milligrams of copper, the Daily Value.

Your body needs copper as well as iron to make hemoglobin. Although it's uncommon, copper deficiency can cause a kind of anemia similar to iron deficiency, Sandon says. Most people get less than 1.6 milligrams a day, the amount considered necessary to maintain proper copper balance in the body. Good food sources include shellfish, nuts, fruits, cooked oysters, and dried beans.

And if you're taking zinc supplements, you'll want to pay special attention to your copper intake. That's because zinc actually interferes with copper absorption. For each 10 milligrams of zinc you take, you should make sure that you're getting 1 milligram of copper. (It's also worth noting that people who

---

A Little Bug'll Do You

Did you know that vitamin B_{12} is produced by bacteria? These "bugs" live in the intestines of animals and in the soil that clings to fresh grains, fruits, and vegetables. If you've ever eaten a carrot straight out of the garden or taken a drink from a fresh mountain stream, you've probably gotten a little B_{12} along with it.

At one time, such contaminants may have added enough vitamin B_{12} to keep a strict vegetarian on the safe side of adequate, says Suzanne Havala Hobbs, DrPH, RD, at the University of North Carolina School of Public Health in Chapel Hill. However, modern sanitation measures make these unreliable sources of vitamin B_{12} today.

Strict vegetarians, known as vegans, eat no meats, fish, poultry, eggs, or dairy products, all good sources of vitamin B_{12}.

Several foods that vegetarians may eat—such as tempeh and miso, which are both fermented soybean products—were once thought to be good sources of vitamin B_{12}. Now, however, it is known that these foods contain inactive forms of the vitamin, which may actually compete for absorption with the form of B_{12} that is needed by the body.

Vegans can protect themselves from shortages of vitamin B_{12} by using B_{12}-fortified soy milk and eating fortified breakfast cereals or simply by taking an over-the-counter B_{12} supplement, Dr. Hobbs says. (The Daily Value for B_{12} is 6 micrograms.)

Because the body uses vitamin B_{12} very slowly, and because most people have considerable stores in their livers, it may take many years of a strict vegan diet for a B_{12} deficiency to appear in adults. One important exception: Breastfed babies of vegan mothers have been reported to show signs of deficiency-related blood and nervous system problems within months of birth. So check with your doctor if you are a vegan and are currently breastfeeding.

take more than 30 milligrams of zinc a day are at increased risk of developing anemia. So don't take more than this amount without medical supervision.)

The B$_{12}$ Anemia

There's no doubt that a little bit of vitamin B$_{12}$ can go a long, long way. The Daily Value is only 6 micrograms, the lowest requirement for any of the vitamins. But a dietary deficit of this nutrient causes major problems.

The anemia associated with vitamin B$_{12}$ deficiency is called pernicious anemia. Until 1934, this form of anemia was invariably fatal. People survived for months or even years while growing ever weaker, but they eventually succumbed. Then in 1934, two Boston doctors won the Nobel Prize in medicine for demonstrating that a diet rich in lightly cooked liver, which contains a lot of B$_{12}$, could ward off the deadly deficiency.

Vitamin B$_{12}$ is needed throughout the body to make DNA, a cell's genetic material. So a shortage leads to impaired cell production. Without adequate amounts of B$_{12}$, red blood cells suffer what is called maturation arrest, Dr. Gerbstadt explains. "They grow big, but they never mature into properly working red blood cells," she says. "Often they never make it out of the bone marrow, where they're made."

Fatigue is only one of several possible symptoms of pernicious anemia. Others include a burning tongue, tingling and numbness in the hands and feet, loss of appetite, irritability, mild depression, memory loss, stomach pains, and nonspecific neurological problems.

Today doctors know that usually it is not a shortage of this nutrient in the diet but an inability of the body to absorb vitamin B$_{12}$ that causes deficiency problems.

As people get older, they may have reduced production in their stomachs of an enzyme called intrinsic factor. Intrinsic factor escorts any vitamin B$_{12}$ that you've eaten across your intestinal lining into your bloodstream. As levels of intrinsic factor drop, less B$_{12}$ gets absorbed, and what's stored in the body gets used up.

"Those who've had stomach surgery or who have Crohn's disease or other stomach or intestinal problems may also lose the ability to absorb vitamin B$_{12}$," Dr. Gerbstadt says.

Most people with vitamin B$_{12}$ deficiencies need injections of B$_{12}$ to bring levels back to normal. "And most will need injections for the rest of their lives," says Dr. Gerbstadt. Only the small percentage of people whose B$_{12}$

deficiencies are caused by dietary shortages, such as strict vegetarians, will benefit from oral supplements or from getting more B_{12} from food to help meet the Daily Value of 6 micrograms.

Folate Shortage Can Cause Problems

They're called tea-and-toasters. And that's a fairly accurate description of the diets of some people who end up with anemia caused by a shortage of folate. Folate is a B vitamin found in brewer's yeast and in spinach and other dark

---

Prescriptions for Healing

Anemia is one disorder that you don't want to self-diagnose. See a doctor if you're tired all of the time. If your doctor determines that you have a nutrition-related form of anemia, he or she may recommend one of these regimens.

Nutrient	Daily Amount
Copper	1.6 milligrams
Folic acid	400 micrograms for older people
	1,000 micrograms for the general population
	2,000–3,000 micrograms for pregnant women
Iron	200–240 milligrams
Vitamin B_{12}	6 micrograms for strict vegetarians

MEDICAL ALERT: Talk to your doctor before taking more than 400 micrograms of folic acid daily, as high doses of this vitamin can mask symptoms of pernicious anemia, a disease due to vitamin B_{12} deficiency.

Most experts recommend that you consult your doctor before taking more than the Daily Value of iron (18 milligrams). Your doctor can prescribe the amount of iron that's appropriate for you based on a blood test. A daily intake of 25 milligrams or more for an extended period of time may cause undesirable side effects.

In people with vitamin B_{12} deficiencies caused by malabsorption problems, doctors give the vitamin by injection to bypass the faulty digestive system.

green leafy vegetables—the foliage foods from which this nutrient gets its name.

The body needs folate to make DNA. As with vitamin B_{12}, when folate is in short supply, blood cells never reach maturity. Instead, they remain large, immature egg-shaped cells that do not function well, Dr. Gerbstadt says.

Unlike vitamin B_{12}, folate is not stored in large amounts in the liver. The liver's supply is used up within 2 to 4 months, so symptoms of folate-related anemia can occur much more quickly than symptoms of vitamin B_{12} deficiency.

Blood tests can determine which vitamin is in short supply. "It's important to make this distinction, since supplementing with folic acid when it's actually vitamin B_{12} that's needed can mask symptoms and lead to B_{12}-related

---

Food Factors

Eating the right kinds of foods is important for healthy blood. Here's what the experts recommend to keep anemia at bay.

Love your red meat. Most doctors advise people to stay away from red meat because it's so high in cholesterol and certain cuts are high in saturated fats. A 3-ounce serving of lean beef offers 14 percent of the Daily Value of easily absorbed iron, along with 37 percent of the Daily Values of vitamin B_{12} and 9 micrograms of folate (the naturally occurring form of folic acid). "If you like lean beef, you can eat it three or four times a week without compromising a cholesterol-lowering regimen," says Lona Sandon, RD, MEd, assistant professor of nutrition at the University of Texas Southwestern Medical Center at Dallas and American Dietetic Association spokesperson.

Choose iron-rich plants. People who prefer to get their iron from nonanimal sources can count on whole-grain and enriched flours and breakfast cereals, dark green leafy vegetables such as kale, turnip greens, and spinach and legumes such as lima beans, chickpeas, and kidney beans to supply at least some of their needs. But strict vegetarians may need supplemental iron, Sandon says.

Chase it down with C. Vitamin C helps the body absorb iron, so include citrus fruits and juices, strawberries, bell peppers, tomatoes, and other vitamin C-rich foods with your meals, recommends Sandon.

Stick to ironware. Select cast-iron pots and pans rather than stainless steel or aluminum, especially for long-cooking dishes such as soups and stews. They can add a little iron to your diet and perhaps provide an edge against deficiency, says Sandon.

nerve damage," Dr. Gerbstadt says. So check with your doctor before taking folic acid as a supplement.

People found deficient are given 1,000 micrograms of supplemental folic acid a day to replenish their tissues' supplies. Pregnant women may need as much as 2,000 to 3,000 micrograms, Dr. Gerbstadt says. Those amounts are much more than you can get from even the best food sources.

Some research indicates that older people, especially those in not-so-great health, are better able to maintain normal blood levels of folate if they get 400 micrograms a day. That's an amount found in many multivitamin/mineral supplements.

Good food sources of folate include spinach, kidney beans, wheat germ, and asparagus. If you're relying on greens to boost your supply of this nutrient, stick to salads and lightly steamed vegetables since lengthy cooking at high temperatures destroys folate.

ANGINA

EASING THE SQUEEZE

Angina is actually a symptom, not a disease. This squeezing or dull, pressurelike pain—a kind of charley horse in the chest—is telling you that your heart muscle isn't getting enough oxygen to meet its needs. The pain is most likely to occur with exercise, stress, or cold weather or after a big meal, when the heart muscle is working its hardest and is in need of more oxygen.

Just like the pain of a heart attack, angina can radiate to the left shoulder and down the inside of the left arm, straight through to the back, and into the throat, the jaw, and even the right arm. The pain typically lasts for only 3 to 5 minutes. If it lasts longer than 15 to 20 minutes, or gets worse, get to a hospital—fast! You could be having a heart attack.

People who get episodes of angina pain usually have coronary heart disease. The spaghetti-size arteries that deliver blood to the heart muscle have been narrowed or clogged by plaque, which forms from cholesterol and scar tissue. Plaque reduces bloodflow to the heart muscle and makes arteries more likely to go into spasm, which reduces the bloodflow even more. And if a fatty deposit ruptures or develops a crevice or fissure where blood can enter, it invites clot-forming platelets to congregate at the scene. The end result of this whole mess can be a full-blown blood clot that obstructs bloodflow and causes a heart attack.

"Drugs such as nitroglycerin, beta-blockers, and calcium-channel blockers offer predictable help," says Robert DiBianco, MD, associate clinical professor emeritus of medicine at Georgetown University School of Medicine in Washington, DC. "These drugs dilate blood vessels and reduce the heart's oxygen needs. Nitroglycerin and beta-blockers may also help protect the heart from the damage associated with oxygen deprivation in the early hours of a heart attack." Cholesterol-lowering drugs are almost always prescribed to prevent future plaques and even shrink the plaques that are already present.

Standard treatment also includes a diet that cuts total fat to less than 30 percent of calories and saturated (animal) fat to under 10 percent of calories—the same fat-trimming diet used to cut your risk of further artery clogging, Dr. DiBianco says.

Some medical experts take these low-fat guidelines even further. They recommend that no more than 10 percent of calories come from fat—a diet that in some cases makes cholesterol deposits shrink and that often reduces muscle spasms and clotting. They also call for nutrients that may help protect the coronary arteries, such as folic acid. And they add other nutrients, such as selenium and magnesium, which are thought to help the heart function better under less than ideal circumstances.

Here's what research shows may help.

Folic Acid: Keeping Things Fluid

One of the many risk factors for coronary heart disease is high homocysteine levels. An elevated amount of this amino acid can damage coronary arteries, making it easier for platelets to clot. Some studies are finding that folic acid supplements can decrease homocysteine levels, allowing blood to flow easily through the blood vessels. Homocysteine levels are usually elevated in people with kidney failure, so researchers at the University of Londrina in Brazil administered 10 milligrams of folic acid three times a year for 2 years to hospital patients. At the end of the study, the homocysteine levels of 92 percent of the patients who received folic acid supplements were normalized. The levels of the patients who received the placebo remained elevated throughout the 2 years. The people who took the folic acid supplement also had a decrease in the thickness of the carotid artery wall, which allowed blood to

flow more easily. The researchers theorized that folic acid may prevent cardiovascular deterioration.

While this and several other studies suggest that folic acid can reduce
homocysteine levels, it hasn't yet been proven that folic acid can reduce the
risk of heart disease. Several clinical trials are under way to get a better

Food Factors

To ax angina, choose foods that help keep your arteries free-flowing.
Here are the details.

Trim fat to the bone. If you can get below 20 percent of calories
from fat and see a big drop in your cholesterol levels, you may even
begin to reverse clogged arteries, says Robert DiBianco, MD, associate
clinical professor emeritus of medicine at Georgetown University School
of Medicine in Washington, DC. The best way to go super low-fat? Eat
mostly vegetarian, with a meal or two of fish each week. Stick to low-fat
or nonfat dairy products, and use olive oil or canola oil sparingly to
season salads and other vegetables. However, before you choose a diet,
get a quick cholesterol check to know which one is right for you.

Eat some mucilage. No, not library paste. It's the gummy soluble
fiber found in flaxseed, oat bran, and many fruits. (The bulk laxative
Metamucil has psyllium, one of these soluble fibers.) Mucilage soaks up
cholesterol-laden bile acids, secreted into the intestines by the liver.
When you eat foods that contain it, your cholesterol levels drop, so
you're less likely to develop blockages in your coronary arteries, Dr.
DiBianco explains.

Get stinky. Scientific studies have shown that the chemical components of onions and garlic help counteract increased platelet stickiness
after a high-fat meal. Platelets are disk-shaped components of blood
that can stick together and to artery walls, causing clots.

Go gingerly. This fiery spice also reduces platelet stickiness. Indian
researchers found that 2 to 3 teaspoons of powdered ginger significantly inhibited platelet stickiness after a fatty meal.

Munch on mackerel. Omega-3 fatty acids, found in oily fish such as
mackerel, tuna, salmon, and sardines, help blood vessels relax, research
suggests. These fatty acids help reduce levels of two potentially harmful types of blood fats: LDL cholesterol and triglycerides. They also
reduce the tendency for blood to clot. "But this is not a food source to
pile on, since fish oil is fat and contains nine calories in each gram," says
Dr. DiBianco.

picture of folic acid's role in cardiovascular health. Until then, rely on green leafy vegetables and fortified breakfast cereals for sufficient folate intake, or make sure to get the Dietary Reference Intake of 400 micrograms through supplements.

Add On Some Selenium

Researchers have long known that without selenium the heart is more prone to plaque buildup. Now researchers know that without adequate amounts of selenium, the heart can suffer in another way as well. Scientists at the Beltsville Human Nutrition Research Center in Beltsville, Maryland, and the University of Buenos Aires in Argentina found that the hearts of selenium-deficient mice didn't pump blood as vigorously.

Fortunately, few Americans are deprived of selenium, so heart damage due to this deficiency is rare in the United States. Unfortunately, far too many Americans have heart disease, which is the single leading cause of death, but there's increasing evidence that selenium may protect coronary vessels.

Prescriptions for Healing

For easing the pain of angina, some doctors recommend both a low-fat diet and these nutrients.

Nutrient	Daily Amount
Folic acid	400 micrograms
Magnesium	400 milligrams
Selenium	55 micrograms

MEDICAL ALERT: *If you have angina, you should be under a doctor's care.*

Taking an excess of 1,000 milligrams of folic acid a day can trigger symptoms of vitamin B_{12} deficiency.

People who have heart or kidney problems should not take magnesium supplements without medical supervision.

Selenium in doses exceeding 400 micrograms daily should be taken only under medical supervision.

Researchers from Johns Hopkins University in Baltimore analyzed 25 observational studies involving selenium and found that the greater the concentration of selenium, the lower the risk of heart disease. Overall, a 50 percent increase in selenium intake was associated with a 24 percent reduction in heart disease risk. It's quite possible that selenium may limit the oxidation of LDL cholesterol, the "bad" cholesterol that encourages a buildup of plaque in the arteries. The authors of the studies caution that larger ongoing studies are needed before a direct link between selenium and reduced risk can be established.

Doctors who recommend selenium supplements to their heart patients generally stick to 50 to 200 micrograms a day. Supplements in excess of 400 micrograms should be taken only under medical supervision, however. (The Daily Value is 70 micrograms.) To up your intake from foods, munch on whole-grain cereals, seafood, garlic, and eggs.

Magnesium May Smooth Things Out

Magnesium is well known for its ability to relax the smooth (involuntarily controlled) muscles. These include the muscles that wrap around blood vessels, bronchial tubes, and the gastrointestinal tract. That's why magnesium seems to be helpful for disorders that may involve muscle constriction, such as high blood pressure, Raynaud's phenomenon, migraines, and at least some kinds of angina.

In several studies, magnesium given intravenously was effective in stopping variant angina, spasms in the coronary arteries not related to a permanent blockage.

"Oral magnesium also seems to be helpful, at least for some kinds of angina," says Burton M. Altura, PhD, a professor of physiology, pharmacology, and medicine at SUNY Downstate Medical Center in Brooklyn, New York, and a leading magnesium researcher.

Unfortunately, magnesium deficiency seems to be all too common in people with heart disease. Studies show that up to 65 percent of all people in intensive care units and 20 to 35 percent of people with heart failure come up short on magnesium.

Magnesium deficiency can be induced by drugs meant to help heart problems, Dr. Altura says. Some types of diuretics (water pills) cause the body to excrete both magnesium and potassium, as does digitalis, a commonly prescribed heart drug. Signs of magnesium deficiency include nausea, muscle weakness, irritability, and electrical changes in the heart muscle.

If you have angina, talk to your doctor to see if your diet is adequate in magnesium. Your doctor might suggest making changes in your diet to increase the magnesium content. If you're still low on magnesium, he or she may recommend magnesium supplementation, Dr. Altura says. How much magnesium you need depends on the results of a magnesium loading test, which involves taking a large dose of magnesium, or a magnesium-specific electrode test, which measures magnesium in bodily fluids, Dr. Altura explains. Either test will reveal how much magnesium your body retains. "Not everyone needs to take the same amount," Dr. Altura says.

Although magnesium is considered to be a fairly safe mineral, even in high doses, don't take supplemental magnesium without medical supervision if you have kidney or heart problems. You could develop a dangerous buildup of magnesium in your blood, or your heart could slow down too much.

The Daily Value for magnesium is 400 milligrams. Based on his research, Dr. Altura has calculated that 70 percent of men get only 185 to 260 milligrams daily, while 70 percent of women get 172 to 235 milligrams daily.

Diets rich in vegetables and whole grains are much higher in magnesium than diets that include lots of meats, dairy products, and refined foods.

ASTHMA

OPENING UP FOR EASIER BREATHING

Want to know exactly what asthma feels like?

"Pinch your nose shut and breathe through a straw," suggests Nancy Sander, president of the Allergy and Asthma Network Mothers of Asthmatics. Then try climbing a flight of stairs or chasing after something fast—say, a frisky toddler. You'll soon be gasping for air the way someone with asthma does during an attack. "It's a frightening experience," Sander says.

The usual setup for an attack combines an allergic (or supersensitive) immune system, an inherited trait, with exposure to environmental allergic triggers such as animal dander, mold spores, and pollen or to environmental irritant triggers such as air pollution, cold air, and cigarette smoke. Other activators can include respiratory infections, colds, laughter, crying, anger, exercise, and stress.

There are two major components of asthma. One is noisy—the wheezing, coughing, choking, can't-catch-your-breath feeling. That's the part most people call an asthma attack, or bronchospasm and congestion.

The second part of asthma is quiet. It is called inflammation—the part of asthma that is always present but not always noticed. Just as a sunburn may not be evident until long after you've come in from the sun, airway inflammation is not noticeable until the damage has become so extensive that an asthma attack begins.

During an asthma attack, the muscles surrounding the lungs' bronchial tubes contract, narrowing airways and making it hard to breathe. People with chronic asthma also have inflammation in their lungs. The membranes lining the inner walls of the air passages become swollen and leaky. And the glands within these walls produce excess mucus. That makes it harder for the lungs to do their job of gas exchange, picking up oxygen from the air and dumping carbon dioxide out of the body.

Asthma is usually treated with drugs that open airways and reduce inflammation as well as by avoiding substances that trigger attacks. For some people, that means finding a new home for a family pet, exchanging the wall-to-wall carpeting for linoleum, or steering clear of cigarette smoke, car and truck exhaust, and chemical fumes.

Dietary counseling for asthma, especially in young children, may include testing for possible problem foods. But it doesn't often include recommendations for vitamin or mineral supplements, experts say. Nevertheless, some research suggests that certain nutrients may play roles in asthma by reducing airway sensitivity and dampening inflammation.

Here's what research shows. (*Note:* If you're feeling well enough to reduce your dosage of asthma medication, do so only under medical supervision, experts warn. Stopping asthma drugs abruptly could lead to problems.)

Magnesium Makes a Difference

The presence of higher magnesium levels seems to correlate with fewer asthma symptoms, says Donald W. Russell, MD, an allergy and immunology specialist and assistant clinical professor at the University of North Carolina School of Medicine in Chapel Hill. In a 2001 cross-sectional study of over 2,500 adults, conducted at the University of Nottingham in England, people who got at least 100 milligrams a day of dietary magnesium had a reduction in airway hyperactivity and reported less wheezing than those who took in less than 100 milligrams a day.

This essential mineral is important for every organ in the body. It's intimately involved in the production of energy and helps regulate levels of vital nutrients. It also has a potential special relevance to asthma sufferers. Large doses of magnesium relax the muscles around blood vessels and airways. Intravenous magnesium is helpful for a person having a life-threatening asthma attack called status asthmaticus, which does not respond to the usual drugs.

A more comfortable way to administer the appropriate dose of magnesium may be on the horizon. Researchers at George Eby Research in Austin, Texas, administered magnesium lozenges to patients in need of asthma res-

Food Factors

Reactions to protein or additives are the strongest links between asthma and food. Additional factors such as salt and caffeine may also play roles. Here's what you need to know.

Aim for an ideal body weight. The rates of obesity in America seem to climb every year. So do the rates of asthma, affecting approximately 7 percent of American adults. Today researchers believe that one could cause the other and vice versa. In fact, obesity raises the risk of asthma by 50 percent. One of the best ways to improve lung capacity is to maintain a healthy weight through exercise. If you have asthma and are overweight, talk to your doctor about how to start an exercise and weight reduction program while maintaining control of your symptoms.

Beware the guacamole. Thanks to laws that require sulfites to be listed on labels, it's fairly easy these days for people with asthma to avoid this potentially deadly food preservative. Dried fruits and vegetables, instant food mixes, and wine are the store-bought foods most likely to contain large amounts of sulfites, says Martha White, MD, director of research at the Institute for Asthma and Allergy in Wheaton and Chevy Chase, Maryland.

It's still possible, however, to get unsuspected sulfites. Potatoes, shellfish, shrimp, salads, and guacamole (avocado dip) are often treated with sulfites. And imported beers and wines may not list sulfites on their labels, Dr. White says. "People are most likely to be unexpectedly exposed to sulfites when eating out," she says. This is because they have no control over food processing or preparation. Call ahead to find out

cue. The throat lozenges, which were formulated with a strong solution of 100 milligrams of a magnesium chloride that releases concentrated ions, prevented and even ended asthma attacks almost immediately and produced a more rapid and stronger response than inhaled or injected magnesium.

The researchers suggest that the promising results of this study warrant further investigations. However, recent clinical trials have yet to show that taking a magnesium supplement produces significant results, says Dr. Russell. Until more studies confirm that magnesium can help control asthma, researchers agree that it's a good idea to get the Daily Value of magnesium, which is 400 milligrams. Studies show that most people fall short.

Your best choices of magnesium-rich foods are nuts, beans, and whole grains. If you are considering trying magnesium supplements, be sure to check with your doctor first if you have heart or kidney problems.

---

which, if any, foods on a restaurant's menu contain sulfites, she suggests.

Stay away from salt. People taking oral steroid drugs for their asthma may need to monitor their sodium intakes because of problems with fluid retention. Your best strategy for cutting back on salt is to avoid processed foods. Canned soups, packaged macaroni and cheese, cottage cheese, and lunchmeats are all high in sodium.

Switch to fish. The oil in fatty fish such as mackerel, salmon, and swordfish has anti-inflammatory effects that may help some people with asthma—and their children, and their children's children. In a study at the University of Aberdeen in Scotland, mothers were asked to complete food questionnaires during their pregnancies and then again when their children were 5 years old. The results revealed that women who had the highest intake of apples and who ate fish at least once a week during their pregnancies had children with less risk of asthma and skin eczema.

Know your trigger foods. Some people, especially children, have asthma attacks soon after eating foods such as peanuts or other nuts, eggs, fish, shellfish, milk, soy, wheat, or bananas, says Dr. White.

People who believe they have such food allergies—or who eliminate certain foods from their children's diets in the hope of improving symptoms—should make sure their diets remain balanced, she emphasizes. "If you are eliminating dairy products, for instance, it's important to take calcium supplements," she says.

Vitamin C May Ease Wheezing

People with asthma sometimes take supplements of vitamin C because they believe in its legendary virus-fighting powers. There's some proof that vitamin C does indeed reduce the duration and severity of colds. Studies of people living in or enduring extreme circumstances, such as soldiers in subarctic conditions, marathon runners, and skiers, claim that vitamin C supplements reduce the risk of developing colds by 50 percent.

But vitamin C may do more than ease sneezing and sniffles.

A study at Cornell University in Ithaca, New York, measured serum levels of vitamin C in 7,500 youths between the ages of 4 and 16. The researchers found that an increase of vitamin C reduced the incidence of asthma by 10 to 20 percent. In children who were exposed to tobacco smoke, the risk reduction climbed to 40 percent. In another study, researchers at Johns Hopkins University School of Medicine evaluated information from more than 4,000 children in a nationwide survey and found that those with low levels of vitamin C were at higher risk of developing asthma.

While these studies suggest that a high dietary intake of vitamin C-rich foods is associated with improved levels of lung capacity, they don't necessarily mean that vitamin C supplements will prevent asthma. They do, though, have intriguing implications.

One of the most commonly prescribed asthma medications is inhaled corticosteroids. British researchers found that vitamin C supplements may decrease the need for asthma sufferers to use them. Adults with asthma who were given 1 gram of vitamin C for 10 weeks were able to maintain control of their symptoms with less reliance on their corticosteroid medications. The results make sense, since vitamin C is said to support the adrenal glands, which produce the body's own corticosteroid hormones. This is promising news for people using inhaled steroids because higher amounts of these medications can have adverse side effects.

Vitamin C may protect the lungs in a number of ways. First, its antioxidant actions protect the lungs from the damaging effects of chemicals in smoke or smog-laden air. It neutralizes these chemicals so that they can't hurt cells. That's important, because exposure to air pollution often makes asthma worse. Vitamin C is also believed to neutralize the harmful chemicals produced by the body as a result of the inflammation that occurs with asthma, helping to prevent a vicious cycle of increasingly severe attacks.

Prescriptions for Healing

Most doctors use drugs, not vitamins and minerals, to treat asthma. Those who do provide nutritional therapy usually combine it with drugs and with recommendations to avoid exposure to substances that can trigger an asthma attack. These are the nutrients that some doctors recommend.

Nutrient	Daily Amount
Beta-carotene	6 milligrams
Magnesium	400 milligrams
Selenium	100 micrograms
Vitamin C	500–1,000 milligrams
Vitamin E	400 IU

MEDICAL ALERT: If you have asthma, you should be under a doctor's care.

If you're feeling well enough to reduce your dosage of asthma medication, do so only under medical supervision, experts warn. Stopping asthma drugs abruptly could lead to problems.

If you have heart or kidney problems, you should check with your doctor before taking supplemental magnesium.

Selenium in doses exceeding 400 micrograms daily should be taken only under medical supervision.

If you are taking anticoagulant drugs, you should not take vitamin E supplements. (Though generally a dose of up to 1,500 IU of vitamin E a day is considered safe, some recent reports suggest that taking more than 400 IU a day could be harmful to people with cardiovascular or circulatory disease or with cancer. If you have such a condition, be sure to consult your doctor before you begin supplementation.)

And, as mentioned earlier, vitamin C also supports the adrenal glands, the body's own personal corticosteroid factory.

Doctors recommending vitamin C to their patients with asthma who exercise prescribe 500 to 1,000 milligrams a day. That amount is considered well within the safe range, but higher doses can cause diarrhea in some people.

Antioxidants Shield Lungs

Researchers who say vitamin C is helpful for asthma point out that other nutrients with similar antioxidant properties could be beneficial. These nutrients include vitamin E, selenium, and beta-carotene, a yellow pigment found in carrots, cantaloupe, and other fruits and vegetables. Laboratory work indicates that all three help reduce inflammation-producing biochemicals.

"So far, however, all we have are primarily case-control studies," says Dr. Russell. Those studies that looked at actual supplementation with micronutrients or vitamins did not show significant improvement of lung function, with the exception of one study, according to Dr. Russell. In that study, by researchers in Sweden, people with asthma who took 100 micrograms of selenium daily for 14 weeks had improved lung function and were less sensitive to airway-constricting inhalants than when they were taking placebos (inactive pills).

Selenium is needed in the body to produce glutathione peroxidase, an enzyme that helps protect cells by breaking down biochemicals associated with inflammation.

It's too soon to say for sure whether supplementing a regular diet with selenium will help people with asthma. People who want to try it can safely take 100 micrograms, the amount found beneficial in the Swedish study. (The Daily Value is 70 micrograms.)

Studies have shown that people generally get about 100 micrograms of selenium a day from the average healthy diet. Don't overdo it with selenium, say nutrition experts. A daily intake of 400 micrograms from foods and supplements is considered the upper limit of the safe range.

People who want to take other antioxidant nutrients can safely supplement with up to 400 IU of vitamin E and 6 milligrams of beta-carotene a day. It's a good idea to talk to your doctor before taking more than 400 IU of vitamin E daily. However, adds Dr. Russell, a diet of fish, whole grains, fruits, and fresh vegetables may be the best approach to prevention of asthma.

Some studies suggest that in addition to the nutrients mentioned above, calcium, zinc, copper, and vitamin D may all play supporting roles in easing the symptoms of asthma. Whew! "There's no doubt in my mind that people with asthma can do better in the long run if they eat a healthy diet, exercise, maintain healthy indoor air environments, and use medications strategically," says Sander.

BEDSORES

NOURISHING SKIN
UNDER PRESSURE

Y ou would think that a couple of thousand years would be enough time
to find a way to beat an ailment as common as bedsores. Evidence of
these painful lesions has been found in ancient Egyptian mummies, but today
we're still struggling to prevent bedsores from forming on people who are
confined to bed.

Clearly, the quality of mattresses has improved since the rule of King Tut.
So why are bedsores still such a problem? Because bedsores, also known as
pressure ulcers, have less to do with beds and lots to do with nutrition, say
the experts. And that, sadly, is something that can still be pretty poor even
in this day and age, especially among the elderly.

"The bottom line is that a malnourished person is predisposed to developing a pressure ulcer," explains Mitchell V. Kaminski Jr., MD, clinical professor of surgery at the Rosalind Franklin University of Medicine and
Science/Chicago Medical School and staff surgeon at Saints Mary and Elizabeth Medical Center in Chicago. Dr. Kaminski has researched and written
extensively on the nutrition-pressure ulcer connection. "In fact, the more
malnourished a person is, the more severe the ulcer. I believe that malnutrition may be the most significant component in the development of the type
of pressure ulcer commonly seen in Americans today," he says.

Anatomy of a Bedsore

Essentially, a bedsore occurs as the result of skin being suffocated beneath
the body's weight. When someone lies or sits in one position for a long time,
as is the case with people who are bedridden with illness or who use wheelchairs, the skin over bony prominences such as the hips and tailbone is
squeezed against hard surfaces. This squeezing cuts off the blood supply that
delivers oxygen and nutrients to the tissues. Eventually the smaller blood vessels clot and a sore red patch appears, which, left unchecked, can crack open

and develop into a craterlike, painful wound. In worst-case scenarios, the tissues can erode deeply, exposing muscle or bone.

One of the best ways to avoid bedsores is by continually changing positions. Doctors recommend moving every 15 minutes, if possible, or at least every 2 hours if you're in a bed or every hour if you're in a chair. It doesn't take much time for a bedsore to develop, especially when skin is thin and frail, when wound healing is slower, and when movement is limited, as is the case with many elderly people.

That's why good nutrition is essential. The healthier and thicker your skin is, the better it can withstand the weight of your body and the less likely you are to get a bedsore.

Food Factors

Though they're called bedsores, your nutrition—along with change of position—is more important than your mattress when it comes to avoiding these painful lesions. Here is what most experts recommend to keep your skin healthy and free of bedsores.

Get protection from protein. "Protein is very, very important for healing skin," says Mitchell V. Kaminski Jr., M.D., clinical professor of surgery at the Rosalind Franklin University of Medicine and Science/Chicago Medical School and staff surgeon at Saints Mary and Elizabeth Medical Center in Chicago. "You really need to increase your protein intake when you're dealing with pressure ulcers."

Researchers at the University of Southampton's Institute of Human Nutrition in the United Kingdom found that pressure sores healed faster in patients given high-protein supplements and feeding tube formulas than in those who received the standard-nutritional supplements and formulas. They also discovered that those high-protein formulas significantly reduced the incidence of pressure sores in patients who were at high risk of developing them.

To prevent or treat bedsores, Dr. Kaminski recommends that people get about 0.68 gram of protein per pound of body weight. That's about double the amount of protein you would typically need. To get enough protein to prevent bedsores, a 140-pound woman who is at risk, for example, would need 95 grams of protein, or about the amount found in four 3-ounce cans of tuna.

"If it's too difficult to get that much protein from foods, liquid protein drinks work just as well," says Dr. Kaminski. These are available in your local pharmacy.

Prescriptions for Healing

Research shows that strong skin and physical activity are your best defenses in the fight against bedsores. Here's what many experts recommend to toughen up and heal your skin.

Nutrient	Daily Amount
Vitamin C	1,000 milligrams
Zinc	15 milligrams
Plus a multivitamin/mineral supplement	

MEDICAL ALERT: It's important that any bedsore be treated under a doctor's supervision.

Note: Though nutritional supplementation may expedite healing, it's very important that any bedsore that develops be treated under a doctor's supervision. And anyone who has diabetes must be especially alert for this condition. Bedsores can get worse very, very quickly.

Multivitamin Protection

Some doctors recommend multivitamin/mineral supplements for most people who are at risk for developing pressure ulcers, because it ensures that they get the appropriate nutrient intake every day.

A multivitamin/mineral supplement is especially important for older people who are confined to bed or to wheelchairs. They are frequently deficient in a wide array of vitamins, notes Dr. Kaminski.

Vitamin C Plays a Major Role

One of the most common single vitamin deficiencies among the elderly is vitamin C. Too little of this vitamin opens the door to thinning skin, capillary fragility, and, consequently, bedsores.

Some studies even indicate that vitamin C deficiency may be the key nutritional factor in bedsore development. Brazilian researchers found that hospital patients with bedsores had lower levels of ascorbic acid, or vitamin C, than those patients without bedsores. Fortunately, studies have also shown that supplements of vitamin C can significantly aid in the healing of bedsores. Doctors at Deakin University in Australia discovered that patients with bedsores who took a regimen of vitamin C, along with zinc and arginine, healed faster than those who took supplements without these nutrients.

"Vitamin C deficiency can double your healing time," says Dr. Kaminski. "I routinely put my patients who are being treated for or who are at risk for pressure ulcers on 1,000 milligrams of vitamin C a day. Vitamin C won't help if there is no deficiency, but the extra vitamin won't hurt, either."

Zinc Speeds Healing

Like vitamin C, zinc has been linked in studies to preventing bedsores and helping them heal.

"If there is a zinc deficiency, healing time is retarded by 50 percent," says Dr. Kaminski. "Like vitamin C, supplemental zinc won't do any good if there is no deficiency. But zinc deficiency is so common that I routinely supplement it as well."

The Daily Value for zinc is 15 milligrams, an amount that you can get from either foods or supplements. To add some superior food sources of zinc to your diet, try eating more seafood and shellfish, wheat germ, and whole-grain breads and cereals.

BERIBERI

GETTING ENOUGH THIAMIN

The legend goes something like this: A 19th-century Dutch shipboard physician, studying the effects of a strange disease in the Far East, calls for his next patient. But instead of seeing someone walking through the door, he hears a faint cry of "Beriberi!"

Roughly translated from Sinhalese, a language of the tiny country of Sri Lanka, the response means "I can't, I can't!" The would-be patient literally

---

Prescriptions for Healing

These days, cases of beriberi are rare in the Western world. When doctors do encounter patients with this thiamin-deficiency disease, they administer the vitamin intravenously or intramuscularly.

Intravenous thiamin is given only in cases of severe deficiency. In less severe cases, doctors prescribe oral thiamin, along with other B-complex vitamins.

Nutrient	Daily Amount
Thiamin	50–100 milligrams, given intravenously or intramuscularly for 7–14 days

MEDICAL ALERT: *If you have symptoms of beriberi, you should see a doctor for proper diagnosis and treatment.*

---

couldn't muster enough muscle to get up to see the doctor. And his response became the name of the mystery disease.

Years later, this disease, which involves a gradual decline in neuromuscular coordination, was linked to a deficiency of thiamin. Although rice and whole grains—dietary staples in that part of the world—naturally contain thiamin, the process of refining them for consumption removes the nutrient. The result: Those folks who live on the devitalized rice and grains become thiamin-deficient. The deficiency soon leads to symptoms such as leg swelling and numbness, fluid buildup in the heart, shortness of breath, memory loss, and coordination problems.

Today beriberi is rare in the United States because most foods are enriched with vitamins, such as thiamin. Eating a balanced, healthy diet will all but ensure an adequate intake of thiamin.

Dealing with Alcohol Abuse

But what fortification eliminates, alcohol precipitates. The most common cause of beriberi in the Western world is alcohol abuse. Thiamin intake is reduced because so many calories are consumed as alcohol, and alcohol can impair thiamin absorption.

As a result, some alcoholics go on to suffer from a beriberi-like disease known as Wernicke-Korsakoff syndrome, which includes symptoms such as severe memory loss, unsteady gait, and loss of appetite, says Gary E. Gibson, PhD, professor of neuroscience at the Weill Medical College of Cornell University in New York City. "If you dramatically reduce thiamin intake, you reduce the ability of the brain to use glucose. And if you reduce that, you have impaired mental ability," he explains. Severe thiamin deficiency not only kills the brain cells responsible for memory but also leads to an increase in a protein that has been linked to Alzheimer's disease. In experimental models, thiamin deficiency exacerbates the formation of amyloid plaques, which are the main characteristic of Alzheimer's disease, says Dr. Gibson. Brains of patients who died of Wernicke-Korsakoff also contain tangles—another characteristic of Alzheimer's disease.

When doctors encounter severe thiamin deficiency these days, they administer the vitamin intravenously or intramuscularly, usually in doses of 50 to 100 milligrams daily for 7 to 14 days. (For the full details on using nutrients to treat alcoholism, see page 72.)

BIRTH DEFECTS

EATING RIGHT FOR TWO

Conception is the quick and easy part. From then on, the fertilized egg has to go through an intricate 9-month-long process of cell growth, division, migration, and specialization, all geared toward producing a living, breathing bundle of joy.

That single fertilized egg cell must grow and divide to produce several billion cells. At the same time, all of the individual cells being formed receive directions to move toward specific regions of the embryo, perhaps where an arm or an eye will be. They also receive signals to differentiate, so some become, say, nerve cells, while others become bone cells. The process is complicated enough that it's a wonder couples turn out as many perfect babies as they do.

When things do go wrong, it's due to any number of different factors. Doctors now know that certain drugs, x-rays, exposure to environmental toxins, certain infections, and inherited genetic abnormalities can all cause a wide range of birth defects if the embryo is exposed at certain critical stages of development. So, too, can nutritional shortages.

Over 120,000 babies (1 in 33) in the United States are born each year with birth defects, and in 70 percent of cases the cause is unknown. However, in many cases, poor nutrition is believed to be one of the factors, acting either directly or in concert with genetic and environmental factors. Though there is still much uncertainly about the different roles that poor nutrition plays in disrupting the normal development of the fetus, the deficiency of one vitamin, folate, has been linked to human birth defects.

"Right now there doesn't seem to be any other nutrient that has as small a margin of safety as folic acid," says Barbara W. Huggins, MD, professor of pediatrics at the University of Texas Health Center at Tyler.

Here's what research shows.

Folic Acid: Right from the Start

As early as 1965, researchers suggested a relationship between folate deficiency and major central nervous system problems. That connection was suspected after reports of very serious birth defects in babies born to women taking anticonvulsant drugs that interfered with folate metabolism.

Those serious birth defects are called neural tube defects (NTDs) and are caused when the spine of the fetus fails to close properly during the early stages of pregnancy.

In a developing baby, the neural tube is a fold of tissue running the length of the embryo. This tube is what develops into the central nervous system, consisting of the brain and spinal cord. The most severe form of NTD is anencephaly. It results when the neural tube fails to close at the top and the baby is born with only a very small brain or with no brain at all. The baby usually dies within a few hours or days.

The common form of NTD is called spina bifida, which results when the neural tube fails to close at the base of the spine. In severe cases, spina bifida causes crippling paralysis of the lower extremities and loss of bowel or bladder control.

Though scientists first suggested a link between NTD and the diet in the 1950s, there was no compelling evidence about a link between folate deficiencies and NTDs. However, in the late 1980s, two separate British studies found that women who had given birth to one baby with an NTD (which put them at high risk for having another) were much less likely to have a second baby with the same problem if they took folic acid supplements prior to becoming pregnant and during pregnancy.

In fact, in the high-risk group of the second study, the incidence of neural tube defects was cut by more than 80 percent.

More recent research indicates that folic acid supplementation, if taken prior to conception and throughout the first trimester, can prevent up to 50 to 70 percent of first-time NTDs. The results of these studies were strong

---

Food Factors

Eating for your baby means paying particular attention to eating right.

Hop on the wagon. The devastating effects of alcohol on a developing fetus are now well known.

The best course of action is to plan your pregnancy and stop drinking all alcohol for at least a few weeks before you conceive, says Barbara W. Huggins, MD, professor of pediatrics at the University of Texas Health Center in Tyler. Fetal alcohol syndrome is 100 percent preventable if the pregnant woman completely abstains from alcohol during her pregnancy. If you use alcohol and are having trouble stopping, consult organizations in your community that can help you.

Don't cut carbs. Researchers have long known that folate deficiencies during pregnancy can lead to serious birth defects of the spine and brain. Up until the late 1990s, birth defects steadily declined as women followed their doctors' advice and increased their folic acid intake through supplements and diet. However, a 4-year study by the Centers for Disease Control and Prevention of 4,500 women in their childbearing years found that folate blood levels declined by 8 to 16 percent over the study period. Some experts speculate that one possible culprit is a booming diet trend— low-carbohydrate diets. Foods that are high in carbohydrates are avoided, but some of those foods, like bread and cereals, are also high in folate.

Women who are pregnant or planning to get pregnant should incorporate enriched breads and cereals with 100 percent of the Daily Value of folic acid into their diet. Before you start any diet that restricts certain foods or nutrients, talk to your doctor.

Forget the franks. A study by researchers at three different cancer centers and hospitals in the United States found that the children of women who ate cured meats, such as hot dogs, bacon, and lunchmeat, at least once a week during pregnancy were more than twice as likely to develop brain tumors as children whose mothers eschewed cured meats.

Although little is known about the cause of these childhood cancers, it is known that certain food preservatives and nitrites are converted to N-nitroso compounds in the body, explains Greta Bunin, PhD, research associate professor at Children's Hospital of Philadelphia. "In animals, nitrosamines (N-nitroso compounds) have been linked to nervous system cancers," she says.

enough that in 1992 the U.S. Public Health Service recommended that all women of childbearing age take 400 micrograms of folic acid daily to reduce their risk of having a pregnancy affected with spina bifida or another NTD. They also recommend that women who have had a baby with NTD take 4,000 micrograms of folic acid before and during pregnancy.

Requirements for this vitamin are much higher in the fetus because of the rapid rate of cell growth and division. Neural tube formation happens early in pregnancy, during the third and fourth weeks. Usually, that's about the time a woman first becomes aware that she's pregnant. "That's why it's important to start taking folic acid before you get pregnant," Dr. Huggins says. Studies show that folic acid offers the most protection when it's started at least 3 months prior to becoming pregnant and is continued for the first trimester.

A recent study published in the *British Medical Journal* has shown that folic acid is also effective in preventing another widespread birth defect: cleft lips and palates. In fact, the consumption of 400 micrograms or more of folic acid prior to conception and during the early stages of pregnancy decreases the risk of having a child with cleft lip or palate by 40 percent.

There is a subtle difference between folate and folic acid. Folate occurs naturally in a variety of foods such as dark leafy vegetables, legumes, citrus fruits and juices, and whole-grain products. Folic acid is the synthetic form of folate. A recent report released by the Institute of Medicine indicates that folic acid may be better absorbed than the folate found naturally in foods. "But because folate-containing foods are packed with so much good nutrition, they should always be part of a healthy diet," says Dr. Huggins.

Since 1998, the FDA has required manufacturers to add 430 to 1,400 micrograms of folic acid per pound of product to refined grain foods, like bread, rice, and noodles. Whole-grain products don't have to be enriched because they contain natural folate, but when the whole grain is refined to other products, like flour, the folate is lost.

Because there is good evidence that women aren't getting anywhere near the recommended daily requirements of 400 micrograms of folic acid, and because 56 percent of all pregnancies are unplanned, the best advice for all women of childbearing age is to supplement their daily diets with 400 micrograms of folic acid.

Taking a Little Insurance

Doctors say that pregnant women need extras of just about every other nutrient as well, including vitamin A, thiamin, riboflavin, vitamin B_{12}, calcium, phosphorus, magnesium, and iron. But dietary surveys indicate that mothers-to-be tend to come up short, consistently getting well below the Daily Values of seven nutrients: vitamins B_6, D, and E, folate, iron, zinc, and magnesium.

Prescriptions for Healing

If you're pregnant or planning to become pregnant within the next year, you should see an obstetrician/gynecologist to plan your course.

Why so far in advance? Because if you're overweight or underweight, you have a higher risk of delivering a baby with birth defects. And if you have diabetes, high blood pressure, or some other chronic disease, you'll want to make sure it's well under control.

If you're not already taking them, you'll need to start taking folic acid supplements 3 months before you stop using contraceptives. You'll also need a multivitamin with iron prescribed by your doctor.

Here's what doctors recommend to help prevent birth defects.

Nutrient	Daily Amount
Folic acid	400 micrograms prior to pregnancy
	800 micrograms during the first trimester of pregnancy
	4,000 micrograms before and during the first trimester of pregnancy for women who've had a baby with a neural tube defect

Pregnant women should also take these nutrients for general health.

Nutrient	Daily Amount
Calcium	1,200 milligrams
Iron	30 milligrams

Plus a multivitamin/mineral supplement containing the Recommended Dietary Allowances for pregnant women or a prenatal vitamin prescribed by your doctor.

MEDICAL ALERT: *High doses of iron, chromium, and selenium should be used with caution, so before taking a supplement with more than 100 percent of the Recommended Dietary Allowances for pregnant women, talk to your doctor.*

That's why Dr. Huggins recommends a multivitamin/mineral supplement that includes no more than the Recommended Dietary Allowances for pregnant women. "Use of a supplement as additional insurance is worthwhile and is not potentially damaging," she says.

If your doctor doesn't recommend a multivitamin/mineral supplement, ask her or him about taking one, especially if you don't eat as well as you should, Dr. Huggins advises. Some doctors also recommend additional amounts of iron and calcium to prevent the anemia and bone loss that can accompany pregnancy. (The Recommended Dietary Allowances for pregnant women are 30 milligrams of iron and 1,200 milligrams of calcium daily.)

On the other hand, it's possible to overdo it with supplements. For instance, women taking more than 10,000 IU of vitamin A daily or eating foods high in vitamin A, such as liver, have a mildly increased risk of having infants with deformities of the head, heart, and brain. You should also use caution with iron, chromium, and selenium. "To avoid high doses, choose a multivitamin that contains no more than 100 percent of the RDA for each vitamin and mineral. Before taking anything other than 100 percent of the RDA, check with your health care provider," says Dr. Huggins. And beware of herbal remedies, which can be toxic if you are trying to get pregnant, are pregnant, or are breastfeeding.

BLADDER INFECTIONS

FLUSHING OUT TROUBLE

For some women, the symptoms are all too familiar: burning and stinging during urination and the persistent urge to go, go, go, even when they have just gone. Their urine may be cloudy, smelly, and sometimes tinged with blood. The usual problem: a urinary tract infection, caused by bacteria that have worked their way up the urethra into the bladder and settled in for the duration.

Urinary tract infections are second only to colds when it comes to infections in women, whose anatomy sets the stage for trouble. (In men, urinary tract infections are much less common but potentially more serious, because they're often tied to prostate problems.)

Women who get bladder infections, particularly women who don't seem to be able to shake them, may have a problem with the cells lining the bladder, says Robert Moldwin, MD, associate professor of clinical urology and director of the Interstitial Cystitis Treatment Center at the Smith Institute for Urology, Long Island Jewish Medical Center, in New Hyde Park, New York. Somehow these cells have undergone a change that makes it easier for bacteria to stick to the bladder wall as well as to the vaginal wall. Once the bacteria are on the vaginal wall, it's easy for them to migrate to the bladder.

Food Factors

Drinking more water is about the only dietary move doctors agree on when it comes to urinary tract infections. Some recommend more acidic foods, since acidic urine can inhibit bacterial growth. Others think this is impractical, because the acid balance of urine can change from hour to hour. "Women may need to experiment with foods to see what sort of diet is least bladder-irritating for them," says Robert Moldwin, MD, assistant professor of urology at Albert Einstein College of Medicine and director of the Long Island Jewish Medical Center's Interstitial Cystitis Center in New Hyde Park, New York. Alkaline foods can help in treating symptoms such as urgency and frequency but can't treat specific bacterial infections, he adds.

Here is what's recommended. (*Note:* These dietary measures won't cure an established infection, but they may help thwart a recurrence or make urinating more comfortable.)

Drink up. Perhaps the single most important dietary measure you can take to prevent urinary tract infections (and to speed your recovery from them) is to drink lots of water—about six to eight 8-ounce glasses a day. Keeping yourself well hydrated helps flush bacteria out of your bladder.

Guzzle cranberry juice. Women have long touted cranberry juice for its ability to prevent bladder infections. Now there's scientific proof for this old wives' tale. But remember, if you have an infection, this won't help much in its treatment, adds Dr. Moldwin.

In a review of two clinical studies by the Cochrane Central Register of Controlled Trials, researchers found that cranberry juice and cranberry products significantly reduced the incidence of urinary tract infections. In a study conducted at Lawson Health Research Institute in London, 15 patients with spinal cord injuries were given cranberry juice twice a day. The results showed that the juice significantly reduced the

"Normally, any bacteria that get into the bladder are flushed right back out, but in this case, they're not," Dr. Moldwin says.

Doctors recommend a number of moves to minimize the risk for women who develop recurrent infections. Urinate before and soon after sex, for example. And think twice about using a diaphragm. Women who rely on this birth control method are two to three times more prone to recurrent infections than nonusers, since the diaphragm causes irritation of the vaginal surface, which allows bacteria to adhere, according to Dr. Moldwin.

---

production of biofilm, a substance that can make bacteria more resistant to antibiotics.

In the past, the theory was that cranberry juice makes the urine more acidic and discourages the growth of bacteria. Today, however, studies are showing that the effectiveness of cranberry juice is more likely to be its ability to prevent bacteria from sticking to interior tissues of the bladder. When bacteria can't hold on, they're easily flushed out by urine. Cranberry juice may be especially helpful to women who tend to have repeated infections. Studies suggest that the more frequent the bladder infections, the easier it is for bacteria to have a foothold on the bladder wall. Cranberry juice may just break that cycle.

Stay neutral. Some doctors believe that acidic foods slow down resolution of a bladder infection because the acid may irritate an already inflamed bladder. So they recommend neutralizing your urine with a low-acid diet, including antacids or a teaspoon of baking soda mixed in a glass of water two times a day. Maintaining a low-acid diet is especially helpful if the bladder infections tend to recur.

Ferret out food foes. If you think something in your diet exacerbates flare-ups, suggests Kristene Whitmore, MD, professor and chair of urology at Drexel University in Philadelphia and coauthor of *Overcoming Bladder Disorders*, try eliminating these possible culprits: caffeine-containing foods (coffee, tea, chocolate, cola, and some drugs), guava juice, citrus fruits, apples, cantaloupe, grapes, peaches, pineapple, plums, strawberries, tomatoes, spicy foods, alcoholic beverages, carbonated beverages, and vinegars. It might also help to eliminate foods that contain the amino acids tyrosine, tyramine, tryptophan, and aspartate. They include aspartame, avocados, bananas, beer, cheeses, chicken livers, chocolate, corned beef, lima beans, mayonnaise, nuts, onions, prunes, raisins, rye bread, saccharin, sour cream, soy sauce, and yogurt.

Spermicidal jellies can also contribute to bladder infections, upsetting the normal balance of "friendly" bacteria in the vagina and the surrounding area. Also, jellies may irritate the vagina, set up inflammation, and let bacteria adhere to the vagina, then migrate to the bladder, adds Dr. Moldwin.

Most doctors treat urinary tract infections with antibiotics, which usually work just fine. "And we often tell patients with recurrent problems to take one antibiotic pill each time they have sex," Dr. Moldwin adds.

In addition to these measures, some doctors suggest the following nutritional therapy.

Acidify with Vitamin C

Some doctors believe that pushing the urine's pH (acid-alkaline) balance a bit toward the acid side helps treat a bladder infection by slowing the growth of bacteria in the bladder. "Some doctors recommend vitamin C supplements for this," Dr. Moldwin says. It is unclear how this has an effect, and there are no studies to prove it, but it seems to help some women, he adds.

"Vitamin C also is likely to be prescribed when a woman is taking a urinary antiseptic drug such as methenamine mandelate (Uroqid-Acid) or methenamine hippurate (Hiprex), which work best when urine is acidified," Dr. Moldwin says. These drugs are most likely to be prescribed as long-term therapy to prevent recurrent or antibiotic-resistant infections.

Doctors who recommend vitamin C to prevent or treat bladder infections usually suggest a daily dose of 1,000 milligrams. You would have to eat about 14

Prescriptions for Healing

Vitamins aren't the first thing most doctors reach for when it comes to treating or preventing urinary tract infections. But some do recommend vitamin C, especially if you're taking a drug that works better when the urine is acidic. You can split the dose and take half two times a day, according to Kristene Whitmore, MD, associate professor and chief of urology at Drexel University in Philadelphia and coauthor of *Overcoming Bladder Disorders*.

Nutrient	Daily Amount
Vitamin C	1,000 milligrams

oranges a day to get that much. In fact, oranges and orange juice aren't your best sources of vitamin C in this case, and not only because you would OD on OJ.

"Because of the way your body metabolizes it, orange juice does not acidify your urine as efficiently as supplements," says Kristene Whitmore, MD, associate professor and chief of urology at Drexel University in Philadelphia and coauthor of *Overcoming Bladder Disorders*.

You can check the acidity of your urine with chemically treated nitrazine strips, a sort of litmus paper that's available in many pharmacies. Follow the directions on the package.

BRUISES

FADING OUT THE BLACK AND BLUE

Trip over a crumpled rug, and you've got one. Bump into the bedpost, and you've got one. Forget you left that bottom drawer open, run right into it as you hurry to answer the phone, and—ouch!—you've got a really bad one. We've all had our share of bruises. It takes just one good, swift blow, and the blood vessels beneath your skin rupture, spilling blood into the surrounding tissues and creating the colorful palette of blacks, blues, purples, yellows, and greens we know as a bruise. For the bruise to heal, the body must reabsorb all of that spilled blood, which, depending on the extent of the damage, could take days or even weeks.

Though bruising is no more than a minor, albeit uncomfortable, inconvenience for most of us, for others, particularly the elderly, it can be a Technicolor nightmare. As skin ages, it becomes thinner and more fragile, a condition that is exacerbated by years of sun exposure. As a result, the underlying blood vessels are more vulnerable to damage. For this reason, older people frequently develop what is known as purpura senilis—bruises on their hands, arms, and sometimes legs that occur from the slightest contact and that take months to heal.

"Virtually everybody in their seventies and eighties develops this problem to some extent," says Melvin L. Elson, MD, medical director of the Dermatology Center in Nashville, coauthor of *The Good Look Book*, and editor of *Evaluation and Treatment of the Aging Face*.

Food Factors

When it comes to bruising, vitamins C and K seem to be getting the lion's share of attention. Some researchers, however, believe that bioflavonoids—chemical compounds related to vitamin C and found in fruits and vegetables—may deserve a second look.

Find your cup of tea. Drinking black tea can boost your level of rutin, a bioflavonoid that was singled out by researchers in the 1950s as one that could help strengthen fragile capillaries and minimize the bruising that often accompanies this condition.

It's important to remember, however, that though this compound may prevent some bruises from occurring, it won't heal a bruise after it has occurred.

Rutin is also found in plentiful supply in buckwheat. So here's a good excuse to enjoy a hearty breakfast of buckwheat pancakes.

If you're prone to bruising, basic first-aid treatment can help you heal. Apply an ice pack, wrapped in a towel, on and off for the first 24 hours, followed by warm compresses the next day. If you really want to give bruises the old heave-ho and make yourself less "bruisable" in the future, however, the mineral zinc and a dollop of cream fortified with vitamin C or vitamin K are the way to go, say many experts. For extra protection, they advise boosting your dietary intake of these nutrients as well.

Vitamin K to Chase the Blues Away

Vitamin K, named for the German word *koagulation*, has long been used to promote blood clotting and prevent bleeding, particularly in cases of aspirin poisoning or blood-thinner overdose. It's also a favorite among plastic surgeons, who use large doses on their patients to prevent postsurgery bruising.

Now these benefits are accessible to the general public as well. Research shows that applying vitamin K topically can prevent and heal bruising from laser surgery and fade away bruises, even those occurring from purpura senilis.

In a study of 12 people with significant bruising, Dr. Elson, a longtime vitamin K investigator, applied vitamin K cream to one arm of each patient and an identical cream without vitamin K to the other. After 1 month, the arms treated with vitamin K had significantly fewer bruises than those treated with plain ointment.

"We also had people use vitamin K cream on one side of a bruise but not on the other and found that the side treated with vitamin K healed in 5 to 7 days, while the untreated side took 11 to 13 days to heal," says Dr. Elson.

Moreover, vitamin K strengthens blood vessel walls, so it also makes you less prone to bruising, explains Dr. Elson, who has developed a 1 percent vitamin K cream called Vitamin K Clarifying Cream. "I've had elderly patients tell me that for the first time since they're older, they can go outside with short sleeves on," he says. Vitamin K Clarifying Cream is available only through a physician, so if you'd like to try some "bruise guard," check with your doctor.

The logical question, of course, is: If vitamin K works when you rub it on, can you also ward off bruises by eating more vitamin K-rich foods such as green leafy vegetables, fruits, seeds, and dairy products? "There's no absolute proof, but studies seem to indicate that you can," says Dr. Elson.

Even though getting plenty of vitamin K—the Daily Value is 80 micrograms—may be helpful, when you have a bruise or an area prone to bruising, you want large doses of vitamin K right where you need them, and the best way to get them there is topically, says Dr. Elson.

Vitamin C Can Help

Vitamin C, the scurvy-fighting nutrient that's abundant in citrus fruits and broccoli, is needed to form collagen, the "glue" within connective tissues that give shape and elasticity to skin and blood vessels. As the body ages and those connective tissues lose strength, skin becomes thinner and blood vessels are more fragile. Sun exposure accelerates the breakdown of connective tissues, making older people who've spent years in the sun more susceptible to bleeding and bruising. The sun's rays also deplete stores of vitamin C, the very vitamin that the body needs to protect cells and tissue from free radical damage.

Eating lots of fruits and veggies high in vitamin C, like citrus fruits, tomatoes, and broccoli, will provide a sufficient amount of vitamin C, but everyone (and their skin) will benefit by taking 60 milligrams of vitamin C every day.

Research has shown that topical products with vitamin C can prevent the damage caused by years of sun exposure and heal bruising in older skin.

And when vitamin C is combined with vitamin E, the effects are even more powerful. "Vitamin E and vitamin C work synergistically to repair tissues, so that same vitamin cocktail should help prevent bruising," says Sheldon Pinnell, MD, distinguished professor emeritus of dermatology at Duke University Medical Center in Durham, North Carolina. In a Duke University Medical Center study, two different formulas were applied to the back skin of nine volunteers who were then exposed to simulated sunlight. Those who received an antioxidant serum containing vitamins C and E had a 96 percent reduction of sunburn cells and up to eight times the antioxidant protection of those who received the control formula.

A topical form of antioxidants along with a broad-spectrum sunscreen will provide maximum protection, says Dr. Pinnell, who has developed three generations of products designed for optimal repairing of photo-aged skin. One such formula, C E Ferulic, helps boost the antioxidant reservoirs the body dips into to help heal itself from bruises. However, since sunscreens and

Prescriptions for Healing

Some experts agree that certain vitamins and minerals can not only heal bruises but also prevent them. Though these nutrients work best at clearing up bruises when applied as topical creams, oral supplements may be helpful in warding off bruising as well. Here's what some doctors recommend.

Nutrient	Daily Amount/Application
Oral	
Vitamin C	60 milligrams
Vitamin K	80 micrograms
Zinc	15 milligrams
Topical	
Vitamin C	15% L-ascorbic acid serum (C E Ferulic serum)
Vitamin K	1% cream (Vitamin K Clarifying Cream)

MEDICAL ALERT: *Frequent inexplicable bruising, although rare, may be a sign of a clotting disorder or an immune problem, or a side effect of some medication. If you find yourself bruising easily and frequently, you should see your doctor.*

antioxidant formulas work in different parts of the skin and through different mechanisms, the formula must be applied to the skin first to neutralize oxidative stress. Once it's absorbed, then the sunscreen can be applied.

C E Ferulic is available without a prescription from dermatologists, plastic surgeons, and other skin care professionals. To find out where to purchase this serum, go to www.skinceuticals.com.

Zinc Lends a Helping Hand

Although its role in bruise healing is not as well researched or well defined as those of vitamins C and K, the mineral zinc is known to lend a hand in wound healing and may help with bruises as well.

"Zinc is important in wound healing and skin repair, but it's probably more important for older people who are most likely to be deficient in this nutrient," says Lorraine Meisner, PhD, professor of population health sciences at the University of Wisconsin School of Medicine and Public Health in Madison.

You can get your Daily Value of zinc (15 milligrams) by filling your plate with shellfish and other seafood as well as with whole grains and lean meats. In fact, just one steamed oyster contains a whopping 12.7 milligrams of zinc.

Note: Frequent inexplicable bruising, although rare, may be a sign of a clotting disorder or an immune problem, or a side effect of some medication. If you find yourself bruising easily and frequently, see your doctor.

BURNS

REPAIRING THE DAMAGE

A roaring fireplace. A cup of hot tea. Glowing candlelight. Ah, the perfect ingredients for quiet conversation, romantic musings . . . and a good burn.

In fact, we burn ourselves so frequently that we even categorize the injury by severity: first-, second-, or third-degree. A burn is first-degree if it is red and painful, with no blisters, and goes away after 7 to 10 days (a minor sunburn, for example); second-degree if it oozes or blisters and has a raw, moist surface that is painful to touch; and third-degree if it leaves the skin charred and white or cream-colored.

Because third-degree burns damage nerve endings, they may be less painful than other burns. But don't be fooled. Third-degree burns can be life-threatening and require immediate medical attention, as do large first- and second-degree burns. First- and second-degree burns that are smaller than a quarter on a child or a silver dollar on an adult, however, can usually be treated at home.

For the best burn treatment outside a hospital, the old standbys still apply: Apply antimicrobial burn ointment and wrap the affected area in a

---

Prescriptions for Healing

Doctors agree that good nutrition is important for healing burns of all sizes. Here are the nutrients they recommend as key helpers when you're nursing a minor burn at home.

Nutrient	Daily Amount/Application
Oral	
Beta-carotene	5,000–25,000 IU
Vitamin C	250–1,000 milligrams
Vitamin E	30 IU
Zinc	15 milligrams
Topical	
Vitamin E	Oil from a capsule or a water-soluble cream applied once a burn has healed to prevent scarring

MEDICAL ALERT: *You should seek immediate medical attention for any serious burn.*

If you are taking anticoagulant drugs, you should not take oral vitamin E supplements. (Though generally a dose of up to 1,500 IU of vitamin E a day is considered safe, some recent reports suggest that taking more than 400 IU a day could be harmful to people with cardiovascular or circulatory disease or with cancer. If you have such a condition, be sure to consult your doctor before you begin supplementation.)

clean bandage. And for even better results, you might consider adding a new twist to this old remedy: nutritional supplements. Research indicates that certain vitamins and minerals can not only speed the healing of a burn but also minimize the scarring once the burn is gone.

The Anatomy of a Burn

To understand the nutrient connection, it helps to first understand what happens when you get a burn.

After a significant burn (one that is roughly 20 percent or more of the body's surface), the body's energy demands increase 1½ to 2 times, tissues deteriorate quickly, fat deposits decrease, and proteins start to break down, all of which leaves the body nutritionally bankrupt.

Burning yourself on a moderately hot pan handle will certainly (and thankfully) not elicit such a tremendous response. But even on the small scale of a minor burn, experts say, it's important to get enough of the proper nutrients—especially vitamins A, C, and E and the mineral zinc—to promote healing.

"There isn't scientific evidence to back up the need for a special diet for people with nonsignificant burns," says Randolph Wong, MD, a plastic and reconstructive surgeon and director of the burn unit at Straub Clinic and Hospital in Honolulu. "But based on common sense, I don't discount the benefits of increasing your intakes of these nutrients to be sure that you're getting the Daily Values."

Burns Eat Vitamin E

When it comes to nutrition, burn studies around the globe are yielding similar results. Certain vitamins known as antioxidants are vital contributors to burn healing because they fight free radicals. Free radicals are unstable molecules that steal electrons from your body's healthy molecules to balance themselves, doing all kinds of damage to your body's cells in the process. Though everyone forms some free radicals through normal activities such as breathing and sun exposure, their production is accelerated by injury, especially burns. Antioxidants such as beta-carotene and vitamins C and E neutralize free radicals by offering their own electrons and so protect healthy molecules from harm.

Although your body is armed with a hefty supply of antioxidants, free radical activity is so rampant after a serious burn that your supply is quickly depleted, giving free radicals free rein. In these cases, supplements may help.

In fact, researchers at the burn unit at Baquba General Hospital in Iraq found that burn patients who received 400 milligrams (600 IU) of vitamin E, along with 500 milligrams of vitamin C and a topical iodine solution, were at significantly less risk of infection and cut their healing time by 2 days.

Sunflower oil, wheat germ oil, and safflower oil are among the best foods for boosting your dietary vitamin E. And if you're nursing a minor burn, you might want to take a multivitamin/mineral supplement to be sure you receive the Daily Value of 30 IU, which experts say is all you need to maintain healthy levels of this antioxidant while treating a minor burn.

For extra protection against scarring, you can also slather vitamin E on your healed burn, says Dr. Wong. It can decrease inflammation and collagen buildup in the burn as it heals. But it should only be used after the skin has stabilized and there are no open wet spots or wounds, cautions Dr. Wong. You can break open a vitamin E capsule and gently rub the oil onto the burn. Any topical application should be discontinued if you experience inflammation or irritation.

Vitamin C Mends Damage

Another free radical scavenger that can help increase healing after a burn is vitamin C. In fact, one of vitamin C's major duties is to build collagen (skin tissue) in the body, says Michele Gottschlich, RD, PhD, director of nutrition services at Shriners Burn Hospital in Cincinnati. And collagen building is just what you need following a burn!

As evidence of vitamin C's skin-healing power, researchers at the Philipps University of Marburg in Marburg, Germany, found that severely burned patients had a lowered risk of shock, fluid loss, and swelling when high doses of vitamin C were administered. Quick healing is especially important because people frequently lose many vital nutrients before a burn heals over. Quick healing also minimizes scarring, says Dr. Gottschlich.

The Daily Value for vitamin C is 60 milligrams. But most experts agree that this amount is woefully inadequate for optimum health, particularly when the body has an added stress such as a burn. Instead, most experts rec-

Food Factors

Because burns speed up your metabolism, your nutritional needs go into overdrive. You need more vitamins and minerals as well as more protein. Here's what doctors use for major burns and what may help for those that are less serious.

Pack in the protein. The best nutritional plan for people with significant burns is a high-calorie, high-protein diet in the hospital. With minor burns, your body doesn't use nearly as much energy for healing as it does with serious burns, so you probably don't need extra calories. But "common sense indicates that you probably want to step up your protein intake," says Randolph Wong, MD, a plastic and reconstructive surgeon and director of the burn unit at Straub Clinic and Hospital in Honolulu. Prime protein sources include tuna, turkey, lean beef, and chicken.

ommend between 250 and 1,000 milligrams as a safe daily intake. Supplementation can help you boost your vitamin C levels, as can eating plenty of broccoli, spinach, and citrus fruits.

Bet on Beta-Carotene

Another nutrient that swings into action following a burn is beta-carotene, an antioxidant that converts to vitamin A in the body. Beta-carotene helps the immune system and accelerates wound healing and repair processes.

In fact, after studying 12 men and women admitted for major burns (burns over 20 percent of their bodies), researchers at the University of Michigan Hospitals in Ann Arbor concluded that people undergoing burn treatment should get supplements of beta-carotene, along with vitamins C and E. When the men and women weren't getting supplements, the researchers found, their beta-carotene levels fell below normal, which lowered their defenses against free radical damage.

Orange and yellow fruits and vegetables, such as carrots and cantaloupe, are packed with beta-carotene. Experts recommend a daily intake of between 5,000 and 25,000 IU. One large carrot contains about 20,000 IU of beta-carotene; one-third cup of mashed sweet potatoes contains about 5,000 IU.

Zinc for Healing

Zinc, a mineral found in foods such as oysters, wheat germ, and Alaskan king crab, has been receiving attention lately for its role as a wound healer. And studies are finding that as with the antioxidant nutrients, levels of zinc decrease after a major burn.

"Zinc is an important mineral in healing burns, large or small," says Dr. Gottschlich, who relies on supplementation for people suffering from serious burns. "For small burns, getting your nutrients by eating the right foods is probably good enough."

The Daily Value for zinc is 15 milligrams, an amount you can easily surpass by treating yourself to a half-dozen steamed oysters. Other zinc-rich foods include beef, lamb, peanuts, wheat germ, and bran flakes.

CANCER

PREVENTION STARTS ON YOUR PLATE

Let's face it: It's really hard to see a light side of cancer. Even jokes about this deadly disease can't help but remind us of our mortality.

But one of the brightest sides of cancer these days is that so much of it seems to be preventable. According to the American Institute for Cancer Research, 30 to 40 percent of all cancers are a direct result of the foods we eat. But because changing diets is not an easy thing for people to do, some experts believe that supplements may be needed to make up for existing nutritional deficiencies.

"There's no one magic bullet to prevent cancer, but there are dietary changes you can make that, when combined, will certainly reduce your risk of cancer," says Patrick Quillin, RD, PhD, certified nutrition specialist; former nutritional director for the Cancer Treatment Centers of America, headquartered in Schaumburg, Illinois; and author of *Beating Cancer with Nutrition*.

The sooner you make those dietary changes, the better your chances of never having to battle this deadly foe, Dr. Quillin says. "Cancer usually develops slowly, over many years, and goes through a number of stages," he adds.

Nutrition is most likely to have an impact on the early precancerous stages known as initiation and progression. These stages include potentially stoppable, even reversible, changes in a cell's genetic material, which are often the result of damage caused by chemical reactions in the body. Once the genetic changes are complete, however, and the now-cancerous cell begins to multiply, nutrition is no longer a sole therapy option.

Researchers are still figuring out the exact details of a cancer-preventing diet, and they probably will be for a long time to come. Sometimes contradictory findings remind us that much remains to be learned about nutrition and cancer. Nevertheless, certain nutrients stand out as valiant warriors in the war against cancer. Here's what research shows.

Vitamin C Shields Cells

Sure they're tasty, but there's another reason that you might want to down a glass of freshly squeezed orange juice, slice a red pepper over your green salad, and nibble a handful of fragrant strawberries. You'll be getting lots of vitamin C, potentially potent protection against cancer.

"Approximately 90 population studies have examined the role of vitamin C-rich foods in cancer prevention, and the vast majority have found statistically significant protective effects," reports researcher Gladys Block, PhD, of the University of California, Berkeley. "Evidence is strong for cancers of the esophagus, oral cavity, stomach, and pancreas. There is also substantial evidence of a protective effect against cancers of the cervix, rectum, and breast."

Low levels of vitamin C have been consistently associated with a higher risk of several types of cancers. In a study of over 600 women conducted by the U.S. Military Cancer Institute in Washington, DC, women with low intakes of vitamin C, along with several other nutrients, were at an increased risk of breast cancer. And the European Prospective Investigation into Cancer and Nutrition (EPIC), an ongoing comprehensive study of the impact of diet on cancer, found a similar effect for stomach cancer. When the researchers compared food diaries and vitamin C blood levels of people with stomach cancer to people without stomach cancer, they discovered that those with the highest levels of vitamin C had a 60 percent lower risk of the disease. The researchers concluded that a diet of vitamin C-rich foods may offer protection against stomach cancer.

Vitamin C has proven itself to be a potent antioxidant. So what is an antioxidant?

(continued on page 138)

Food Factors

Just about everything that goes in your mouth can play a role, positive or negative, when it comes to cancer. Vitamins and minerals are only part of the story. Experts offer these additional dietary suggestions to reduce your risk.

Change the fat rule. Doctors used to tell us to eat a low-fat diet. But today they know that what really matters isn't how much fat is in your diet, but the type of fat in your diet. The damaging effects of saturated fats and trans fats have been consistently implicated in spiking the risks of non-Hodgkin's lymphoma and prostate and colon cancer. Conversely, studies have shown that monounsaturated fats—usually in the form of olive oil—reduce the risk of breast cancer.

Saturated fats, which are hard at room temperature, include animal fats—lard and butter, for example—and hydrogenated vegetable oils, the white stuff that comes in a can. (Lots of processed foods are made with hydrogenated vegetable oils; make sure you read the labels carefully.) Since January 2006, it's become easier to identify foods made with trans fats since food manufacturers are required to list the content on the label. According to the Institute of Medicine, there is no safe level of trans fats. Fortunately, there are plenty of "trans fat-free" products to choose from.

Polyunsaturated fats include most vegetable oils, such as corn, safflower, sunflower, and soy. Monounsaturated fats include olive oil, canola oil, and the fat found in avocados.

You can increase your use of monounsaturates by switching to olive oil or canola oil or by mixing them equally with polyunsaturated oils when you cook.

Use the freshest oils you can find, at least one expert recommends. Never use rancid oil; if it smells "off," toss it. Oils become rancid as they oxidize and produce damaging free radicals. Buy your oil in small quantities and keep it refrigerated.

Go on green . . . and yellow, and red. One of the easiest ways to cut your risk of cancer, and all other diseases, is to eat five to seven servings of fruits and vegetables a day. If you think that sounds like a lot, consider this: One serving size is small enough to fit into the palm of your hand, so eating a fruit salad, for instance, could account for several servings.

When choosing which fruits or vegetables to eat, try to think in terms of color. The greater the variety of hues, the broader the range of powerful cancer-fighting compounds, called flavonoids, you'll get. A study at the University of North Carolina at Chapel Hill found that post-menopausal women with the highest intake of flavonoids had a 45 percent lower risk of breast cancer than women with the lowest intake. So stock up on flavonoid-rich produce like red apples, red cabbage, red grapes, broccoli, kale, leeks, and yellow onions.

Hit the sauce. Tomato sauce, that is. It's chock full of lycopene, possibly a more powerful cancer-fighter than its close relative, beta-carotene. Studies suggest it reduces the risk of breast, esophageal, and prostate cancer. It's best absorbed from cooked or processed tomato products, like tomato sauce and paste, tomato soup, or ketchup. Lycopene is also found in sweet red peppers, watermelon, papaya, guava, and pink grapefruits.

Be a tea tippler. It turns out that tea contains antioxidants called catechins that, in laboratory animals at least, have been proven to have cancer-preventing properties. Catechins may inhibit the growth of certain cancers, says the National Cancer Institute. They appear to scavenge oxidants before they have a chance to damage cells, and reduce the number and size of chemically induced tumors in mice. Some human studies look promising. A study of over 18,000 men in China found that the tea drinkers were about half as likely to develop stomach and esophageal cancer than were men who didn't drink much tea. Studies on humans have been inconsistent, though, so the National Cancer Institute is investigating this further.

Both green and black tea are rich in antioxidants. However, green tea contains higher levels, perhaps because it is less processed. No matter what variety of tea you choose, be sure to steep the tea a while before you drink it. One study found that after 5 minutes of steeping, 80 percent of the catechins were released.

Stock up on garlic and onions (and breath mints). These pungent bulbs ward off more than evil spirits. Researchers in Milan, Italy, found that people who ate a diet rich in garlic and onions had a lower risk of several types of cancers than people who avoided those foods. Garlic consumption was associated with a lower risk of colorectal and kidney cancers. Onions seemed to protect against colorectal, ovarian, oral, and esophageal cancers.

Compounds in garlic, onions, and chives—all members of the allium vegetable family—are involved in the production of enzymes that neutralize cancer-causing chemicals.

Fill up on fish. There are plenty of studies that associate omega-3 fatty acids from fish such as mackerel, salmon, and sardines with lower rates of cancer. In one Swedish study, women who ate fatty fish at least once a week had a 44 percent lower risk of kidney cancer than women who ate very little fish. And in another study, prostate cancer was two

(continued)

Food Factors (*cont.*)

to three times more common in men who didn't eat fish than in men who ate moderate to large amounts of fish.

Save the red meat for rare occasions. Red meat is already known to increase the risk of colon cancer. Now researchers are finding that it can double the risk of breast cancer as well. In a follow-up study of the Nurses' Health Study, Harvard researchers found that higher intake of red meats was strongly related to an increased risk of a common type of breast cancer that's fueled by estrogen and progesterone.

Don't throw one on the bar-be. When you *do* indulge in a juicy steak, don't make a habit of grilling, barbecuing, or smoking it. A study at the University of North Carolina at Chapel Hill suggested that women who consistently ate diets high in grilled, barbecued, or smoked meats and low in vegetables and fruits had a whopping 74 percent greater risk of postmenopausal breast cancer than women who ate less meat and more vegetables and fruits. The findings were based on the calculated amount of exposure to carcinogens produced by frequent grilling and smoking of meats. Interestingly, grilled chicken and fish didn't appear to cause an increased risk. This doesn't mean your picnicking days are over. The researchers say that these carcinogens exert their influence over decades worth of grilling, not just a few summers.

Have a soyburger. Animal and human cell studies have shown that soybeans contain several chemicals that have proven anti-cancer activity. One such chemical, genistein, may protect against cancer by inhibiting the growth of cancerous blood vessels and killing cancer cells. Large population studies show that soy may help prevent breast, colon, endometrial, and prostate cancers. In addition to tofu, try soy milk or cheese, miso, and tempeh.

Fiber up. In the bowel, fiber bulks up the stool, increases acidity, and reduces the concentration of potential cancer-causing bad guys. When fiber intake goes up, colon cancer rates go down. A high-fiber diet also seems to fight hormone-related cancers such as prostate and breast cancers. The Recommended Dietary Allowances of dietary fiber are between 30 and 38 grams a day for men and between 21 and 25 grams a day for women. Unfortunately, Americans only consume about half of those amounts daily. You'll be well on your way to reaching those ranges if you eat a bowl of high-fiber cereal, a serving of beans, three slices of whole-grain bread, four servings of fresh vegetables, and two pieces of fruit a day.

Add oregano. This spice jump-starts your spaghetti sauce *and* your resistance to cancer. A study by the U.S. Department of Agriculture found that oregano offers the most antioxidant activities of all herbs—

42 times more activity than apples, 30 times more than potatoes, and 12 times more than oranges, to be exact. Oregano's health-giving properties may be due to quercetin, which may protect against breast, ovarian, and endometrial cancers. Try oregano on chicken and potatoes as well as Italian foods.

Don't get too sweet. Diets rich in sugar can increase your risk of cancer, studies show. Experts point out that a high-sugar diet is likely to also be high in fat and low in fiber and other nutrients.

Go easy on the alcohol. Drinking by itself can increase the risk of cancer two to three times. But mix even moderate levels of alcohol with smoking, and your risk of mouth and throat cancers skyrockets 15-fold, according to one study. Alcohol may directly irritate tissues, and it may induce marginal nutritional deficiencies that drop the body's defenses against cancer.

According to the American Institute for Cancer Research, men should limit their drinking to less than two drinks a day and women should limit themselves to one.

Be a cabbage head. Compounds found in cruciferous vegetables such as cabbage, broccoli, brussels sprouts, and cauliflower may rev up production of cancer-blocking enzymes. The beneficial compounds in these vegetables are associated with a lower incidence of lung, stomach, and colorectal cancers.

Find apples appealing. Eating an apple a day may not keep the doctor away if you peel it first. Researchers found that one of the best sources of phenolics, cancer-fighting compounds in fruits and vegetables, is apple skin. In a study at Cornell University in Ithaca, New York, researchers extracted the chemical content of four different varieties of apple peels—Idared, Roman Beauty, Cortland, and Golden Delicious. They found that the peels, regardless of variety, had far more antioxidant activity and cancer-fighting properties than the flesh of the apple. Idared and Roman Beauty had the highest levels of phenolics. The researchers concluded that the skin may be responsible for much of apples' health-giving abilities.

Spice up your life. The Asian spice turmeric may be yellow, but don't be fooled by the color—it's anything but cowardly. Researchers at Wake Forest University School of Medicine in Winston-Salem, North Carolina, found that curcumin, an antioxidant in turmeric, prevents the growth of several types of cancerous tumors in lab animals. While studying the effects of different natural products, they observed that curcumin binds and isolates iron, a mineral that tumors thrive on. Researchers are doing more studies to explore turmeric's anti-cancer potential in humans.

Vitamin C, along with certain other nutrients, has the ability to protect cells from free radicals, harmful molecules in the body that can be produced during chemical reactions that involve oxygen. Free radicals steal electrons from your body's healthy molecules to balance themselves, and in the process, they can harm a cell's membrane and genetic material. Antioxidant nutrients such as vitamin C save cells from oxidative damage. Free radical damage can occur as the result of normal body processes as we age and can also be the result of exposure to cancer-promoting chemicals.

Vitamin C helps prevent mouth, throat, stomach, and intestinal cancers by neutralizing cancer-promoting nitrosamines. Nitrosamines are produced during the digestion of nitrites and nitrates. Nitrites are preservatives found in especially high concentrations in meats such as hot dogs and ham, while nitrates are naturally present in vegetables.

Vitamin C helps maintain a healthy immune system, an additional cancer-fighting talent. It may also help build up vitamin E, another anti-cancer nutrient, to proper fighting form. Experts agree that eating vitamin C-rich fruits and vegetables, like oranges, strawberries, broccoli, and cauliflower, is the best way to reap vitamin C's preventive benefits. These foods not only supply vitamin C, they also deliver the powerful teamwork of phytochemicals to all tissues of the body, something that supplements can't do. But vitamin C supplements appear to have a protective, maybe even a confrontational, role in the presence of cancer cells.

When researchers from Korea, where breast cancer is becoming increasingly common, treated human breast cancer cells with vitamin C, proliferation was reduced by 23 percent. When vitamin C was combined with retinoic acid, a derivative of vitamin A, it reduced cell growth by an impressive 75 percent.

In an intriguing study at the Molecular and Clinical Nutrition Section at the National Institute of Diabetes and Kidney and Digestive Diseases, researchers found that vitamin C appeared to increase the production of hydrogen peroxide, which killed cancer cells and left healthy cells unharmed. The levels of vitamin C that were used were so high that they could only be given intravenously. The scientists caution that it's not yet clear what the implications are for humans, since the study was conducted on human cells, not people. However, the Cancer Treatment Centers of America is currently conducting a safety trial of intravenous vitamin C on patients with advanced cancer.

Most experts believe that the reference values of vitamin C, 90 milligrams for men and 75 milligrams for women, aren't enough to provide optimum cancer protection. Although vitamin C supplements can easily boost your intake, eating vitamin C-rich foods, such as citrus and other tropical fruits, broccoli, and brussels sprouts, provides additional cancer protection with nutrients such as folate (the naturally occurring form of folic acid), beta-carotene, bioflavonoids, and fiber. In fact, evidence of anti-cancer activity is considerably stronger for vitamin C-rich fruits and vegetables than for vitamin C itself.

Vitamin C supplements simply can't take the place of nutrient-dense foods when it comes to optimizing the potential for cancer prevention. Vitamin C supplements are usually only recommended for people who are deficient in this vitamin or who don't have access to fresh produce. To be on the safe side, however, some doctors recommend a multivitamin with 100 percent of the Daily Value of vitamin C (60 milligrams). If you have cancer, talk to your doctor before taking any single-nutrient supplements.

Vitamin E for Extra Protection

Wheat germ, almonds, and sunflower seeds: Sure, they're crunchy and delicious, and great on yogurt or hot cereal, but they also provide healthy amounts of yet another nutrient that may help protect against cancer—vitamin E.

Studies using experimental animals have consistently shown that vitamin E can help protect cells from damage that can lead to cancer. "Population studies have had mixed findings, however, probably because most people don't get enough vitamin E from foods to get much cancer protection," Dr. Quillin says.

Most studies show a benefit of vitamin E in the prevention and treatment of cancer, says Dr. Quillin. In a large-scale study of over 900,000 men and women conducted by the American Cancer Society in Atlanta, researchers studied the association between bladder cancer and vitamin E supplements. They observed that regular use of vitamin E supplements was linked to a reduced risk of bladder cancer deaths. Another study by researchers at the National Cancer Institute found that male smokers who said they regularly used vitamin E supplements had a reduced risk of prostate cancer.

Experts who have looked at blood levels of vitamin E have also found evidence of protective effects. British researchers, for example, found that women who had the highest blood levels of vitamin E had only one-fifth of the risk of breast cancer compared with women who had the lowest blood levels of vitamin E.

For years, much of the nutritional research being done focused on one dietary or supplemental nutrient. Today, scientists are putting combinations of supplements to the test and studying how nutrients can work synergistically to prevent disease. "It's the total balance of antioxidants, not one single nutrient, that's important," says Roberd Bostick, MD, professor of epidemiology at Emory University in Atlanta.

Prescriptions for Healing

If you have cancer, you should be under a doctor's care. The high doses of vitamins and minerals recommended here should be taken only under knowledgeable medical supervision and are not substitutes for standard cancer treatment.

Some doctors recommend these nutrients, in a range of amounts, as part of a program to prevent or treat cancer.

Prevention

Nutrient	Daily Amount
Beta-carotene	6 milligrams through a multivitamin
Fish oil	1–3 grams
Folic acid	400–800 micrograms
Selenium	50–200 micrograms (l-selenomethionine)
Vitamin B$_{12}$	1,000 micrograms for folic acid absorption
Vitamin E	400–600 IU

Plus a multivitamin/mineral supplement that contains 100% of the Daily Value of vitamin C (60 milligrams)

Treatment

This program is used by the Cancer Treatment Centers of America, a national health care organization headquartered in Schaumburg, Illinois, and dedicated exclusively to the treatment of cancer. The centers combine nutritional, psychological, and pastoral programs with traditional and innovative therapies in developing comprehensive, individualized treatment regimens for their patients.

Researchers at Oregon State University in Corvallis discovered that when vitamin E is partnered with vitamin C, it is able to sustain its ability to resist depletion from cigarette smoke. They asked a group of smokers and nonsmokers to maintain a diet of low-level vitamin C. After 3 months, participants received either 1,000 milligrams of vitamin C supplements or a placebo every day for 2 weeks. Smokers who received the supplements had the

Nutrient	Daily Amount
Beta-carotene	100,000 IU (60 milligrams)
Fish oil	3–10 grams
Folic acid	400 micrograms
Selenium	800 micrograms (l-selenomethionine)
Vitamin B$_{12}$	1,000 micrograms
Vitamin C	2,000–12,000 milligrams
Vitamin E	400 IU (mixed natural tocopherols), plus additional amounts of dry vitamin E (tocopherol succinate)
Plus a multivitamin/mineral supplement	

MEDICAL ALERT: *Talk to your doctor before taking more than 400 micrograms of folic acid daily, as high doses of this vitamin can mask symptoms of pernicious anemia, a disease due to vitamin B$_{12}$ deficiency.*

Selenium supplements in excess of 400 micrograms should be taken only under medical supervision.

Start with a low dose of vitamin C and work up to the higher amount. Large doses can cause diarrhea in some people.

If you are taking anticoagulant drugs, you should tell your doctor if you are taking fish oil supplements.

If you are taking anticoagulant drugs, you should not take oral vitamin E supplements. (Though generally a dose of up to 1,500 IU a day is considered safe, some recent reports suggest that taking more than 400 IU a day could be harmful to people with cardiovascular or circulatory disease or with cancer. If you have such a condition, be sure to consult your doctor before you begin supplementation.)

same levels of vitamin E in their bloodstream as the nonsmokers. But smokers who received the placebo had 25 percent less vitamin E levels than the nonsmokers.

Vitamin E is one of the first lines of defense your body uses against lung cancer. It tries to neutralize free radicals that target the tissue of the lungs. However, as cigarette smoke depletes stores of vitamin E and levels begin to drop, some experts believe that vitamin E has the potential to join with the enemy and become a destructive, rather than a productive, oxidant. In 2005, researchers from Johns Hopkins Medicine School in Baltimore published a controversial analysis of vitamin E claiming that vitamin E supplements in doses above 400 IU a day caused a higher risk for early death. The differences in outcome may stem from different forms of vitamin E, explains Dr. Quillin. There are alpha, beta, gamma, and delta forms of vitamin E, all of which are found in whole foods like wheat germ. Yet synthetic alpha-tocopherol acetate has been the vitamin E of choice in many clinical trials.

Researchers at East Tennessee State University in Johnson City, however, conducted a study on gamma-tocopherol and found a link between this form of vitamin E and a reduced incidence of colon cancer. Vitamin E, like vitamin C and other antioxidants, is thought to protect against cancer by strengthening cell membranes, which may be particularly important in the colon, says Dr. Bostick. "The bacteria there produce a lot of free radicals, the unstable molecules believed to harm DNA and promote tumor growth," he adds. Vitamin E may also stimulate and enhance the immune system so that it attacks budding cancer cells and inhibits the production of nitrosamines, Dr. Bostick says.

Based on its possible protective effects against some types of cancer, a growing number of researchers believe that vitamin E may prove to be a key player in any cancer prevention plan. Many recommend 400 to 600 IU a day, but you should consult your doctor before taking more than 400 IU daily. Such large amounts are difficult to get through dietary sources alone. Even a diet that contains good sources, such as wheat germ and safflower oil, provides only about 30 to 40 IU of vitamin E a day. "Only supplements can provide these large amounts," Dr. Quillin notes. In taking vitamin E supplements, look for "mixed natural tocopherols" or at least try to get some gamma-tocopherol along with the commonly available alpha-tocopherol. Vitamin E succinate is another form of vitamin E that has shown considerable benefit in animal studies to treat cancer. According to research papers published in numerous respected journals, vitamin E succinate seems to induce "suicide" or apoptosis in cancer cells, says Dr. Quillin. It may become an ideal agent to consider as a selective anti-cancer drug, he says.

Be sure to ask your doctor what the health implications of vitamin E supplements will be before you add them to your daily regimen, especially if you are being treated for cancer.

Selenium: Vitamin E's Partner in Protection

Lots of evidence points to the fact that when selenium intake goes down, cancer rates go up. It seems that getting enough of this essential mineral cuts your risk of several kinds of cancer.

Many observational studies have suggested that the incidence of lung, colorectal, and prostate cancer is lower in people with high blood levels of selenium. When it comes to a healthy intake of selenium, sometimes location is everything! The selenium content found in food depends a great deal on the selenium content of the soil. For example, people living in northern Nebraska and the Dakotas generally have high levels of selenium because the plants and livestock thrive on selenium-rich soil. Conversely, people living in areas of selenium-deficient soil have low levels of selenium and, perhaps not coincidentally, are at a higher risk of nonmelanoma skin cancer.

In one study, people with the lowest blood levels of selenium were more than four times as likely to develop skin cancer as people with the highest levels. The question of whether supplements can help pick up the slack of a selenium-deficient diet is one that scientists are on a quest to answer. So far, research results are mixed. A large study at the Arizona Cancer Center in Tucson looked at 1,312 patients over the course of 10 years. The researchers discovered that selenium supplements didn't offer extra protection from skin cancer, perhaps because skin cancer begins with sun damage that occurs decades before tumors appear. However, in that study, supplemental selenium decreased deaths due to cancer by 50 percent. Lung, colorectal, and prostate cancers were also reduced by 45 percent, 58 percent, and 63 percent, respectively.

In a more recent long-term population study of cancer and selenium called the Nutritional Prevention of Cancer (NPC) study, researchers found that participants taking 200 micrograms of selenium a day had reduced their prostate cancer incidence by 52 percent and their total cancer incidence by 25 percent.

"Selenium acts as an antioxidant, which means that it helps protect cells from harmful free radical reactions that occur when skin is exposed to sunlight or when lungs are exposed to cigarette smoke and pollutants," reports Karen E. Burke, MD, PhD, a dermatologic surgeon and dermatologist in private practice in New York City. Selenium acts together with vitamin E, with selenium protecting within the cells and vitamin E protecting the outer cell membranes, she adds.

The Daily Value of selenium for adults is 70 micrograms. The average daily intake from food is slightly more than 100 micrograms.

Calcium Takes On Colon Cancer

Generally, any vitamin or mineral that's good for fighting one kind of cancer is good for all kinds. Occasionally, however, one nutrient earns star status for its ability to prevent just one form of cancer. Such is the case with calcium. This mineral seems to be emerging as something of a hero in the fight against colon cancer. That's because population studies suggest that people who get lots of calcium-rich foods in their diets are less likely to develop precancerous polyps of the colon and colon cancer.

Calcium may help reduce the risk of colon cancer by binding with cancer-promoting fats and acids contained in bile, the digestive fluid secreted by the liver, says Bernard Levin, MD, professor of medicine and population sciences at the University of Texas M. D. Anderson Cancer Center in Houston. This neutralizes their toxic effects and causes them to be excreted without harming intestinal cells, he says.

Several studies of people at high risk for colon cancer, such as those with a history of polyps, benign growths that can lead to cancer, also suggest that calcium may help reduce the possibility of abnormal growth in the cells lining the colon.

Don't count on miracles, however, Dr. Levin warns. "The effects are fairly modest and occur only at amounts well above normal intake," he says. Most studies used 1,250 milligrams a day, while the average daily intake of calcium is less than 800 milligrams. The Recommended Dietary Allowance for calcium is 1,000 milligrams for most adults up to the age of 50, and 1,200 milligrams for those over the age of 50.

Dr. Levin advises eating a diet low in fat, high in fiber, and loaded with fruits and vegetables. Then, if you like, he says, you can add enough calcium-rich foods (and supplements, if necessary) to push you over the 1,000- or 1,200-milligram mark. He also suggests that you avoid any tobacco and excessive alcohol.

Incidentally, fortified dairy foods such as milk may provide additional protection. Fat-soluble vitamin D, best known for helping to escort calcium into the bloodstream, may also play a role in protecting cells from cancer-inducing genetic damage, says Dr. Levin.

For cancer prevention, nutrition-oriented doctors, including Dr. Burke, recommend 50 to 200 micrograms of selenium a day (depending on what part of the country you live in and your personal and family history of cancer), taken in the form of l-selenomethionine. This is the organic form of selenium, which means it is more easily absorbed, with less possibility of adverse side effects.

To treat cancer, doctors at the Cancer Treatment Centers of America use up to 800 micrograms of selenium daily. In very large amounts, selenium can be toxic. Experts recommend that selenium supplements in excess of 400 micrograms be taken only under medical supervision. Children shouldn't take extra selenium until they have their adult teeth.

Good food sources of selenium include whole-grain cereals, seafood, Brazil nuts, garlic, and eggs. "Foods that are processed lose their selenium," Dr. Burke says. Brown rice, for example, has 15 times the selenium content of white rice, and whole-wheat bread contains twice as much selenium as white bread.

The Beta-Carotene Connection

The real heroes in the war against cancer are fruits and vegetables, hands down. "Studies consistently show that people who eat plenty of fruits and vegetables are less likely to develop cancer than those who avoid fruits and vegetables," Dr. Block reports.

And when fruits and vegetables are broken into their individual nutrients, several components seem to stand out as particularly protective against cancer. One of them, beta-carotene, is the yellow pigment found in a variety of fruits and vegetables.

Beta-carotene is just one of the disease-fighting compounds known as carotenoids. Plentiful in fruits and vegetables, carotenoids are potent antioxidants. They help thwart the harmful ways of those pesky free radicals just as vitamins C and E do.

In the body, some of the beta-carotene we eat is converted to vitamin A, an important regulator of cell growth and differentiation. Vitamin A holds promise as a cancer therapeutic agent and has been used for decades in high doses in European cancer clinics with good success and low toxicity, says Dr. Quillin. (High-dose vitamin A administration should be monitored by a health care professional, he cautions.)

Over 30 case-control studies have shown that people who eat foods rich in beta-carotene or who have high blood levels of beta-carotene have lower risks of lung, oral, esophageal, stomach, and colon cancer. An increasing number of studies are finding that certain foods offer specific benefits for different types of cancer. For instance, according to an expansive analysis of the top studies on fruits and vegetables conducted by the International

What If You Already Have Cancer?

Most research regarding nutrition and cancer is geared toward preventing the disease. Some doctors, however, believe that optimum nutrition can help people with cancer live longer and better.

Doctors who consider nutritional therapy an important addition to cancer treatment tend to go far beyond the usual three squares a day recommended by hospital dietitians. Many recommend a low-fat, low-sugar, low-salt, mostly vegetarian diet for their cancer patients who are doing well.

"Those who are losing muscle weight, however, may not do well on such a diet and may need additional protein and fat," says Patrick Quillin, RD, PhD, certified nutrition specialist; former nutritional director for the Cancer Treatment Centers of America, headquartered in Schaumburg, Illinois; and author of *Beating Cancer with Nutrition*. In hospitals, people with cancer who are losing weight get either protein-rich "whey shakes" or total parenteral nutrition (feeding via a tube inserted into a vein).

Most nutrition-oriented doctors also recommend vitamin and mineral supplements. Doctors at the Cancer Treatment Centers of America, for instance, recommend that all of their patients take a multivitamin/mineral supplement that contains several times the Daily Values of numerous nutrients. One such supplement, Immunomax, is available by calling 800-295-8333 or by ordering online at www.cncahealth.com, the Web site for the Cancer Nutrition Centers of America. Doctors at the Cancer Treatment Centers of America also prescribe a daily regimen of 2,000 to 12,000 milligrams of powdered buffered vitamin C; 400 IU of vitamin E as mixed natural tocopherols and additional amounts of dry vitamin E (tocopherol succinate); 100,000 IU of beta-carotene; 800 micrograms of a low-toxicity form of selenium, l-selenomethionine; and 2 grams of eicosapentaenoic acid and 400 milligrams of gamma-linolenic acid, both fatty acids that in laboratory studies have been found to slow tumor growth.

Some doctors at the centers also prescribe non-nutrient supplements such as 200 milligrams of coenzyme Q10, 2 to 12 grams of arginine, 1 to 5 grams of glutamine, and a large assortment of herbs. If you wish to add supplements to your cancer therapy, consult your doctor or health care provider and let her or him know about the kinds and amounts that you are taking.

Agency for Research on Cancer, eating more fruit may reduce the risk of esophageal, stomach, and lung cancer. Eating more vegetables appeared to reduce the risk of esophageal and colon/rectum cancer. Vegetables, not fruit, were associated with a slight reduction of ovarian cancer, and fruits, not

There's a small but growing body of scientific literature on the benefits of nutritional supplementation in reversing established cancers. One intriguing study, however, did find longer life spans in people who received nutritional therapy similar to that offered by the Cancer Treatment Centers of America.

That study, by Abram Hoffer, MD, PhD, and Linus Pauling, PhD, looked at people with cancer who were receiving state-of-the-art treatment such as chemotherapy or radiation.

Those who continued eating as they had before they found out they had cancer had an average life span of 5.7 months. Of those receiving nutritional therapy (high-dose vitamins and minerals as well as information on food selection), 80 percent lived an average of 6 more years after diagnosis. The remaining 20 percent who didn't respond as well to nutritional therapy still survived almost twice as long as the patients not receiving nutritional support.

"This group included people with tough-to-treat cancers—lung, pancreas, and liver," Dr. Quillin points out. Women with cancer of the breast, ovaries, cervix, or uterus did best; the average life span was 10 years for women with these cancers who received nutritional therapy, a 21-fold improvement over those who did not.

In another study, conducted by researchers at West Virginia University School of Medicine in Morgantown, men with bladder cancer who took large doses of vitamin A (40,000 IU), vitamin B_6 (100 milligrams), vitamin C (2,000 milligrams), vitamin E (400 IU), and zinc (90 milligrams), in addition to a multivitamin/mineral supplement that provided the Recommended Dietary Allowances and their regular treatment, had a 40 percent reduction in tumor recurrence compared with men getting only the Recommended Dietary Allowances of these nutrients. This study also showed that after 5 years, the men taking large amounts of nutrients went for a significantly longer time without tumor recurrence.

"The take-home lesson in all of this," Dr. Quillin says, "is that nutrition is not a magic bullet against all cancers. Nutrition should not be used as a sole therapy. But nutrition can dramatically improve the quantity and quality of life and chances for complete remission for people with cancer."

vegetables, had a protective effect against bladder cancer. However, experts agree that no one single food group or one sole nutrient is likely to ward off diseases. Eating a variety of fruits and vegetables is the key to overall cancer prevention.

What doesn't earn an across-the-board consensus among researchers is the issue of beta-carotene supplements. For the past 2 decades, the role of beta-carotene supplements in the fight against cancer has been fraught with debate. Five large-scale studies conducted in the 1990s found conflicting effects among different people. One of those studies, known as the Chinese Cancer Prevention Study, showed that beta-carotene, along with other anti-oxidant supplements, significantly reduced the incidence of gastric cancer and cancer overall. Two more studies concluded that beta-carotene increased the incidence of lung cancer, and the remaining two showed no benefit or harm from beta-carotene supplements.

The mixed results of ongoing studies continue to confound scientists today. Researchers at Dartmouth Medical School in Hanover, New Hampshire, discovered that nonsmoking, nondrinking participants who took 25 milligrams of beta-carotene daily had a 44 percent decrease in the risk of reoccurring colorectal polyps. The drinkers and smokers who took beta-carotene actually doubled their risk of a recurrence. To add to the confusion, a large population study of over 29,000 men conducted by the Division of Cancer Epidemiology and Genetics at the National Cancer Institute found that those with low levels of beta-carotene who were given 2,000 micrograms a day of beta-carotene supplements were at less risk for prostate cancer.

Many scientists have speculated about the reasons for such conflicting results. It's possible that the answer lies in the varying doses used in different studies. Participants in the human trials were taking 20 to 30 milligrams of beta-carotene supplements a day, a considerably higher amount than the average dietary intake of 2 milligrams per day. Researchers at the Nutrition and Cancer Biology Laboratory of the Jean Mayer USDA Human Nutrition Research Center on Aging at Tufts University in Boston set out to discover how doses affect the experimental outcomes. They conducted studies using animals with health statuses mimicking those of smokers and administered high, low, and no doses of beta-carotene. In both the high-dose and no-dose groups, precancerous lesions were found in lung tissues. However, the low-dose group, which received 6 milligrams of beta-carotene (equivalent to a day's worth of fruits and vegetables), had fewer signs of cancer. And this dose appeared to protect against lung cancer. The researchers speculated that too much beta-carotene led to a depletion of retinoic acid, a form of vitamin A that may have anti-cancer capabilities.

Since the line between too much and too little beta-carotene is a fine one, most experts recommend getting no more than 6 milligrams a day through a multivitamin. However, the best way to enjoy all the health-giving benefits of beta-carotene is to make sure your diet includes a variety of beta-carotene-rich fruits and vegetables, like cantaloupe, carrots, sweet potatoes, and spinach.

If you have lung cancer, make sure to talk to your doctor before taking any vitamin and mineral supplements.

Nutrition and Cancer Medications

When it comes to nutrition, cancer can do a double whammy on your body. The disease itself can cause nutritional deficiencies, and so can the medications used to treat it.

Both cancer and its treatments can cause loss of appetite, nausea, intestinal absorption problems, and increased metabolism (calorie burning), all of which can lead to malnourishment and weight loss. "If you have cancer, it's important that your doctor recognize these problems and correct them if possible," says Patrick Quillin, RD, PhD, certified nutrition specialist; former nutritional director for the Cancer Treatment Centers of America, headquartered in Schaumburg, Illinois; and author of *Beating Cancer with Nutrition*. Malnutrition causes 40 percent or more of deaths in cancer.

Studies show that certain nutrients can help protect the body's healthy cells from the damaging effects of chemotherapy without interfering with, and sometimes even enhancing, these drugs' antitumor activity. In one animal study, vitamin E given prior to treatment with bleomycin, a common cancer drug, helped prevent the lung tissue scarring this treatment can cause.

In animal and human studies, niacin, vitamin C, and selenium also showed promise in reducing chemotherapy's toxicity and tissue damage. So did the supplements cysteine and coenzyme Q10. These two are nonessential nutrient factors, and they protect the body against free radicals, naturally occurring unstable molecules that damage your body's healthy molecules by stealing electrons to balance themselves. If you are slated for chemotherapy, you may wish to discuss taking these nutrients with your health care professional. Don't start nutritional therapy on your own without informing your doctor.

Folic Acid's Cancer-Stopping Power

Kale, spinach, romaine lettuce: These leafy greens are packed with a number of cancer-crushing nutrients. One in particular, folate, appears to help protect cells from cancer-inducing genetic damage from certain chemicals. However, the precise actions of folate are still a matter of speculation.

Some experts believe that folate deficiency can induce damage to the genetic material in a cell, which in turn can lead to cancer and make the cell more vulnerable to cancer-causing chemicals. Folate deficiency may also make it harder for a cell to repair its genetic material, which also sets the stage for cancer.

In one study at the Vanderbilt-Ingram Cancer Center in Nashville, researchers tracked the dietary habits of over 1,300 women with breast cancer and almost 1,400 women without breast cancer in Shanghai, China, between 1996 and 1998. The 20 percent of women with the highest folate intake had a significantly lower risk of breast cancer than the 20 percent of the women with the lowest folate intake. The risk was even lower for women who had the highest intakes of vitamin B_6, vitamin B_{12}, and other nutrients that help the body absorb folate.

Folate supplements may be especially suited to offer protection for women at high risk of breast cancer due to alcohol. In Harvard University's 16-year Nurses' Health Study, a low-folate diet combined with alcohol led to folate deficiency and a high risk of breast cancer. Incorporating more folate into the diet appeared to reduce the risk of breast cancer in women who drank about 15 grams of alcohol a day, an amount equivalent to 12 ounces of beer or 5 ounces of wine. The women received their folate in a multivitamin, but it was enough to compensate for the approximately 9 percent higher risk that even moderate alcohol consumption can cause.

Today, research indicates that our bodies require more folate as we get older to combat the diseases that become more prevalent as we age. Scientists at Tufts University's Jean Mayer USDA Human Nutrition Research Center on Aging set out to discover whether folate levels and aging affect the development of cancer and, if so, whether folic acid supplements can reverse the process. Groups of both old and young rats were fed a diet high in folate, a diet low in folate, or a diet lacking folate. The older rats had lower amounts of folate in their colons prior to the experiment than the younger ones did. Even when the aged rates were given diets with normal folate levels, they had 35 to 40 percent lower levels at the end of the study than the young rats following the same diets did. The researchers concluded that aging does affect the metabolism of folate. The good news was that the aging rats who received a diet high in folate were actually able to reverse impaired functions. It appeared as though the supplements reversed the folate deficiency.

Some doctors believe people should be getting at least 400 to 800 micrograms of folic acid a day to prevent cancer. To get that amount, you'd have to fill up on the very best food sources: dark green leafy vegetables, oranges, beans, rice, and brewer's yeast.

Doctors who treat cancer with nutrition recommend about 400 micrograms of folic acid, along with 1,000 micrograms of vitamin B_{12}, every day, Dr. Quillin says. Vitamin B_{12} is available from food sources such as seafood and green leafy vegetables. Supplements may also be helpful.

Finding a doctor who uses folic acid to treat rather than prevent cancer can be difficult. Because methotrexate, an early anti-cancer drug, worked by interfering with folate metabolism, there has been concern among cancer specialists that folic acid could fuel cancer growth. Not so, says Dr. Quillin. In animal studies, folic acid did not increase cancer growth. And according to him, a folate deficiency increases the likelihood that a cancer will spread to other parts of the body. Doctors at the Cancer Treatment Centers of America include 400 micrograms of folic acid in their treatment regimens.

Be aware that high doses of folic acid can mask symptoms of pernicious anemia, caused by vitamin B_{12} deficiency. It's best to work with a doctor if you plan to take much more than the Daily Value of folic acid.

CANKER SORES

SOOTHING A SORE MOUTH

Never is the statement "Out of sight, out of mind" less true than in the case of a canker sore. From the outside, you can't see that little white ulcer with the red border on the inside of your mouth. Others can't tell anything is amiss. But you sure know it's there every time you open your mouth to talk or—ouch!—eat.

Aphthous ulcer, the technical name for a canker sore, is a bit of a medical mystery. No one really knows why some people frequently get these stinging lesions on their tongue and gums and inside their cheeks. What is known is that they occur more often in women than in men and they can appear for the first time anywhere between the ages of 10 and 40. Heredity does seem to play a role, as do stress, vitamin deficiencies, certain foods, and abrasions, such as those caused by dentures.

Left alone, the pain of canker sores will generally lessen within 7 to 10 days, and they'll usually clear up completely anywhere between 1 and 3 weeks, but there's no need to suffer in silence that long. Doctors can recommend an over-the-counter ointment such as Orajel to numb the pain. For especially

---

Food Factors

You already know about certain foods from experience. That salty, sharp-edged potato chip, for example, is sure to hurt when it bumps up against a canker sore. And you wouldn't think of giving it that opportunity. But do you know that some foods can actually trigger a new sore? Here's what oral health experts recommend eating (or not eating).

Avoid citrus. Acidic foods such as tomatoes and citrus fruits can both aggravate an existing sore and stimulate an outbreak, according to research gathered by the American Academy of Otolaryngology-Head and Neck Surgery. If you're prone to canker sores, go easy on things such as grapefruit and lemonade.

Eat more yogurt. Eating yogurt each day might just keep canker sores away. Ukrainian researchers studying children with recurrent canker sores found they had less lactobacillus cultures in their mouths than children without canker sores. So eating yogurt with active *Lactobacillus acidophilus* cultures every day may prevent outbreaks and perhaps treat existing canker sores. There hasn't been much research in this area, but dipping into an 8-ounce container of yogurt every day is certainly worth a try. Just be sure the yogurt contains active *Lactobacillus acidophilus* cultures. (If it does, it will say so on the label.)

Try this honey of a deal. When it comes to the sting of canker sores, some cultures have been stinging them right back for centuries with a bee product called propolis. Researchers at the Harvard School of Dental Medicine decided to put this remedy to the test and evaluate the effectiveness of propolis in a pilot study. Patients who suffered with recurrent canker sores were given 500 milligrams of propolis a day or a placebo (inactive pill). The scientists found that the group taking propolis had significantly fewer outbreaks of canker sores, and they even reported an improved quality of life.

Bee propolis supplements should not be taken if you are pregnant; have asthma; or are allergic to pollen, bee stings, or any plants.

painful or severe canker sores, doctors can prescribe an antibiotic or antiviral medication that will speed healing.

If you're prone to canker sores, then a nutritional deficiency could be at the root of the problem. A diet lacking certain nutrients can cause some people to have canker sores as much as 50 percent of the time. A recurrence of canker sores or a canker sore that doesn't heal within 10 days warrants a visit with the doctor to find out what the underlying cause is. Here are some nutritional strategies that may prevent these nasty critters from becoming repeat offenders.

Vitamin C for Relief

Though studies have not yet been done to prove their effectiveness, vitamin C supplements get their share of kudos. Some oral health experts tout this vitamin as an effective means of preventing canker sores.

Dentists have reported that patients plagued with recurring canker sores find that daily supplements of vitamin C help lessen the healing time if they take the supplement at the first sign of a lesion. To treat a new sore, take 500 milligrams of vitamin C four times a day until the sore has cleared up. (Some people may experience diarrhea when taking more than 1,200 milligrams of vitamin C a day.)

Although oranges and grapefruit are excellent sources of both vitamin C and bioflavonoids, too much citrus can backfire and trigger canker sore outbreaks in people prone to these pesky lesions. Oral health experts say that for this group, supplementation is the best bet.

Take a Multi for Your Mouth

If you find that your canker sores have become more like intrusive weekend guests than occasional party crashers, you may need more than just a boost of vitamin C. According to the National Institutes of Health, canker sores can be caused by a number of different nutrient deficiencies.

Several studies have linked deficiencies of folate, iron, and vitamin B_{12} to recurrent canker sores, and some doctors believe that upping your intake of these nutrients might be beneficial for prevention.

Your best bet, say oral health experts, is to cover all your bases by taking a multivitamin/mineral supplement that includes the Daily Values of these nutrients.

Prescriptions for Healing

Only time is guaranteed to make canker sores go away. But if you want to speed healing and avoid new outbreaks, some experts say these nutrients might help.

Nutrient	Daily Amount
Vitamin C	500 milligrams 4 times a day until the sore heals
Zinc	Lozenges 4 to 6 times a day or supplements of 10 to 50 milligrams a day for 1 month
Plus a multivitamin/mineral supplement containing the Daily Values of folic acid, iron, and vitamin B_{12}	

MEDICAL ALERT: *Vitamin C in excess of 1,200 milligrams a day may cause diarrhea in some people.*

If you have liver or kidney disease, talk to your doctor before taking zinc supplements. Zinc in excess of 150 milligrams a day for more than 2 weeks can cause gastrointestinal problems in some people and interfere with the absorption of other minerals.

Zap 'Em with Zinc

Zinc may be just what the dentist orders. In a study of zinc supplementation, 40 people with recurring canker sores were all found to have low zinc levels. Half of them were given 220 milligrams of zinc supplements once a day for 1 month, while the other half received a placebo. The group taking zinc supplements had fewer canker sores and fewer outbreaks for 3 months after completing treatment.

The curative power of zinc may not be limited to canker sores. This mineral might just ensure overall good oral health. Turkish researchers discovered that laboratory rats fed a diet rich in zinc not only had fewer canker sores but also had healthier gums and teeth than rats that were given a zinc-deficient diet. The scientists concluded that zinc deficiencies could be a risk factor for oral and periodontal diseases.

Some people have found that sucking on zinc lozenges four to six times a day provides relief and reduces the healing time of canker sores. Others ease recurring outbreaks with zinc supplements of 10 to 50 milligrams a day for 1 month. If you are taking zinc for more than 3 months, be sure to include 2 or

3 milligrams of a copper supplement to your regimen since zinc can deplete levels of copper.

CARDIOMYOPATHY

HEART-PROTECTING NUTRIENTS

Cardiomyopathy is a special form of heart disease. It's a breakdown of the muscle tissue in the heart. This muscle tissue, known as the myocardium, becomes inflamed, then scarred and fibrous. As a result, the walls of the heart may become thick and hard, often when blood pressure is too high, or thin and weak, after a viral infection, heart attack, or too much alcohol. The heart sometimes enlarges and beats faster, trying to play catch-up because it isn't pumping blood efficiently.

People with cardiomyopathy may become breathless when they're active and sometimes even when they're doing nothing at all. They may tire easily, develop ankle swelling, and have chest pains.

Compared with coronary heart disease, which is the most common form of heart disease, cardiomyopathy is rare. But it's one of the main reasons people become candidates for heart transplants. That's because traditionally, there hasn't been a whole lot available for cardiomyopathy. Most doctors use drugs to provide some relief by reducing demands on the heart.

"These drugs are indispensable and have been shown to be remarkably effective in some people," explains Robert DiBianco, MD, associate clinical professor emeritus of medicine at Georgetown University School of Medicine in Washington, DC.

Unlike coronary heart disease, cardiomyopathy isn't always caused by fat-clogged arteries, although it can be, Dr. DiBianco says. It may be caused by a virus or another type of infection, such as Lyme disease or AIDS; an inherited metabolic disorder; exposure to toxic chemicals such as cobalt, lead, or carbon monoxide; sensitivity to commonly used drugs; toxins such as alcohol or cocaine; or heart damage caused by a disease such as diabetes.

Poor nutrition also seems to play a role in the development of some forms of cardiomyopathy or in worsening its symptoms.

Food Factors

Other than eating a well-balanced diet that's high in whole grains, fruits, and vegetables, there's just one more thing you need to be concerned about if you have cardiomyopathy. Here's what experts recommend.

Don't get pickled. Alcohol abuse can cause cardiomyopathy by depleting the body of nutrients and having a direct toxic effect on the heart, says Robert DiBianco, MD, associate clinical professor emeritus of medicine at Georgetown University School of Medicine in Washington, DC. Limit yourself to no more than two drinks a day. And don't "save up" your drinks for the weekend. Binge drinking is particularly hard on hearts, not to mention friends and family.

Several of the "classic" deficiency diseases—pellagra (niacin deficiency), beriberi (thiamin deficiency), and kwashiorkor (protein deficiency)—can cause cardiomyopathy. So can imbalances of calcium and magnesium, which play important roles in proper heart function.

And shortages of other nutrients, particularly selenium and thiamin, make the heart more vulnerable to damage.

Here's what research shows can help this potentially life-threatening problem.

Selenium Shields Hearts

Until 1979, researchers didn't know for sure that the mineral selenium is essential for human nutrition. That year, evidence came from Chinese scientists who reported an association between low selenium intake and a condition called Keshan disease, a form of cardiomyopathy that affects primarily children and women of childbearing age.

People in certain parts of China were getting little selenium in their diets because the soil in their regions contains almost none. Since plants don't require selenium, they can grow in selenium-poor soil. But they offer no selenium to the people and animals who eat them, so there is simply no good food source, plant or animal, in the region. In fact, some animals suffered from the same heart condition, and it was Chinese veterinarians who first made the connection between human cardiomyopathy and selenium. Chinese doctors soon found that selenium supplements could prevent this potentially fatal problem.

Selenium deficiency doesn't cause cardiomyopathy. It does, however, make the body more vulnerable to viruses that zero in on the heart muscle.

Scientists at the University of North Carolina at Chapel Hill found that a particular kind of virus called coxsackie remained mild-mannered in laboratory animals that were getting enough selenium. But in selenium-deficient lab animals, it caused extensive heart damage.

Selenium seems to help protect the heart muscle from viral damage, perhaps through its antioxidant properties. Viral invasions cause the generation of free radicals, unstable molecules that steal electrons from healthy molecules in your body's cells to balance themselves, thus damaging the cells. Antioxidants disarm free radicals by offering up their own electrons, saving cells from harm.

Selenium deficiency is not the only condition that contributes to cardiomyopathy. Severe high blood pressure, lupus, celiac disease, and alcoholism can weaken the heart muscle as well. But in cases where poor intake of selenium results in a laboring heart, selenium is just the ticket for the ticker.

Many experts don't think Americans are deficient enough in this mineral to develop cardiomyopathy. Chinese researchers found it takes only a small amount, about 20 micrograms a day, to prevent cardiomyopathy. Most Americans get well above that amount, averaging 130 micrograms a day.

But some research shows that so-called adequate amounts of selenium may not be high enough to provide optimum antioxidant or immunity-stimulating protection. That's why some doctors recommend selenium supplements of 50 to 200 micrograms a day.

If you're concerned about deficiency, ask your doctor to check your blood level of selenium. If your blood level is low, you may need to take supplements. Supplements of more than 400 micrograms a day should be taken only under medical supervision, however, since selenium can be toxic in large amounts. Stop taking selenium if you develop a persistent garlic odor on your breath and skin, loss of hair, fragile or black fingernails, a metallic taste in your mouth, or dizziness or nausea with no apparent cause. These symptoms mean that you're getting too much.

The selenium content of food can vary greatly depending on where it's grown. Generally, fruits and vegetables don't contain much selenium. On the other hand, seafood and, to a lesser extent, meats are rich in easily absorbed selenium. Grains and seeds, garlic, and mushrooms also offer some selenium.

Keep Things Thumping with Thiamin

A failing heart is deficient in so many different antioxidants, but most notably thiamin, or vitamin B_1. In fact, thiamin deficiency is one of the known causes of cardiomyopathy.

Every living organism needs thiamin to survive. It's involved in muscle function, the transport of electrolytes, and the metabolism of carbohydrates. As vital as this vitamin is, though, very little of it is stored in the body. Depletion can occur in as little as 14 days. Fortunately, most Americans get sufficient amounts of thiamin through beef, milk, whole grains, and white flour. However, some conditions, such as chronic alcoholism, can increase the risk of thiamin deficiencies. Excessive amounts of alcohol can deplete stores of B_1 and B_6 vitamins by as much as 33 and 25 percent, respectively, so

Coenzyme Q10: Good for Your Heart?

Many cardiologists would consider it unproven, and harmless at best, but a growing number of nutrition-oriented doctors say that supplements of coenzyme Q10 (it isn't exactly a vitamin) are absolutely essential for people with heart failure. They say it has allowed their patients to live longer, more active lives; has saved some people who would otherwise have died waiting for donor hearts; and has even allowed some to take their names off the transplant list.

"In some people, the improvement is clear, often dramatic," says coenzyme Q10 researcher Peter Langsjoen, MD, a cardiologist in private practice in Tyler, Texas, who has a special interest in nutrition.

Some studies, mostly from Japan, have looked at coenzyme Q10's role in cardiovascular disease. They include two double-blind, placebo-controlled studies, which are considered the most reliable. The studies showed that coenzyme Q10 had clinical benefits for 70 percent of patients with congestive heart failure. Coenzyme Q10 is normally concentrated in the heart muscle, and levels drop when the heart begins to fail.

"Bear in mind, however, that some studies done in the United States found no benefits with coenzyme Q10 and were never published," says Robert DiBianco, MD, associate clinical professor emeritus of medicine at Georgetown University School of Medicine in Washington, DC. "Unless more studies showing a positive effect are done and published, American doctors will remain rightly skeptical."

Coenzyme Q10 is an essential ingredient in the body's production of energy. It has "bioenergetic activity," meaning that it participates in bio-

alcoholics are at an especially high risk of developing cardiomyopathy. Scientists at the University of North Dakota School of Medicine and Health Science in Grand Forks studied the effects of vitamins B_1, B_6, and B_{12} on the alcohol-damaged hearts of lab animals. Vitamin B_1 was the only nutrient that appeared to repair mechanical defects and protein damage.

People with cardiomyopathy due to thiamin deficiency reportedly respond well to thiamin supplements. Several animal studies have demonstrated that replacing thiamin through supplements can bring those depleted levels back up and even improve the structure and function of the heart. However, some studies are showing that thiamin supplements may help treat cardiomyopathy caused by other conditions as well.

The number one cause of heart failure in people with diabetes is cardiomyopathy. Experts aren't sure of the exact mechanics yet, but they do know that

chemical reactions that provide energy. In cardiomyopathy and other kinds of heart failure, supplements of coenzyme Q10 are thought to help the remaining muscle cells do their jobs more efficiently, Dr. Langsjoen says.

Coenzyme Q10 is manufactured by the body and stored in your organs: liver, kidneys, and, you guessed it, heart. It's possible that people with low levels of coenzyme Q10 aren't getting enough of the vitamins necessary to convert the amino acid tyrosine to coenzyme Q10. These vitamins include niacin, vitamin B_6, vitamin B_{12}, vitamin C, and folate.

There are also coenzyme Q10 supplements, available in drugstores and health food stores. Dr. Langsjoen typically prescribes 300 to 600 milligrams of coenzyme Q10 a day, taken in doses of no more than 200 milligrams at a time. (This means that if you are taking more than 200 milligrams a day, you need to divide the dose.) This fat-soluble nutrient needs to be taken with a bit of fat or oil (although some supplements are in an oil base, similar to vitamin E capsules). Dr. Langsjoen has his patients chew the tablets along with a spoonful of peanut butter. Dosage is determined by measuring blood levels of coenzyme Q10. (Your doctor can order this test by sending your blood to a lab for analysis.)

If you're interested in taking coenzyme Q10, find a doctor who's familiar with its use or ask your own doctor to study up, Dr. Langsjoen suggests. Those using this nutrient in research or practice report no toxicity.

Prescriptions for Healing

Even if you decide to try certain nutrients for your heart condition, don't toss away your heart drugs! Doctors who use nutritional therapy for cardiomyopathy say drugs are still necessary for some people. Here are the nutrients they recommend.

Nutrient	Daily Amount
Magnesium	400 milligrams
Selenium	50–200 micrograms

Plus a multivitamin with the recommended daily amounts of antioxidants

MEDICAL ALERT: *If you have cardiomyopathy, you should be under a doctor's care.*

If you have a kidney problem or heart disease, it's important to take magnesium supplements only under medical supervision.

Selenium supplements of more than 400 micrograms a day should be taken only under medical supervision. In large amounts, selenium is toxic.

like all people with cardiomyopathy, diabetics with this condition have high levels of oxidative stress in the heart. Researchers at the University of Wyoming in Laramie gave diabetic mice a derivative of thiamin called benfotiamine. After 14 days, the benfotiamine treatment alleviated the oxidative stress and improved heart functioning. The results suggested that thiamin supplements may protect the heart against the oxidative stress that causes cardiomyopathy.

Since a heart beleaguered with cardiomyopathy is lacking so many vital nutrients, many experts suggest supplementing treatment with a daily multivitamin that contains the Recommended Dietary Allowances of all antioxidants to lessen free radical damage. To boost your thiamin levels, include thiamine-rich foods like beef, legumes, white rice, and brewer's yeast in your diet.

Magnesium May Aid Weakened Hearts

In animals, the evidence is clear. When put on a low-magnesium diet, young animals develop heart muscle damage that leads to heart failure.

"In humans, the picture isn't so clear," says William Weglicki, PhD, professor of physiology and experimental medicine at George Washington University in Washington, DC. "For people, there's no good proof that magnesium deficiency causes cardiomyopathy."

Magnesium is so intimately involved in heart function, however, that getting enough may help a compromised heart work better for a number of reasons.

Magnesium affects heart muscle contraction, and magnesium deficiency can cause abnormal heart rhythms and/or irregular beats. Adequate amounts can help prevent constriction of isolated blood vessels, which can affect the blood supply to the heart muscle.

If you are a heart patient concerned about magnesium, have your doctor monitor levels of the mineral in your red blood cells. This is the best indicator of a magnesium deficiency—though be aware that it's possible to have "borderline" or "normal" levels on a test and still experience heart problems related to a deficiency. If you have kidney problems or heart disease, it's important to take magnesium supplements only under medical supervision.

If you're simply concerned about heart health, experts suggest that you make sure to get the Daily Value of 400 milligrams. Nuts, beans, and whole grains are your best food sources, and green vegetables also provide a fair amount. Studies show that most people fall short of the Daily Value.

CARPAL TUNNEL SYNDROME

OPENING UP TO RELIEF

They were awkward, all right. But Richard Comstock wasn't about to part with his doctor-prescribed wrist splints, weapons in the fight against his painful, hand-numbing case of carpal tunnel syndrome (CTS).

He wasn't about to abandon hope for a vitamin cure, either. So when the Scotia, New York, resident read that vitamin B_6 might be the answer to his CTS pain, he combined treatments.

That was more than 2 decades ago. He's still taking his trusty vitamin B_6, but Comstock's severe carpal tunnel pain is long gone. And so are the wrist splints. "Every once in a while, I'll have a little problem, but it doesn't keep me awake at night like it used to," says the retired utility supervisor.

Comstock may have been way ahead of his time. Even though over 100,000 carpal tunnel surgeries are performed each year, some doctors who prefer a less drastic solution recommend daily supplements of 200 milligrams of vitamin B_6 along with wearing splints at night and taking an anti-inflammatory for less serious cases. Doctors have reported that 40 to 50 percent of their patients with CTS experience some improvement using this therapy.

Some doctors are even more enthusiastic about the use of vitamin B_6 for CTS.

Touring the Tunnel

Just inside your wrist is a narrow, bony passage called the carpal tunnel. Anything but empty, this tunnel contains nine tendons as well as a nerve called the median nerve, all of which are encased, sausagelike, in a slippery sheath called the synovium. When the synovium and tendons become inflamed and swollen, they squeeze the median nerve, which runs to the fingers.

Ever watch a live electrical wire rub metal? The pinched median nerve can send angry sparks of pain, numbness, and tingling from your fingertips to your shoulder. More often the pain is in the thumb and the index and middle fingers. Sometimes the ring finger is also involved. Many people who suffer

---

Food Factors

The pain hits your wrist, your hand, and sometimes even your shoulder. But carpal tunnel syndrome can start in your stomach. Here are some things to consider.

Hold the reins on cocktails. Alcohol is known to deplete the body of nutrients, especially the B vitamins, which are vital for preventing carpal tunnel syndrome.

Drop those pounds. Many doctors have noted that people who lose weight sometimes also lose their symptoms of carpal tunnel syndrome. If you're on a weight-reducing diet, be sure to eat foods that contain vitamin B_6, such as bananas and avocados.

from CTS say it feels like their hands have fallen asleep; others complain of weak grips and stiff fingers.

Women seem to suffer from CTS more often than men. Changes in female hormones caused by pregnancy, taking birth control pills, and menopause somehow make the synovium swell. And because women generally have small wrists, just a little swelling is enough to cause carpal tunnel pain, experts say.

Surgeons agree that CTS should not be treated with surgery during pregnancy. In studies, vitamin B_6 helped relieve CTS in 11 percent of pregnant women with severe CTS signs and symptoms during their pregnancies. These women were treated with 50 to 300 milligrams of B_6 daily for at least 60 to 90 days before giving birth. And there was no harm to either the mother or the child. If you'd like to try this therapy, you should discuss it with your doctor.

Obesity creates a similar situation. "There is about a fivefold increase in CTS in people who are obese and couch potatoes. So we encourage them to be in better shape and lose weight," says Morton Kasdan, MD, clinical professor of plastic surgery at the University of Louisville in Kentucky and clinical professor of preventive medicine and environmental health at the University of Kentucky in Lexington.

CTS has also become the unofficial health complaint of the modern age, the result of an increase in cases among people in manufacturing jobs. In fact, according to the Bureau of Labor Statistics, carpal tunnel syndrome is the most frequently reported occupational illness.

The most common culprit is repetitive activities that put pressure on the median nerve, such as typing on the computer or performing assembly line-type work like meat packaging or sewing. The repetitive activity produces inflammation, and this leads to swelling.

The Benefits of B_6

Doctors are divided on why vitamin B_6 seems to provide relief from CTS. On the basis of early research, experts contend that synovium swelling and inelasticity are caused by a B_6 deficiency. In one study at the Institute for Biomedical Research at the University of Texas at Austin, 22 of 23 people with CTS were healed just by taking 50 to 300 milligrams of vitamin B_6 daily for at least 12 weeks. And a number of them had already undergone surgery without experiencing relief.

Other doctors believe vitamin B_6 acts as a diuretic, helping the body to eliminate excess fluid. The swelling that many women experience during

Prescriptions for Healing

Many doctors recommend B vitamins for carpal tunnel syndrome. Because even the foods richest in vitamin B_6, such as bananas, avocados, brewer's yeast, and beef, provide barely a single milligram, you'll probably need to take a supplement. B-complex capsules often include all of the recommended vitamins below.

Nutrient	Daily Amount
Biotin	300 micrograms
Riboflavin	50–100 milligrams
Vitamin B_6	50–100 milligrams

MEDICAL ALERT: *Take vitamin B_6 in amounts above 100 milligrams only under the supervision of your doctor.*

pregnancy can increase the tissue surrounding the carpal tunnel and squeeze the nerves around the wrist and fingers. For some women, the problem worsens when they lie down, as fluid that makes the ankles swell during the day is redistributed throughout the body, including to the wrists. Some preliminary studies show that B_6 reduces swelling in tissues.

Another theory, backed up by two European studies, suggests that vitamin B_6 somehow short-circuits an angry nerve's ability to transmit pain signals. "We don't know the mechanism, but we do know B_6 reduces the amount of pain that animals feel, and that may be what's happening here," says Allan L. Bernstein, MD, chief of neurology at Kaiser Permanente Medical Center in Santa Rosa, California. "In my practice, it's very effective in reducing pain, tingling, and swelling in patients with mild cases," says Dr. Bernstein. "It allows people time to modify their activities that set up the irritation in the first place and, hopefully, avoid the need for surgery."

There is also a less appreciated effect of vitamin B_6, and that's its ability to increase serotonin levels in the central nervous system, says Dr. Bernstein. Some research has shown that it may increase serotonin levels in the spinal fluids of children with attention deficit hyperactivity disorder. "The clinical effect on adults is an antidepressant effect, a natural Prozac, if you will," explains Dr. Bernstein. "Often depression makes pain symptoms worse, so just monitoring the emotional effect of the pain allows for a more constructive approach to treating carpal tunnel syndrome."

Medical experts do agree on one thing: No matter how vitamin B_6 gets the job done, you have to be careful not to take too much. In studies using laboratory animals, researchers found that excess B_6 can harm your central nervous system.

Researchers at the U.S. Department of Agriculture Western Human Nutrition Research Center in Davis, California, fed 12 experimental animals 1, 10, 100, 200, or 300 times their requirement of vitamin B_6 for 7 weeks. At the three highest levels of B_6 intake, the animals' reaction time to a loud noise was reduced. Signs of a B_6 overdose also include an oversensitivity to sunlight, which produces a skin rash and numbness.

Taking too much vitamin B_6 can cause nerve damage in the arms and legs. Fortunately, toxicity symptoms are rarely seen, but when they do occur it's usually as a result of taking massive amounts of vitamin B_6 supplements over the long term. A multivitamin/mineral supplement with 50 to 100 milligrams of vitamin B_6 is considered safe.

Some Recommend Riboflavin and Biotin

There's some evidence that vitamin B_6 won't work properly unless you're getting adequate amounts of riboflavin and biotin, other B vitamins. Each one of these vitamins is synergistic, working in concert with the other. Doctors suggest aiming for 300 micrograms of biotin and 25 milligrams of riboflavin daily.

By law, most cereals, flours, and other grain products are fortified with riboflavin; milk, yogurt, and cheeses are good sources, too. Biotin is found in brewer's yeast, soy flour, cereals, egg yolks, milk, nuts, and vegetables.

Older adults, alcoholics, and those with nutritionally poor diets are at particular risk for deficiencies in these vitamins. Generally, the elderly have poor diets, so taking a B-complex supplement is a good idea. That is, unless they have Parkinson's disease, in which case vitamin B_6 may interfere with the absorption of their levodopa medication.

"My patients are getting between 50 and 100 milligrams of vitamin B_6 and riboflavin a day, using a B-complex supplement," says Dr. Kasdan. "And 60 percent of them have gotten better."

Most doctors agree that catching CTS early is a key to successful treatment. "If you have severe carpal tunnel, the vitamin B_6 isn't really going to reverse it," says Dr. Bernstein. "But if you catch it early, when you're just starting to have pain and tingling, and if there's no weakness and it bothers you at night but not during the day, you'll do extremely well."

CATARACTS

CHASING AWAY THE CLOUDS

Crack open an egg and drop it into a hot frying pan. You'll see the egg white turn cloudy, then white, as normally clear proteins in the egg are irreversibly altered by the heat.

Well, something similar to that happens when you get cataracts. Proteins in the lens of the eye lose their crystal-clear properties, becoming yellowish, cloudy, and about as easy to see through as a fried egg. Of course, cataracts take not seconds but many years to form. And it's not heat but cigarette smoking, a buildup of sugar in the lens (usually associated with diabetes), and especially years of exposure to sunlight that eventually pull the shades on vision for many people.

Many doctors think that the main cause of cataracts is oxidative damage to cells in the eye's lens. Oxidative damage is the same chemical process that rusts iron and makes cooking oil turn rancid. In the lens, the oxidative process can occur as part of normal metabolism as well as in the presence of light, which creates harmful unstable molecules called free radicals. These free radicals grab electrons from your body's healthy molecules to balance themselves, causing an ever-escalating molecular free-for-all that ends up hurting perfectly innocent cells.

Nutrients Shield the Lens

The lens can partially protect itself from this free radical damage, and it relies on certain nutrients to keep its defense system strong. Some vitamins and minerals such as vitamin C, vitamin E, and selenium may all play roles in protection. Even B vitamins such as thiamin and riboflavin may be involved.

Unfortunately, research supporting the use of some supplements to prevent cataracts is slim. "Not all of the facts are in, but the evidence to date is mixed that nutrients such as vitamins C and E and beta-carotene are helpful," says Randall Olson, MD, professor and chair of the department of ophthalmology at the University of Utah School of Medicine and director of the John A. Moran Eye Center, both in Salt Lake City. Several small studies suggest that people who take multivitamin/mineral supplements are less likely to develop cataracts than those who do not. A Harvard University study, for instance, found that doctors who regularly took multivitamin/mineral supplements cut by about one-fourth their risk of developing cataracts compared with those not taking supplements. And a study by Canadian researchers found that supplements reduced cataract formation by about 40 percent.

However, a rigorous 10-year nationwide study now largely completed called the Age-Related Eye Disease Study (AREDS) has evaluated whether a mix of vitamins and minerals, including E, C, beta-carotene, zinc, and copper, really does keep lenses clear. Unfortunately, the results of this study didn't document either beneficial or harmful effects. On the other hand, the study did find that antioxidant and zinc supplements reduced the risk of advanced macular degeneration by about 25 percent.

Researchers are trying to pinpoint why various studies yield such different outcomes. It could be that the criteria for defining cataracts and their various stages differ from one study to the next. Until science has identified the most effective strategy to preserve vision, doctors at the Laboratory of Nutrition and Vision Research at the Jean Mayer USDA Human Nutrition Research Center on Aging at Tufts University in Boston suggest that a healthy lifestyle, proper diet, and, in some cases, nutritional supplements may be the least costly and most practical way to delay the onset of cataracts.

Food Factors

Doctors may recommend these additional dietary tips to people concerned about cataracts.

Save alcohol for special occasions. Daily drinkers up their odds for cataracts by about one-third compared with people who rarely drink.

Pretend you're Popeye. Spinach is chock-full of lutein and zeaxanthin, two antioxidants that happen to be the only carotenoids found in the lens. So perhaps it wasn't so surprising when researchers doing a 5-year follow-up of the Beaver Dam Eye Study found that people who got the most lutein and zeaxanthin in their diets had a much lower risk of developing new cataracts than people who got the least. If spinach doesn't strike your fancy, try other lutein- and zeaxanthin-rich foods like tangerines, persimmons, orange peppers, peas, broccoli, and other colorful fruits and vegetables.

Take C and See

Researchers have known for some time that the lens of the eye can concentrate vitamin C. Concentrations of vitamin C in the lens and in the aqueous humor, the watery fluid surrounding the lens, are about 10 to 30 times the concentrations in other parts of the body.

"We're very interested in a possible protective effect, especially since vitamin C is a water-soluble antioxidant and the lens is composed mostly of water and proteins," says Allen Taylor, PhD, director of the Laboratory for Nutrition and Vision Research at the Jean Mayer USDA Human Nutrition Research Center on Aging at Tufts University in Boston.

In studies using laboratory animals, vitamin C seems to help protect the lens from oxidative damage from light, sugar, and certain drugs, Dr. Taylor says.

And what about people? One of the strongest predictors of cataracts is a low level of vitamin C, so it's possible that people who are not getting enough vitamin C in their diets are at a higher risk for cataracts. And there are a couple of studies that suggest vitamin C supplements can help protect against cataracts.

In the Nutrition and Vision Project (NVP), a substudy of the federally funded Nurses' Health Study, the development of cataracts in almost 500 women over the age of 50 was measured over a period of 13 to 15 years. Women with higher vitamin C intakes and who had taken vitamin C supplements for over 10 years were less likely to have cataracts than those with lower levels of vitamin C. What was considered a "low" level? The women who had comparatively less vitamin C were taking as much as 140 milligrams a day, over twice the Reference Daily Intake. It's been estimated that eye tissue only becomes fully saturated with vitamin C at levels somewhere between 200 and 300 milligrams. So even though the women with the least amount of vitamin C intakes were taking in more than the RDI, it still wasn't enough to guard against cataracts.

Doctors who recommend vitamin C to people at risk for cataracts suggest from 500 to 3,000 milligrams a day. (Some people may experience diarrhea when taking more than 1,200 milligrams of vitamin C daily.) "Research has yet to determine an optimum amount of vitamin C to take to prevent cataracts, but several observational studies are consistent with benefit at significantly lower levels," says Dr. Taylor.

It may be wise to get at least some of your daily vitamin C from citrus fruits. That's because chemical compounds called bioflavonoids, which are closely related to vitamin C and are found in the white membranes of oranges and grapefruit, also seem to offer antioxidant protection and may even be more important.

A Bright Future for B Vitamins

There is some evidence that B vitamins, which include thiamin (B_1), riboflavin (B_2), and niacin (B_3), may help you maintain clear, healthy vision. Australian researchers at the University of Sydney studied the diets of almost 3,000 participants, ages 49 to 97, and found that those with higher intakes of B vitamins had reduced their risk of cataracts by 50 percent. Thiamin, riboflavin, and niacin appeared to protect the nucleus, or the center of the lens,

---

Prescriptions for Healing

Doctors sometimes recommend these nutrients to help delay the development of cataracts.

Nutrient	Daily Amount
B vitamins	Multivitamin with between 1.6 and 2.2 milligrams of thiamin and riboflavin
Selenium	50–200 micrograms
Vitamin C	500–3,000 milligrams
Vitamin E	200 IU

MEDICAL ALERT: *If you have cataracts, you should be under a doctor's care.*

Don't take more than 400 micrograms of selenium daily without medical supervision.

Some people may experience diarrhea when taking more than 1,200 milligrams of vitamin C daily.

If you are taking anticoagulant drugs, you should not take vitamin E supplements. (Though generally a dose of up to 1,500 IU of vitamin E a day is considered safe, some recent reports suggest that taking more than 400 IU a day could be harmful to people with cardiovascular or circulatory disease or with cancer. If you have such a condition, be sure to consult your doctor before you begin supplementation.)

which seems to be the most vulnerable to nutritional deficiencies. And in more recent findings, researchers for the USDA Human Nutrition Study discovered that women with higher intakes of riboflavin and/or thiamin over the course of 5 years showed less age-related cataracts than women with lower intakes.

While the results of studies on age-related cataract and nutrition are frustratingly inconsistent, the one finding they all share is that oxidation within the eye damages vision. Vitamins in the B family play a role in preserving glutathione, an enzyme that guards the eye against oxidation. Fortunately, incorporating thiamin, riboflavin, and niacin into your diet is simple. They are all widely available in dairy products, meats, and fortified cereals. A multivitamin supplement will also supply you with sufficient stores of B vitamins. Population studies show that thiamin and riboflavin in doses of 1.6 to 2.2 milligrams a day, a range generally provided by most multivitamins, may prevent age-related cataracts.

E Is for Eyes

What do wheat germ and sunflower oil have to do with healthy eyes? Both are good sources of vitamin E, an antioxidant nutrient that works its way into cell membranes and disarms free radicals before they have a chance to attack cells.

"Research in animals and test tube studies indicates that vitamin E may help protect the lens from oxidative damage from light, sugar, and cigarette smoke," Dr. Olson explains.

In humans, the story may be the same. While AREDS didn't show beneficial effects of vitamin E, in another study at the National Epidemiology Program at the Jean Mayer USDA Human Nutrition Research Center at Tufts University in Boston, women who supplemented their diets with vitamin E for 10 years or more had significantly less cataract progression at the 5-year follow-up exam.

"Vitamin E is a powerful antioxidant," Dr. Olson explains. "There's reason to believe that combined with other nutrients, it may help slow the progress of lens clouding."

You'd have to plow your way through bowls and bowls of wheat germ to get 400 IU of vitamin E, the amount found in some capsules. So supplementation is in order. "Recent studies have suggested that vitamin E at 400 international units a day may increase the possibility of sudden death by increasing our clotting risk, so I recommend 200 international units a day," Dr. Olson says. The Daily Value for vitamin E is 30 IU, but most people get only about 10 IU a day from their diets.

Selenium Adds Antioxidant Power

Doctors sometimes round out their antioxidant prescriptions with selenium, a mineral involved in the body's production of glutathione peroxidase, another protective enzyme found in the eye and other parts of the body.

Dr. Olson does not recommend individual selenium supplements but does sometimes recommend multivitamin/mineral products that contain selenium, such as ICaps and Ocuvite (available in health food stores).

Doctors who recommend selenium supplements suggest 50 to 200 micrograms a day, no more. In even small amounts, selenium can be toxic, so don't take more than 400 micrograms daily without medical supervision.

If you're a fan of garlic, you'll be getting a healthy amount of selenium with each bite. Other selenium-rich foods include onions, mushrooms, cabbage, grains, and fish.

CELIAC DISEASE

FIGHTING TO ABSORB ENOUGH NUTRITION

Weak and pale from fatigue, a woman waits patiently in the examination room for her doctor to return. She thinks she's just tired. But he has seen these symptoms before, and he knows better. His diagnosis: iron-deficiency anemia caused by celiac disease.

Triggered by a sensitivity to grains, most notably wheat, rye, and barley, celiac disease also often causes a variety of problems ranging from gas, diarrhea, and constipation to anemia osteoporosis and dental enamel defects. The culprit: gluten, an ingredient of these grains that damages the small intestine, causing inflammation and impaired absorption of nutrients, explains Jerry S.

Trier, MD, professor emeritus in the department of gastroenterology, hepatology, and endoscopy at Harvard Medical School in Boston. Researchers have identified an enzyme resulting in an immune-mediated response that damages the mucosal lining of the small intestine, says Jean Guest, RD, dietary advisor to the Celiac Sprue Association and former pediatric clinical dietitian at the University of Nebraska Medical Center in Omaha.

Like a sponge that no longer absorbs, the damaged mucosal lining can't soak up key nutrients, including fat and fat-soluble vitamins such as A, E, D, and K, triggering diarrhea and fatigue, explains Guest. Even iron, zinc, folic

---

Food Factors

Because celiac disease is caused by specific proteins found in certain grains, avoiding the offender is the top priority. Here is how it's done.

Go on a grain watch. Tossing out your sandwich bread and pasta is a big step toward becoming gluten-free. But maintaining your independence from grains like wheat, rye, and barley also requires careful reading of food labels. Many processed foods use wheat for a variety of purposes, such as for filler and flavoring. It may appear on the label as "hydrolyzed vegetable protein" or "textured vegetable protein," explains Jerry S. Trier, MD, professor emeritus in the department of gastroenterology, hepatology, and endoscopy at Harvard Medical School in Boston.

New labeling laws make it easier to tell if wheat is an ingredient in food, says Jean Guest, RD, dietary advisor to the Celiac Sprue Association and former pediatric clinical dietitian for the University of Nebraska Medical Center in Omaha. Right now if a food contains wheat, it's listed on the label, but barley, rye, and oats are not. This will change in 2008 when sources of gluten will also have to be listed on the label. However, foods cooked in restaurant deep fryers and grills that have been used to cook other foods with wheat-containing breadings and coatings can provoke a reaction, she says.

Since some medications contain gluten, ask your doctor or pharmacist whether your drugs, both prescription and over the counter, are safe to take.

Mind your moo. Many people with celiac have yet another food sensitivity: They are unable to digest a sugar in milk called lactose. For this reason, some doctors suggest going easy on dairy products until your recovery is complete, says Dr. Trier.

Some people may have a broader intolerance to all carbohydrate sugars, including fructose, which is found in sweetened milks, table sugar, fruit, and some cereals. Your doctor can make specific recommendations about what foods to restrict based on your symptoms.

Prescriptions for Healing

The key treatment for anyone with celiac disease involves eliminating gluten-containing foods. Many experts also advise taking these nutrients.

Nutrient	Daily Amount
Calcium	1,000–2,000 milligrams
Vitamin D	200–400 IU

Plus a gluten-free multivitamin/mineral supplement containing the Daily Values of all essential vitamins and minerals

MEDICAL ALERT: If you have celiac disease, you should be under a doctor's care.

---

acid, magnesium, and calcium pass through the body with only a portion of them being used, she says. In children, growth failure, gastrointestinal problems, and mood swings are the most common problems. In someone who has had celiac disease for a long time without the problem being diagnosed, calcium deficiency can result in the bone-thinning disease osteoporosis, she adds.

Dietary Detective Work Pays Off

In most cases, treatment involves avoiding gluten, which isn't always easy. Even communion wafers and the glue on some envelopes contain gluten. "Some people are exquisitely sensitive to gluten, and even a minute amount can cause a reaction, although that's not usually the case," says Dr. Trier.

But the effort needed to avoid gluten can be worthwhile. About 70 percent of people who start a gluten-free diet will notice an improvement of their symptoms after 2 weeks. Once gluten is no longer included in the diet, nutrient absorption problems quickly improve. In a yearlong study that looked at whether a gluten-free diet could help children with celiac, researchers found that the bone growth of those on a gluten-free diet was faster than that of healthy children. Since the children with celiac were behind their counterparts in bone growth, the exclusion of certain grains prompted their bodies to play catch-up.

Since a gluten-free diet is strict, it's wise to take a gluten-free multivitamin/mineral supplement to make sure you get all of the nutrients you need, says Guest.

The Case for Extra Calcium

And since calcium absorption can be dramatically reduced by celiac disease, patients are at a higher risk of developing osteoporosis. Some doctors may recommend taking extra calcium to rebuild calcium stores along with vitamin D to help your body absorb calcium. Ask your doctor if you'll need to supplement your diet with more than the Daily Value of 1,000 milligrams of calcium.

"It's a good idea," says Dr. Trier. "People are often calcium-depleted when they're diagnosed."

CERVICAL DYSPLASIA

GETTING YOUR CELLS IN LINE

It gets scraped during a Pap test, bumped during intercourse, stretched open during childbirth, and occasionally covered with latex or squirted with foam when you're trying to avoid pregnancy. But other than that, your cervix is not really a focal point of your life. Out of sight, out of mind, right?

Right. Until your gynecologist says that something is wrong.

For somewhere between 250,000 and 1 million women every year, that something is cervical dysplasia, or cervical intraepithelial neoplasia (CIN), a condition in which cells lining the cervix stop organizing themselves into nice, neat horizontal layers that reflect their maturity from youngest to oldest.

Instead, a few older cells apparently decide to hang out with the younger crowd, then become disruptive when their increasing growth no longer allows them to neatly fit in among their younger siblings. They push the other cells around, which eventually disrupts the rows.

Fortunately, the fact that these cells are out of line signals itself on a Pap test. Depending on how many of these juvenile delinquents there are, a lab technician will label the test as "low-grade squamous intraepithelial lesion" (CIN I) for the minor disruptions of mild dysplasia, moderate dysplasia (CIN II), or "high-grade squamous intraepithelial lesion" (CIN III) for the more significant disruptions of severe dysplasia. Carcinoma in situ, which is also a high-grade squamous intraepithelial lesion, is not a form of cancer, despite its name. Dysplasia becomes cancer when the delinquent cells quit jostling their brothers and sisters and invade the cervix itself.

And that, of course, is what most women who find out they have cervical dysplasia are afraid of. Although not all dysplasia progresses to cervical cancer, most doctors surgically remove or otherwise destroy the cells involved because they feel that dysplasia is the first step down the road to cancer.

There is a strong link between cervical cancer and the human papillomavirus (HPV). "Recent evidence has shown that many women are transiently infected with [HPV], so the question has become why some women clear the virus while others go on to have chronic infections and cervical dysplasia," says Judith Stanton, MD, a professor of primary care medicine at Alameda County Medical Center in Oakland, California, and a physician at the California Healing Institute in Berkeley. "Anything that weakens the immune system, like excessive alcohol, stress, poor nutrition, and sleep deprivation, will increase the risk of chronic infections and cervical dysplasia. Anything that helps strengthen the immune system, like good nutrition and adequate sleep, will help clear the virus," she says.

Certain nutrients, especially antioxidants and the B vitamin folate, are thought to enhance immune function and help the cervix return to a healthier state.

Antioxidant Power

Evidence that low levels of antioxidants can increase the risk of cervical dysplasia is impressive.

In a study at Albert Einstein College of Medicine in New York City, researchers took blood samples from 37 women with cervical dysplasia and compared them with blood samples taken from women who did not have the condition. The comparison revealed that lower levels of vitamin E corresponded to a significantly increased risk of cervical dysplasia.

In other words, say the researchers, the lower the concentration of vitamin E in a blood sample, the more oxidative stress was present in the cervix of women with dysplasia.

Another study of vitamin C, done in Brazil, showed similar results when researchers looked at oxidative stress and its role in cervical cancer. In that study, researchers figured out the amount of vitamin C in the diets of 46 patients with untreated cervical cancer and patients with premalignant disease, then compared it with the amount of vitamin C in the diets of women

Food Factors

Beta-carotene, a precursor of vitamin A, is important in the prevention and treatment of cervical dysplasia. But it's not the whole story. There are other members of the carotenoid family—lycopene, lutein, zeaxanthin, beta-cryptoxanthin, and alpha-carotene, for example—that may be equally important. Medical researchers say that many of these carotenoids, which are responsible for the yellow and red pigments found in foods, may have healing properties.

Advances in technology have given scientists the tools to measure these carotenoids individually. Here are some carotenoid-rich foods that may be beneficial.

Eat tomatoes. In a study conducted at Albert Einstein College of Medicine in New York City, researchers found that lycopene, a carotenoid found in tomatoes, has a direct effect on the development of cervical dysplasia. Studies are ongoing, but right now it looks as though the more tomatoes you eat, the less cervical dysplasia you get.

Reach for the leafy greens. Kale, raw spinach, and fresh parsley are good sources of the carotenoids lutein and zeaxanthin.

Get more fruits. Fresh papaya, tangerines, and dried peaches are good sources of the carotenoid beta-cryptoxanthin.

Eat deep orange vegetables. Carrots and pumpkin are good sources of alpha-carotene.

without cancer. They found that the patients had lower levels of vitamin C than women who were healthy. The researchers theorized that decreased amounts of vitamin C could play an important role in progression of cancer cells. But will increasing your intake of antioxidants help heal dysplasia and head off cervical cancer?

Perhaps. A few small clinical studies and several population studies demonstrate that a diet rich in beta-carotene, vitamin C, and vitamin E can prevent cervical cancer.

Researchers at the Gifu University School of Medicine in Japan evaluated the relationship between carotenoids and vitamins and the risk of cervical dysplasia in 156 women. They found that higher serum levels of alpha-carotene were significantly associated with a decreased risk of cervical dysplasia.

In a study in four Latin American countries of 748 women with cervical cancer, researchers found that women who got more than 300 milligrams of vitamin C and 6,000 micrograms (about 10,000 IU) of beta-carotene a day from fruits and fruit juices were roughly 30 percent less likely to develop cervical cancer than women who got less of these nutrients.

How antioxidants might keep cervical dysplasia in check is still unknown. Some researchers suspect that these nutrients enhance the ability of your immune system to fight off attackers such as HPV, which is known to increase your risk of dysplasia. Others feel that the nutrients work by increasing the amount of vitamin A available to your cells.

It appears that the antioxidant properties are important, but depending on supplements alone is not the best way to guard against cervical dysplasia, says Dr. Stanton. That's because cervix-protecting nutrients are delivered to the tissues more efficiently when they're ingested as fresh fruits and vegetables.

But supplements can provide added benefits to a diet that already gets five servings of fruits and vegetables a day. Many nutrition experts do recommend taking daily supplements that include 50,000 IU of beta-carotene, 500 milligrams of vitamin C, and 100 IU of vitamin E.

Folic Acid Fixes

Although antioxidants such as carotenes, vitamin C, and vitamin E clearly play important roles in protecting your cervix from dysplasia, folate (the naturally occurring form of folic acid) may actually be more important.

In a study at the University of Alabama at Birmingham, researchers tested whether folate concentrations affect the risk of CIN in 345 women. They found that women who tested positive for HPV had low levels of folate and were significantly more likely to develop CIN than women without HPV, who had higher folate levels. The researchers suggested that, based on these findings, folate supplementation may lower the risk of CIN and thus the risk of cervical cancer. Another study from Thailand found similar results but noted that the dysplasia group had a much higher incidence of HPV, a higher frequency of a family history of cancer, and greater exposure to multiple sex partners. Grain foods are not enriched with folic acid in Thailand, and all of the women had low folic acid levels.

Researchers have been studying the effects of folate on cervical dysplasia for years, yet the relationship between folate levels and dysplasia is so complex that study results have been equivocal. Some studies indicated that a low level of folate in the body increases the risk of dysplasia; others indicated that it doesn't.

Besides HPV infection and low folate levels, several other factors can promote the viral invasion in susceptible women. Smoking, family history,

Prescriptions for Healing

A broad array of nutrients found in fruits, fruit juices, green leafy vegetables, and orange and red vegetables have been shown to reduce the risk of cervical dysplasia.

Some experts also recommend that you get the following nutrients from foods or supplements on a daily basis to protect your cervix.

Nutrient	Daily Amount
Beta-carotene	50,000 IU
Folic acid	400 micrograms
	Up to 800 micrograms for pregnant women
Vitamin C	500 milligrams
Vitamin E	100 IU

MEDICAL ALERT: *If you have been diagnosed with cervical dysplasia, you should be under a doctor's care.*

If you are taking anticoagulant drugs, you should not take vitamin E supplements. (Though generally a dose of up to 1,500 IU of vitamin E a day is considered safe, some recent reports suggest that taking more than 400 IU a day could be harmful to people with cardiovascular or circulatory disease or with cancer. If you have such a condition, be sure to consult your doctor before you begin supplementation.)

sexual exposure, and early sexual intercourse have all been linked to cervical dysplasia. But "folic acid deficiency is most likely one of the promoters of dysplasia," says Bruce Young, MD, professor of obstetrics and gynecology at New York University School of Medicine and member of the medical advisory board of the Grain Foods Foundation.

According to the National Institutes of Health Office of Dietary Supplements, folate is involved in the synthesis and repair of DNA. Research suggests that folate deficiencies may increase DNA damage, which can lead to cancer. It's possible that cervical cells that have had unrepaired DNA damage related to low folate levels in the presence of an HPV infection could become dysplastic and may not be able to repair themselves. As a result, they may very well be blocked from returning to normal and instead progress to cervical cancer.

Given that possibility, it may be more risky to be low in folate than to be low in antioxidants. "Research suggests that a diet with plenty of enriched cereals, fruits and green leafy vegetables, as well as orange and red vegetables, beans, and peas, will help prevent cervical dysplasia," says Dr. Young. So there's yet another reason to learn to love those colorful veggies. Enriched grain foods, such as cereals, pastas, and breads, have folic acid added to them and are another excellent of folic acid.

The recommended Daily Value for folic acid is 400 micrograms, although pregnant women should get up to twice that amount. Unfortunately, most American women get only about 236 micrograms a day. "Every woman should be eating a diet rich in folate before pregnancy to prevent dysplasia and prevent abnormalities of the baby's spine and brain, which can occur before she is aware that she is pregnant. When women have low folic acid levels, both cervical dysplasia and congenital abnormalities of the newborn are more common. Don't wait until the pregnancy test is positive to start a diet high in folic acid. Start now," Dr. Young says.

CHRONIC FATIGUE SYNDROME

BUILDING ENERGY WITH NUTRIENTS

Everyone gets tired. But not everyone gets chronic fatigue syndrome (CFS).

People with this disease aren't just tired. They're constantly exhausted, not just for a few days but day in and day out for 6 months or longer.

And the fatigue is only the beginning. Many people with CFS also have flulike symptoms, such as sore throat, painful lymph nodes, and aching muscles. Others have problems concentrating and bouts of confusion and forgetfulness. And many people with CFS have no tolerance for exercise: Imagine a woman who used to run several miles a day being so exhausted by a walk around the block that she stays in bed for the next couple of days. That's CFS.

While children and older people aren't immune, CFS is most common in middle-aged adults. "About 90 percent of my CFS patients are between ages 25 and 50," says Charles Lapp, MD, clinical associate professor of family and community medicine at Duke University and a CFS specialist at the Hunter-Hopkins Center in Charlotte, North Carolina. "The median age is about 40 years," says Dr. Lapp.

Once it hits, CFS is hard to get rid of. Doctors don't know what causes CFS or how to cure it. And while many people recover on their own within a year or two, some never fully recover.

The Illness behind the Headlines

While CFS has probably been around for a long time, it wasn't until the mid-1980s that a mysterious flulike illness that hit mostly young professional

---

Food Factors

When it comes to battling chronic fatigue syndrome (CFS), supplements are only part of the picture. Medical experts agree that the overall quality of your diet also makes a big difference in how you feel. Here are a few dietary changes that might prove helpful.

Go easy on sugar. "Eating too much refined sugar weakens the immune system and may inhibit the ability of white blood cells to stay active," says Allan Magaziner, DO, director of the Magaziner Center for Wellness and Anti-Aging Medicine in Cherry Hill, New Jersey. "Both of those factors play roles in CFS."

Some research suggests that people with CFS are deficient in an enzyme needed to metabolize sugar, says Charles Lapp, MD, clinical associate professor of family and community medicine at Duke University and a CFS specialist at the Hunter-Hopkins Center in Charlotte, North Carolina. The result is a buildup of lactic acid in the bloodstream, which can lead to muscle pain, vascular headaches, and neuropsychiatric disorders such as panic attacks, all of which are associated with CFS.

"We recommend avoiding sugar as much as possible, but if you're going to have an indiscretion, have dessert after a meal instead of eating something sweet on an empty stomach," says Dr. Lapp. "That slows down the absorption of the sugar, so you don't get a sharp elevation in lactic acid."

Don't depend on caffeine. When you're exhausted all the time, there's a great temptation to depend on caffeine to make you more alert. "But it's also important to avoid or cut back on foods that may cause loss of minerals. Caffeine is one example," says Dr. Magaziner.

women made headlines. Nicknamed the yuppie flu, it was often written off as burnout or depression. Many people who had CFS looked so healthy that they were told that their symptoms were "all in their heads."

Today most doctors are familiar with CFS, but they still have a hard time diagnosing it. Symptoms vary widely from person to person and often resemble the flu, mononucleosis, or depression. And because no one knows what causes CFS, medical science has not yet developed a definitive test that can prove whether a person has it. In the 1980s, some researchers believed CFS, like mononucleosis, was caused by the Epstein-Barr virus; while that theory has been rejected, some experts still suspect that a virus may play a role.

These days, many experts consider CFS an immune activation (autoimmune) disorder similar in some respects to lupus and rheumatoid arthritis. In

---

Trim the fat. By now just about everyone has gotten the message that a low-fat diet is essential for overall health. This advice takes on new importance for the person with CFS, since fatty foods are difficult to digest and can cause a general sluggish feeling, the last thing a person with CFS needs. "There's also some evidence that too much fat in the diet can have an adverse effect on immunity," says Dr. Magaziner.

Eat healthy. The optimum diet for a person with CFS is the same as for anyone who's aiming for optimum health: high in fiber and complex carbohydrates, with lots of fruits, vegetables, beans, and whole grains. Dr. Magaziner also tells people with CFS to avoid processed foods, which are often full of additives, preservatives, and artificial colorings and flavorings.

Get tested for food allergies. People with CFS are particularly prone to food allergies and often improve significantly when the allergies are detected and treated, says Dr. Lapp. "It seems to be a combination of difficulty digesting protein and increased gut permeability," he says. In other words, he explains, often the intestines of a person with CFS absorb substances from foods that would pass right through the digestive tract in a healthy person.

Dr. Lapp treats the problem with enzymes to improve protein digestion and, in extreme cases, by eliminating the foods that cause the most problems. "Generally speaking, red meat, wheat, and dairy seem to be the most problematic," says Dr. Lapp.

If you suspect that food allergies are making your symptoms worse, discuss the problem with your physician.

immune activation disorders, the immune system is so cranked up to defend the body against invaders that it actually attacks the body's own tissues. Doctors also see a high incidence of allergies among people with CFS, another sign that their immune systems tend to overreact.

CFS resembles other immune activation disorders in another way: A disproportionate share of people with CFS—probably around 75 percent—are women, says Dr. Lapp. "It could be that women's immune systems are just stronger than men's," he says. Like most aspects of this mysterious disease, the reasons that women are more susceptible are subject to much debate. But one thing doctors do agree on is that CFS isn't all in the patient's head. Today CFS is widely regarded as a physical illness, not a mental one.

Getting the Big Picture

No one knows for sure how many people have CFS. The Centers for Disease Control and Prevention (CDC) in Atlanta estimates that more than 1 million Americans are affected by it, but tens of millions have similar illnesses that don't meet the CDC's strict definition of this disease. Unless an individual has the right number and combination of symptoms, the case isn't reported as CFS. Many researchers believe the disease is far more common than the figures indicate.

In a random sampling of over 18,500 individuals, approximately 0.42 percent were believed to have CFS, with rates being higher for Latino and African American people than white people. "The results of this epidemiological study suggested that this illness may affect approximately 800,000 people in the United States," says Leonard Jason, PhD, professor of psychology at DePaul University in Chicago, who conducted the study. Since women, Latinos, middle-aged individuals, and those of middle to lower socioeconomic status were found to be at a higher risk, "the findings directly contradicted the perception that middle to upper-class Caucasian women were the primary individuals with this illness," Dr. Jason says.

While no one has found a cure for CFS, dietary changes and nutritional supplements can help strengthen the immune system, improve energy levels, and ease some of the symptoms, says Allan Magaziner, DO, director of the Magaziner Center for Wellness and Anti-Aging Medicine in Cherry Hill, New Jersey. Dr. Magaziner has been treating people with CFS for more than 20 years.

"Of course, taking a supplement isn't going to cure CFS," he cautions. "People need to understand that they also have to eat right, exercise appropriately, and work with a physician who's knowledgeable about CFS."

Fighting Back with Coenzyme Q10

For those doing daily battle with chronic fatigue syndrome (CFS), their doctors may just prescribe coenzyme Q10, according to Charles Lapp, MD, clinical associate professor of family and community medicine at Duke University and a CFS specialist at the Hunter-Hopkins Center in Charlotte, North Carolina.

Coenzyme Q10 is available in supplement form in drugstores and health food stores. This little-known nutrient isn't exactly a vitamin, although its chemical makeup is similar to that of vitamins E and K. Experts believe that like vitamin K, coenzyme Q10 can be manufactured by the body, though it's also found in soybeans, vegetable oils, and many meats.

Like vitamins C and E, coenzyme Q10 is a member of the antioxidant family, a group of nutrients that protect your body's tissues from everyday wear and tear by disarming destructive free radicals. Free radicals are unstable molecules that wreak havoc at the cellular level by stealing electrons from your body's healthy molecules to balance themselves.

Besides being a potent antioxidant, coenzyme Q10 has an important function in energy production: It reacts with another enzyme to let cells convert protein, fat, and carbohydrates into energy.

While people with CFS aren't deficient in coenzyme Q10, they seem to have functional shortages of the enzyme it reacts with, explains Dr. Lapp. Taking extra coenzyme Q10 prompts the body to improve the function of this partner enzyme. And the better the partner enzyme works, the better the body's ability to convert food into energy.

For people with CFS who'd like to try coenzyme Q10 on their own, he recommends a daily dose of 200 milligrams, taken in a divided dose. And since this nutrient is fat-soluble, it should be taken with a little bit of fat or oil (although some supplements are in an oil base, similar to vitamin E capsules).

Muscling Up with Magnesium

Some people with CFS have benefited from taking supplements of magnesium, a mineral that is involved in the cells' energy production.

One study of 32 people with CFS found that most of those who received magnesium injections had increased energy, a better emotional state, and less pain than the patients who didn't have injections.

Some people with CFS have been shown to have low blood levels of magnesium. But even if their blood tests don't show magnesium deficiencies, people can still benefit from extra doses of the mineral, according to Dr. Lapp. "Their blood levels of magnesium may be normal, but that doesn't tell the whole story," he says. "Magnesium, like potassium, is pumped into the cell, so normally there's a higher concentration inside the cell than there is in the blood. And that pump mechanism may not work very well in people with CFS, so their magnesium levels can be normal in the blood and low in the cell."

Dr. Magaziner also finds that most people with CFS notice improvement in their symptoms after starting magnesium supplements. "It doesn't work for everyone," he says. "But many of my patients find it eases their muscle aches and makes them feel less fatigued."

This is probably because people with CFS have enzyme deficiencies that hamper the cells' ability to convert food into energy, according to Dr. Lapp. And extra magnesium improves enzyme function, which results in greater energy production on the cellular level.

If you're interested in trying magnesium, Dr. Magaziner recommends starting with 500 milligrams a day. "This level is perfectly safe, although occasionally a person will develop loose bowels or diarrhea," he says. "If that happens, I would simply reduce the dose to the point where the diarrhea goes away." If you have heart or kidney problems, however, you should check with your doctor before taking magnesium supplements.

Dr. Lapp recommends a chelated form of magnesium called magnesium glycinate. "It's rapidly absorbed in the gastrointestinal tract, so it doesn't cause digestive problems," he explains. "And it tends to be drawn into the cell, where it's needed."

And because taking more magnesium increases the body's need for calcium, Dr. Magaziner suggests taking calcium supplements as well. "I usually recommend taking them in a two-to-one ratio—1,000 milligrams of calcium if you're taking 500 milligrams of magnesium," he advises.

A Boost from B-Complex

The B-complex vitamins help support the adrenal glands, which are among the major organs in the body connected with stress, says Dr. Magaziner. "B vitamins also support the central nervous system, to help us cope with stress in general," he explains. "We lose a lot of B vitamins when we're stressed, so we need to replenish them." These nutrients are also involved in energy production, which makes them essential for people with CFS.

Dr. Magaziner recommends a supplement containing the entire B complex. Thiamin, pantothenic acid, and vitamins B_6 and B_{12} are especially important for people with CFS, he says.

Prescriptions for Healing

Nutrients can play roles in treating chronic fatigue syndrome. Here's what some doctors recommend.

Nutrient	Daily Amount
Antioxidant-complex supplement containing . . .	
Coenzyme Q$_{10}$	200 milligrams, taken in a divided dose
Selenium	50 micrograms
Vitamin C	500 milligrams
Vitamin E	400 IU
B-complex supplement containing . . .	
Pantothenic acid	50 milligrams
Thiamin	50 milligrams
Vitamin B$_6$	50 milligrams
Vitamin B$_{12}$	50 micrograms
Calcium	500 milligrams
Magnesium	500 milligrams (magnesium glycinate)
Vitamin C	4,000 milligrams (ester-C), taken as 2 divided doses

MEDICAL ALERT: *If you have been diagnosed with chronic fatigue syndrome, you should be under a doctor's care.*

Selenium in doses exceeding 400 micrograms daily should be taken only under medical supervision.

If you are taking anticoagulants, you should not take vitamin E supplements. (Though generally a dose of up to 1,500 IU of vitamin E a day is considered safe, some recent reports suggest that taking more than 400 IU a day could be harmful to people with cardiovascular or circulatory disease or with cancer. If you have such a condition, be sure to consult your doctor before you begin supplementation.)

If you have heart or kidney problems, you should always check with your doctor before taking magnesium supplements.

Doses of vitamin C in excess of 1,200 milligrams a day can cause diarrhea in some people, so it's a good idea to check with your doctor before taking more than that amount.

If you're using ester-C as your vitamin C source, you won't need a separate calcium supplement, since ester-C contains mainly calcium carbonate.

You can get the B-complex vitamins in most multivitamin/mineral supplements, says Dr. Lapp. Check the label to make sure the supplement contains at least 50 milligrams each of thiamin, pantothenic acid, and vitamin B_6 and 50 micrograms of vitamin B_{12}. He also recommends taking a separate B-complex supplement whenever you're under stress.

Higher doses of vitamin B_{12}, given through injection by a physician, can also be helpful in cases of enzyme deficiency, says Dr. Lapp. Injected B_{12} doses may be 1,000 times higher than the normal daily dose.

Arm Yourself with Antioxidants

Also helpful in treating CFS are the so-called antioxidant nutrients, which include vitamin C, vitamin E, and the mineral selenium.

These nutrients form a veritable SWAT team that helps defend your cells against free radicals, unstable molecules that occur naturally in the body and that are also produced by bad habits such as smoking, sunbathing, and drinking alcohol. Free radicals steal electrons from your body's healthy molecules to balance themselves, damaging cells in the process. Antioxidants neutralize free radicals by offering their own electrons, protecting healthy molecules from harm.

"Antioxidants protect the body from deterioration, degeneration, and environmental stresses," says Dr. Magaziner. "And since many people with CFS are unusually sensitive to environmental factors such as household chemicals, food additives, and artificial fragrances, taking antioxidants makes sense."

Damage from free radicals is such an important factor in CFS that some researchers consider CFS a free radical-generated disease, says Dr. Lapp. "I don't think it's caused by free radical damage, but that seems to be one of the factors that maintains it," he says.

To help bolster the immune system and improve stamina, both doctors recommend an antioxidant-complex supplement, available in most drugstores and health food stores. Because dosage varies widely from brand to brand, read the label to make sure you're getting about 500 milligrams of vitamin C, 400 IU of vitamin E, and 50 micrograms of selenium.

People with CFS may also want to try a vitamin C supplement in the form of ester-C, says Dr. Lapp. "Ester-C is much more bioavailable than regular vitamin C," he explains. "Your body absorbs twice as much." Taking more than 1,200 milligrams of vitamin C can cause diarrhea in some people, however, so it's a good idea to check with your doctor before exceeding that amount. Ester-C is available in health food stores.

COLDS

COMMON NUTRIENTS FOR
A COMMON CONDITION

You've probably heard it said at least a million times: There's no cure for the common cold.

The reason the cure continues to elude our greatest minds is due in part to the sheer multitude of viruses that cause colds. More than 200 different strains of viruses can trigger sneezes and sniffles, and often two or more provoke a single cold! "Finding a vaccine to incorporate all of these is impractical," says Ray Sahelian, MD, a physician in private practice in Marina del Rey, California, and author of *The Common Cold Cure*. "It wouldn't be worth the trouble for a condition that's mildly annoying and not the least bit life-threatening."

Regardless of which strain gets hold of you, though, you know the symptoms when they hit: A phlegm-filled cough. Nose blowing that rivals any air horn blast. Sneezes so severe that even good china in the next room isn't safe.

Not only are these cold symptoms, but experts think that they're also cold senders, launching tiny droplets of mucus into the air with every wheeze, hack, and honk. Inside these specks of mucus are soccer ball-shaped organisms called rhinoviruses, so tiny that 15,000 lined up side by side would barely span the space between two words on this page. Whether carried on a finger as you scratch your nose or inhaled through your nose or mouth, some of these malevolent microbes may eventually get the break they're looking for: the chance to get inside your body.

It's all downhill from there, literally. The wavelike downward motion of the tiny hairlike projections that line your throat pushes the virus as well as your normal throat mucus toward your esophagus. If you're fortunate, powerful digestive acids destroy the virus before it can do any harm.

When you do become infected, however, the virus's cold-producing plan begins to unfold. Finding a warm spot in your throat where your own mucus layer is thin and offers little protection, a single virus attaches itself to a cell and commandeers the cell's own replicating capability. Office copiers should work so well: Within a few hours, over 100,000 viruses are created.

And all of that awful sneezing, snorting, and coughing? That's called the host response, your body's way of fighting this unwanted guest from within. Before long, white blood cells, the avenging angels of your immune system, are rushed to the scene of the infection to kill the cells containing the virus. That influx of blood causes swelling in the sinuses. Stepped-up mucus pro-

Food Factors

These dietary tips may help you keep your cold under control.

Get souped up. The word is still out on whether or not it really helps your soul, but chicken soup definitely can help fight a cold. Researchers at Mount Sinai Medical Center in Miami Beach, Florida, have found that hot chicken soup apparently increases the flow of mucus. Although researchers aren't sure whether it's the aroma or the taste, they say chicken soup helps make your nose run, which shortens the amount of time cold germs spend inside your nose. In a test, hot chicken soup worked better than hot water alone.

Historians say chicken soup was first recommended for colds 800 years ago by Maimonides, court physician to Saladin, the caliph of Egypt.

Drink plenty of fluids. The next time you come down with a cold, you can help banish that pesky virus to a digestive grave by drinking lots of liquids. When the mucus that lines your throat is moist, it traps viruses and sends them down to the stomach, where powerful digestive acids destroy them. Normally 6 to 8 cups of water, milk, juice, lemonade, or soup a day is enough to meet your liquid quota, but you can easily lose a quart or more of fluids a day when you're sick. The recommendation: Double your fluids. And avoid alcohol, which depletes your body of immune-boosting nutrients and causes dehydration.

Grab some garlic. Long championed by garlic lovers for fighting off colds, the odorous bulb is gaining new respect in, of all places, the laboratory. Studies with laboratory animals showed that garlic actually helps protect them from flu viruses while boosting their production of immune system antibodies. And preliminary studies showed that people who ate garlic for 3 weeks had enhanced immune system activity.

Turn up the heat. Spicy foods containing hot peppers, curry, and chili powder get your mucus flowing, which can help unplug your nose and make your cough more productive, experts say. In fact, if you're really brave, you may just want to try adding some garlic and hot peppers to your chicken soup.

duction designed to trap the virus makes for a running nose and eventually a hacking cough.

When it comes to treating your cold, the natural route to relief may be your best bet. Antibiotics are a no-no. "By giving antibiotics too regularly, all you're doing is showing the bacteria these drugs repeatedly so that they learn how to be resistant," says Ben Kligler, MD, medical director of the Continuum Center for Health and Healing in New York City. And over-the-counter drugs may provide quick relief, but their interference with the body's normal defenses can actually prolong the illness. "Unless they're incredibly uncomfortable, I usually just have my patients take over-the-counter medications at night to get to sleep," says Dr. Kligler.

While conventional medicines might drag a cold out longer, some natural medicines, if used at the onset of a cold, can shorten its duration. Here are the vitamins and foods that may help.

The Mystery of Vitamin C

Taking vitamin C to treat a cold is about as common as . . . well, the common cold.

And yet the controversy over its effectiveness continues, with the general public serving as its strongest advocate.

Ever since the late chemist Linus Pauling, PhD, shocked the medical community with his book *Vitamin C and the Common Cold*, doctors have debated the merits of his recommendations. Among them: taking 500 to 1,000 milligrams of vitamin C every hour for several hours to reduce the length and severity of a cold. Dr. Pauling certainly walked his talk: For 6 years prior to his death at age 93, the two-time winner of the Nobel Prize reportedly took 12,000 milligrams of vitamin C a day.

Dozens of studies of varying professionalism and reliability followed Dr. Pauling's pronouncements, with mixed results. At last count, roughly half supported his megadose claim. The others, testing much lower doses, showed that vitamin C is of little help in ending a cold in progress.

And that is precisely what vitamin C advocates have claimed all along: If you're going to take vitamin C for a cold, you have to take a lot. In fact, a review conducted by a British researcher found that all of the studies done since 1970 in which people were taking 1,000 milligrams or more of vitamin C a day to reduce the symptoms of their colds showed positive results, including a 72 percent reduction in the duration of cold symptoms.

Take Vitamin C for Symptoms

Dr. Kligler believes the best approach is to begin taking vitamin C when you first feel the scratchy throat, stuffy nose, or congested chest of a cold coming on. "The evidence with vitamin C has more to do more with the immune system than the lungs," he says. "It increases our ability to fight viral illnesses, so someone experiencing upper respiratory infections might do well to take vitamin C early on in the stages of their respiratory problem."

A number of studies over the years have examined the efficacy of taking a large dose of vitamin C every day to actually *prevent* the symptoms of a cold before they start. But Dr. Kligler feels that the evidence that this is helpful is dubious at best. "Personally, I feel that the literature about vitamin C for prevention is a lot weaker than vitamin C for treatment," he says. "A lot of people take vitamin C for the prevention of respiratory illness. Although many people feel that this helps them, the research doesn't really support that."

Dr. Kligler believes that taking this much vitamin C on a daily basis may actually be harmful rather than helpful. "There are some people who feel that in higher doses, vitamin C may actually be pro-oxidant," he says. "This is still the subject of some controversy, but a number of studies seem to indi-

---

Prescriptions for Healing

Some doctors recommend taking these nutrients to help banish cold symptoms.

Nutrient	Daily Amount
Vitamin C	2,000 milligrams a day at the first sign of symptoms, for no more than 7 days
Selenium	100 micrograms, taken along with 20 micrograms of zinc, daily (for those age 65 and older)
Zinc gluconate	24 milligrams, dissolved in your mouth every 2 hours (up to 8 lozenges a day)

MEDICAL ALERT: *Doses of vitamin C larger than 1,200 milligrams a day can cause diarrhea in some people.*

Selenium in doses exceeding 400 micrograms daily should be taken only under medical supervision.

cate that a dose of vitamin C on a long-standing basis of over 500 milligrams a day is not necessarily good for you. If it were to turn from an antioxidant into a pro-oxidant, it greatly increases your risk of tissue damage."

Keeping this in mind, the best approach may be to stick to mega-dosing vitamin C only when you feel the symptoms of a cold first taking hold. "Dr. Andrew Weil recently revised downward the maintenance dose of vitamin C that he recommends, and a lot of people are going that way," says Dr. Kligler. "You should take at least two grams as soon as you feel an upper respiratory illness developing, continue for a finite period of time, like five to seven days, and then stop. This would have to be in a pill, as you can't get this much vitamin C from food."

The Daily Value for vitamin C is only 60 milligrams. Doses larger than 1,200 milligrams a day can cause diarrhea in some people.

Zinc: Another Cold Controversy

Long appreciated for its immune-boosting power, zinc attracted considerable attention in the 1980s as a cold remedy, and in a remarkable way.

George Eby of Austin, Texas, observed a 3-year-old girl who suffered repeated severe colds. He reported giving her a 50-milligram zinc gluconate tablet at the start of one of her colds in a bid to boost her immune system. But she refused to swallow the tablet, instead dissolving it in her mouth. Her symptoms were gone within a few hours, far faster than usual. After observing zinc's cold-stopping effect several more times, Eby wondered whether sucking, not swallowing, zinc might actually be the long-sought cure for the common cold.

Eby conducted a scientific study to see if he was on to something. Published in a medical journal, the results of the study were promising. Those who took plain, awful-tasting zinc gluconate tablets reported that their symptoms were gone after an average of 4 days, while those taking better-tasting placebos said that their colds lasted an average of 11 days.

Fast-forward to today, and zinc gluconate (and zinc acetate, which works equally well) lozenges have been refined to eliminate the awful taste. They are now readily available over the counter at most major drugstores and grocery stores. (The most common brand is Cold-EEZE.)

And there's a good reason that zinc lozenges are now so widely available: They really seem to shorten the duration of a cold. "There have been quite a number of studies with zinc that support its role in treating the common cold," says Dr. Sahelian. "It's unfortunate that more people don't know about it, and even more unfortunate that most doctors still do not recommend it."

Dr. Sahelian says that just like vitamin C, the best time to begin taking zinc lozenges is at the very first signs of a cold. "Immediately place a zinc lozenge in the mouth, and keep it there long as possible. Then take another zinc lozenge every hour for five hours," he says. "After that, I recommend the zinc every two to four hours, depending on the symptoms. And if you wake up during the night, go ahead and use the zinc lozenge again. Sometimes I've found that it's quite helpful during the day, and then a patient will go eight to ten hours without using it. By morning some of the symptoms will have returned."

Dr. Sahelian adds that the way you take the zinc lozenge is also critical. "The important thing with the zinc is that some people make the mistake of swallowing it too quickly," he says. "It doesn't work systemically, which means the zinc is not going to work in the stomach or the bloodstream. It's going to work directly in the throat, so by keeping it in the oral pharynx area as long as possible, it helps to directly kill the cold."

Zinc lozenges do cause some minor side effects in some, but the results are often worth it, adds Dr. Sahelian. "Usually the most common side effects are nausea from the zinc," he says. "And if the zinc is used frequently, people will report soreness in the throat and a raw feeling on the tongue."

Zinc plus Vitamin C: The Power Combination

Dr. Sahelian believes it's no mistake that vitamin C and zinc appear to be the two most effective nutrients for treating the symptoms of a cold. In fact, he believes that using the two in combination makes for a simple surefire cold stopper. At the very earliest onset, be it a tingle in the nose, a mild sore throat, or the sinuses filling up, take 2,000 milligrams of vitamin C in one dose. Then, suck on a zinc lozenge, keeping it in your mouth for at least 5 minutes, followed by another lozenge every hour for 5 hours. Then space them out every 2 to 3 hours after that. "In most cases, I find that this combination is able to stop a cold dead in its tracks," says Dr. Sahelian. "It appears that the zinc is able to act locally to kill the virus, and vitamin C probably stimulates the white blood cells to fight off infection. Two-thirds to three-quarters of the time, it goes away before it has a chance to start." If the cold does continue, Dr. Sahelian recommends continuing to take 1,000 milligrams of vitamin C a day in divided doses, but the first large dose is most important.

For the Elderly, Try Zinc and Selenium

A recent study seems to indicate that low-dose supplementation of zinc and selenium may help seniors fight respiratory infections and reduce the duration of their symptoms. The study found that the seniors who received 100 micrograms of selenium along with 20 milligrams of zinc daily experienced a lot fewer infections over a 2-year period than they did prior to receiving the supplements.

COLD SORES

MINOR MIRACLES FOR YOUR MOUTH

It usually starts with that all-too-familiar tingle. Then 2 or 3 days later, it rears its ugly head in the form of one or more red, painful blisters on or around your lips.

Though your greatest wish is for these painful intruders to go away as soon as possible, they likely have other plans. Over the next 7 to 10 days, you can expect the sores to swell up until they rupture and ooze fluid before finally going away.

You probably wouldn't want even your greatest enemy to undergo this unpleasant scenario. But if you get cold sores, then you've likely experienced it countless times yourself. And since an estimated 90 percent of the population gets cold sores . . . well, your greatest enemy probably gets them, too.

Cold sores, also called fever blisters, are caused by the herpes simplex virus, the same virus that's responsible for genital herpes (see page 263). But while genital herpes are known as "type 2" and occur in almost 30 percent of the population, cold sores are "type 1" and commonly attack the mouth, lips, nose, chin, or cheeks.

You can get cold sores by kissing or coming in contact with the skin of someone who has an active outbreak. And even worse, towels, utensils, razors, and other items that come in contact with blisters can also spread the virus.

Most of the time, the virus stays dormant in the body. But by taxing your body with a cold, flu, fever, lack of sleep, or general stress, you can cause it to rear its ugly head. Sunburn can also cause a cold sore outbreak. On average, people with cold sores experience two to three outbreaks every year.

Fortunately, as bad as the cold sore virus can be, you don't have to be completely at the mercy of this blistering beast. By controlling stress and using sunscreen, you can help prevent cold sores, says Craig Zunka, DDS, past president of the Holistic Dental Association and a dentist in Front Royal, Virginia. And, say doctors, over-the-counter ointments containing zinc oxide can speed the healing of the cold sores that do occur.

Some doctors have also found nutritional strategies that, though they aren't clinically proven, may ward off herpes outbreaks as well as speed up their departure. Here's what these doctors recommend.

Food Factors

Since the herpes simplex virus often waits until you're stressed out or falling ill to strike, doctors say that keeping your cool and eating a nutritious diet to stay healthy are always good deterrents. Also, some experts have found that certain foods may actually prevent or trigger outbreaks. Here's what they recommend.

Love lysine. Lysine is an amino acid that suppresses the growth of the herpes simplex virus and therefore limits the number of outbreaks, says Craig Zunka, DDS, past president of the Holistic Dental Association and a dentist in Front Royal, Virginia.

You can boost your lysine intake by eating potatoes, milk, brewer's yeast, fish, chicken, and beans. Since the optimum dose to prevent herpes outbreaks may be higher than the amount you can get from foods, however, some doctors also recommend supplements.

"I recommend taking one or two 500-milligram supplements a day, depending on the severity of the case," says Dr. Zunka. Lysine supplements are available in health food stores.

Go easy on arginine. The flip side of lysine is arginine, an amino acid found in foods such as chocolate, peas, cereals, peanuts, beer, gelatin, and raisins. The herpes virus apparently needs a certain amount of arginine to grow. You might try limiting these foods in general and eliminating them during an outbreak, suggests Dr. Zunka.

Nip 'Em with Vitamin C

You may be able to stop a cold sore before it appears by zapping it with a high dose of vitamin C at the first tingle, say the experts.

"As soon as you start to feel the burning and tingling of a cold sore coming on, take vitamin C with bioflavonoids. The two together inhibit the progression of the virus," says Dr. Zunka. He recommends taking 1,000 milligrams of both vitamin C and bioflavonoids as soon as you feel the tingling, then 500 milligrams of each three times a day for the next day or two. (Bioflavonoids are chemical compounds related to vitamin C. Some vitamin C supplements contain them, but bioflavonoids are also available as a supplement alone.)

Medical research seems to reinforce Dr. Zunka's recommendation: One study found that 40 people who took vitamin C and bioflavonoid supplements experienced less severe blisters and shorter outbreaks than 10 people who took placebos. (The duration of the outbreaks was 4 days versus 10 days, respectively.) The researchers also concluded that the therapy achieved the best results when people took the supplements as soon as they experienced cold sore symptoms.

Some people may experience diarrhea when taking more than 1,200 milligrams of vitamin C a day. You can also introduce more vitamin C and bioflavonoids into your daily diet by eating fruits (especially citrus), vegetables, nuts, and seeds.

In other vitamin C news, vitamin C can also work topically to bring relief. To speed along healing, try applying a topical vitamin C solution to the blisters three times for 2 minutes each at 30-minute intervals.

Zap It with Zinc

In test-tube studies, zinc has been shown to block the reproduction of the herpes simplex virus, so using zinc might help reduce the frequency, duration, and severity of cold sore outbreaks. Here are three ways it can help.

Once a cold sore has made its not-so-grand appearance, you can dry it up and heal it more quickly by applying a dollop of an ointment containing zinc oxide directly to the sore, some experts suggest.

If a cold sore is really getting under your skin, you might consider asking

Prescriptions for Healing

If recurrent cold sores have your lips in their grip, some oral health experts suggest that you might find relief from these nutrients.

Nutrient	Daily Amount/Application
Oral	
Vitamin C and bioflavonoids	1,000 milligrams of each, taken at the first sign of an outbreak; then 1,500 milligrams of each, taken as 3 divided doses for 1 or 2 days
Zinc	50 milligrams a day taken in divided doses with food during an outbreak, and 20 milligrams a day as a preventive measure
Topical	
Vitamin C	A topical solution, applied three times for 2 minutes each at 30-minute intervals on the first day of the outbreak
Vitamin E	Oil from 1 capsule, applied directly to a cotton swab and then dabbed on the sore every 8 hours as needed
Zinc oxide	As an ingredient in an over-the-counter ointment

MEDICAL ALERT: *Some people may experience diarrhea when taking more than 1,200 milligrams of vitamin C a day.*

Do not take more than 15 milligrams of zinc a day unless under medical supervision.

your doctor or dentist about getting a shot of protamine zinc, a protein-zinc compound, says Dr. Zunka.

"I use it all the time for healing lesions in the mouth," he says. "You just inject a small amount at the site of the herpes sore, and it clears up the sore very quickly. Zinc is known for reducing healing time up to 30 or 40 percent."

Finally, it might be worth trying an oral zinc supplement to put an end to the outbreak. Some experts recommend 50 milligrams a day in divided doses with food during an active outbreak, or 20 milligrams a day as a preventive measure. However, zinc supplements can cause copper deficiency, and doses over 15 milligrams a day require medical supervision, so you'll want to ask your doctor if this is the right approach.

Add a Dash of Vitamin E

Finally, some doctors have found that the topical application of vitamin E can also take the bite out of a painful cold sore. To try this treatment, just crack open a vitamin E capsule, apply the oil to a cotton swab, and dab it onto the blisters every 8 hours as needed.

Note: If the cold sore is on or around your eyes, see a doctor immediately. This could be a far more dangerous complication.

CYSTIC FIBROSIS

NUTRITION FOR A LIFE-THREATENING CONDITION

Mucus, sweat, and saliva are not the most pleasant substances produced by our bodies, but they play critical roles in keeping us healthy. They provide lubrication for vital bodily functions, shield the body from noxious intruders, and even help remove toxins.

For the 30,000 Americans who suffer from cystic fibrosis, though, these seemingly benign substances become deadly. In this genetic disorder, the cells that produce mucus, sweat, and saliva, as well as digestive juices, work improperly. These substances are usually thin and slippery, allowing them to perform their bodily functions properly. But in those with cystic fibrosis, the secretions become thick and clumpy.

Though this sounds like a mere nuisance, the condition is deadly. These thick, clumpy secretions make their way to vital ducts and passageways in places like the pancreas and lungs and block them. In the lungs, they can cause respiratory failure and death. And in the pancreas, they block the body from absorbing key vitamins, which is why nutrition is so critical for those with cystic fibrosis.

New Hope for a Difficult Disease

Despite the seemingly grim prospects for cystic fibrosis sufferers, the news about the disease isn't all bad. In recent years, researchers have made great strides in improving the quality of life of those living with the disease. According to the Cystic Fibrosis Foundation, life with the disease, though challenging, is far better than it was 50, 30, or even 10 years ago.

In years past, most children born with cystic fibrosis never made it to adulthood. Today, 40 percent of the cystic fibrosis population is age 18 or older. This is a testament to improved therapies and methods of care that have not only lengthened lives but improved them as well.

"Everybody who is working with cystic fibrosis children and their families today does it with a different sense of hope than we had a few years ago," says Virginia Stallings, MD, professor of pediatrics at Children's Hospital of Philadelphia. "This used to be thought of as a fatal disease. Now we know that the more years we can add to the window of excellent health, the better the chance at one of the new therapies."

Starving in a Land of Plenty

One critical aspect of cystic fibrosis treatment is making sure patients get enough nutrients to sustain good health. And considering some of the challenges they face, this can often be difficult.

In healthy people, mucus in the digestive tract is thin and slippery, so food can easily slide along the digestive tract and nutrients can pass from digested food through the intestinal wall, into the bloodstream, and on to the rest of the body, explains Donna Mueller, RD, PhD, associate professor of nutrition and foods at Drexel University in Philadelphia. But in people with cystic fibrosis, the digestive tract sometimes is covered with such thick mucus that many, if not most, nutrients can't get through the intestinal wall and into the bloodstream. That's why people with cystic fibrosis are frequently at risk for malnutrition. They are literally starving in a land of plenty.

Complicating the situation is the fact that the pancreas, which produces enzymes that help the body digest protein, fat, and carbohydrates, also is affected by the thick mucus. "The enzymes produced in the pancreas's cells leave the pancreas through little canals that empty out into the small intestine," explains Dr. Mueller. But in people with cystic fibrosis, the canals sometimes get so clogged with mucus that most enzymes never reach the food, so most of the food they eat simply is not digested.

"Some nutrients are going to get through," says Dr. Mueller. "But cystic fibrosis is a textbook on nutrition, because every nutrient is affected: protein, fat, carbohydrates, vitamins, and minerals."

Meeting the Body's Increasing Demands

Unfortunately, just as the body is least likely to get the nutrients it requires, its need for those nutrients will increase by 20 percent or more.

This is a chronic, progressive disease that hits the airways particularly hard, explains Dr. Mueller. The lungs worsen. People get sicker and sicker while their bodies work harder and harder. That's why nutrition is always important. As the lungs become more involved and the body is working harder, energy requirements increase.

"Unfortunately, when someone doesn't feel well, one doesn't feel like eating, either," says Dr. Mueller. "So just when there are greater body needs, there's less of an appetite."

But tough as it is for adults with cystic fibrosis to meet their daily nutritional needs, children with cystic fibrosis also have to meet the demands of growing bodies.

Prescriptions for Healing

To keep the body as strong as possible while new scientific and medical therapies are under development, a person with cystic fibrosis is encouraged to (1) eat a well-balanced diet, (2) take specially prepared supplemental pancreatic digestive enzymes (these break down food so nutrients can be better absorbed), (3) add specially formulated multivitamin/mineral supplements provided by their doctor or nutritionist, and (4) take other vitamin and mineral supplements based on individualized blood tests and in consultation with a cystic fibrosis nutrition specialist, says Donna Mueller, RD, PhD, associate professor of nutrition and foods at Drexel University in Philadelphia.

MEDICAL ALERT: *Anyone who has cystic fibrosis should be taking vitamin and mineral supplements only after discussing it with both a physician and registered dietitian who are cystic fibrosis specialists.*

"You know the growth charts doctors use?" asks Dr. Stallings. Children with cystic fibrosis are often at the bottom, somewhere around the 10th percentile, she says. That means that 90 percent of everybody else their age is bigger. That's why the goal of most doctors, including Dr. Stallings, is to give kids the nutritional support they need to grow as big as their brothers and sisters and to get them through these growth phases, so they go into adulthood as strong and as well-nourished as possible.

On average, Dr. Stallings is successful. "We have a little trouble with adolescent girls because of the body image issues in our society," says Dr. Stallings. With all of the cultural emphasis on thinness as an ideal, "they don't mind being the skinniest kids in class," she says. "But of course, that may be harmful to their health."

Winning with Prevention Power

Once children with cystic fibrosis have completed their adolescent growth spurts, doctors and nutritionists generally breathe a sigh of relief. But only for a moment. They still need to help them store up enough nutritional support as adults to withstand the frequent infections associated with the disease without losing ground.

To help meet the nutritional demands of their bodies, people with cystic fibrosis are encouraged to eat a well-balanced diet. For the lucky few who do not have a genetic problem with digestion, that might be enough. However, for the majority of people with cystic fibrosis, that balanced diet gets combined with other nutritional therapies determined by their doctors and nutritionists. Often, these therapies include supplemental pancreatic digestive enzymes, as well as specialized multivitamin/mineral supplements, says Dr. Mueller.

"The major issue is calories," adds Dr. Stallings. "If anything affects growth, energy, quality of life, and being able to fight off infection, the big thing is absorbing adequate calories. If you can get enough calories to keep up your body weight, then almost everything else that you can do nutritionally follows."

In fact, she adds, "if someone with cystic fibrosis is consuming adequate calories and has maintained normal body weight, I try to not prescribe any extra supplements besides what has been determined to be absolutely necessary. Since these are people who may be taking 60 pills a day, they don't need to be taking another pill if they don't have to."

Dr. Mueller agrees with the need to keep the food and pill regimens as simple as possible. But she also feels that "even with a well-balanced diet and pancreatic enzyme replacements, most people with cystic fibrosis need extra vitamins and minerals."

Dr. Mueller explains that there are a number of reasons why supplements are necessary. For one, the pancreatic digestive enzymes are not always 100 percent effective, and "there's no good way of knowing exactly how much of these enzymes is necessary at any particular time," she says. Also, people's diets vary quite a bit from day to day and are not always nutritionally balanced. And finally, the thickness of mucus in the digestive tract—and hence the amount of vitamins and minerals being absorbed—constantly varies.

Luckily, adds Dr. Mueller, our understanding of the nutrients that those with cystic fibrosis need has grown exponentially in recent decades. Now, there are specially designed vitamin and mineral preparations for babies, children, and adults.

Even with these specialized supplements, though, people with cystic fibrosis face a number of challenges that can create additional nutritional demands. That's why it's so important to have blood levels of target nutrients checked at least once a year, says Dr. Mueller. People with cystic fibrosis have changing needs, and what was fine last year may not be so this year. Some vitamins and minerals might need to be decreased, and some might need to be increased. And because deficiencies of these nutrients may make the body even more vulnerable to infection and disease, "vitamin and mineral levels are as important as drug level tests," says Dr. Mueller. Keeping people with cystic fibrosis healthy longer is in large part a matter of optimal nutrition.

It is important to remember that anyone with cystic fibrosis should be under a doctor's care. Only a doctor or nutritionist with extra training in cystic fibrosis can recommend the right types and amounts of vitamin and mineral supplements for each person. To locate a cystic fibrosis center near you, contact the Cystic Fibrosis Foundation by writing to 6931 Arlington Road, Bethesda, MD 20814, calling 800-FIGHTCF, or logging on to www.cff.org.

DEPRESSION

DISPELLING THE DARKNESS

It's debatable that few words in the English language are misused more than *depression*. Just as an example, if you've ever had a friend or family member who's felt a little down in the dumps, chances are they've described themselves as depressed.

The problem with this, of course, is that it undermines just how serious depression can truly be, says Harold Bloomfield, MD, a retired psychiatrist and author of numerous books on the topic, including *How to Heal Depression* and *Making Peace with Your Past*.

"Depression isn't the same as being sad or discouraged," says Dr. Bloomfield. "Those feelings are just part of being alive. Depression is an illness, one that can be controlled with proper treatment or that can ruin your life if you don't get the help you need."

Are You at Risk?

Depression may look and sound like the blues, but it lasts longer and has a more profound impact on a person's life. If you're clinically depressed, you live in a state of sadness and hopelessness so severe that it makes normal activities seem impossible. You may lose interest in friends or hobbies, have suicidal thoughts, or feel overwhelming guilt because you can't "snap out of it." Depression can kill your appetite or make you want to eat all the time. Sleeping more or less than usual and having problems concentrating can also be warning signs.

Depression can happen to anyone. Sometimes it's triggered by an emotional blow such as a divorce or the death of a loved one, but it can also appear out of nowhere.

A family history of depression can also put you at risk. "We see depression running in families just as diabetes and high blood pressure run in families," says Dr. Bloomfield. "That doesn't mean there aren't other causes, but a family history of depression makes a person more prone to it."

Depression often surfaces during times of transition, such as the teenage years, midlife, and retirement. The elderly are particularly vulnerable: Dr. Bloomfield estimates that people over age 60 are four times as likely to be depressed as younger people.

Hormones can also play a role. Some women who take birth control pills or hormone replacement therapy may experience depression as an effect of their pills and should see their doctors for guidance. Premenstrual and post-partum depression are also common.

Not much has changed in our understanding of depression over the last decade except for this: Its incidence is rising. The National Institute of Mental Health estimates that depression is the leading cause of disability among Americans ages 15 to 44. In any given year, about 15 million Americans—or nearly 7 percent of the population—suffer from depression. But what's most frightening is that children are the fastest-growing group that suffers from clinical depression—already, 23 percent of American children are considered depressed.

Feed Your Head

Studies examining the role of nutrition in depression are surprisingly sparse, but if you read between the lines, the connection is definitely there. "Most professionals still do not focus on nutrition as a contributing factor to depression," says Larry Christensen, PhD, chair of the department of psychology at the University of South Alabama in Mobile and author of *The Food-Mood Connection*. "The primary emphasis is still on issues such as a neurochemical aberration, stress, and the like. But from my own perspective, I believe that nutrition is a factor in about 25 percent of depressed individuals."

Moreover, nutritional deficiencies are common in depressed people, adds Dr. Bloomfield, though which comes first—deficiency or depression—isn't entirely clear. "If people haven't been eating right their whole lives, it can start to catch up with them in their forties or fifties. And if they have a tendency toward depression, it often shows up around the same time," he says.

While poor nutrition probably doesn't cause depression, correcting a deficiency can be beneficial if you're battling it, says Dr. Bloomfield. But nutritional supplements are no substitute for professional evaluation. "If you think you're depressed," he advises, "it's crucial that you see a physician or psychiatrist for help."

A Boost from the B Vitamins

A healthy intake of the B-complex vitamins is important for anyone who wants to keep depression at bay, says Dr. Bloomfield. While the whole B complex apparently plays a role in keeping you emotionally and physically healthy, a few members of the family seem to have particularly strong effects on depression.

Perhaps the biggest depression fighter of the B-vitamin family is folic acid. Studies have shown that more than 30 percent of people with depression may have low levels of folic acid in their bodies. In addition, a study at

Food Factors

When it comes to healing depression, individual nutrients are only part of the story. Some experts feel that what you're eating and drinking also plays an important role. Here are some tips from Larry Christensen, PhD, chair of the department of psychology at the University of South Alabama in Mobile and author of *The Food-Mood Connection*.

Cut back on sugar. While a sweet treat may temporarily boost your mood, the lift doesn't last. This slump is especially pronounced in people who are depressed to begin with, says Dr. Christensen. He estimates that up to 30 percent of his depressed patients show some sensitivity to sugar. To find out if sugar is contributing to your depression, cut out sweets and added sugars for a few weeks, says Dr. Christensen. Artificial sweeteners are okay, he adds.

If the thought of never eating another Oreo only contributes to your depression, take heart. While a minority of people are so sensitive to sugar that they shouldn't have it at all, others can handle a little bit, according to Dr. Christensen. Gradually reintroduce sweets to your diet—while at the same time carefully monitoring your mood—to find out how much you can tolerate.

Avoid the caffeine crash. Studies show that some depressed people depend on caffeine to improve their mood and get them through the day. Dr. Christensen advises his patients to eliminate coffee, tea, cola, and chocolate as well as pain relievers containing caffeine to see if caffeine is contributing to their depression. "Depressed people who are sensitive to caffeine generally notice improvement after about four days without caffeine," he says.

If you do find that you're sensitive to caffeine, he adds, it usually isn't an all-or-nothing proposition. "There are some people who can tol-

the University of Toronto indicated that depressed individuals with higher levels of folic acid seemed to get over their depression more quickly than those with lower levels. The newest evidence also seems to indicate that high levels of folic acid cause people to be more receptive to prescription antidepressant medicine, which makes folic acid supplementation a great addition to your doctor's recommendations.

Two other B vitamins that appear to play a role are thiamin and riboflavin. "There has been lots of evidence that if you're deficient in thiamin or riboflavin, over time it's going to lead to a depression of the whole functioning of the body, both physically and emotionally," says Dr. Bloomfield.

erate a cup of tea a day, but not more than that. People need to experiment to find their own limits."

Go low-fat. Some research suggests that besides improving your overall health, a low-fat diet may help stabilize your mood. In a 5-year study at the State University of New York at Stony Brook, 305 men and women followed a diet that got only between 20 and 30 percent of its calories from fat. The diet didn't just lower their cholesterol. They actually showed less depression and hostility after adopting the leaner diet.

Cutting the fat from your diet isn't complicated. Avoid fried foods, switch to leaner cuts of meat, and remove the skin from poultry. Swap whole milk for 1 percent or fat-free milk, and choose low-fat or nonfat cheeses and yogurt. And if you make an effort to eat more fruits, vegetables, and whole-grain cereals, you'll be less likely to fill up on fatty fare.

Feel good with fish. Not all fats are bad, however. A growing amount of research seems to support the notion that the omega-3 fatty acids found in fish such as salmon and mackerel play a role in combating the symptoms of depression. And this has been shown to be the case whether the omega-3s come from the diet or supplements. In addition, other studies have shown that individuals with abnormally low levels of omega-3s are more likely to suffer from depression to begin with. To up your intake of omega-3 fatty acids, strive to eat fish such as salmon or mackerel at least three times a week, or take 1.5 to 6 grams of a fish oil supplement daily. Consult with your physician to determine the dose that is right for you.

Beef up on L-carnitine. A handful of studies seem to indicate that L-carnitine, an amino acid derivative found in meats and dairy products, can combat serious depression, particularly in elderly populations that may be deficient in the compound to begin with.

Symptoms of thiamin deficiency include fear, uneasiness, confusion, and mood changes, which can be signs of depression. A study at the University of California, Davis, found that thiamin supplements improved sleep, appetite, and mood in older women who were only slightly deficient in the nutrient.

Experts advise that it's also important to make sure you're getting enough vitamin B_6. People with depression often don't, according to a study of 101 depressed men and women evaluated by the New York State Psychiatric Institute in New York City. Your body needs B_6 in order to manufacture the hormone serotonin, which seems to play a role in regulating your mood.

Many drugs, including those containing estrogen, can interfere with the absorption of vitamin B_6. This may be why some women experience depression after starting oral contraceptives or hormone replacement therapy. Vitamin B_6 may be particularly helpful for women on the Pill or for those who grapple with premenstrual depression, says Dr. Bloomfield.

Some researchers suggest that the B vitamins are even more effective when taken as a group. One study found that elderly people with depression who took supplements of thiamin, riboflavin, and vitamin B_6 along with antidepressant medication showed more improvement than those taking medication alone.

The safest, most convenient way to get all of your Bs is to invest in a B-complex supplement, says Dr. Bloomfield. Look for a supplement that contains at least 10 milligrams each of thiamin, riboflavin, and vitamin B_6 and 100 micrograms of folic acid, he suggests, and take it twice a day.

Staying Up with Vitamin C

If your diet fails to supply all of the vitamin C you need, doctors know that your mental as well as physical health may be at stake. Depression is a well-documented symptom of scurvy, a disease that results from severe deficiency of vitamin C. And while scurvy is relatively rare in developed countries, there's reason to believe that even a minor deficiency of vitamin C can affect your mental health.

Vitamin C is important for strengthening the immune system, which isn't in top form in depressed people. "We know that depressed people are more vulnerable to illness, so anything that strengthens the immune system is beneficial," says Dr. Bloomfield. He recommends vitamin C supplements in

Prescriptions for Healing

To make sure your body is getting the nutrients it needs to combat depression, Harold Bloomfield, MD, a retired psychiatrist and author of numerous books on depression, including *How to Heal Depression* and *Making Peace with Your Past*, recommends this daily supplement program.

Nutrient	Daily Amount
B-complex supplement, taken twice a day, containing . . .	
Folic acid	100 micrograms
Riboflavin	10 milligrams
Thiamin	10 milligrams
Vitamin B$_6$	10 milligrams
Selenium	100–200 micrograms
Vitamin C	1,000–4,000 milligrams

MEDICAL ALERT: If you have symptoms of depression, you should see your doctor for proper diagnosis and treatment.

Selenium in doses exceeding 400 micrograms daily should be taken only under medical supervision.

Doses of vitamin C exceeding 1,200 milligrams a day can cause diarrhea in some people, so it's a good idea to check with your doctor before taking more than that amount. Also, since vitamin C can interfere with the absorption of tricyclic antidepressants, you should discuss vitamin C supplementation with your doctor if you are taking this type of medication.

generous doses, up to 4,000 milligrams a day. This amount is many times the Daily Value, but since excess vitamin C is excreted in the urine, Dr. Bloomfield says that this large dose is safe.

Some people may experience diarrhea from this much vitamin C, however, so experts say it's a good idea to check with your doctor before taking more than 1,200 milligrams a day. Also, since vitamin C can interfere with the absorption of tricyclic antidepressants, you should discuss vitamin C supplementation with your doctor if you are taking this type of medication.

Dr. Bloomfield recommends that vitamin C supplements be taken early, first thing in the morning or at lunch, because some people might have difficulty falling asleep if they take the supplements later in the day.

Mind Your Minerals

A growing amount of evidence seems to be supporting the role of the mineral selenium in controlling or even combating the symptoms of depression. Researchers at Swansea University in Wales found that people who took supplements of 100 micrograms of selenium daily felt less fatigue, anxiety, and depression than those who didn't. A similar study looking at the amount of selenium in the diet showed that those with high-selenium diets experienced less depression, confusion, uncertainty, and anxiety than individuals with low-selenium diets. And finally, another study showed that selenium substantially improved mood in people after a period of 2 to 5 weeks.

To achieve your Daily Value of 70 micrograms of selenium, eat a balanced diet, and make sure your daily multivitamin contains selenium. It also might be worth taking 100 to 200 micrograms daily of a separate selenium supplement. Just make sure not to exceed 400 micrograms of selenium daily.

DERMATITIS

SUPPLEMENTS TO SAVE YOUR SKIN

Other than weight, perhaps no aspect of the body draws our obsession more than the skin. One only has to peruse the covers of women's magazines to see the perceived importance our culture places on healthy, youthful-looking skin. With this in mind, few conditions can be more distressing than dermatitis, also called eczema.

Dermatitis isn't life-threatening, or contagious. But for those who suffer from the itchy, red rashes and lesions that result from the condition, it can be quite distressing. Sometimes, the itching can be so bad that some children with dermatitis cause permanent skin damage and leave themselves prone to infection. And in extreme cases, the skin can grow thick and leathery in affected areas from over-itching.

In most people, dermatitis is an allergic reaction, which is why many people with dermatitis also have hay fever and asthma. But other irritants, such as soaps, detergents, perfume, and jewelry, among others, can also trigger an outbreak. The condition is common among children—10 percent of all children suffer from it at some point, and the number is as high as 17 percent in some parts of the United States and Europe, says Stephen Schleicher, MD, clinical instructor of dermatology at King's College and Arcadia University in Pennsylvania and director of the DERMDx Centers for Dermatology. But in some, it can linger on well into adulthood.

In addition to the allergens and irritants that cause dermatitis, doctors are now aware that vitamin and mineral deficiencies can also help launch dermatological tirades. Deplete your body of vitamin A, biotin or any of the other B vitamins, vitamin E, or zinc, and it won't be long before a skin rash appears.

"Vitamin deficiency is an extremely rare occurrence in the United States, and the vast majority of dermatoses have no relationship to vitamins," says Dr. Schleicher. "A rare genetic disease (acrodermatitis enteropathica) is associated with decreased zinc absorption and dermatitis. Deficiency of vitamin C leads to scurvy characterized by skin bruising and fragility. And pellagra is the disorder caused by a deficiency of niacin (vitamin B_3) and is also characterized by a rash."

Zero In on Zinc

Perhaps the best-understood deficiency-dermatitis connection is the link to zinc. Imagine your roof without shingles to protect against the elements, and you get a picture of your skin without zinc.

Take in less than the Daily Value of 15 milligrams of zinc for a few weeks, and the shingles of your skin—your top layer of skin cells—begin to dissolve. Without this protective layer, your skin becomes rough and crusted, opening up opportunities for bacteria, yeast, and other infections to take hold. "Zinc is critically important in skin function," says Thomas Helm, MD, clinical associate professor of dermatology and pathology at the University at Buffalo in New York and director of the Buffalo Medical Group Dermatopathology Laboratory. "This is because zinc-based enzymes and proteins are important for skin renewal and allowing for normal barrier functions. When you have a zinc deficiency, it manifests itself as dermatitis, or inflammation of the skin."

As a result, zinc deficiency can cause dermatitis around the mouth and rectum of young children. Such deficiencies aren't exactly common, but they

Food Factors

It's rare that a food will cause a case of dermatitis, but experts say certain foods are more likely than others to do so. Here are the most common culprits.

Consider your moo. A great source of protein for young bodies, milk can occasionally worsen atopic dermatitis in allergic children, says Jon Hanifin, MD, professor of dermatology at Oregon Health & Science University in Portland. "This allergy to milk and dairy products seems to subside as the individuals grow older," he says.

If you suspect that an allergy is the culprit behind your dermatitis and you want to try eliminating milk and dairy products from your diet, you have to learn to read food labels carefully. Milk can appear as an ingredient where you least expect it, says Dr. Hanifin.

Go easy on the eggs. During a Japanese study of 27 people with dermatitis, researchers found that 11 had outbreaks within 2 hours of eating eggs. If you think eggs are causing your dermatitis or eczema, avoid them, and when your skin is clear, test yourself by eating eggs again. If your dermatitis returns, then it would be a good idea to avoid eggs, says Dr. Hanifin.

Say good-bye to wheat. For an unfortunate few, an ingredient in wheat called gluten is enough to give them itchy red rashes on the arms, the legs, and sometimes the scalp. But in this case at least, knowing the source of the problem is only part of the solution. "They have their work cut out for them. It's very hard to avoid wheat products," says Stephen Schleicher, MD, clinical instructor of dermatology at King's College and

occur more frequently than other nutrient-related skin problems, says Jon Hanifin, MD, professor of dermatology at Oregon Health & Science University in Portland.

Other people who are most susceptible to this kind of dermatitis are those with irritable bowel syndrome (a distressing digestive disorder), those undergoing chemotherapy, alcohol-dependent people, and some moms-to-be. "In all of these cases, their zinc levels may actually go below the normal range even if they are eating enough zinc," says Dr. Helm. "It's just not being absorbed properly."

Fortunately, alleviating problems caused by a zinc deficiency is as simple as adding more zinc to your diet; you should aim for the Daily Value of 15 milligrams. Even when there is a problem with zinc absorption, zinc deficiency can usually be overcome by increasing dietary zinc, Dr. Helm says.

Arcadia University in Pennsylvania and director of the DERMDx Centers for Dermatology. Fortunately, more and more companies are making gluten-free products for people who are sensitive to wheat, he says. (Gluten is also found in rye, barley, and oats, but in much smaller amounts.)

Shy away from shellfish. Shrimp and squid provoke dermatitis in some people that's bad enough to scare Davy Jones back to his locker. Don't be surprised if lobster, clams, mussels, and other shellfish also bring on the itch, experts say. These often contain the same dermatitis-causing chemicals.

Search out soy. This inexpensive protein source, which pops up in all kinds of prepared foods, is another trigger for atopic dermatitis in some people, says Dr. Hanifin.

Note those nuts. Peanuts round out the list of foods that most often cause dermatitis or eczema, says Dr. Hanifin.

Go fishing for fish oil. According to the most current research, people with eczema seem to have low levels of omega-3 fatty acids, and several studies have shown that getting more omega-3s in the form of fish oil capsules led to a reduction in the severity of eczema inflammation and other symptoms. Try to get more omega-3 fatty acids from food sources like salmon, sardines, and herring, or take 2 to 4 grams of fish oil capsules daily. Make sure the capsules you purchase contain both eicosapentaenoic acid (EPA) and docosahexaenoic acid (DHA).

"Foods high in zinc are also foods high in protein, such as beef and pork," says Dr. Schleicher. "Peanuts are also a good source, but, interestingly, the zinc found in most plants is poorly absorbed." As far as supplementation goes, "this is only required in rare circumstances," says Dr. Schleicher. "It should also be noted that zinc supplements can cause abdominal pain and diarrhea and may interfere with copper absorption."

Give Vitamin E a Go

You probably won't find a scientific study to confirm it, but clinical reports seem to show vitamin E's effectiveness against some kinds of dermatitis.

One such case, published in the British medical journal *Lancet*, described

Prescriptions for Healing

Finding out what is irritating your skin and avoiding it are, of course, the keys to dealing with dermatitis. There are also a few nutrients that can help some people. Here's what some doctors recommend.

Nutrient	Daily Amount
Vitamin C	60 milligrams
Vitamin E	400 IU
Zinc	15 milligrams

MEDICAL ALERT: *If you are taking anticoagulant drugs, you should not take vitamin E supplements. (Though generally a dose of up to 1,500 IU of vitamin E a day is considered safe, some recent reports suggest that taking more than 400 IU a day could be harmful to people with cardiovascular or circulatory disease or with cancer. If you have such a condition, be sure to consult your doctor before you begin supplementation.)*

an otherwise healthy 38-year-old man who suffered from dermatitis on his hands for 4 years. Under the supervision of his doctor, he tried all kinds of approaches to get rid of it, including changing soaps, watchbands, and the wrap on his steering wheel, as well as wearing gloves to the gym and taking a multivitamin/mineral supplement. Then he began taking 400 IU of vitamin E a day. Nine days after he started the supplement, the man's dermatitis cleared.

Despite this evidence, Dr. Schleicher recommends a bit of caution when it comes to vitamin E. "Although vitamin E has been recommended for many skin conditions, controlled studies that document benefit have not been performed," he says. "Vitamin E supplementation is in general safe, but megadoses have been linked to coagulation abnormalities and possibly to increased risk of death." Because of this, experts recommend not exceeding 400 IU of vitamin E daily.

Vitamin C Might Help

Most dermatologists don't suggest vitamin C for dermatitis, but there are reasons that it might work, says Dr. Helm. For one thing, doctors are just learning that vitamin C seems to protect the skin from sun damage. Vitamin C speeds wound healing and prevents ultraviolet-induced free radical damage to the skin. Studies show decreased photoaging and susceptibility to sunburn in animals given vitamin C supplementation, Dr. Helm reports. "It's not unreasonable to suspect that vitamin C can help the skin stay healthy when exposed to harmful stresses other than ultraviolet light," he says.

Dr. Schleicher, however, doesn't recommend going overboard when it comes to your vitamin C intake. "Vitamin C is necessary for normal skin," he says. "But this does not mean that excess vitamin C will produce an added beneficial effect."

DIABETES

HELPING THE BODY
HANDLE SUGAR

When she finally went to the doctor, 3 months after she first noticed her symptoms, Allene Harris of Valley Mills, Texas, was surprised to learn she has diabetes. It doesn't run in her family.

"I just didn't feel right," she recalls. "I was very tired, and I thought it was because of the stress I'd gone through when my mother died. But I was happy to hear it could be controlled by diet. My doctor said that as long as I was willing to make some changes, I probably wouldn't need to take insulin."

Her diet—a careful balance of carbohydrates, protein, and fat that's heavy on fiber and light on saturated fat and sugar, with just enough calories to maintain her weight—perked her up as fast as it dropped her blood sugar. She was feeling better in a matter of days.

"I knew this was something that wouldn't get better on its own, so I found out as much as I could about taking care of it and started doing it," she says. Much of her nutrition information comes from a diabetes support group that includes a nutritionist.

This sort of take-charge approach can make the difference between living a long, healthy life despite diabetes and suffering the potential consequences: heart disease, blindness, nerve and kidney damage, and poor circulation in the hands and feet.

"There's absolutely no doubt that diet is the cornerstone of diabetes care," says Mary Dan Eades, MD, author of *Protein Power* and *The Protein Power Lifeplan*. "The change in a person's condition as a result of proper nutritional guidance can be dramatic."

Double Trouble with Sugar

Most of us know that people with diabetes have problems with too much sugar in their bodies. But there's a bit more to be aware of in understanding this complex disease. For one thing, diabetes comes in two different forms.

Type 1 diabetes, formerly called juvenile diabetes, results from a lack of insulin, the hormone that allows cells to take up glucose circulating in the bloodstream. Glucose is the simple sugar that the body uses for fuel. Type 1 diabetes is also called insulin-dependent diabetes mellitus. (*Mellitus* means "honeyed" in Latin.) The lack of insulin comes about because of damage to insulin-secreting cells in the pancreas. The damage may be caused by a virus or by an autoimmune reaction, in which the body's immune system attacks cells in the body.

Type 2 diabetes, or non-insulin-dependent diabetes mellitus (formerly called adult-onset diabetes), results because sugar can't get inside cells, a condition called insulin resistance. Most people with type 2 diabetes have plenty of insulin, at least in the beginning stages of the condition. But receptor sites, or portals, on the membranes of the cells don't work properly to allow sugar inside. Exactly why that happens nobody knows, but research indicates that the defect in the receptors probably occurs from damage brought about by chronic exposure to high levels of insulin.

In both types, the end result is too much sugar in the blood. "Excess sugar causes tremendous oxidative stress in the body, which leads to all sorts of problems," explains Joe Vinson, PhD, professor of chemistry and nutrition at the University of Scranton in Pennsylvania. That simply means sugar molecules react with oxygen to form unstable molecules called free radicals, which cause havoc by stealing electrons from your body's healthy molecules to balance themselves.

This electron pilfering damages cells and sets the stage for heart disease as well as for kidney, eye, and nerve damage. "Oxidative damage is thought to be associated with all of the complications of diabetes," Dr. Vinson says.

Excess sugar also sticks to proteins, causing their structural and functional properties to be significantly changed. "This is another major cause of diabetes complications," Dr. Vinson explains. "It's one reason people with diabetes often have a hard time healing from wounds or surgery. They have trouble making quality collagen, the connective tissue that is the major structural protein in the body."

Diabetes as Epidemic

Our basic understanding of diabetes, how it affects the body, and how important diet is in managing the condition has remained largely unchanged for several years now. What's discouraging is that despite our understanding of the disease, diabetes levels have skyrocketed recently. According to the American Diabetes Association, over 20 million Americans have the disease. And 90 to 95 percent of those have type 2, a fact that's directly related to the rise in obesity in the United States.

"While our knowledge about diabetes is about the same, the urgency surrounding the disease has grown," says David L. Katz, MD, MPH, director of the Yale-Griffin Prevention Research Center in Derby, Connecticut, and author of *The Way to Eat*. "It's one of the major health scourges facing America today."

Luckily, the news about diabetes isn't all bad. The newest studies have proven just how powerful diet can be in controlling the condition and keeping it under control. One major study, the Diabetes Prevention Program, directly compared the effects of diet, exercise, and behavior modification to medication in over 3,200 people at high risk of developing type 2 diabetes.

The Diabetes Prevention Program divided its participants into three groups: those that would undergo significant training in diet, exercise, and behavior modification, with the goal being to lose 7 percent of their body weight and keep it off; those that took the drug metformin to control symptoms; and those that took a placebo.

"The results were substantial," says Dr. Katz. "The group who took the drugs reduced their risk of developing type 2 diabetes by 31 percent. But the group that made lifestyle changes reduced their risk by 58 percent."

Food Factors

Diet is considered the cornerstone of treatment when it comes to diabetes. But don't count on your doctor to fill you in on all the details. Several experts recommend that, in addition to your doctor, you should also be working with a dietitian to fill out your diabetes "prescription." Here are some of the highlights you should keep in mind.

Check the glycemic index. As explained on page 218, the glycemic index is changing how we look at foods when it comes to diabetes. In the simplest of terms, the index rates foods with carbohydrate content on a scale of 0 to 100, based on how much and how rapidly they raise blood sugar levels. Foods at the high end of the scale (55 to 100) raise blood sugar fairly quickly and can pose problems for those with diabetes. By contrast, foods at the low end of the scale are digested and absorbed into the bloodstream slowly. This not only improves blood glucose and lipid levels, but it can help with weight loss by delaying and reducing hunger.

Recently, another number, the glycemic load, has provided a clearer picture of the overall quality of the carbohydrates in food. But while it's useful in scientific research, most experts advise not getting bogged down in the differences between the glycemic index and the glycemic load. And at www.glycemicindex.com, they have a database where you can easily look at both numbers side by side.

For the most part, the glycemic index aligns itself with what most doctors recommend as a healthy diet. Most whole grains, nuts, fruits, vegetables, beans, legumes, and other sources of fiber are low on the glycemic index. By contrast, high-sugar foods and drinks, sweets, white bread, and other refined sources of carbohydrates are quite high. Some foods, such as meats, aren't ranked by the glycemic index. That's because a food that doesn't have carbohydrates is not ranked by the scale.

Count down calories. If you're overweight and diabetic, the best thing you can possibly do is drop some pounds. "In diabetics, the greatest improvements were related to a seven percent weight loss in studies," says David L. Katz, MD, MPH, director of the Yale-Griffin Prevention Research Center in Derby, Connecticut, and author of *The Way to Eat*. "This has been proven to be iron-clad advice."

If your blood sugar is high, it will drop within a day or two of starting a reduced-calorie diet. (So if you're using insulin, your doctor will need to adjust your dose downward.) In fact, in the days before insulin was available, people were sometimes treated with low-calorie, low-carbohydrate diets or intermittent fasting, after doctors observed that their diabetes patients did better during times of relative famine.

Fill up on fiber. In addition to losing weight, Dr. Katz says that increasing your intake of soluble fiber may be the best way to fight diabetes. Most experts recommend that people with diabetes double their fiber intakes to 30 grams a day, or even more.

Fiber is helpful for a number of reasons. It reduces cholesterol and triglyceride levels in the blood. It also may help the body use insulin more efficiently. In studies, it has been shown to be as effective as some medicines in lowering blood sugar. And it makes you feel fuller longer, preventing you from overeating.

"I try to get patients to add fiber to every meal, such as oatmeal or an oat-based cereal for breakfast, and beans and lentils along with lunch and dinner," says Dr. Katz. Other good sources of fiber are whole grains, beans, fruits, and vegetables. Top fiber sources are dried pears (11.5 grams in five halves), corn bran (7.9 grams in 2 tablespoons), blackberries (7.2 grams in 1 cup), and chickpeas (7 grams in a half-cup).

Pick the right fats. Choosing monounsaturated fats over saturated fats whenever possible is one key to reducing diabetes symptoms, says Fred Pescatore, MD, a traditionally trained physician practicing nutritional medicine and author of numerous books, including, most recently, *The Hamptons Diet.* "Fat causes slower blood sugar release, feelings of satiety, and, therefore, better blood sugar control," he says. "Clearly, all fats are not created equal, so people should learn to decrease the amount of saturated fats in their diet and increase the amount of monounsaturated fats. Eating more avocadoes, olives, and macadamia nuts could easily accomplish that and maintain better glycemic control."

In addition, Dr. Katz adds that the omega-3 fatty acids found in fish like salmon, sardines, and mackerel also seem to play a role in helping people with diabetes. And their healthy effects on heart health are well documented. If you can't eat enough fish, take 3 grams of a fish oil supplement daily in divided doses with meals.

Go extra-easy on the hard stuff. People with diabetes used to be told not to drink at all, period. After all, alcohol is empty calories that most folks with this disease don't need.

But since there is no convincing evidence to show that moderate drinking causes significantly higher blood sugar, and since many people with diabetes are at least occasional social drinkers, the American Diabetes Association offers these guidelines.

- Don't drink more than two drinks two times a week. One drink equals 1½ ounces of distilled spirits, 4 ounces of dry wine, 2 ounces of dry sherry, or 12 ounces of beer.

- Drink only when you're also eating food.

- Avoid sugared drinks such as liqueurs, sweet wines, and sweet mixes.

- Sip slowly. Make your drink last a long time.

A Word on the Glycemic Index

One tool that has helped those with diabetes make more intelligent food choices in recent years is the glycemic index. In essence, the glycemic index ranks foods by the impact they have on your blood glucose (or blood sugar) levels. So the foods that create the smallest changes in blood sugar levels are some of the smartest choices for keeping your diabetes symptoms under control.

Dr. Katz explains that the system has become more sophisticated in recent years with the addition of the concept of glycemic load. "When the glycemic index first came out, some foods high in natural sugars like carrots were almost as bad as ice cream," he says. "But the glycemic load looks beyond just sugar content to the distribution of sugars within the foods. When you look at foods by their glycemic load, it gives you a better picture of how healthy they are."

For more information on eating with the glycemic index and glycemic load, see "Food Factors" on page 216. You can also search a thorough database of foods by their glycemic index and glycemic load at www.glycemicindex.com. Also, see the tips below to learn how individual nutrients play a role.

Chromium Helps Insulin Work Better

Chromium is a trace mineral. The very same mineral used to put a shine on car bumpers, it is a key player in the body's use of sugar. It hooks up with insulin to help escort sugar through the cell membrane and into the cell. Deficiencies of chromium make cells resistant to insulin and lead to high blood sugar levels.

In one study, people with diabetes who took 200 micrograms of chromium or 9 grams of high-chromium brewer's yeast a day had lower blood levels of sugar, insulin, triglycerides, and total cholesterol and higher levels of heart-healthy HDL cholesterol than they did before they started taking chromium.

"Chromium is vital in diabetics, as it has been shown to help control blood sugar," says Fred Pescatore, MD, a traditionally trained physician practicing nutritional medicine and author of numerous books, including, most recently, *The Hamptons Diet*. And lowering blood sugar may not be the only way chromium helps with diabetes. "Deficiency of chromium not only worsens sugar metabolism but also may contribute to development of the numbness, pain, and tingling in your feet, legs, and hands that diabetes causes," Dr. Eades says.

Additionally, "there is some evidence that chromium also acts as an appetite suppressant," says Dr. Katz. "Since weight loss is so important in controlling diabetes, this is a secondary way that the supplement can help."

It should be known that chromium only improves glucose tolerance, which is the body's ability to maintain normal levels of blood sugar after eating, in people who are low in this trace mineral. But plenty of people fit that category: Most people get only 25 to 30 micrograms a day, which is much less than the Daily Value of 120 micrograms. You'd need to eat at least 3,000 calories a day to get 50 micrograms of chromium and 7,200 calories a day to get 120 micrograms.

"It's impossible to get enough from foods, as our soil has been depleted of chromium," says Dr. Pescatore. "The only other place to find it in a food source is brewer's yeast, which most people will not eat."

Dr. Pescatore recommends chromium picolinate supplementation, which is the variety cited in most studies, at a level of 200 micrograms, three times per day.

If you have diabetes and you want to try chromium supplementation, you should do so only under your doctor's supervision. He or she may need to adjust your insulin dosage as your blood sugar level drops.

A Question Mark for Vitamin E

In years past, vitamin E supplementation at levels ranging from 100 to 400 IU was often recommended for diabetes patients. Part of the reason was the strong evidence that vitamin E seemed to prevent heart disease (for more on this, see Heart Disease on page 290).

Beyond that, vitamin E appeared to offer specific help for those who are diabetic. In the early 1990s, studies conducted by Sushil Jain, PhD, professor of pediatrics, physiology, and biochemistry in the department of pediatrics at Louisiana State University Health Sciences Center in Shreveport showed that people with diabetes who took 100 IU of vitamin E daily had 25 to 30 percent lower blood levels of harmful triglycerides. Vitamin E also reduced the tendency for sugar to stick to proteins in the blood, Dr. Jain says.

Though the initial study results looked promising, recent research has cast doubt on the effectiveness of vitamin E. Once vitamin E was isolated from other potentially heart-healthy factors in randomized clinical trials, it didn't fare any better than a placebo at reducing the risk of heart disease associated with diabetes. One strong example of this was the Heart Outcomes Prevention Evaluation (HOPE), which determined that vitamin E had no more impact on the risk of heart disease than a placebo in more than 10,000 patients.

Other recent evidence has called even the safety of vitamin E supplementation into question. In 2004, researchers from the American Heart

Prescriptions for Healing

Doctors agree that good nutrition is important for people with diabetes. What they consider good nutrition varies, however. Doctors who do recommend nutritional supplements suggest these amounts.

Nutrient	Daily Amount
B-complex	100 milligrams
Biotin	15,000 micrograms
Chromium	200 micrograms of chromium picolinate, three times daily
Magnesium	500 milligrams
Vitamin E	100–400 IU

Plus a multivitamin/mineral supplement containing the Daily Values of all essential vitamins and minerals

MEDICAL ALERT: It's best to work with a doctor knowledgeable in nutrition when you're adding nutritional supplements to your diabetes treatment program. Your blood sugar and drug dosage need to be carefully monitored.

If you have diabetes and you want to try chromium supplementation, you should do so only under your doctor's supervision. He or she may need to adjust your insulin dosage as your blood sugar level drops.

People who have heart or kidney problems should talk to their doctor before beginning magnesium supplementation.

If you are taking anticoagulants, you should not take vitamin E supplements. (Though generally a dose of up to 1,500 IU of vitamin E a day is considered safe, some recent reports suggest that taking more than 400 IU a day could be harmful to people with cardiovascular or circulatory disease or with cancer. If you have such a condition, be sure to consult your doctor before you begin supplementation.)

Association analyzed the results of 14 studies of vitamin E from 1993 to 2004. Their conclusion was that those who take more than 400 IU of vitamin E a day have a slightly greater risk of death than those who don't take it.

This one-two punch against vitamin E's effectiveness and safety has led many health professionals to withdraw their vitamin E recommendation for diabetes. The experts we spoke with agreed: "After you take a look at all the recent data surrounding vitamin E, the story doesn't look good," says Howard N. Hodis, MD, director of the atherosclerosis research unit at the University of Southern California School of Medicine in Los Angeles. "In fact, if vitamin E were a drug, the FDA would have halted its production by now."

For this reason, it's best to get the Daily Value of vitamin E (30 IU) through foods such as nuts, seeds, oils, and whole grains, or from a daily multivitamin.

Magnesium Offers Secondary Benefits

Magnesium supplementation has traditionally been recommended for its blood pressure-lowering benefits. Since lowering blood pressure helps ease diabetes symptoms—and both lowering blood pressure and easing diabetes symptoms help prevent heart disease—magnesium is helpful by association.

"Magnesium helps in preventing nerve damage and in keeping the heart healthy," says Dr. Pescatore. "The heart needs magnesium in order to function properly."

And magnesium has another connection with diabetes as well, says Dr. Eades. People with diabetes, especially those taking insulin or those whose blood sugar is not well controlled, tend to come up short on magnesium, studies show. One in four may have the kind of marginal deficiency that often goes undetected, even when they seem to be eating a healthy diet, because it's quite difficult to get magnesium in food. "People with diabetes tend to lose magnesium through their urine," Dr. Eades explains.

"If they can tolerate the dose, I have people take 600 to 1,000 milligrams of magnesium a day for four weeks to assess their responses," Dr. Eades says. But she cautions against taking these amounts unless you discuss it with your doctor first. This is especially important if you have heart or kidney problems. During this therapy, most people experience some improvement in blood sugar and blood pressure and have less fatigue. After 4 weeks, Dr. Eades reduces the dose to 500 milligrams a day (100 milligrams more than the Daily Value).

Dr. Eades adds that she will sometimes add 1,000 milligrams of calcium supplementation to this recommendation, but only for people who aren't getting enough calcium through their diet. "If people regularly consume dairy products, such as cheese and yogurt, then they shouldn't need calcium supplementation," she says.

Foods rich in magnesium include whole grains, almonds, cashews, spinach, beans, and halibut.

B-Complex May Help Nerves

It's old news that the B-complex vitamins—niacin, thiamin, folic acid, vitamin B_6, and others—are essential for your body to convert sugar and starches to energy. These vitamins are involved in many of the chemical reactions necessary for this process, which is known as carbohydrate metabolism.

A shortage of any one of the B-complex vitamins can cause problems. Vitamin B_6 deficiency, for instance, has been linked to something called glucose intolerance, which is an abnormally high rise in blood sugar after eating. This deficiency has also been linked to impaired secretion of insulin and glucagon. Both of these hormones are essential in regulating blood sugar levels.

Shortages of B vitamins can also lead to nerve damage in the hands and feet. Some studies indicate that people with diabetes experience less of the numbness and tingling of diabetes-caused nerve damage if they get supplemental amounts of B vitamins such as B_6 and B_{12}.

"One of the biggest problems in diabetes is the nerve damage that can occur," says Dr. Pescatore. "And the B vitamins seem to play a critical role in keeping the nerve endings healthy."

The whole family of B vitamins seems to play a role in diabetes health, so your best bet for a supplement might be a B-complex vitamin. "In general, my recommendation is 100 milligrams of a B-complex vitamin daily," Dr. Eades says. "Then I'll determine whether someone may need bigger doses of particular B vitamins, such as thiamin, B_6, and B_{12}, if there are symptoms of diabetic nerve damage."

In such cases, she may prescribe up to several hundred milligrams a day, or injections in the case of vitamin B_{12}, until symptoms wane, then cut back.

For vitamin B_{12}, she prescribes injections of 300 to 500 micrograms weekly until symptoms respond, then monthly doses of 500 micrograms indefinitely. (If you can't get B_{12} injections, she suggests 500 to 1,000 micrograms taken under the tongue. These supplements are available over the counter.)

Check with your doctor before taking an amount above the Daily Value of any B vitamin, since high dosages may lead to side effects. Doses of 200 milligrams or more of vitamin B_6 a day, for example, have caused nerve damage.

Some people may also benefit from taking biotin, another B vitamin, in amounts of up to 15 milligrams (15,000 micrograms) a day, Dr. Eades adds. A study by Japanese researchers found that this vitamin helps cells in muscle tissue use sugar more effectively.

Covering All the Bases

In addition to these particular vitamins, doctors may also recommend that people with diabetes take a multivitamin/mineral supplement that contains the Daily Value of every essential nutrient. That might not be such a bad idea. Research suggests that a multitude of nutrients—zinc, copper, manganese, selenium, calcium, vitamin D, and vitamin A—may be in short supply in people with diabetes.

DIARRHEA

FOODS THAT CAN STOP THE FLOW

Diarrhea is one of those unfortunate conditions that we all have to live with. Since the average American has a run-in with the runs at least four times a year, that means even the most intestinally fortitudinous of us probably can't escape its slippery grasp at one time or another.

And as distressing as diarrhea can be, what's even more distressing is that you may never know what's really causing the condition in the first place. Sure, it could be those 3-day-old leftovers you forced down last night, but it could also be an allergy, a virus or bacteria, medication, an intestinal disease, or something else.

"There are a million and one causes of diarrhea," says Joel B. Mason, MD, associate professor of medicine and nutrition at Tufts University in Boston. But fortunately, most short-term cases of diarrhea—those lasting for a day or two or three—will not deplete your body's nutritional reserves enough to harm you.

Food Factors

Acute diarrhea may last for only a couple of days, but it can make you feel as weak and vulnerable as a kitten. Here are a few tips to get you back on your paws and in roaring good health.

Listen to your body. Diarrhea should begin to slow 24 hours after you start sipping liquids, says William B. Ruderman, MD, practicing physician at Gastroenterology Associates of Central Florida in Orlando. When it does, start paying attention to what your body is telling you. When your body says . . . well, maybe it's a little hungry, that's the time to reintroduce food.

Go for the bland. In addition to the B.R.A.T. diet (see opposite page), the first foods you should reach for are bland complex carbohydrates such as noodles, white bread, and applesauce, says Dr. Ruderman. Start with one-fourth of what would be a normal serving for you, then see how it goes down. If your abdomen feels comfortable and diarrhea does not resume, then increase the amount of food at your next meal.

Go easy on yourself. Gradually increase food until you're back to full portions, says Dr. Ruderman. If your abdomen feels uncomfortable at any point or if diarrhea resumes, go back to the previous levels. Reintroduce your normal diet after you're able to consume normal kinds of foods such as whole grains, says Dr. Ruderman.

Try some garlic. If you're certain that your diarrhea is the result of a bacterial infection, then a bit of garlic can help fight it. To fight bacteria with garlic, just crush a clove of raw garlic and take it two to three times a day. Mixing it with a bit of applesauce or yogurt will help it go down more easily.

"Acute infectious diarrhea, what people call gastrointestinal flu, is usually related to a viral or bacterial infection," says Dr. Mason. "It is self-limiting and usually runs its course in several days to a week. The only immediate danger to an otherwise healthy person is the loss of fluid and electrolytes, including salt, magnesium, potassium, and calcium."

When to Seek Help

Diarrhea often goes hand in hand with other symptoms such as nausea, bloating, stomach cramps, abdominal pain, and sometimes fever. Most of the time, you don't need to seek the care of a doctor when you have diarrhea, but you do want to watch out in a few specific instances.

"It's not of great concern if you can't absorb this or that nutrient for a few days," says Dr. Mason. But there are two prominent exceptions: the very young and the very old. Both groups—preschoolers, for example, and those over age 70—tend to feel the effects of electrolyte and fluid loss very quickly.

"Remember that between 500 and 1,000 children in the United States still die of acute diarrhea every year," adds Dr. Mason. "And that's largely because small children, preschool children, are very susceptible to dehydration."

"Whenever diarrhea lasts more than six to eight hours in the very young or the very old or more than twelve hours in healthy adults, you should add fluids and electrolytes to the diet," says William B. Ruderman, MD, practicing physician at Gastroenterology Associates of Central Florida in Orlando. The same goes for anyone who develops signs of dehydration, such as dry mouth, sunken eyes, dry skin, decreased urination, and skin that tents when pinched.

"When these symptoms occur, you can assume that levels of electrolytes and fluid need to be supplemented," says Dr. Ruderman.

Fortunately, electrolytes are easily replaced. "Sodium and potassium losses are the most important, so you want to get sodium, potassium, fluids, and a simple sugar in first," says Dr. Ruderman. "The sugar helps your body absorb the fluids and nutrients. The easiest way to get these in our busy lives is to go to the store and buy one of those sports drinks, such as Gatorade."

"If there's nausea or vomiting with the diarrhea, wait until it clears," says Dr. Ruderman. "Then begin rehydration. Start with a small amount: four ounces every hour for as long as the diarrhea lasts." That should combat the nutritional effects of most short-term cases of diarrhea, he adds.

If you don't have a taste for sports drinks, another approach is to simply boil vegetables like celery, carrots, and spinach or broccoli in a pot of water for an hour. The broth that results will help rehydrate you while at the same time replenishing your levels of sugar, sodium, and potassium.

In addition to the rehydration process, a bland diet that excludes sugar and dairy products has a better chance of staying down as you make your recovery from diarrhea, says Gerard E. Mullin, MD, director of integrative GI nutrition services and capsule endoscopy in the division of gastroenterology and liver disease at Johns Hopkins Hospital in Baltimore "I recommend the B.R.A.T. diet," he says. "That stands for bananas, rice, apples, and toast."

Prescriptions for Healing

For most people, a bout of diarrhea is not harmful. The exceptions are preschoolers and people over age 70. As a general rule, medical experts say, diarrhea lasting more than 8 hours in the very young or the very old or more than 12 hours in an otherwise healthy adult requires replacement of fluid as well as of essential nutrients known as electrolytes. Here's what these experts recommend.

Nutrient	Daily Amount
Potassium and sodium	4-oz. sports drink, taken every hour for as long as diarrhea lasts (the idea is to sip constantly)

MEDICAL ALERT: If diarrhea lasts for more than 12 to 24 hours in an infant or an older person, you should seek medical help.

If you're an otherwise healthy adult, you should see your doctor if diarrhea persists for more than 3 days; if it is accompanied by fever or lethargy; if there is blood or pus in the stool; if any signs of dehydration continue despite efforts to replace fluid; or if the diarrhea is paired with chills, rash, vomiting, severe headache, or fainting.

If the diarrhea lasts for more than 12 to 24 hours in an infant or an older person, you should seek medical attention. And if you're an otherwise healthy adult, you should see your doctor if the diarrhea lasts for more than 3 days; if it is accompanied by fever or lethargy; if there is blood or pus in the stool; if signs of dehydration continue despite efforts to replace fluid; or if the diarrhea is paired with chills, rash, vomiting, severe headache, or fainting.

EATING DISORDERS

MENDING THE MIND-BODY CONNECTION

Lisa thought college would be the perfect opportunity to lose some weight. Typically about 5 or 10 pounds overweight, she had always felt fat and wanted to take advantage of her newfound independence to shed a few pounds.

At first she just restricted her eating: no snacks, no fat, just salads. Then she discovered that if she occasionally wavered, she could "undo the damage" by vomiting. Before long she was planning daily binges and purges that sometimes consisted of a dozen doughnuts, pizza, cookies, and candy bars. Weighing herself five or six times a day, she became so afraid of gaining weight once she hit 100 pounds that she could barely eat anything without purging.

Two years later she knew she was in trouble. "I was so weak that I would skip classes because I couldn't make it across campus. I had heart palpitations, my teeth were rotting, I couldn't stand the cold, I had terrible mood swings, I couldn't concentrate, and my hair was breaking off and falling out," she recalls. "It sounds ridiculous in retrospect, but the only thing that made me get help was having too many bad hair days."

Lisa didn't realize then that her "bad hair" was just one sign of what had become severe malnutrition. Though her body could digest some food during a binge, the high-fat foods she binged on didn't stay with her long enough to provide much nutrition.

Diseases of Depletion

Lisa suffered from a combination of related eating disorders: bulimia nervosa and anorexia nervosa. Although these disorders primarily affect females in their teens and twenties, they can also affect men, older women, and young children.

Of the two, anorexia is easier to spot. People with this disease have an intense fear of being fat, causing them to starve themselves to emaciation. In women, it also causes amenorrhea, or the cessation of the menstrual cycle. People with bulimia are generally closer to normal weight, but they are also obsessed with body size. Bulimia is characterized by frequent binge-purge episodes, which involve eating a large amount of food in a short period of time and then trying to prevent weight gain by vomiting, using laxatives, dieting, fasting, or exercising vigorously. It is common for people to have symptoms of both disorders.

Medical experts don't know exactly why some women dive headlong into this pool of self-destruction, though they generally agree that the cause includes an intricate web of social, psychological, and biological factors. Some of the newest research seems to indicate that eating disorders are, in fact,

Food Factors

Part of the recovery process for people with eating disorders is making peace with food instead of battling with it. Here are some tips that many experts believe might prove helpful.

Avoid alcohol. The newest research indicates that eating disorders are addictions and should be treated as such. So it's no surprise that eating disorders and alcohol addiction are so closely linked. According to the most recent surveys, 72 percent of alcoholic women younger than age 30 also have eating disorders. Considering the close link, abstaining from alcohol is critical in successful rehabilitation.

Don't lean on supplements. One of the primary goals of eating disorder treatment is to restore a healthy weight, so nutritional supplements should be viewed as just that—supplements, and not replacements for food.

Eat only with help. An eating disorder is a disease, and it's not one that you should try to fix on your own through your diet. The complicated road to recovery must be overseen by experts to be successful. "Get counseling from a nutritionist and a psychologist working as a team," says Cheryl L. Rock, PhD, RD, a professor of medicine at the University of California, San Diego. "Also get a full medical evaluation from a psychiatrist knowledgeable about pharmacotherapy."

addictions. "The complex topics of eating disorders and food addictions have recently become more clearly defined with the evolution of functional MRIs and PET scans," says Sam Sugar, MD, of the Pritikin Longevity Center and Spa in Aventura, Florida. "As it turns out, these disorders are closely linked to diseases like drug and alcohol addiction and may require interventions like they do."

Experts also agree that malnourishment exacerbates the condition, rendering women less receptive to treatment. "It's a vicious cycle," says Amy Tuttle, RD, LCSW, a nutrition therapist in private practice and former director of nutrition services at the Renfrew Center of Philadelphia. "Malnutrition creates a physical and emotional shutdown, and the lethargy that results makes reaching out for physical and emotional nourishment even more difficult."

But there are signs of hope in the downward spiral of an eating disorder. "Today's medications and therapy, as well as the newest treatment programs, have been showing a continuously increasing record of success in treating eating disorders," says Dr. Sugar.

Feeding Your Brain and Your Body

One of the major problems with an eating disorder is that experts have a difficult time even defining the condition: Is it a mental illness, or a physical one? Evidence seems to indicate that it's both.

"Eating disorders are definitely mental illnesses," says Cheryl L. Rock, PhD, RD, a professor of medicine at the University of California, San Diego. "The mind-body connection, if it suggests that the physical consequences of starvation explain much of the behavior, is true, however. People cannot respond to psychological counseling if they are starved. Achieving improved nutritional status is a crucial step necessary to enable good response to counseling."

Dr. Rock is not alone in this line of thinking. Contrary to the old practice of first putting people in therapy and then slowly reintroducing food, treatment specialists now know that re-establishing proper nutrition is critical before psychological therapy can be effective. Many use vitamin and mineral supplements to help pave the way.

Generally, the supplement of choice is a multivitamin/mineral that provides 100 percent of the Daily Values of all essential nutrients while people are relearning to eat real food. Doctors do not recommend exceeding the Daily Values; they may, however, recommend supplements of certain individual nutrients, particularly potassium, calcium, iron, zinc, vitamin A, vitamin E, and the B vitamins.

Experts do warn that supplements cannot take the place of food, however. "Vitamins contain no calories; they are not food," advises Dr. Sugar. "Other than the trace elements, they have no dietary value as such and cannot be a substitute for food."

Moreover, Dr. Rock says these supplements may be more helpful once a person has regained his or her health nutritionally. "Low-dose (100 percent Daily Value) multivitamins are not a risk," says Dr. Rock. "However, there are studies suggesting that these nutrients are better utilized in a person who is not starving."

Considering our society's obsession with thinness, it's not surprising that eating disorders have become so common, particularly among women. Surveys indicate that around 1 percent of female adolescents in the United States have anorexia, and 4 percent of college-age women have bulimia. And if left untreated, 20 percent of women with serious eating disorders die. With anorexia, that number rises to 25 percent.

But an eating disorder doesn't have to be a death sentence. With treatment, the mortality rate falls to 2 percent, and about 60 percent will make a full recovery. The key is to work with a specialist to learn how to eat normally again, and the tips that follow will help show you how.

Balancing Electrolytes

One of the consequences of eating disorders is a potentially life-threatening electrolyte imbalance. Electrolytes are minerals that, when dissolved in the body's fluid, become electrically charged. They are responsible for controlling heart rate and blood pressure.

The two major causes of this imbalance, says Dr. Rock, are purging and laxative abuse. "Purging especially causes the loss of vital nutrients and electrolytes such as sodium, potassium, calcium, and magnesium," says Dr. Sugar. "Serious heart problems, as well as metabolic and kidney problems, can ensue if they are not replaced properly."

Because too much potassium can make you ill, it is best to get the Daily Value of this mineral (3,500 milligrams) by eating fruits and vegetables such as bananas, oranges, spinach, and celery. You can get 885 milligrams just by eating half of a cantaloupe. Magnesium supplements are available in various forms, but eating seafood and green leafy vegetables can help you easily get your Daily Value of 400 milligrams.

Also, our experts warn that any supplements of these electrolytes be administered and monitored only by a physician. "These should be diagnosed and managed medically, not self-diagnosed," says Dr. Rock. "Excessive amounts of these nutrients can be just as harmful as deficiencies."

Calcium to Protect Bones

Calcium, an essential mineral in the development and maintenance of bone health, is one of the nutrients most likely to be deficient in people with eating disorders. Those who treat eating disorders say the impact of severe calcium deficiency, especially when combined with amenorrhea, can be devastating.

"We see 28-year-old women with the bones of 80-year-olds," says Tuttle. "They already have osteoporosis. It's sad, but fortunately, sometimes this serious medical issue is the alarm that helps a woman choose to move forward in her recovery." Tuttle notes that doctors often give women with eating disorders calcium supplements of 1,000 milligrams (the Daily Value) or more while also attending to the amenorrhea.

Prescriptions for Healing

Although eating food is absolutely essential to preventing the damage that eating disorders can do to the body, some doctors believe that vitamin and mineral supplements can expedite the process of recovery and healing. These are the nutrients that doctors recommend.

Nutrient	Daily Amount
Calcium	1,000 milligrams
Iron	18 milligrams
Magnesium	400 milligrams
Potassium	3,500 milligrams
Vitamin A	5,000 IU
Vitamin E	30 IU
Zinc	15 milligrams

Plus a multivitamin/mineral supplement containing the Daily Values of all essential vitamins and minerals

MEDICAL ALERT: Experts warn that supplements cannot take the place of food in someone who has an eating disorder. The body will not properly absorb and use vitamins and minerals without also receiving adequate calories. It is important to be under a doctor's care when treating this condition.

People who have heart or kidney problems should check with their doctor before taking magnesium supplements.

Potassium supplements should not be taken by those with diabetes or kidney disease or by those using certain medications, including nonsteroidal anti-inflammatory drugs, potassium-sparing diuretics, ACE inhibitors, and heart medications such as heparin.

If you are taking anticoagulant drugs, you should not take vitamin E supplements. (Though generally a dose of up to 1,500 IU of vitamin E a day is considered safe, some recent reports suggest that taking more than 400 IU a day could be harmful to people with cardiovascular or circulatory disease or with cancer. If you have such a condition, be sure to consult your doctor before you begin supplementation.)

Dr. Rock, however, is quick to point out that calcium deficiency is not the only contributing factor to bone loss. "Bone loss in anorexia is caused by many factors, and inadequate calcium intake is only a contributing or permissive factor," she says. "Replacement of calcium will not reverse the problem if the other factors, such as hormonal issues, are not addressed. This has been shown in randomized clinical trials."

Dr. Rock adds that calcium supplementation under your doctor's supervision is advisable if dietary intake is inadequate, but it's best to up your intake of calcium-rich foods. Drinking fat-free milk is a good way to increase your dietary calcium, as just 3 cups packs more than 1,000 milligrams. Other sources include broccoli, tofu, and fortified orange juice.

Breaking the Cycle with Zinc

Because zinc deficiency causes symptoms that are similar to those seen in people with anorexia and bulimia, including weight loss, depression, stomach bloating, and amenorrhea, many researchers believe that low zinc intake, which is common in people with eating disorders, helps to perpetuate the illness.

Fortunately, studies have found that zinc supplementation can help turn the tables. In fact, researchers studying 35 girls with anorexia at St. Paul's Hospital in Vancouver found that those who took just 14 milligrams of zinc a day were able to achieve their target weight gains twice as fast as those not taking zinc.

Dr. Rock says that the best approach here is to rely on a low-dose multivitamin to provide your daily supply of zinc, along with foods. "Excess zinc has been associated with adverse effects, and a specific role in recovery has not been established," she says.

A and E to the Rescue

Because vitamins A and E are fat-soluble, if you don't have fat in your body, you don't have enough of these vitamins. So in people with eating disorders, these important nutrients can be in short supply. "With prolonged malnutrition and nonreplacement of these stored vitamins, their availability becomes greatly decreased," says Dr. Sugar. "Abnormalities in numerous body organs, including the eyes and skin, can ensue."

One study, by researchers at Hebrew University of Jerusalem in Israel, found that women with anorexia had significantly lower levels of both vitamin A and vitamin E in their bodies than women without anorexia.

"We generally supplement the fat-soluble vitamins in the beginning of treatment, because these women have no fat," says Kathryn J. Zerbe, MD, professor of psychiatry and obstetrics/gynecology at Oregon Health & Science University in Portland and author of *The Body Betrayed: Women, Eating Disorders, and Treatment*. "Fortunately, you don't have to get your fat stores up too high before your body is able to store the vitamins again."

If you want to get your Daily Value of 5,000 IU of vitamin A and build your stores of this important vitamin, two of the best food sources are spinach and pumpkin. And you can get plenty of beta-carotene, which turns to vitamin A in the body, by eating carrots, sweet potatoes, and other bright orange and yellow fruits and vegetables as well as dark green leafy vegetables.

The Daily Value for vitamin E is 30 IU, and good dietary sources include whole-grain cereals, eggs, and green leafy vegetables.

Iron against Anemia

Because people with eating disorders generally shun red meat and don't eat enough to get iron elsewhere, they sometimes develop iron-deficiency anemia.

"Anemia is caused by not having the fuel to produce energy, which adds to the fatigue and general lack of interest," says Dr. Zerbe. She prefers that women get iron from foods but notes that supplementation can be helpful for reaching the Daily Value.

Though red meat is one of the best sources of iron, you can also get the Daily Value of 18 milligrams by eating clams, chickpeas, tomato juice, raisins, Cream of Wheat, tofu, and soybeans.

ENDOMETRIOSIS

LIVING WITHOUT PAIN

For most women, the cramping, swelling, bleeding, and irritability at that time of the month are bad enough as it is. But for an unfortunate 5.5 million American women, the pain of a period can become so excruciating that it almost becomes unbearable. And what's worse, this frustrating condition causes more than pain. More than 30 percent of the women who have it end up infertile, and for 25 to 50 percent of American women who have trouble getting pregnant, this condition is the reason.

This painful condition is endometriosis. It affects many women in their childbearing years, and its cause remains a mystery. But what we can do is explain what is happening in the body during endometriosis—and how nutrition can help with the painful symptoms. Read on to find out.

An Understanding of Endometriosis

In the simplest of terms, endometriosis is tissue growing where it doesn't belong. During a typical menstrual cycle, hormones cue your body to begin thickening the lining of the uterus, the endometrium, to prepare for a possible pregnancy. If pregnancy doesn't occur, this lining is shed and expelled from the body through the vagina—a phenomenon you recognize as your monthly period.

But in endometriosis, endometrial tissues wander outside their typical domain of the uterus. Instead, they begin building up in the fallopian tubes, ovaries, and the tissue lining your pelvis. (Some cases of endometriosis exhibit tissue extending even beyond the pelvic region, but these are extremely rare.)

These foreign tissues act just like their cousins in the uterus: Every month, they build up, and then break down prior to menstruation. The problem is that the tissues in other parts of the body have nowhere to go. Trapped within the body, they continue to accumulate and agitate the surrounding tissue, hence the source of the pain. Eventually, they form cysts and then scar tissue that can damage reproductive organs and cause fertility problems.

Help through Nutrition

Endometriosis can be quite frustrating for the young women who suffer from it. But there is hope. Pain medication can help control the monthly pain of the condition, and hormone therapy can force the cysts into remission. Hormones can also be controlled through nutrition, which is why diet and supplements can also play a role.

"We've found that adopting a healthy lifestyle goes a long way in preventing and relieving the symptoms of endometriosis," says Susan M. Lark, MD, a physician specializing in women's health; editor of *Women's Wellness Today*;

president of DrLark.com in Forrester Center, West Virginia; and author of *Fibroid Tumors and Endometriosis*. As part of her practice, Dr. Lark helps women with endometriosis live pain-free through a wide variety of dietary regimens and herbal and nutritional supplements.

Food Factors

The best line of dietary defense for women with endometriosis is a healthful diet full of fruits, grains, and vegetables and devoid of fatty foods, which can aggravate the disease. Here's what many experts recommend.

Stick to low-fat dairy products. One of the most common recommendations made by endometriosis experts is to eliminate or limit consumption of dairy products.

Dairy products contain saturated fat, which puts stress on the liver and increases circulating estrogen, says Susan M. Lark, MD, a physician specializing in women's health; editor of *Women's Wellness Today*; president of DrLark.com in Forrester Center, West Virginia; and author of *Fibroid Tumors and Endometriosis*. Saturated fat also produces a muscle-contracting component in the body called prostaglandin F2-alpha, which can make the cramps and inflammation of endometriosis much worse, says Dr. Lark.

Because dairy products also are a vital source of calcium, however, your best bet may be to stick to very low-fat sources, such as fat-free milk or nonfat yogurt. Or strive to get more calcium from nondairy sources like calcium-fortified cereals and orange juice.

Stick to veggies. Because meats also contain saturated fat, experts recommend getting your nutrients from whole-grain and vegetable sources whenever possible.

Go organic. When shopping for veggies, buy organic whenever you can; when you can't, scrub or peel your fruits and vegetables before eating them. Several studies show a direct correlation between exposure to dioxin, a chemical found in pesticides, and the incidence of endometriosis in laboratory animals.

Cut caffeine. Caffeine depletes the body's B vitamin stores and hampers healthy liver function, which can increase estrogen levels and worsen endometriosis symptoms. Women with endometriosis should limit coffee, black tea, chocolate, and caffeinated soft drinks, says Dr. Lark.

Banish alcohol. Since optimum liver function is essential for mopping up excess estrogen and controlling endometriosis, imbibing alcohol is a definite no-no, says Dr. Lark. Eliminating alcohol from the body stresses the liver, she explains. Dr. Lark recommends that women with endometriosis avoid alcohol entirely, if possible.

Hormone Helpers

Whether estrogen or immunity is to blame, all of your body's systems need to be operating at maximum efficiency to properly regulate your hormones, maintain your immunity, and keep endometrial implants at bay.

This is not to say that medical treatments such as estrogen-blocking hormones and surgical removal of endometrial growths aren't effective, says Dr. Lark. They are. But too often endometrial implants recur even after surgical removal.

"Nutritional plans are particularly successful for women who have recently undergone traditional treatment," says Dr. Lark. "I don't suggest that

Prescriptions for Healing

Increasingly, endometriosis specialists are discovering the power of nutritional healing. But since the necessary doses can be high and vary from woman to woman, they recommend consulting a physician before starting a vitamin and mineral regimen.

Because getting the Daily Values of all of the essential nutrients is important if you have endometriosis, doctors who use nutritional regimens recommend starting with a general multivitamin/mineral supplement and adding other supplements as needed.

Nutrient	Daily Amount
Beta-carotene	25,000–50,000 IU
Biotin	200 micrograms
Calcium	500 milligrams, 2 or 3 times daily
Iron	30 milligrams, twice daily
Folic acid	400 micrograms
Magnesium	500–800 milligrams
Niacin	50 milligrams
Pantothenic acid	50 milligrams
Riboflavin	50 milligrams
Selenium	25 micrograms

women not use medications, because hormone treatments can really help lessen endometriosis. But to prevent the pain from recurring, nutritional programs work very well."

The following are nutrients that many experts recommend for controlling endometriosis.

Note: Because the required doses are high and vary from woman to woman, be sure to consult your doctor before starting a nutritional regimen. Because getting the Daily Values of all of the essential nutrients is important if you have endometriosis, doctors who use nutritional regimens recommend starting with a general multivitamin/mineral supplement and adding additional supplements as needed.

Nutrient	Daily Amount
Thiamin	50 milligrams
Vitamin B_6	30 milligrams
Vitamin B_{12}	50 micrograms
Vitamin C	1,000–4,000 milligrams
Vitamin E	400–2,000 IU

MEDICAL ALERT: *If you have symptoms of endometriosis, you should see a doctor for proper diagnosis and treatment.*

People who have heart or kidney problems should check with their doctor before taking magnesium supplements.

Selenium in doses exceeding 400 micrograms daily should be taken only under medical supervision.

Doses of vitamin C exceeding 1,200 milligrams a day may cause diarrhea.

Before taking the amount of vitamin E recommended here, you should discuss it with your doctor. If you are taking anticoagulant drugs, you should not take vitamin E supplements. (Though generally a dose of up to 1,500 IU of vitamin E a day is considered safe, some recent reports suggest that taking more than 400 IU a day could be harmful to people with cardiovascular or circulatory disease or with cancer. If you have such a condition, be sure to consult your doctor before you begin supplementation.)

B Vitamins Lower Estrogen Levels

If you're looking for a natural way to keep your estrogen levels low and thus reduce recurrent episodes of endometriosis, try boosting your intake of B-complex vitamins.

"The liver is responsible for breaking down and disposing of excess estrogen," explains Dr. Lark. "The B vitamins are important in regulating estrogen because they promote a healthy liver. Studies dating back to the 1940s show that if you remove B vitamins from animals' food, they can no longer metabolize estrogen." Studies have also shown that B vitamin supplementation helps alleviate other symptoms of excess estrogen, such as premenstrual syndrome and fibrocystic breasts, she says.

Dr. Lark recommends that women with endometriosis take considerably more than the Daily Values of the B vitamins. She suggests approximately 50 milligrams each of thiamin, riboflavin, niacin, and pantothenic acid; 30 milligrams of vitamin B_6; 50 micrograms of vitamin B_{12}; 400 micrograms of folic acid; and 200 micrograms of biotin.

Always speak with your doctor before taking such high levels of these nutrients on your own, however. You can also fortify your diet with B vitamins by eating whole-grain cereals, pastas and rice, fish, legumes, and green leafy vegetables.

Antioxidant Onslaught

Another way to thwart the effects of endometriosis is by upping your intake of these antioxidant nutrients: vitamins C and E, beta-carotene (which converts to vitamin A in the body), and the mineral selenium. Antioxidants are best known for their ability to fight free radicals, the naturally occurring unstable molecules that cause tissue damage in the body by stealing electrons from healthy molecules to balance themselves. Doctors know that antioxidants can also build immunity, lessen cramping, and reduce excessive menstrual bleeding. All of these are useful functions in treating endometriosis.

"While you can't just pop these supplements and expect instant relief from acute pain, I've found that doses of antioxidants, along with dietary changes, can treat the chronic problem of endometriosis," says Dr. Lark.

Dr. Lark recommends a daily regimen of 1,000 to 4,000 milligrams of vitamin C; 25,000 to 50,000 IU of beta-carotene; 400 to 2,000 IU of vitamin

E; and 25 micrograms of selenium. She has arrived at these dosages during her many years of treating women's health problems.

Because these recommended doses of vitamin C and vitamin E are many times the Daily Values of these nutrients, you should check with your doctor before trying this therapy. Vitamin C can cause diarrhea when taken in doses exceeding 1,200 milligrams a day.

And just because symptoms improve, that doesn't mean you can stop taking supplements, cautions Dr. Lark.

Antioxidants can have a dramatic effect on the regulation of bleeding as well as on the reduction of pain and cramps that may accompany endometriosis, says Dr. Lark. "Vitamin C is good for controlling excessive bleeding," she explains. "Vitamin A has also been shown to lessen profuse menstrual bleeding. And vitamin E has antispasmodic effects, which help in pain management."

To get more antioxidants in your diet, start by hitting the farmers' market. Broccoli, spinach, and cantaloupe are excellent sources of vitamin C and beta-carotene; cabbage, celery, and cucumbers are great sources of selenium. For more vitamin E, try sautéing these veggies in sunflower oil or safflower oil. Or reach for a handful of almonds, another good source of vitamin E.

Minerals Offer Liver Aid

Along with the B family of vitamins and antioxidants, two minerals may play a role in endometriosis support. Calcium and magnesium help the liver metabolize hormones properly, which can promote healthy endometrial growth and menstruation.

Good food sources of calcium are low-fat dairy products, such as fat-free milk and low-fat yogurt. Some vegetables like broccoli are also good sources, as are calcium-fortified foods like cereal and orange juice. You can get more magnesium from foods such as brown rice, spinach, baked potatoes, beans, and yogurt, among others. Talk to your doctor before adding calcium or magnesium to your supplement regimen.

Add Some Iron

One side effect of endometriosis is excessive menstrual bleeding, which can lead to iron deficiency in some women. To get more iron, try to eat more soy foods, or talk to your doctor about iron supplementation.

EPILEPSY

QUIETING A
SHORT-CIRCUITED BRAIN

When one thinks of epilepsy, the first symptom that comes to mind is seizures. And while the two are undeniably linked, there's a lot more going on with this relationship than most people realize.

First of all, a seizure does not necessarily indicate epilepsy. Many children have nonepileptic seizures, usually associated with a high fever. Overall, 1 in 10 people will likely experience a seizure at some point.

When the seizure recurs once or more, however, that's when a diagnosis of epilepsy is likely. And the source of the problem is somewhere between your ears.

Like all nerve tissue, our brains rely on electrical impulses to receive and send messages. Electrical currents that enter our brains through the spinal cord or optic nerves allow us to process billions of pieces of information and react to our environment, scratching an itch here, swerving to avoid a confused groundhog there, or adding a comma here . . . or is it there?

Normally, electrical currents move through the brain in an orderly and limited fashion. In epilepsy, however, the currents get short-circuited or out of sync for a variety of reasons. The result is a burst of electrical activity that causes a seizure, which can be anything from a staring spell, called an absence seizure, to a full-fledged grand mal, complete with jerking arms and legs and loss of consciousness.

One interesting thing about epilepsy is that it typically occurs in the very young or the very old. A deeper look into the causes of epilepsy helps explain just why this is. In the old, the likely cause is stroke or other conditions that restrict bloodflow to the brain. This in turn can cause a small scar in the brain, which is often the source of the "short circuit."

In the young, epilepsy can sometimes be traced back to head trauma from an accident in early childhood. But with frustrating frequency, the cause is unknown. Recent research does suggest a genetic disposition to epilepsy, however. So if you have it, your children could be at an increased risk.

Nutrients Can Play a Role

Nutrition can have a hand in causing, and controlling, epilepsy in a couple of ways. Recent research has shown the importance of a diet high in antioxidants for protecting the body against heart disease, cancer, and numerous other common conditions. But lost in the headlines is the fact that antioxidants also play a crucial role in controlling epilepsy.

"Epilepsy is a form of oxidative stress—that is, damage to the brain cells can occur through aggressive chemical species derived from oxygen," says Georg F. Weber, MD, PhD, an associate professor and researcher at the University of Cincinnati College of Pharmacy. "A strong antioxidant defense, built through proper nutrition, can help protect [against] epilepsy-induced brain damage."

Nutrition's second role in epilepsy is tied to the genetic link mentioned earlier. Part of this genetic link stems from metabolic diseases, inherited disorders that result in an inability to properly utilize a particular nutrient in the body, such as a vitamin or an amino acid. "Seizures associated with metabolic disorders usually begin soon after birth and rarely start after age six," says Robert J. Gumnit, MD, president of MINCEP Epilepsy Care in Minneapolis.

In about half of these cases, the metabolic disorder can be figured out. "A specialist, a pediatric neurologist, may consider 20 to 80 different metabolic disorders that are most commonly associated with seizures," Dr. Gumnit says. Sometimes seizures can be controlled by a diet that restricts certain foods. Children with a condition called phenylketonuria, for instance, need to avoid the amino acid phenylalanine, found in large amounts in aspartame (a sugar substitute).

Adding more of a nutrient may help others. Children who develop seizures because their bodies have a hard time using vitamin B_6, for instance, may take 25 to 50 milligrams of B_6 each day, an amount large enough to overcome metabolic roadblocks.

If you think your child has seizures because of a metabolic disorder, see a specialist for a diagnosis, Dr. Gumnit urges. Don't try to treat a metabolic disorder on your own.

Seizures can also be caused by nutritional deficiency. "Most doctors, however, think that nutritional deficiency is only rarely the cause of repeated seizures," Dr. Gumnit says.

Shortages of magnesium, thiamin, vitamin B_6, and zinc have been reported to be associated with seizures in some individuals. These nutrients, among numerous others, are needed for normal chemical reactions in the brain.

Nutritional support for people with seizure disorders, then, involves correcting metabolic problems and nutritional deficiencies. In some cases, it may

Food Factors

Most cases of epilepsy are not treated with dietary changes, but some are. Here are a few things that might prove helpful.

Ask your doctor about a ketogenic diet. A diet virtually devoid of starches and sugars and high in fat has been used as a treatment for children whose epilepsy cannot be controlled with drugs or who have to take such high doses of drugs that side effects become intolerable.

"The diet makes the body burn fat, not sugar, for energy and produces waste products called ketones that are thought to help suppress seizures," explains John M. Freeman, MD, professor of pediatric neurology at Johns Hopkins Medical Institutions in Baltimore.

Over the last 10 years, perhaps the greatest breakthrough in epilepsy treatment has been the acceptance and success of this diet. In March 2007, Dr. Freeman and his colleagues published a comprehensive review of the use of the diet over the last decade in the scholarly journal *Pediatrics*. Among its findings were that 30 percent of children who try the diet have their seizures completely controlled; another 40 percent have enough benefit to warrant staying on the diet. Some are able to reduce medication, some have fewer seizures, and some function better.

In addition, the ketogenic diet has caught on worldwide, and there are now 75 centers in 45 countries that offer the treatment. And most of the results seem to indicate that the diet may be even more effective than most of the newer epilepsy medications. Researchers are now looking into other promising benefits of the diet, such as its modified use in adults, and even its benefits in treating other conditions.

Most children who benefit stay on this very restrictive diet for 2 years, then gradually begin to eat more starches and sugars. Often the children eventually stop the diet and find their seizures do not recur.

Vitamin and mineral supplements are necessary during this diet, since it is low in fat-soluble vitamins and calcium. Critics say the diet is too high in fat and is unhealthy for growing children. But, says Dr. Freeman, "we've seen no evidence of heart disease or growth problems."

Avoid aspartame. The official word from the FDA's Center for Food Safety and Applied Nutrition is this: Aspartame is not likely to cause seizures. (An important exception: It will cause seizures in people with phenylketonuria, a metabolic disorder that makes it difficult to break down phenylalanine, an amino acid found in aspartame.) Nevertheless,

also involve taking larger amounts of certain nutrients to help protect against drug-related damage and, in theory at least, against damage caused by the seizures themselves.

The final piece of the nutritional puzzle when it comes to epilepsy is the

there are scattered reports of seizures associated with this food additive in apparently healthy people.

A report from Ralph G. Walton, MD, medical director of Safe Harbor Behavioral Health in Erie, Pennsylvania, describes a woman who switched from sugar to aspartame to sweeten her iced tea. Since she drank about a gallon of tea a day, she was exposed to large amounts of aspartame. After a few weeks of the artificially sweetened drink, she began having seizures. Doctors could find nothing wrong. The seizures stopped when she switched back to sugared tea.

The best approach here is to try eliminating aspartame from your diet for at least a week to see if it helps. If it doesn't, you can gradually reintroduce it.

Go easy on alcohol. People who drink too much have three times the normal risk of developing epilepsy, a risk similar to that of people who've had head injuries or central nervous system infections. In adults newly diagnosed with epilepsy, alcohol abuse accounts for symptoms in one in four, report researchers from Columbia University in New York City.

Ease up on coffee. "Although most can tolerate two to three cups of coffee or tea a day without trouble, a small percentage of people with epilepsy are very sensitive to caffeine and shouldn't take it at all," says Robert J. Gumnit, MD, president of MINCEP Epilepsy Care in Minneapolis.

Check for food triggers. Food sensitivities may cause seizures, especially in people with personal or family histories of food allergies or sensitivities. Such people might have additional symptoms such as migraines, recurrent stomach pains, diarrhea, and hyperactivity.

Pinpointing trouble foods can be difficult, so find a specialist in food allergy testing. It's possible to be sensitive to a food and not know it. It's also very common for a person to eat the very food he or she is sensitive to on a daily basis.

In a study by researchers at the Hospital for Sick Children in London, doctors found that cow's milk; cheeses; citrus fruits; wheat; and two food additives, tartrazine (a food dye known as FD&C Yellow #5) and benzoic acid (a preservative), are mostly likely to cause seizures in children with epilepsy. Tartrazine and benzoic acid are found in thousands of foods, and the best way to avoid them is to read food labels.

ketogenic diet, and perhaps the greatest advances in epilepsy treatment in the last decade have come in this area. This very low-carbohydrate, high-fat diet has proven extremely helpful in reducing seizures in some children with epilepsy. (For more information on the ketogenic diet, see "Food Factors" on page 242.)

Conflicting Evidence on Vitamin E

There is good reason to believe that vitamin E could be helpful for some kinds of seizures. Animals given vitamin E are more resistant to seizures induced by pressurized oxygen, iron, and certain chemicals. And clinical studies show that people taking antiseizure drugs have reduced blood levels of vitamin E.

That's why researchers at the University of Toronto decided to test vitamin E in 24 children with epilepsy whose seizures could not be controlled by medication.

They found that the frequency of seizures was reduced by more than 60 percent in 10 of 12 children taking vitamin E supplements. (They took 400 IU a day for 3 months in addition to their regular medication.) Six of them had a 90 to 100 percent reduction in seizures. By comparison, none of the 12 children who took placebos (inactive substances) along with their medication improved significantly.

What's more, when the children who were taking placebos were switched to vitamin E, seizure frequency was reduced 70 to 100 percent in all of them. The researchers noted that there were no adverse side effects.

"Vitamin E is a fat-soluble antioxidant vitamin," says Dr. Weber. "It can protect cell membranes, which are lipids, from oxidative stress. If taken at moderate doses, it may help to limit epilepsy-induced damage to the brain."

However, Dr. Weber adds that recent research has called the safety of high doses of vitamin E, particularly in children, into question. "At high doses, fat-soluble vitamins can accumulate in the body to potentially harmful levels," he says. "In particular, the benefit of large quantities of vitamin E has recently been called into question. The Daily Value is 30 international units per day. High doses of vitamin E (400 IU per day) are sold over the counter but are not advisable, specifically not for children."

Considering the conflicting information, Dr. Weber recommends that the best approach to vitamin E is to have a conversation about its helpfulness with your doctor.

Prescriptions for Healing

There are a number of nutrients that have proven useful in helping to prevent seizures. But please note: These supplements are meant to provide optimum nutritional support, not to be treatments in and of themselves. It's important to work with a doctor knowledgeable in nutrition, especially if you are giving nutritional supplements to children. These are the nutrients that doctors recommend.

Nutrient	Daily Amount
Folic acid	No more than 2,500 micrograms for children ages 5–15
	400–5,000 micrograms for adults
	1,600 micrograms for women of childbearing age on antiseizure drugs
	3,000 micrograms for women on antiseizure drugs who are planning to become pregnant, taken for 3 months before stopping birth control (requires a prescription)
Selenium	50–150 micrograms for children
	50–200 micrograms for adults
Vitamin E	400 IU for children ages 3 and over (d-alpha-tocopherol acetate)
	400–600 IU for adults (d-alpha-tocopherol acetate)

Plus a multivitamin/mineral supplement containing the Daily Values of all essential vitamins and minerals

MEDICAL ALERT: *If you have been diagnosed with epilepsy, you should be under a doctor's care.*

Make sure you are under a doctor's supervision when taking more than 400 micrograms of folic acid daily. High amounts can mask the symptoms of vitamin B_{12} deficiency, also known as pernicious anemia.

Selenium in doses exceeding 400 micrograms daily should be taken only under medical supervision.

Infants under 1 year of age should not be given more than 50 IU of vitamin E daily. If you are taking anticoagulant drugs, you should not take vitamin E supplements. (Though generally a dose of up to 1,500 IU of vitamin E a day is considered safe, some recent reports suggest that taking more than 400 IU a day could be harmful to people with cardiovascular or circulatory disease or with cancer. If you have such a condition, be sure to consult your doctor before you begin supplementation.)

Selenium May Stop Seizures

The mineral selenium, another nutrient with antioxidant properties, also appears to help control seizures in some children, says Dr. Weber.

Dr. Weber has found that some children with severe, uncontrollable seizures and repeated infections have low blood levels of glutathione peroxidase, a selenium-dependent antioxidant enzyme. "Glutathione is the most abundant natural antioxidant within our cells, and selenium is essential in helping glutathione perform its functions," he says. "If measurements of blood glutathione or selenium levels indicate that they are low, supplementation of selenium is advisable. It can help the brain cells cope with the oxidative damage of a seizure attack."

Specifically, in the course of his research Dr. Weber has found that giving children 50 to 150 micrograms of selenium a day significantly reduces the occurrence of seizures. "We believe that these children have a metabolic problem that prevents them from using selenium properly and that the problem may be far more frequent than has been believed," he says.

Talk to your doctor if you're thinking about taking selenium supplements yourself and especially if you're considering giving them to your child with epilepsy, Dr. Weber says. Although he has found amounts of up to 150 micrograms a day to be safe for children with severe deficiency, children's needs can vary greatly depending on the amount of deficiency they have, and giving too much selenium could be detrimental to their health.

For adults with epilepsy, experts who use nutritional therapy recommend 50 to 200 micrograms of selenium daily to control seizures. But be sure not to take more than 400 micrograms daily without medical supervision. You can get more selenium from foods if you eat lots of garlic, onions, whole grains, mushrooms, broccoli, cabbage, and fish.

Fill Up on Folic Acid

Deficiency of folate (the naturally occurring form of folic acid) isn't thought to often play a role in the development of seizures. But some antiseizure drugs deplete this B-complex vitamin, sometimes leading to abnormalities in red blood cell formation.

"Folate deficiency can also lead to serious birth defects called neural tube defects," explains Dr. Gumnit. "These birth defects happen very early in the pregnancy, often before a woman knows she is pregnant." (For more information on birth defects, see page 114.)

That is why any woman of childbearing age who's taking antiseizure drugs should also take 1,600 micrograms of folic acid a day, Dr. Gumnit says. And any woman who's taking antiseizure drugs and planning to become pregnant should also take 3 milligrams (3,000 micrograms) of folic acid every day for 3 months before she stops using birth control, he says. (That high amount requires a prescription supplement.)

Other people taking antiseizure drugs should simply take 400 micrograms, the amount of folic acid found in ordinary multivitamin/mineral supplements, Dr. Gumnit says. A few doctors recommend up to 5,000 micrograms a day for adults.

Make sure that you are under a doctor's supervision when taking more than 400 micrograms, because high amounts of folic acid can mask the symptoms of vitamin B_{12} deficiency, also known as pernicious anemia.

Some experts say that children ages 5 to 15 may safely take up to 2,500 micrograms of folic acid daily, but it's best to talk to a doctor about this, Dr. Gumnit says.

Many doctors also recommend a multivitamin/mineral supplement for their patients with epilepsy, and that's probably not a bad idea. Some research suggests that deficiencies of vitamin B_6, zinc, and magnesium may also play roles in seizure disorders.

FATIGUE

PUT THE PEP BACK IN YOUR STEP

Zombies are more than just a frightening image from the latest horror movie. If the most recent statistics about fatigue in the United States are to be believed, you are walking among them—or might even be one yourself.

Survey results released by the National Sleep Foundation in March 2007 indicate that over 60 percent of American women say they get a good night's sleep only "a couple of nights per week," and an incredible 80 percent say they experience sleepiness during the day but just go on with their business, even if it puts them in danger. Another study showed that 20 percent of fatal road accidents involve driver fatigue, and 30 percent of single-car accidents in rural areas also involve fatigue.

Surveys also indicate that fatigue is one of the most common reasons that we consult our family doctors. And for 500,000 Americans, this fatigue can evolve into a far more serious condition: chronic fatigue syndrome.

When you consider the number of conditions, both major and minor, that have fatigue as a symptom, these numbers become less surprising. Stress, depression, thyroid problems, anemia, and food allergies can all cause persistent tiredness, says Susan M. Lark, MD, a physician specializing in women's health; editor of *Women's Wellness Today*; president of DrLark.com in Forrester

---

Food Factors

When it comes to beating fatigue, what you don't eat is just as important as what you do eat.

Keep yourself on the wagon. "Alcohol is a central nervous system depressant, which is the last thing you need if you are feeling chronically tired," says Susan M. Lark, MD, a physician specializing in women's health; editor of *Women's Wellness Today*; president of DrLark.com in Forrester Center, West Virginia; and author of *Chronic Fatigue and Tiredness*.

Don't lean on caffeine. It's tempting to reach for a cup of strong coffee when you can barely keep your eyes open, but if you're mainlining coffee, tea, or cola from morning to night, you're doing yourself more harm than good, says Dr. Lark. Caffeine may give you a temporary jolt of energy, but in a few hours, you'll be just as tired as before—if not more tired.

Master your carb cravings. Simple sugars, such as those found in cookies, candies, and sweet desserts, and other refined carbohydrates, like those in bread and crackers, cause sharp increases in your blood sugar level, which may make you feel temporarily energized. But after the initial rush, blood sugar drops sharply, says Dr. Lark, which can result in an energy crisis.

Lighten up on fat. "Fatty foods, including most meats, are very hard to digest," says Dr. Lark. "Eating meat two or three times a day is like eating Christmas dinner 21 times a week. You're spending all of your energy digesting rich, heavy foods." She recommends a low-fat diet high in whole grains, legumes, and fresh fruits and vegetables, the same type of diet that is recommended for preventing heart disease and some types of cancer.

More omega-3s, please. Low levels of omega-3 fatty acids have been found in some people with chronic fatigue syndrome. To up your intake of these fats, eat more fish like salmon and herring, or take 2 to 3 grams of a fish oil supplement in divided doses with meals.

Center, West Virginia; and author of *Chronic Fatigue and Tiredness*. Many women also have premenstrual fatigue or fatigue that's related to menopause.

If your fatigue continues for 6 months or longer and is so severe that you can't function normally, you may have chronic fatigue syndrome, a mysterious illness that causes flulike symptoms, persistent muscle pain, and problems remembering or concentrating. Chronic fatigue syndrome hits mostly people between ages 25 and 50 and is relatively rare. Experts estimate that of all of the people who are fatigued enough to see a doctor about it, only 1 in 30 has chronic fatigue syndrome.

Luckily, there are a number of vitamins and minerals that play roles in helping to keep you fatigue-free. Read on to see how.

Iron: The Usual Suspect

One of the most common causes of fatigue is iron-deficiency anemia, says Dr. Lark. She estimates that 20 percent of women who menstruate are anemic because of the blood they lose each month. "Women with heavy menstrual flow have the greatest risk," she adds. Anemia is also common among teenagers, pregnant women, and women nearing menopause.

Even if you're not anemic, a slight iron deficiency can affect your energy level, and you may benefit from getting more iron in your diet, says Dr. Lark. Experts who recommend iron to combat fatigue generally suggest between 12 and 15 milligrams a day. The best source of iron is animal products, so go for lean meats, cooked oysters, and clams. Some vegetables, such as spinach, as well as legumes, such as green beans, lima beans, and pinto beans, are also rich in iron, but the type of iron found in them is not as easy to absorb as the iron found in animal sources.

If you're a vegetarian, drinking some orange juice or taking a vitamin C supplement of at least 75 milligrams along with iron-rich vegetables will help your body absorb more iron from your food, says Dr. Lark. Many commercial breads and breakfast cereals are also fortified with iron.

Potassium and Magnesium: A Potent Combination

Two other minerals that may be beneficial for people with persistent fatigue are potassium and magnesium, says Dr. Lark. "In studies where potassium and

Prescriptions for Healing

Here's what experts recommend to help you banish fatigue.

Nutrient	Daily Amount
B-complex vitamins	Take a B-50, B-75, or B-100 supplement daily
Iron	12–15 milligrams
Magnesium	100–200 milligrams
Potassium	100–200 milligrams
Vitamin C	1,000 milligrams, in 4 divided doses

MEDICAL ALERT: *People with heart or kidney problems should consult their doctors before taking supplemental magnesium.*

Potassium supplements should not be taken by those with diabetes or kidney disease or by those using certain medications, including nonsteroidal anti-inflammatory drugs, potassium-sparing diuretics, ACE inhibitors, and heart medications such as heparin.

High doses of vitamin C may cause diarrhea in some people.

magnesium were given together, 90 percent saw improvements in their energy levels," says Dr. Lark. She recommends trying between 100 and 200 milligrams of each mineral for up to 6 months to see if they alleviate fatigue. It's safe for anyone in good health, she says, although people with heart or kidney problems or diabetes shouldn't take these minerals without consulting a doctor first.

Rev Up with Vitamin C

Some older studies suggest that low vitamin C intake can also contribute to fatigue. A 1976 study of 411 dentists and their spouses found that those with low vitamin C intakes reported twice as many fatigue symptoms as those who got the most vitamin C. And studies of adolescent boys showed that even those with slight vitamin C deficiencies had more stamina after taking vitamin C supplements for 3 months.

To see if a high dose of vitamin C might help, some experts suggest taking 1,000 milligrams of vitamin C daily, in four divided doses. High doses of vitamin C can cause temporary diarrhea in some people, so cut back on the dose if this occurs.

Beat Fatigue with B Vitamins

Carbohydrates can't become energy in the body without adequate levels of the B family of vitamins. So if you're deficient in folic acid (vitamin B_9), pantothenic acid (vitamin B_5), thiamin (vitamin B_1), and cobalamin (vitamin B_{12}), the result can be fatigue.

The best way to up your intake of all these supplements at once is with a B-complex vitamin. And if you suffer from chronic fatigue syndrome, some experts recommend extra pantothenic acid.

FIBROCYSTIC BREASTS

LESSENING THE LUMPS

From an early age, women learn that a lump found in the breast during self-examination could be a sign of breast cancer.

It's a testament to the effectiveness of breast cancer awareness that this fact is so widely known. But at the same time, most people don't realize that—while a lump should absolutely *not* be taken lightly—there's a better-than-average chance that this lump is not a sign of breast cancer but rather fibrocystic breast disease, also known as cyclic mastalgia.

Fibrocystic breast disease is one of those medical conditions that create more fear than they probably should. Part of that fear, as addressed above, stems from the stigma associated with the risks of breast cancer. Couple this with the fact that the cysts that are the symptom of fibrocystic breasts are difficult to tell apart from cancerous cysts during a mammogram, and you can begin to understand the fear.

But though they can be frightening, and sometimes painful, fibrocystic breasts are not uncommon. In fact, more than 50 percent of women will experience them at some point in their lives, usually between the ages of 30 and 50. The condition begins as small lumps and gets classified as fibrocystic breast disease when these lumps grow large enough to be considered cysts. In addition to the cysts, women with fibrocystic breasts may also experience fullness of the breasts, pain and tenderness, and even bloody discharges from the nipples.

Causes and Treatments

The changes in hormones that occur during a woman's menstrual cycle are believed to be the most common cause of fibrocystic breasts, and high levels of the hormone prolactin have also been implicated in some studies. In fact,

Food Factors

Ever wish that the food you eat would go straight to your bustline instead of your waistline? For women with fibrocystic breasts, that's often what happens, only not in a way they appreciate. Here are some dietary changes that doctors recommend to lessen the pain and lumpiness of fibrocystic breasts.

Cool the coffee habit. Some experts consider reducing caffeine consumption to be the best, most cost-effective treatment for fibrocystic breasts. That's because caffeine apparently stimulates estrogen production and promotes swollen, painful breasts.

According to researchers at Michigan State University College of Human Medicine in East Lansing, women who ingest more than 500 milligrams of caffeine a day, the amount in about 4 cups of coffee, are at 2.3 times greater risk of fibrocystic breasts than those who abstain. And those who eliminate caffeine from their diets, the researchers say, experience a 60 to 65 percent reduction in symptoms.

Other sources of caffeine include tea, chocolate, and cola.

Trim the fat. "Eating too much saturated fat increases estrogen levels and stimulates fibrocystic changes," says Susan M. Lark, MD, a physician specializing in women's health; editor of *Women's Wellness Today*; president of DrLark.com in Forrester Center, West Virginia; and author of the *Premenstrual Syndrome Self-Help Book*. Dr. Lark recommends that women avoid animal fat whenever possible. That means cutting back on meats and eating nonfat dairy products.

Several scientific studies seem to back up Dr. Lark's advice. In one recent study, women cut their fat intake down to 15 percent of their usual levels and experienced significant reductions in breast pain. In another, women cut down to 20 percent of their usual intake over a 3-

many women with fibrocystic breasts actually see the cysts literally disappear once they reach menopause.

Some researchers also believe that nutritional factors can play a role. Caffeine, for example, could cause the tenderness and pain associated with fibrocystic breasts. And an imbalance of essential fatty acids in the body may cause the cysts in the first place. In addition, some studies indicate that reduced fat intake overall may reduce the symptoms. (See more information on all these in "Food Factors.")

Nutrition can also play a role in treating the cysts, as well as the pain, associated with the condition. But before you try these methods of self-care,

---

month period, and their levels of lactogenic hormone dropped substantially. This is particularly good news, as this hormone has been linked to increased breast cancer risk in other studies.

Power up with bran. While you're cutting fat, you may also want to consider boosting your fiber intake. Among other things, fiber can absorb estrogen and excrete it from the body. Women should aim for 25 to 30 grams of fiber a day. You can increase your fiber intake by eating more whole grains, fruits, and vegetables.

Lean toward teetotalism. "The liver is responsible for detoxifying circulating estrogen, and alcohol is toxic to the liver," says Dr. Lark. "I suggest that women with fibrocystic breasts avoid drinking or limit their alcohol intakes."

Lower the sodium. Doctors have found that benign breast cysts are affected by how much fluid you retain. Since sodium makes you hold water, many doctors recommend limiting salt intake to less than 1,500 milligrams a day. (That's not much salt; 1 teaspoon contains 2,000 milligrams of sodium.)

Eat your diuretics. A diuretic is a substance that helps your body get rid of excess water. As a sodium-cutting complement, Dr. Lark recommends that women increase their intakes of naturally diuretic foods such as parsley, celery, and cucumbers, which can help decrease fluid retention.

Try some flax. A few studies have suggested that flaxseed oil, when used along with evening primrose oil (see sidebar, page 254), can bring women relief from the pain and tenderness associated with fibrocystic breasts. Try taking 1 to 4 tablespoons daily, divided into three or four doses.

one point is critical: See your doctor *whenever* you feel a lump during a self-examination. Your physician can perform the necessary steps to determine whether the condition is fibrocystic breasts or something more serious.

And remember: If the diagnosis you receive from your doctor is fibrocystic breasts, you should feel relieved, not fearful. Though they present similar lumps, fibrocystic breasts are in no way associated with breast cancer or an increased risk of breast cancer.

Fibrocystic breasts can be challenging, however, in that they can make it difficult to detect new lumps when performing your regular self-examination. According to many experts, the key is to perform the examinations more often to become familiar with your breasts. Then, see your doctor if you find a new change or lump that persists for two menstrual cycles.

Though hormone therapy is one approach that's often recommended for treating fibrocystic breasts, some experts, including Susan M. Lark, MD, a physician specializing in women's health; editor of *Women's Wellness Today*; president of DrLark.com in Forrester Center, West Virginia; and author of the *Premenstrual Syndrome Self-Help Book*, maintain that nutritional regimens can work just as well without the side effects of hormone therapy. Here's what they recommend.

Evening Primrose Relief

Want relief from swollen, tender fibrocystic breasts without the side effects of hormone therapy? Evening primrose oil—a rich source of gamma-linolenic acid, which your body uses to regulate its salt and water balance—could be your answer. Welsh researchers who have studied the supplement for nearly 20 years now recommend it as the first line of treatment to relieve the pain of fibrocystic breasts without side effects.

"Evening primrose oil is a common treatment," says Susan M. Lark, MD, a physician specializing in women's health; editor of *Women's Wellness Today*; president of DrLark.com in Forrester Center, West Virginia; and author of the *Premenstrual Syndrome Self-Help Book*. "It's a good source of essential fatty acids, and it has a diuretic and anti-inflammatory effect on the body."

For relief from breast pain and lumps, some experts recommend taking 1,000 milligrams three times daily for a period of 3 months. Before you start with supplementation, check with your doctor.

The Intriguing Effects of Iodine

Though it's hardly the first nutrient that comes to mind for treating illnesses, iodine has shown some remarkable results when it comes to reducing benign breast cysts, as well as the pain associated with those cysts. Before you reach for the saltshaker, however, you should know that iodized salt will likely not be of much help. The iodine experts are recommending is an oral iodine supplement.

When it comes to using iodine to treat the pain associated with fibro-cystic breasts, the results look promising. In one 5-year study at Hotel Dieu Hospital at Queen's University at Kingston in Ontario, more than 1,000 women were supplemented with sodium iodide (that's what is in iodized salt), protein-bound iodide, or diatomic iodine. Researchers found that diatomic iodine reduced breast pain in the most women, with the fewest side effects.

In addition, more recent research seems to indicate that iodine can play a role in preventing, and even reducing, the growth of cysts. "Iodine research has become a scientifically impressive area in breast disease," says Bernard A. Eskin, MD, MS, a professor at Drexel University College of Medicine in Phil-adelphia. "Studies on human cancer cultures show a positive or improved effect with iodine. This is indicated by a reduction of the cancerous tissue and protection from further growth as long as it is used. And clinically, basic research has indicated that iodine generally appears to be even more effective in treating benign disease in humans."

The only iodine supplement currently on the market is Iodoral, a formu-lation that contains 5 milligrams of iodine and 7.5 milligrams of potassium iodide. The recommended dosage is one to four tablets daily, but Dr. Eskin recommends working with your physician to determine the proper dosage.

Note: The iodine in your medicine cabinet is not recommended for con-sumption for any reason.

Extra Help from Vitamin A

Pointing to a promising pilot study of the effects of vitamin A on fibrocystic breasts as well as her own work with her patients, Dr. Lark believes that this potent nutrient may also be effective for soothing sore, lumpy breasts.

In this study, which was conducted at the University of Montreal, 12 women with moderate to severe breast pain were given high doses of vitamin

Prescriptions for Healing

Doctors can't promise that anything will lessen breast pain and lumpiness for sure, but some experts have had some success with these nutrients.

Nutrient	Daily Amount
Beta-carotene	20,000 IU
Iodine	1–4 tablets of Iodoral
Vitamin B_6	100 milligrams, taken as 2 divided doses

MEDICAL ALERT: *If you feel any new or unusual lump in your breasts, check with your doctor for a complete diagnosis.*

If you are at risk for heart disease or osteoporosis, talk with your doctor before taking beta-carotene supplements.

Do not take Iodoral without your doctor's supervision.

If you have liver disease, you should talk to your doctor before taking more than 50 milligrams of vitamin B_6. Also, don't take this much vitamin B_6 for more than 6 months, and discontinue use immediately and consult your doctor if you experience numbness in the hands or feet.

A for 3 months. Nine of the women experienced significant pain relief, and five of the women experienced decreases in breast lumps. The bad news is that the dosage in that study was 150,000 IU a day, an amount 30 times the Daily Value and one with which few experts feel comfortable, since vitamin A is toxic in high doses.

Thankfully, another recent study showed that vitamin A can also be effective at lower levels. In this study, women were given 20,000 IU of beta-carotene every day, starting 7 days before menstruation. A significant number of these women felt relief from their breast pain without experiencing any negative side effects.

Beta-carotene supplementation does have some inherent risks, especially for those with heart disease and osteoporosis. So your best bet may be to get your daily intake of beta-carotene from food. Focus on eating plenty of orange and yellow fruits and vegetables. One sweet potato alone, for instance, packs a beta-carotene punch of 10,000 IU.

Better Breasts with B$_6$

According to some doctors we spoke with, their patients experienced a reduction of pain and swelling from fibrocystic breasts when taking vitamin B$_6$. But the scientific studies done on the subject have shown mixed results.

"Recent studies with vitamin B$_6$ have been published that show a reduction of fibrocystic breast symptoms in patients," says Dr. Eskin. "However, the improvement is not significantly greater than the placebo." Taking 100 milligrams of vitamin B$_6$ daily is considered safe for most. However, if you have liver disease, you should talk to your doctor before taking more than 50 milligrams of vitamin B$_6$. Also, don't take this much vitamin B$_6$ for more than 6 months, and discontinue use immediately and consult your doctor if you experience numbness in the hands or feet.

To increase your vitamin B$_6$ intake from foods, try slicing a banana on your morning cereal and adding a baked potato to your evening meal.

FINGERNAIL PROBLEMS

BEATING BRITTLE NAILS

If the eyes are the windows to the soul, then the fingernails just might be the windows to the body.

Before you laugh, consider this: Many doctors actually look to the fingernails first to determine if you may be suffering from a serious nutritional deficiency, or even a condition such as heart disease or diabetes. Yellow nail syndrome, for example, can be a telltale sign of a respiratory condition such as chronic bronchitis. And "spoon nails," nails that curve outward in a scoop shape, are a sign of iron-deficiency anemia.

These are just two of the many ways that fingernails can show you something more serious is going on. Brittle or otherwise abnormal nails also have been associated with deficiencies of calcium and zinc, as well as with too much selenium.

Nail problems are often related to thyroid dysfunction, so you may want to ask your doctor about that first. Then, look into the following foods and supplements, which might help restore your healthy nails.

Prescriptions for Healing

Only one nutrient, biotin, has been shown in scientific studies to help fingernails.

Nutrient	Daily Amount
Biotin	2,500 micrograms

Also take a multivitamin/mineral supplement every day

MEDICAL ALERT: *While biotin is considered one of the safest of all nutrients, the dosage recommended here is extremely high and should be taken only under medical supervision.*

Biotin Banishes Brittle Nails

A study by Swiss researchers looked at people with apparently normal intakes of biotin: 28 to 42 micrograms a day. Researchers found that people in the study with thin, frail, and split nails who took extra amounts of biotin—2.5 milligrams (2,500 micrograms), or roughly 70 times the average daily intake—experienced a 25 percent increase in nail thickness.

"Biotin is absorbed into the matrix of the nail, where it may help correct brittle nails," explains Richard K. Scher, MD, dermatologist and head of the nail section at Columbia-Presbyterian Medical Center in New York City. (The matrix is the part embedded in the finger where nail cells are generated.) Dr. Scher recommends biotin supplements to his patients with weak nails. "It seems to help about two-thirds of them," he says.

The amount of biotin used in the Swiss study is very high. This dose should not be taken except under medical supervision.

Top dietary sources of biotin are egg yolks, soybean flour, cereals, and yeast. Cauliflower, lentils, milk, and peanut butter also provide decent amounts.

Go for Total Protection

Since fingernail problems are associated with a number of nutritional deficiencies, your best bet is to take care of them all with a daily multivitamin/mineral supplement. This will fulfill your dietary needs of iron, zinc, calcium, and any other nutrient that can adversely affect your nail health.

GALLSTONES

HEALTHY WAYS
TO PREVENT THE PAIN

The gallbladder is one of those organs that usually gets classified with the tonsils, in the "What does it do?" category. This tiny sac that's located under the liver has the less-than-appetizing job of storing bile produced by the liver. When your body is trying to digest fat, the gallbladder then releases its slimy contents into the small intestine to aid in its breakdown. Your body then continues the digestive process, and everything heads for the exit. The gallbladder also has a more notorious reputation, however: as the producer of gallstones. Most of the time, gallstones stay put in the gallbladder or nearby bile ducts and produce no symptoms at all. But if you ever experience the nausea, vomiting, or intense abdominal pain that's associated with a gallstone-instigated gallbladder attack, you won't soon forget it.

The Not-So-Romantic Stone

Whether or not a doctor has ever looked you in the eye and announced the presence of a pea-size pellet wandering through your digestive system, there's a good chance that you have at least one. More than 20 million Americans do. Most of these people are overweight, over age 40, and women—and most of them don't even know the gallstones are there.

The stones are formed when a grain or two of calcium arrives in the gallbladder and hangs around long enough to become coated with either cholesterol or bilirubin, a substance that is part of the hemoglobin in your blood. Eighty to 85 percent of all stones are coated with layer upon layer of waxy-looking cholesterol, although many stones are coated with both substances. A few are made exclusively of yellowish green bilirubin.

Exactly what causes this buildup of cholesterol or bilirubin on the calcium is not totally clear. What is known is that something goes wrong in the gallbladder's typical process of releasing bile, and the organ's sludgelike contents crystallize. This provides the opportunity to layer thicker and thicker coats of cholesterol or bilirubin around a calcium speck, thus forming a gallstone.

Naturally occurring female reproductive hormones are known to encourage that process by delaying gallbladder emptying, such as during pregnancy and dieting. What's more, birth control implants that contain progesterone may do the same, while birth control pills containing estrogen seem to increase the cholesterol content of bile—not a helpful situation, either.

Blame Your Genes and Diet

All told, hormones, pregnancy, dieting, and birth control may help explain why two-thirds of all gallstones belong to women. But aside from being a woman, what else puts you at risk for gallstones? (After all, many men get them, too.)

"Diet and genetics," replies Henry Pitt, MD, professor of surgery at the Indiana University School of Medicine in Indianapolis. And it's difficult to sort out which is responsible for what. So far, many scientific studies of populations only add to the confusion.

In Chile, for example, 60 percent of people have gallstones by the time they're 80 years of age. Yet in Africa, gallstones affect only 1 to 2 percent of the population.

Is that diet or genetics?

It could be one or the other or both, says Dr. Pitt. Studies of ethnic groups who rarely get gallstones indicate that when they move from a geographic location in which they have consumed a low-fat, low-cholesterol diet to a location in which they consume a high-fat, high-cholesterol diet, they start getting gallstones.

Aside from calories and fat, another dietary factor may have an impact on gallstone formation, and it involves a mineral: calcium.

The Calcium Controversy

A low-fat, low-cholesterol diet may help prevent gallstones, agrees Alan Hofmann, MD, PhD, professor emeritus at the University of California, San Diego, but the most important aspect of the diet is that it doesn't have too many calories, so a person stays slender. But Dr. Hofmann also feels there is reason to believe that supplementing the diet with calcium may act to prevent gallstones.

Food Factors

Dietary strategies are crucial in reducing gallstone formation, according to medical experts. Here's what they recommend.

Cut out the carbs. The last decade has shown us how well carbohydrates can become fat in the body, says Henry Pitt, MD, professor of surgery at the Indiana University School of Medicine in Indianapolis. Obesity is one of the biggest risk factors for gallstone formation, and that puts refined carbohydrates high on the list of foods to avoid. Choose healthy whole-grain sources of carbohydrates in favor of refined sources like white bread and crackers. Also, be sure to cut back on any sweets and sugar-loaded foods.

Can the cholesterol. Stick closely to the American Heart Association's recommendation to consume no more than 300 milligrams of dietary cholesterol a day, advises Dr. Pitt. Reducing the amount of cholesterol in your blood may reduce your body's ability to incorporate it into gallstones.

Dietary cholesterol comes exclusively from animal sources: meats and dairy products. To reduce your cholesterol levels, you need to cut back on these foods as well as on saturated fat. (That's any fat that is solid at room temperature.)

Cut those calories. Studies indicate that women who consume so many calories that they become obese can have up to six times the risk of gallstones of women of normal weight. That's why Dr. Pitt suggests maintaining a healthy weight and following the American Heart Association's recommendation to get less than 30 percent of your calories from fat.

Eat your omega-3s. A number of recent studies have indicated that the omega-3 fatty acids found in fish like salmon, as well as fish oil supplements, may reduce the formation of gallstones. "We're not saying that we can dissolve gallstones," says Dr. Pitt. "But we can slow the rate at which they form. So people at high risk, such as those who diet frequently, might want to incorporate fish as a regular part of their diets." It also might be worth looking into taking 3 to 5 grams of a fish oil supplement daily.

"In addition to helping your bones, calcium has a good effect on bile acid metabolism," explains Dr. Hofmann. "What has been found is that large doses of oral calcium form calcium phosphate in the gut." This sets off a chain of chemical events that eventually lowers the amount of cholesterol in the gallbladder, thus reducing the possibility that gallstones will form, he explains.

It also seems to explain why a study of 872 Dutch men between the ages of 40 and 59 found that the more calcium the men consumed over a 25-year period, the fewer gallstones they were likely to have.

In fact, one study in the Netherlands revealed that men who had more than 1,442 milligrams of calcium in their diets every day had a 50 percent lower prevalence of gallstones.

"Since most individuals have stopped drinking much milk by the time they're 45 years old, it makes good sense to take calcium supplements," says Dr. Hofmann.

Nonetheless, the view that large doses of supplemental calcium can prevent gallstones has not yet been tested experimentally. Normal doses of calcium do not increase the risk of kidney stones, however, and are likely to be good for both bones and bile. Studies are needed to prove this point as well as to prove that there are no important risks associated with long-term use of oral calcium supplements, says Dr. Hofmann.

Experts who recommend calcium to help prevent gallstones suggest aiming for the Daily Value, which is 1,000 milligrams. And in some cases, even more may be needed, for both men and women, adds Dr. Hofmann. Just be sure to check with your physician first.

Dr. Pitt, however, sees calcium's role in a different light. "Calcium may have something to do with the origin of most of the gallstones in this country," says Dr. Pitt. "It's at the center of almost every stone we find. And in our

Prescriptions for Healing

Although reducing dietary fat and cholesterol and keeping your weight down are clearly the two most important strategies that you can choose to prevent gallstones, there is one mineral that may help as well, according to Alan Hofmann, MD, PhD, professor emeritus at the University of California, San Diego.

Nutrient	Daily Amount
Calcium	1,000 milligrams

MEDICAL ALERT: *If you have a gallstone, you should be under a doctor's care.*

Dr. Hofmann considers calcium supplementation to be fine for both men and women.

animal studies, diets with high calcium seem to enhance the formation of pigment stones," the stones made of bilirubin.

And keep in mind all of the hormonal factors that affect women, says Dr. Pitt. It may turn out that calcium prevents gallstones in men but actually contributes to their formation in women.

So while men can feel comfortable taking calcium supplements, women should ask their family physicians to help evaluate individual risks and benefits, particularly in light of their family medical histories, says Dr. Pitt.

"If all of the women in your family get gallstones and none of them gets osteoporosis, then I'd stay away from calcium," he advises. But if all of the women get osteoporosis and only an occasional stone rolls down someone's duct, then calcium should be okay, he adds.

Beef Up on Iron

When it comes to gallstone formation, another nutrient that has received more attention in recent studies is iron.

"Part of the reason more women of childbearing age get gallstones is because they are often anemic," says Dr. Pitt. "Iron makes smooth muscles, such as those in the gallbladder, function well, and studies have shown that animals that are deficient in iron have more gallstones and decreased gallbladder function."

The Daily Value of iron for women in their childbearing years is 18 milligrams, so you'll want to focus on foods such as red meat, chicken, and beans, as well as a multivitamin, to reach that level. Also, speak with your doctor about the possibility of an iron supplement if anemia continues to be a problem.

GENITAL HERPES

PUT A STOP TO THE SORES

Despite all the health breakthroughs of recent decades, one disease that we have not been able to stop—let alone slow down—is genital herpes.

Ten years ago, new cases of herpes were growing at a rate of 500,000 a year in the United States. That number has remained unchanged. In fact, it's now estimated that close to 30 million Americans have herpes, and if new cases continue at their current rate, some day half of all American adults could have the disease. It's far and away the most common sexually transmitted disease: There are more cases of herpes than all other viral STDs combined.

But perhaps the most frightening fact about genital herpes is that most people don't even know they have it. Most experts estimate that somewhere between 80 to 90 percent of herpes cases go undiagnosed. Couple this fact with the fact that there's no cure for genital herpes, and you can begin to understand why the disease continues to spread at such an alarming rate.

How It Happens

The culprit is the herpes simplex virus, a relative of the Epstein-Barr virus that causes mononucleosis and the varicella zoster virus that causes chicken-pox and shingles. The virus can take two forms in the body: type 1, which includes cold sores and other "fever blisters," though it can on rare occasions become a genital infection, and type 2, which is genital herpes.

In most cases, genital herpes is contracted by having sex with someone who has it. The initial outbreak is often the worst and causes painful blisters on and around the genitals, as well as flulike symptoms. Though subsequent outbreaks are usually more subdued, they occur about four to five times a year in the average person with herpes.

Hope for Herpes

A diagnosis of genital herpes does not have to mean a life of solitude. Though there is no cure, the symptoms and occurrence of outbreaks can be controlled with antiviral medication. One medication, Valtrex (valacyclovir HCl), has been shown to reduce the chance of spreading the disease when combined with other safe sex practices, such as using condoms and abstaining from sex during an active outbreak.

Nutritional therapies for genital herpes exist, but experts have found them to be less than consistent: Some people have considerable success with them, while others have none at all. "None of these treatments is well researched, and we can't recommend them across the board because the suc-

Food Factors

Along with keeping your stress levels under control, there are a number of dietary approaches that many medical experts say can help prevent genital herpes from recurring.

Here's what they say helps.

Load up on lysine. Researchers have found that lysine, an amino acid that your body needs in order to function, interferes with reproduction of the herpes virus. And apparently, increasing your intake of lysine just might help reduce your number of outbreaks. Good sources of lysine include fish, chicken, cheeses, potatoes, milk, brewer's yeast, and beans.

Additionally, supplementing your lysine intake with a 500-milligram tablet daily during an outbreak has also been shown to help. And lysine topical cream, applied twice a day, may also provide some relief.

Lighten up on arginine. They say that for every force, there's a counterforce. Well, in the case of lysine, that counterforce is arginine, another amino acid that your body needs.

Arginine, which has been linked to herpes outbreaks, is found in abundance in foods such as peanuts and other nuts and seeds as well as chocolate and gelatin. You don't have to eliminate these foods completely, but some doctors suggest that when you're under stress, it might be a good idea to cut back on them.

cess rates are so random," says Stephen Tyring, MD, PhD, professor of dermatology, microbiology and immunology, and internal medicine at the University of Texas Medical School in Houston. "If it's safe and it seems to help a person, however, then I don't discourage it."

That said, here's what some doctors recommend as potential nutritional treatments.

Boost Immunity with Vitamin C

Since herpes tends to become reactivated when your defenses are down, some doctors recommend upping your intake of vitamin C, which is known to help your body's infection-fighting white blood cells do their duty.

"There is strong scientific evidence that vitamin C can boost the immune system, and therefore it should help. But people who take megadoses of vitamin C are sometimes helped and sometimes not," cautions Dr. Tyring. "It'll probably have the biggest effect if you're not getting enough in your diet to begin with."

To reduce the healing time of herpes blisters during outbreaks, or just before symptoms develop, try taking 250 to 500 milligrams twice a day in

---

Prescriptions for Healing

While there are no guarantees when it comes to treating genital herpes, some people experience fewer, less severe outbreaks by boosting their intakes of certain nutrients. Here's what many experts recommend.

Nutrient	Daily Amount/Application
Oral	
Copper	1–3 milligrams (1 milligram for every 10 milligrams of zinc, up to 3 milligrams)
Vitamin C	500–1,000 milligrams, taken as divided doses during the active part of the infection
Zinc	30–60 milligrams
Topical	
Vitamin C	Apply a topical vitamin C solution to lesions 3 times for 2 minutes each at 30-minute intervals
Vitamin E	Apply the oil from a vitamin E capsule onto a cotton swab and dab on affected areas every 8 hours as needed
Zinc oxide	As an ingredient in ointment, applied directly to the blisters (for men only)

MEDICAL ALERT: *If you have symptoms of genital herpes, you should see your doctor for proper diagnosis and treatment.*

Do not take more than 3 milligrams of copper per day without medical supervision.

Doses of vitamin C above 1,200 milligrams a day can cause diarrhea in some people.

You should not exceed 15 milligrams of zinc a day without first discussing it with your doctor.

divided doses. A topical solution containing vitamin C may also help. To use this, apply it three times, for 2 minutes each at 30-minute intervals, on the first day of the outbreak to speed healing.

If you suspect that you're among those who don't get enough vitamin C, you can give your diet a boost of this important nutrient by eating more fruits and vegetables, particularly oranges, broccoli, and red bell peppers.

Think Zinc for Relief

The mineral zinc acts as a double agent in the fight against herpes, working both from the inside out and from the outside in.

Like vitamin C, zinc is a frontline player in boosting the immune system, especially the production of T-lymphocyte cells, which are important body defenses against viral infections. Though they admit that zinc's effect against herpes is speculative, doctors who recommend nutritional regimens for preventing recurrent herpes outbreaks often suggest taking zinc supplements.

How much you should take varies depending on whom you ask, but the recommended range is somewhere between 30 and 60 milligrams a day, well above the Daily Value of 15 milligrams. (You should consult your doctor before exceeding 15 milligrams of zinc a day.) And because zinc can interfere with the absorption of copper, doctors also suggest taking 1 milligram of copper for every 10 milligrams of zinc, up to 3 milligrams.

If you want to get more zinc through your diet, then soup up your intake of seafood. Just six steamed medium oysters pack about 76 milligrams of zinc.

Also, if you're a man with genital herpes, some doctors recommend having a topical preparation containing zinc oxide on hand. Applied directly to the blisters, the ointment will ease the burning and dry out the blisters more quickly. Doctors warn women not to use zinc oxide ointments for vaginal herpes, however, because drying agents shouldn't be used on mucous membranes.

"This doesn't work as an antiviral agent," says Dr. Tyring. "But it may numb the pain and itching."

Try Topical Vitamin E

Another nutrient that may help in a topical form is vitamin E. Vitamin E oil, which can be taken straight from a vitamin E capsule, should be squeezed onto a cotton swab and applied directly to herpes lesions every 8 hours during an outbreak. Not only can it reduce the pain of an outbreak, but it can also speed along the healing process.

GINGIVITIS

NUTRITIONAL SECRETS TO HEALTHY GUMS

From an early age, few tidbits of health advice are reinforced more often than those of your dentist—to brush and floss regularly.

And your dentist has a very good reason to be so persistent about this. What's at stake if you neglect your brushing and flossing duties is gingivitis, and it's definitely cause for concern.

Left for even a short time along your gum line, food particles and bacteria combine to form plaque, which hardens on your teeth and irritates your gums. Irritated gums bleed and eventually start to recede, creating pockets next to your teeth that collect even more junk. Before long, the plaque starts attacking the roots of your teeth and your jawbone; this is the point at which gingivitis turns into a more serious gum problem known as periodontal disease. If periodontal disease progresses too far without proper medical intervention, you might even lose some teeth.

When it comes to healthy gums, most dentists rightly focus on clearing out the crud with frequent flossing and brushing. But there's no doubt that diet also plays a role. "After all, the mouth is attached to the rest of the body," says Cherilyn Sheets, DDS, a spokesperson for the Academy of General Dentistry and a dentist in Newport Beach, California. "Anything that improves health overall and the body's ability to resist disease will affect the mouth positively." Eat badly enough, or indulge in damaging behaviors such as smoking and excessive drinking, and your whole body suffers, including your mouth, says Dr. Sheets.

In recent years, this connection between the health of your teeth and gums and the rest of your body (called the "oral-systemic connection") has become even stronger, adds Dr. Sheets. A number of studies have shown that gingivitis and periodontal disease are more common in patients who also

Food Factors

Keeping these dietary tips in mind may keep your gums in the pink.

Reduce your sugar. In addition to promoting dental decay, sugar has been shown to harm gums in numerous studies. Although the exact reason why sugar damages the gums is not known, many dentists believe that sugar feeds the bacteria that cause the infection leading to gingivitis.

Phase out soft drinks. Soft drinks are cause for concern because of the high levels of sugar alone. But they also contain phosphorus, a mineral that could lead to the leaching of calcium from your bones. This one-two punch of sugar and phosphorus makes soft drinks worth avoiding when it comes to gingivitis.

Try coenzyme Q10. Recent research has shown that this supplement is helpful for gum health. "I generally recommend 100 milligrams to 300 milligrams a day for people with gum disease," says Mary Dan Eades, MD, author of *Protein Power* and *The Protein Power LifePlan*. "The nutrient is an oil-soluble one, so it should be either taken with some fat in the meal or in an oil-based gel cap."

suffer from heart disease, diabetes, or pneumonia. And though it's not known whether one condition actually causes the other, or if they simply share a similar cause, the fact exists that there is definitely some relationship between the conditions. This makes nutrition more important to your oral health than we previously believed.

Take Vitamin C and See Improvement

"Certainly, vitamin C is the one nutrient that has been shown to have quite a positive effect on the mouth when in adequate levels in the body and a negative effect on the mouth when in low levels in the body," says Dr. Sheets. People with vitamin C deficiencies can have some of the worst gum and dental problems that dentists see.

To measure the effect of vitamin C deficiency on gum health, researchers at the University of California, San Francisco, School of Dentistry fed 11 men rotating diets that purposely excluded fruits and vegetables for 14 weeks. Vitamin C, in the form of a supplement dissolved in grape juice, was added to their diets only during certain weeks.

At the end of the study, researchers found that as vitamin C levels in the men went down, their gums bled more. When they received more vitamin C, their gums bled less.

Further research with laboratory animals confirmed that vitamin C deficiency causes gum swelling, decreased mineral content of the jawbone, and loose teeth.

Why the damage? As it turns out, vitamin C is vital for production of collagen, the basic protein building block for the fibrous framework of all tissues, including gums, explains Mary Dan Eades, MD, author of *Protein Power* and *The Protein Power Lifeplan*. "Vitamin C strengthens weak gum tissue and makes the gum lining more resistant to penetration by bacteria," she says.

Dr. Eades recommends using vitamin C in two ways—as a mouthwash and as a supplement—to fight gingivitis. "Mix a half-teaspoon of crystalline vitamin C with a sugar-free citrus beverage, swish the mixture in your mouth

---

Prescriptions for Healing

You may see substantial improvement in the health of your gums by making sure you brush, floss, and get adequate levels of vitamin C each day, says Mary Dan Eades, MD, author of *Protein Power* and *The Protein Power LifePlan*. Here are her recommendations for a healthier mouth.

Nutrient	Daily Amount
Vitamin C	1,000–2,000 milligrams (slow-release capsules), taken as 2 divided doses
	½ teaspoon crystalline vitamin C, mixed with a sugar-free citrus beverage and used as an oral rinse twice a day (swish in your mouth for 1 minute)
Coenzyme Q10 100–300 milligrams per day	

MEDICAL ALERT: *If you have gingivitis, you should be under a dentist's care.*

Chewable and powdered vitamin C have been found to erode tooth enamel, which is a big problem and can also cause tooth sensitivity. Because of this, it's best to use the crystalline form in a mouth rinse. Some dentists prefer using the oral rinse for 3 to 5 days at a time. Follow the rinse with plenty of fresh water. Vitamin C can also cause diarrhea in doses exceeding 1,200 milligrams.

for one minute, then swallow, twice daily," she advises. Follow each rinse with plenty of fresh water. Crystalline vitamin C is also called powdered pure ascorbic acid and is available in health food stores and through vitamin supply houses. Your doctor could help you find a supply. (Chewable or powdered vitamin C can erode tooth enamel. So it's best to stick to the crystalline form if you're using it as a mouth rinse.)

You can also take 500-milligram slow-release vitamin C capsules, one or two in the morning and one or two in the evening, says Dr. Eades. (Some people may experience diarrhea when taking vitamin C in doses exceeding 1,200 milligrams a day.) Meanwhile, keep on brushing and flossing!

GLAUCOMA

EASING EYE PRESSURE NATURALLY

We live in a highly visual society. And as computers and televisions play a greater role in how we communicate with one another, it's a trend that shows no sign of slowing. With this in mind, few things are more important than the health of those little orbs that make it all possible: your eyes.

Considering just how critical your eyes are, nothing is more frightening to most of us than the prospect of losing our vision. And that's what makes a condition like glaucoma so scary. Not only can the group of diseases known as glaucoma rob you of your vision, but they can do it without you even knowing it's happening. That's why glaucoma is sometimes called "the silent thief."

When your eyes are working properly, a flow of fluid called aqueous humor is constantly running through them, providing nourishment and keeping them clean. But when you have glaucoma, something prevents this fluid from draining properly. The result is increased pressure that, with time, can damage the delicate cells of the optic nerve and cause peripheral vision loss or total vision loss.

Glaucoma comes in several forms, but the most common is open-angle glaucoma, a condition that takes years to develop and doesn't present itself until you begin to lose vision. The populations at the greatest risk of developing glaucoma are African-Americans over age 40, or anyone over age 60.

The most common traditional treatment of glaucoma includes the use of pressure-reducing eye drops and, in some cases, surgery. But Benjamin C. Lane, OD, director of the Nutritional Optometry Institute in Lake Hiawatha, New Jersey, says that nutrition can play a large role in preventing and controlling the symptoms of glaucoma. In fact, many people can experience some improvement through measures as simple as changing what they eat.

"It's not going to help everyone," he says. "But if they get the right nutrients over a period of a few years, many people with glaucoma are able to be weaned off medication or to use much less medication."

Taking a Shine to Chromium

Aside from making sure that your reading prescription is up-to-date, one of the best ways to lower pressure inside the eyeballs is to talk to your eye doctor about a chromium test. Chromium deficiency has a strong connection with glaucoma, says Dr. Lane.

In a study done at Columbia University in New York City, Dr. Lane asked more than 400 patients with eye disease to detail the foods they had eaten during the previous 2 months. Then Dr. Lane did tests to measure the vitamin and mineral content of the patients' blood. Among the findings: Those people who didn't get enough chromium and who ate too many vanadium-containing foods were at higher risk for glaucoma. (Vanadium is a common trace mineral. It occurs naturally in many foods, including kelp, dulse, and other seaweed, as well as in large marine fish and in marine-phosphate and fishmeal-supplemented poultry.)

"What set of muscles do we use more today than ever before in recorded history? The focusing muscles in our eyes," says Dr. Lane. "And what nutrient helps facilitate the ability of our eye muscles to focus? The bottom line is that most of us need more chromium, especially if we have been eating refined and sugar-supplemented foods." Adequate chromium levels are necessary to help deliver needed energy to your eye-focusing muscles, he says.

And what's the connection between eye muscles and glaucoma? When we perform tasks that require prolonged, intense "binocular accommodation" focusing, such as reading, too much fluid can be produced inside the eyeballs, Dr. Lane explains. In some people, he says, the fluid doesn't drain properly and pressure builds. This in turn leads to less nutrients and circulation reach-

Food Factors

Try these tips to help knock out glaucoma.

Veer away from vanadium. Vanadium is a commonly occurring trace mineral that can deplete your body of chromium. And chromium is important in normalizing the pressure inside your eyeballs. Vanadium is found in kelp, dulse, and other kinds of seaweed, as well as in shark, swordfish, tuna, commercially raised chicken and turkey (they're often fed a seafood-based meal), vinegar, mushrooms, pickles, chocolate, and carob.

Cut the sugar. Chromium stores that could be used to keep the pressure inside your eyeballs stable are diverted to handle added sugar in the diet, says Benjamin C. Lane, OD, director of the Nutritional Optometry Institute in Lake Hiawatha, New Jersey.

Eat your omega-3s. Early studies seem to indicate that omega-3 fatty acids decrease intraocular pressure with age by increasing aqueous outflow, says Dr. Lane. So it certainly couldn't hurt to increase your intake of omega-3 fatty acids by eating more fish like salmon, sardines, and herring. You could also try taking 2 to 3 grams of a fish oil supplement daily, in divided doses with meals.

Get more greens. Dr. Lane's most recent research seems to indicate that foods high in the natural antioxidants lutein and zeaxanthin, especially when eaten raw, seem to be helpful in normalizing intraocular pressure. These foods include turnip greens, kale, collard greens, spinach, corn, yams, and broccoli.

Watch the protein powders. Recently, Dr. Lane has seen a lot more seemingly healthy men in their thirties and forties with glaucoma. The culprit, it seems, may be the large doses of protein powders these men are taking to build muscle. This protein, explains Dr. Lane, is stripped of all the nutrients, like vitamin B_6, that are essential for it to form high-quality eye proteins in the body. As a result, these lower-quality proteins seem to be contributing to restricted fluid movement in the eyes and the development of pigmentary glaucoma.

Dr. Lane adds that other proteins in our diet also contribute to this problem. But because these powders deliver protein in such high levels, it seems to be accelerating the process in some men.

ing the cells at the optic nerve head and in the retina, contributing to glaucoma.

People who suffer from type 2 (non-insulin-dependent) diabetes seem more likely to develop glaucoma, says Dr. Lane. And that's not surprising, he says, because both people with diabetes and those with glaucoma have been found to be low in chromium.

The best sources of chromium include Concord grape juice, red wine, egg yolks, brewer's yeast, and most unrefined foods rich in energy content. Consequently, ripe fresh sweet and starchy fruits and vegetables also contain more than adequate chromium, says Dr. Lane.

The Daily Value for chromium is 120 micrograms.

If you want to try chromium supplementation, discuss it with your doctor. This is especially important if you have diabetes, since chromium may cause your blood sugar level to drop and reduce your need for insulin. Your doctor should monitor your insulin level carefully while you're taking supplements.

Dr. Lane also notes that many people make the mistake of taking chromium at the same time that they take vitamin C. Vitamin C interferes with the uptake of chromium.

Prescriptions for Healing

It's important to be under a doctor's care if you have glaucoma. Uncontrolled, the disease can lead to blindness.

Doctors generally prescribe medication in the form of eye drops to treat glaucoma. If you'd like to try supplements as an adjunct to your treatment, discuss it with your ophthalmologist.

Some doctors recommend these nutrients to help treat glaucoma.

Nutrient	Daily Amount
Chromium	120 micrograms
Vitamin C	500–1,500 milligrams, taken as 2 divided doses

MEDICAL ALERT: *Nutritional therapy for glaucoma is not commonly practiced, nor is it for everyone. It is important to remain under a doctor's care if you have glaucoma and to continue using whatever medication your doctor prescribes.*

If you want to try chromium supplements, discuss it with your doctor. This is especially important if you have diabetes, since chromium may affect your blood sugar level. Also, many people make the mistake of taking chromium at the same time that they take vitamin C. Vitamin C interferes with the uptake of chromium.

Taking more than 1,200 milligrams of vitamin C daily can cause diarrhea in some people.

Vitamin C Lets Up on Pressure

Like chromium, vitamin C also seems to reduce intraocular pressure, but by a different method. Studies show that it apparently raises the acidity of the blood, explains Dr. Lane. "That in and of itself seems to help normalize intraocular pressure," he says. (Intraocular pressure is the pressure inside the eyeballs. In people with glaucoma, the pressure is too high, which eventually damages the blood circulation to and from the neural tissues in the eye.)

Vitamin C delivers yet another benefit for your eyes. Like chromium, it increases the efficiency of fuel utilization by the eye muscles, says Dr. Lane. Between 500 and 1,500 milligrams of vitamin C daily seems to work best. Any more than that increases the risk that the jellylike substance in your eye may gradually become more liquefied when exposed to too much sunlight, causing it to be pulled away from the retina and related structures at the back of the eye. (The retina contains a light-sensitive layer of cells that receives images.) "This is known as a posterior vitreous detachment, or PVD," says Dr. Lane. Taking more than 1,200 milligrams of vitamin C daily, however, can cause temporary diarrhea in some people.

Take part of your vitamin C with juice or fruit before breakfast in the morning, then allow at least one meal to go by before taking the rest, advises Dr. Lane. Vitamin C has a tendency to block the absorption of other essential nutrients such as copper and chromium, he says.

Nutritional therapy for glaucoma is not commonly practiced, nor is it for everyone. It is important to remain under a doctor's care if you have glaucoma and to continue using whatever medication your doctor prescribes. But do discuss your concerns with your doctor.

GOUT

FIGHT FOOT PAIN WITH FOOD

Gout is a funny condition in that its primary target is the big toe. But if you've ever suffered from a bout of this strange form of arthritis, you know that it's no laughing matter.

The pain of a gout attack is so intense that it defies mere words. Some have described gout as the feeling of your big toe being "on fire," but even that doesn't quite do it justice. What we do know about gout is that it often strikes in the middle of the night, and the pain is often strong enough that it will wake you up—and make even the weight of your blanket feel unbearable.

Interestingly enough, gout is one of the oldest recognized diseases in the world. In days gone by, gout was called the "disease of kings" because it was believed to be contracted by men who overindulged in rich foods and beverages.

Over the years, this belief has proven to be true in many cases. People who have more than two drinks every day are of particular risk for developing gout, and so are individuals who eat foods high in purines, a type of

Food Factors

Even if drugs control your gout, some doctors believe that it's wise to change your eating habits to avoid future attacks. That way, you can avoid taking drugs, with their unpleasant side effects. Plus you'll be eating heart-healthy fare.

In most cases, gout responds well to dietary changes. Here's what many doctors recommend.

Purge purines from your platter. Liver, beef, lamb, veal, shellfish, yeast, herring, sardines, mackerel, and anchovies are all high in purines, protein components that break down to form uric acid. Some legumes, such as lentils, peas, beans, and soybeans, also contain small amounts of purines. Doctors recommend avoiding these foods during a gout attack and limiting your intake of them between attacks.

Say good-bye to booze. Drinking alcohol causes a buildup of uric acid in the body because it increases uric acid production at the same time that it reduces uric acid excretion. That's why so many gout sufferers pay the price for a single episode of overindulgence. "Eliminating alcohol is all many people need to do to avoid attacks," says Joseph Pizzorno Jr., ND, president emeritus of Bastyr University in Seattle. If you do drink occasionally, stick to hard liquor or wine, both of which have fewer purines than beer.

Try cherries. Many people with gout swear that eating cherries helps quickly resolve attacks. Only one study, though, published in 1950, found that eating about a half-pound of fresh or canned Royal Ann or black Bing cherries a day helps lower uric acid levels. But it's worth a try.

"Cherries, hawthorn berries, blueberries, and other dark red-blue berries are rich sources of anthocyanidins and procyanidins," Dr. Piz-

protein that gets converted to uric acid in the body. These foods include rich meats such as veal and game; organ meats such as liver and kidneys; seafood like anchovies and scallops; and legumes like lentils, peas, and beans.

But rich food and drink aren't the only causes of gout. People with high blood pressure and heart disease (or those on high blood pressure medication) are more likely to suffer from gout, and about one in five people with gout can blame it on their genes. Men are also more likely than women to get the disease, but after menopause, a women's chances of developing the condition get closer to those of men. Gout is also not limited just to the big toe—in some people, the pain strikes the feet, ankles, wrists, and hands.

zorno explains. These compounds apparently help strengthen and prevent the destruction of the connective tissue that forms joints as well as inhibit tissue-destroying enzymes secreted by immune cells in the course of inflammation, he explains.

If a half-pound of cherries a day seems a bit extreme, you can also try drinking 8 to 16 ounces of cherry juice a day.

Go for the H$_2$O. Drinking lots of water keeps urine diluted and promotes the excretion of uric acid, says Jeffrey Lisse, MD, professor of medicine at the University of Arizona and the interim director of the Arizona Arthritis Center in Tucson. Drinking lots of nonalcoholic fluids during a bout of gout is particularly important. It prevents your kidneys from forming uric acid crystals, which can lead to damage and kidney stones.

Peel off the pounds. If you're overweight, reducing will lower uric acid levels, Dr. Pizzorno says. "A high-fiber, low-fat diet—fruits, vegetables, whole grains, beans, and the like—is the best way to go," he says.

Gradual weight loss is mandatory, however. Losing weight too fast also increases uric acid levels and can trigger an attack, says Dr. Lisse.

Try fish oil. The omega-3 fatty acids found in fish oil have been shown to be effective in controlling the pain and inflammation associated with gout. But since many of the fish that contain omega-3s naturally, like salmon and mackerel, also have purines, your best bet may be to try a fish oil supplement. Strive for 3 to 6 grams a day in divided doses with meals.

Eat pineapple. Pineapple contains high amounts of bromelain, an anti-inflammatory enzyme that can reduce the inflammation caused by gout.

The source of the pain is uric acid. Usually this is removed from the body through the urine, but the risk factors mentioned previously can sometimes cause too much of it to accumulate in the body. When this occurs, the acid sometimes gets deposited in the form of shardlike needles in the joints between the bones, where it causes the not-so-pleasant pain described earlier.

Since gout is often caused by dietary choices in the first place, the good news about the disease is that most cases respond nicely to dietary changes, says Joseph Pizzorno Jr., ND, president emeritus of Bastyr University in Seattle. "Dietary changes are all that many people need to control their symptoms," he says. For some, avoiding alcohol is all that's necessary. Others may need to cut back on both alcohol and certain foods, such as the aforementioned meats and legumes that are rich in purines.

Ironically, gout can also be induced by very-low-calorie diets—starvation diets, for example—which also increase blood levels of uric acid as the body begins to break down tissues, explains Jeffrey Lisse, MD, professor of medicine at the University of Arizona and the interim director of the Arizona Arthritis Center in Tucson.

Although individual nutrients are not the main dietary treatments for gout, there are a few that can prove helpful.

Folic Acid Dissolves Crystals

Some doctors recommend folic acid, a B vitamin that in large doses inhibits xanthine oxidase, the enzyme responsible for the body's production of uric acid. In fact, one prescription drug used to treat gout, allopurinol (Zyloprim), also inhibits this enzyme. "I wouldn't use folic acid alone, but it may be helpful to some people as part of a complete package of dietary changes and nutritional supplements," says Dr. Pizzorno. The vitamin won't resolve an acute attack, when uric acid crystals have already formed in a joint. But it may help ward off further attacks.

The recommended dosage, 10,000 to 40,000 micrograms of folic acid a day (25 to 100 times the Daily Value of 400 micrograms), is far more than is available from even the best food sources. "People must take supplements to get this large amount," Dr. Pizzorno says. And supplements in this large amount are available only by prescription. So if you'd like to try folic acid as a preventive measure, you'll have to discuss it with your physician.

Here's another good reason for taking large doses only under medical supervision: Not all studies find side effects at large doses, but in one that did,

Prescriptions for Healing

Dietary changes and drugs, not vitamins, are considered the primary strategies for preventing gout attacks. But some experts believe that these vitamins may provide an additional edge.

Nutrient	Daily Amount
Folic acid	10,000–40,000 micrograms
Vitamin E	400–800 IU

Plus a supplement containing the Daily Values of all the B-complex vitamins

MEDICAL ALERT: If you have symptoms of gout, you should see a doctor for proper diagnosis and treatment.

This dosage of folic acid is way beyond the Daily Value of 400 micrograms and is available only by prescription. Take this much folic acid only under medical supervision. Large doses of folic acid can mask symptoms of pernicious anemia, a disease resulting from vitamin B$_{12}$ deficiency.

If you are taking anticoagulant drugs, you should not take oral vitamin E supplements. (Though generally a dose of up to 1,500 IU of vitamin E a day is considered safe, some recent reports suggest that taking more than 400 IU a day could be harmful to people with cardiovascular or circulatory disease or with cancer. If you have such a condition, be sure to consult your doctor before you begin supplementation.)

people taking 15 milligrams (15,000 micrograms) of folic acid a day complained of nausea, bloating, problems sleeping, and irritability. Large doses of folic acid can also mask symptoms of pernicious anemia, a disease resulting from vitamin B$_{12}$ deficiency.

Since some experts contend that large doses of any one of the B-complex vitamins can cause shortages of others, your doctor probably will also have you take a supplement containing the entire B complex.

Vitamin E Adds Anti-Inflammatory Power

Some doctors add vitamin E to their gout-relieving prescriptions. While there are no studies to show that vitamin E alone can abort or prevent a gout attack, this vitamin has properties that may help dampen inflammation, Dr. Pizzorno says. He suggests 400 to 800 IU daily, both during and between attacks. (*Note:* If you are considering taking more than 400 IU of vitamin E daily, it's a good idea to discuss it with your doctor first.)

Vitamins to Banish

Two vitamins that you'll want to avoid in excess during a bout of gout are vitamin C and niacin. "Both increase uric acid levels in the body," Dr. Pizzorno says. By the way, low doses of aspirin, a commonly used anti-inflammatory drug, also increase blood levels of uric acid, says Dr. Lisse. So you'll want to avoid using it to relieve gout pain. "Any other nonsteroidal pain reliever is safe," he adds.

HAIR LOSS

KEEPING WHAT YOU HAVE

For some men, the search for a baldness cure is akin to the age-old search for the fountain of youth. The virility, attractiveness, and just overall masculinity associated with a full head of flowing hair is understandably something that many men would do anything to hold on to . . . and the insecurity associated with losing your hair is the reason so many hair loss products have been so successful.

But in reality, we're all losing our hair—all the time. On average, you lose 50 to 150 hairs a day. The difference between Fabio and your bald Uncle Frank is that people with full heads of hair are constantly regrowing new ones to fill in the empty spaces. With hereditary baldness, known medically as androgenetic alopecia, though, about one-third of men will someday notice that new hair is not growing back, sometimes as early as their teens. And they have nobody to blame but their family—specifically their mother's side of the family.

When it comes down to it, baldness is just something most men have to learn to live with. A couple of drugs, Rogaine (minoxidil) and Propecia (finasteride), can help some men regrow hair or prevent the loss of what they

Food Factors

What you eat may well have an effect on how good your hair looks, but there's little you can do in terms of diet that will have an impact on how much hair you have. Here are a couple of things that doctors say you can do for healthier hair.

Steer clear of crash diets. Trimming pounds gradually not only is healthier than crash dieting but also keeps your hair on your head. "Any woman who has lost 20 pounds or more in a period of three months is going to have a problem with hair loss," says Wilma Bergfeld, MD, a dermatologist and director of the section of dermatopathology and dermatological research at the Cleveland Clinic.

Pump up your iron. To boost iron absorption, some doctors also recommend drinking orange juice, which is high in vitamin C, whenever you eat foods high in iron, such as broccoli and red meat, says Alexander Zemtsov, MD, professor of dermatology at the Indiana University School of Medicine in Muncie.

Feed on fatty acids. Since hair loss is often related to hormonal imbalances, a diet rich in fatty acids, which form the biological backbone of many hormone molecules, may help. Strive for two or more servings of salmon, herring, and other fatty fish every week, or try a fish oil supplement.

have. But the results are mixed, and the effects of the drugs stop as soon as people stop taking them.

And unfortunately for men, the fountain of youth cannot be found through nutrition. (Sorry, guys. Except in cases of extreme malnutrition, no amount of vitamins or minerals will regrow hair.) But for some women who have experienced hair loss related to physical trauma, crash dieting, or heavy menstrual flow, certain nutrients can help.

Iron and the Maiden

When a woman loses iron because of something such as trauma, poor diet, or heavy menstruation, several things happen. Among them: Her body literally stops producing hair until she gets more iron.

"I've been practicing medicine for more than 30 years now, and it's my experience that in most females who are menstruating regularly, there is mild to severe iron deficiency anemia," says Wilma Bergfeld, MD, a dermatologist and director of the section of dermatopathology and dermatological research at the Cleveland Clinic. Dermatopathology is the study of the causes and effects of skin diseases and abnormalities.

But getting enough iron is only part of the picture, says Alexander Zemtsov, MD, professor of dermatology at the Indiana University School of Medicine in Muncie.

Because iron absorption is boosted by vitamin C, he recommends talking to your doctor about a prescription for Niferex with vitamin C. Each capsule contains 50 milligrams of iron and 100 milligrams of vitamin C. Or you can get over-the-counter Niferex, which has 50 milligrams of iron, and take it with 100 milligrams of vitamin C. "I recommend taking one of these capsules a day until the hair is back to normal, usually in two to three months," says Dr. Zemtsov.

High daily intake of iron can cause iron overload in some people. For this reason, doses exceeding the Daily Value (18 milligrams) should be taken only under medical supervision.

Prescriptions for Healing

Except in cases of starvation, it doesn't seem that vitamins and minerals affect hair growth in men. On the other hand, nutrients may prove helpful for some women who have experienced hair loss. Here's what the experts recommend.

Nutrient	Daily Amount
Iron	50 milligrams (Niferex)
Vitamin C	100 milligrams
Zinc	30 milligrams

Plus a multivitamin/mineral supplement containing the Daily Values of all essential vitamins and minerals

MEDICAL ALERT: *High daily intake of iron can cause iron overload in some people. For this reason, doses exceeding the Daily Value (18 milligrams) should be taken only under medical supervision.*

Do not take more than 15 milligrams of zinc a day unless under medical supervision.

Taking a Little Insurance

In rare cases, nutritional deficiencies in certain vitamins can lead to hair loss. "Biotin deficiency is characterized by brittle hair and nails," says Stephen Schleicher, MD, clinical instructor of dermatology at King's College and Arcadia University in Pennsylvania and director of the DERMDx Centers for Dermatology. "And dietary zinc deficiency will produce a skin rash, hair loss, and diarrhea."

In particular, if your hair loss is related to a zinc deficiency, taking 30 milligrams of zinc daily may help hair begin growing back in as little as a week. You'll want to talk to your doctor before taking this much zinc, however.

Other nutrients, such as vitamin C, iron, and folate, among others, also seem to play a role in hair growth. So the best advice may be to take a multivitamin/mineral supplement to cover all your nutritional bases.

"Biotin, for example, appears to enhance hair growth, thicken fibers, and diminish shedding. But all of these nutrients sort of do the same thing," says Dr. Bergfeld. "What we're talking about is fitting multiple pieces together. There are just so many factors that it's hard to isolate which one is the most important."

Further strengthening the argument for taking a multivitamin/mineral supplement is that many older people get fewer nutrients, says Dr. Bergfeld. "As women get into their forties and fifties, medical conditions that exaggerate hair loss include reduction of female hormones, thyroid disorders, and diabetes. The frequent necessity for drug therapy for medical conditions can also exaggerate hair loss," she says.

Some Promises Don't Wash

What about feeding your hair from the outside? Some ads for shampoos and conditioners that contain nutrients make it sound like your hair needs an infusion of what these products provide to stay lush and healthy.

"These really aren't very helpful," says Dr. Bergfeld. "They can help hair have the appearance of body and fullness by temporarily swelling the hair shafts, but that's about it."

Hair care products can't help hair grow because the hair on your head is dead. The only way nutrients can affect hair growth is if they make it to the scalp, where hair is produced, explains Dr. Zemtsov. "You can put whatever you like on there," he says. "But if it doesn't penetrate about a half-centimeter or deeper into the scalp to reach the hair follicle—and it never will—it doesn't work." Nutrition must come from the inside.

HEART ARRHYTHMIA

SUBDUING THE ELECTRICAL STORMS OF THE HEART

No biological action within the body is more integral to your life and your health than the heartbeat. And most of us hardly give it a second thought as it beats away—70 or so times a minute, 4,200 times an hour, and 108,000 times a day—delivering blood to the body's 62,000 miles of arteries, veins, and capillaries.

Yet as critical as a heartbeat is, it's an incredibly intricate, highly coordinated event. For things to go off without a hitch, a number of things have to go right—over and over again.

It all starts with the sinus node, a small grouping of cells in your right atrium. (The atria are the upper two chambers of the heart; the ventricles are the lower chambers.) This node sends an electrical impulse to the atria, which causes them to contract and in turn force blood into the relaxed ventricles.

From the atria, this electrical impulse travels downward to the atrioventricular node in the center of the heart. It then travels further into the ventricles, causing them to contract and release blood into the body, where it travels to all your vital organs.

As you can see, there are a lot of things that can go wrong in the seemingly simple process of a heartbeat. And when they do, the results can vary wildly—from nonthreatening conditions that cause painful symptoms to life-threatening events with no symptoms. And all these various types of irregular heartbeats are classified under the name "arrhythmia."

There are dozens of different types of arrhythmias, but doctors divide up the conditions in a couple of different ways. One method of classification is the speed at which the heart is beating. Tachycardia refers to a heart rate greater than 100 beats per minute, and bradycardia refers to a resting heart rate less than 60 beats per minute.

Arrhythmias are also subdivided based on where they occur in the heart: the atria or the ventricles. While both can cause symptoms and discomfort at times, the most dangerous arrhythmias occur in the ventricles. In fact, over 300,000 Americans die every year from ventricular fibrillation, a frightening condition in which the ventricles stop contracting properly and cease pumping blood.

"People with serious arrhythmia are usually under a doctor's care," says Michael A. Brodsky, MD, a staff cardiologist and cardiac electrophysiologist at Kaiser Permanente in Honolulu. Indeed, it's often a doctor who discovers the problem, since arrhythmia frequently has no apparent symptoms, he adds.

But sometimes an arrhythmia will give you a clue that something is wrong, such as chest fluttering, a racing heartbeat, a slow heartbeat, or chest pain. An arrhythmia can also reduce the bloodflow throughout the body, in which case you may experience symptoms such as dizziness, shortness of breath, and even lightheadedness or fainting.

What makes the heart get out of sync? In serious cases, disease of the coronary arteries or heart muscle is the most likely cause, Dr. Brodsky says. But in some cases, and often in conjunction with heart disease, mineral imbalances interfere with the heart's normal nerve function.

Nutritional therapy for arrhythmia focuses on two minerals in particular: magnesium and potassium. Nerve cells make use of both to help fire off messages, and a shortage of either one can cause life-threatening problems.

Here's what research has to say about these two heart-healthy minerals.

Magnesium Helps Hearts Stay Regular

Several studies have shown that when it comes to certain types of arrhythmia, magnesium can save lives.

One study found that the risk of developing potentially fatal ventricular arrhythmia was reduced by more than half in people with heart failure who received large intravenous doses of magnesium compared with those who did not receive the mineral.

Intravenous magnesium is now considered standard therapy for two types of arrhythmia: torsades de pointes, an unusual type of ventricular arrhythmia, and ventricular arrhythmia induced by digitalis, a commonly prescribed heart drug.

And researchers are doing preliminary work to see if people with heart disease who take oral magnesium supplements can reduce their chances of developing arrhythmia.

In the meantime, Dr. Brodsky tests all of his heart patients for magnesium deficiency. He prescribes oral magnesium supplements or intravenous magnesium when blood levels are low and sometimes oral supplements when blood levels are normal but symptoms suggest it might help. "If blood levels are low, you can be pretty sure someone is deficient," Dr. Brodsky says. "But people can have low tissue stores of magnesium and still have normal blood levels."

One thing on which more doctors than ever apparently agree is that a fair number of people with heart problems can benefit from getting enough

Food Factors

Mineral balance plays an important role in regulating heartbeat. But other dietary factors can also throw your heart out of sync. Here are two items to avoid and two to add to your anti-arrhythmia diet.

Go fish. Howard N. Hodis, MD, director of the atherosclerosis research unit at the University of Southern California School of Medicine in Los Angeles, says that the omega-3 fatty acids found in fatty fish like salmon and mackerel, as well as fish oil supplements, have shown great promise in promoting regular heartbeat and preventing arrhythmia.

"There's quite a bit of evidence around the world that those with a high intake of fish have a low incidence of heart disease," says Dr. Hodis. "When that was taken into randomized trials, it appears that the protection may be from sudden death, which is an arrhythmia-induced event, not a coronary disease event. So it looks like fish may be effective in preventing arrhythmic death. But the exact mechanism is not known."

Nevertheless, what is known is that fish rich in omega-3s not only seem to be helpful for overall heart health but also may play a role in preventing arrhythmia.

To derive the benefits of omega-3 fatty acids, Dr. Hodis recommends replacing the beef, chicken, and dairy products in your diet with fish like salmon and mackerel a few times a week. You also may want to consider taking 1 to 4 grams a day of a fish oil supplement, in divided doses with meals.

"Omacor is a reliable fish oil supplement to try," says Dr. Hodis. "It's been approved by the FDA, so you can at least be assured that the levels of fatty acids in this product are fairly consistent."

magnesium. "I'd say 50 to 60 percent of the people I see have at least mild magnesium deficiencies," Dr. Brodsky says.

Getting Enough Magnesium

Magnesium deficiency can be induced by the very drugs meant to help heart problems. Some types of diuretics (water pills) cause the body to excrete both magnesium and potassium, as does digitalis. And magnesium deficiency is often at the bottom of what's called refractory potassium deficiency, Dr. Brodsky adds. "The amount of magnesium in the body determines the amount of a particular enzyme that determines the amount of potassium in the body,"

Hold on to heart-healthy foods. Though arrhythmias have many causes, clogged arteries and other heart disease symptoms are strong risk factors. So doctors recommend the basic tenets of a heart-healthy diet to their arrhythmia patients as well. Those include eating plenty of fruits and vegetables; choosing whole grains that are high in fiber; and reducing red meat, dairy, and other sources of saturated fat in favor of heart-healthy fish. For more information on eating a heart-healthy diet, see the Heart Disease chapter on page 290 and the High Blood Pressure chapter on page 301.

Stick to herbal brews. A small amount of caffeine (less than 300 milligrams a day, about 3 cups of brewed coffee) doesn't seem to cause many problems. But more than this amount may aggravate heartbeat irregularities, some experts say.

Be a party pooper. When it comes to heavy drinking, evidence is firm: People who abuse alcohol not only have a higher than normal risk of heartbeat irregularities but are also more likely to die suddenly and unexpectedly, a fate that may be linked to fatal arrhythmia. Even moderate drinking—no more than a drink or two a day—may increase your risk by depleting body stores of magnesium and potassium.

Not everyone with arrhythmia needs to stop drinking entirely, says Michael A. Brodsky, MD, a staff cardiologist and cardiac electrophysiologist at Kaiser Permanente in Honolulu, Hawaii. "I tell people to keep diaries of the foods they eat and drink, their activities, and their symptoms," he explains. "If we see a trend develop, they may have to make some behavior changes, such as cutting back on alcohol."

he explains. "So if you are magnesium-deficient, you may in turn be potassium-deficient, and no amount of potassium is going to correct this unless you are also getting enough magnesium."

If you have arrhythmia, talk to your doctor about the possibility of magnesium supplementation, Dr. Brodsky suggests. Have your blood level of magnesium checked, and if you start taking magnesium supplements, have your blood levels of magnesium and potassium checked regularly, especially if you are taking large amounts of either of these minerals.

"How much magnesium you need to take depends on the results of your blood tests," Dr. Brodsky says. "Not everyone needs to take the same amount."

Dr. Brodsky gives his patients supplements of magnesium lactate. Both magnesium lactate and magnesium gluconate are easily absorbed and are less likely to cause diarrhea than magnesium oxide and magnesium hydroxide, the other forms of magnesium. (Magnesium hydroxide is found in Phillips' Milk of Magnesia, Mylanta, and Maalox.)

Prescriptions for Healing

To prevent potential problems with heart arrhythmia, experts recommend aiming for the Daily Values of these two nutrients.

Nutrient	Daily Amount
Magnesium	400 milligrams
Potassium	3,500 milligrams

MEDICAL ALERT: If you have been diagnosed with a heart arrhythmia, you should be under a doctor's care.

Mineral balance is important to a beating heart, but people with irregular heartbeats should take mineral supplements only under medical supervision. That's because the amounts of minerals they need to take depend on their blood levels, which must be carefully monitored.

People with heart or kidney problems should check with their doctor before taking supplemental magnesium.

Potassium supplements should not be taken by those with diabetes or kidney disease or by those using certain medications, including nonsteroidal anti-inflammatory drugs, potassium-sparing diuretics, ACE inhibitors, and heart medications such as heparin.

"I generally give my patients either Slow-Mag or Mag-Tab, up to about six tablets—about 450 milligrams—a day," Dr. Brodsky says.

He has found that magnesium can help heart medications such as digoxin work better. "Most people won't be able to go off their drugs completely, but they may be able to cut their dosages," Dr. Brodsky says. It's important to cut dosage slowly, over time, with your doctor's supervision, he adds. Stopping abruptly could make your heart problems worse.

Although magnesium is considered to be a fairly safe mineral, even in high doses, don't take supplemental magnesium without medical supervision if you have kidney or heart problems. Your heart rate or breathing could slow down too much.

Studies have shown that men get about 320 milligrams of magnesium daily, while women average 230 milligrams. The highest concentrations of magnesium are found in whole seeds such as legumes, nuts, and unmilled grains. Bananas and green vegetables are also good sources.

Potassium Powers Healthy Hearts

There's no doubt that potassium is just as important as magnesium for regular heartbeat. And doctors know it. In heart patients, low potassium levels are likely to be recognized and quickly corrected. Heartbeat irregularities, along with muscle weakness and confusion, are among the classic signs of potassium deficiency.

"Unlike magnesium, potassium levels are carefully regulated in the kidneys, and the body normally conserves potassium," Dr. Brodsky says. People who have normal kidney function and healthy hearts usually have adequate blood levels of potassium, even if they eat only a serving or two of fruits and vegetables a day.

People run into severe potassium deficiency that causes heart arrhythmia only when something interferes with the kidneys' potassium-hoarding tendency. "People who take thiazide diuretics or digitalis, who have poorly functioning kidneys, or who are alcoholics often become low in potassium unless they take supplements," Dr. Brodsky says. Prolonged diarrhea or vomiting and laxative abuse can also cause dangerously low potassium levels.

Here again, the amount of potassium each person should take depends on blood levels of this mineral. Too much potassium is as bad as too little, which is one reason potassium supplements containing more than 99 milligrams per tablet (the amount found in a bite or two of potato) are available only by prescription. Potassium supplements should not be taken by those with diabetes or kidney disease or by those using certain medications, including nonsteroidal anti-inflammatory drugs, potassium-sparing diuretics, ACE inhibitors, and heart medications such as heparin.

The Daily Value for potassium is 3,500 milligrams. Studies show that among the general population, intakes vary widely—anywhere from 1,000 to 3,400 milligrams a day. Eating lots of fruits, vegetables, and fresh meats and drinking juices is the way to pack in the most potassium. A medium banana supplies 451 milligrams of potassium, 1 cup of cubed cantaloupe supplies 494 milligrams, and 1 cup of cooked cabbage supplies 146 milligrams.

Other Electrolytes

Along with magnesium and potassium, imbalances of sodium and calcium in the body have also been implicated in arrhythmias. Though supplementation of these two minerals is not usually recommended, it's worth asking your doctor about the role that these two minerals can play in your arrhythmia.

HEART DISEASE

KEEPING YOUR HEART'S PATHWAYS CLEAR

Few diseases are the subject of more study, research, and press than heart disease. And despite everything we have learned about the disease, one simple fact remains: No disease kills more people every year. In the year 2004 alone, more than 650,000 people in the United States lost their lives to heart disease.

Though heart disease is often considered a "man's disease," the statistics seem to suggest otherwise. In the United States, 41 percent of deaths in women are attributable to heart disease. In fact, women are more than 10 times more likely to die of heart disease than of breast cancer.

Okay, enough bad news: The good news is we know more than ever before about your heart health. And the nutrients you take in through diet and supplements can play a major role in keeping it healthy.

The Basics of a Healthy Heart

For several years now, doctors have known that the most important ways to prevent a heart attack are to avoid tobacco smoke, eat a low-cholesterol diet, keep dietary fat to a minimum, strive for 30 minutes of physical activity every day, and reduce stress across the board.

But researchers are learning a lot more beyond just eating a healthy diet about how specific nutrients in food impact the health of your heart and circulatory system. In particular, the antioxidants vitamin C, vitamin E, and selenium seem to play a role in neutralizing free radical molecules that are linked to some forms of heart disease. And zinc is necessary to promote the absorption of these antioxidants. The B vitamins (B_6, B_{12}, and folic acid), keep the body's levels of homocysteine in check, thus preventing the formation of plaque. And excess iron may play a role in the formation of free radicals and may contribute to heart problems.

Over the next few pages, we'll explain how these nutrients and others found in common foods can help you shape a heart-healthy diet regimen, thus keeping your ticker going strong for years to come.

Understanding the Disease

To comprehend just how powerfully nutrients protect your arteries, you need to take a look at what causes heart disease to begin with.

Most heart disease, including angina and electrical problems that are responsible for sudden cardiac death, is actually caused by atherosclerosis, a condition in which cholesterol and cells roaming your bloodstream build up along the walls of coronary arteries and cause them to narrow. Narrowing reduces the flow of blood to the heart and increases the chance that a bunch of blood cells might clump together and get wedged in the artery. When that happens, or if an artery suddenly spasms, bloodflow to the heart is cut off, triggering a heart attack.

Sometimes referred to as hardening of the arteries, atherosclerosis is a silent process that can begin in childhood. It starts when the cells lining an artery are damaged by constant pounding from high blood pressure, by repeated exposure to toxic chemicals such as those in cigarette smoke, by repeated exposure to high concentrations of LDL cholesterol, or even by a bacterial or viral infection.

Once the damage occurs, the body tries to repair it. LDL cholesterol and blood cells called monocytes are attracted to the site, where they try to patch

Food Factors

What you eat—and what you don't eat—in large part determines whether you eventually develop heart disease. Here are a few tips to help you keep the number one killer in this country at bay.

Cut the fat. "We need to follow the American Heart Association's Step I guidelines," says Howard N. Hodis, MD, director of the atherosclerosis research unit at the University of Southern California School of Medicine in Los Angeles. "In general, that means a total cholesterol intake of less than 300 milligrams a day and a total fat intake of less than 30 percent of total calories a day."

Most Americans get approximately 40 percent of their calories from fat. You can lower the amount of fat in your diet by cutting back on fatty meats and whole-fat dairy products; avoiding fast foods, candies, and most baked goods; and eating more fruits and vegetables.

Get hooked on fish. Of all the foods for saving your heart, fish may show the most promise, says Dr. Hodis. The omega-3 fatty acids found in fish such as salmon and mackerel can reduce abnormal blood clots, improve blood vessel function, decrease triglyceride levels, and lower the risk of irregular heartbeat. "Omega-3 fatty acids appear to be effective in preventing a second heart attack in men who have already had one," says Dr. Hodis. "Also, a number of epidemiological studies have shown that populations that eat a lot of fish have lower symptoms of heart disease."

In addition to striving to eat fish rich in omega-3s at least twice a week, experts also recommend taking 3 to 5 grams of a fish oil supplement every day, in divided doses with meals.

---

the damage. When that fails, cells from other areas of the arterial wall move in and form a protective mat, usually referred to as plaque, over the injury. The plaque hardens as it takes up calcium, and it continues to grow until it protrudes into the artery's hollow interior.

This condition gradually develops into the most common form of heart disease: coronary artery disease. Eventually, the plaque can narrow the artery's interior enough to slow the flow of blood to your heart and cause chest paint, or angina. When the blockage becomes so severe that blood no longer flows through the heart, you can experience a heart attack. Common symptoms of a heart attack include chest pain that lasts more than a few minutes or extends to the shoulder, arm, back, teeth, or jaw; sweating; shortness of breath; nausea and vomiting; and lightheadedness.

Eat your fruits and veggies. A Dutch study of more than 800 men between the ages of 65 and 84 found that the more bioflavonoids these guys consumed (they got them from tea, onions, and apples), the less likely they were to die of heart disease.

Bioflavonoids, chemical compounds related to vitamin C that may neutralize "bad" LDL cholesterol and reduce the tendency of red blood cells to stick together and block arteries, are found in nearly all plants, so fruits and vegetables are likely to be good sources.

Another easy tip for getting more bioflavonoids is that the deeper the color of the fruit or vegetable, the more bioflavonoids it probably has. So spinach, carrots, and berries are often better choices than potatoes or corn.

Dine on soy. Soy products such as tofu contain isoflavones, which are naturally occurring substances that may prevent the formation of plaque on artery walls.

Don't forget the garlic. Several studies indicate that one-half to one clove of garlic, eaten daily, can significantly lower total cholesterol. High cholesterol is a major risk factor for heart disease.

Have a glass. Although alcohol is considered a no-no for many conditions, a glass of red wine for heart health is generally smiled upon. That's because it contains 640 micrograms of resveratrol, a substance that studies have shown to have heart-protecting effects. It's not only a strong antioxidant, but it seems to prevent inflammation in blood vessels as well. If you're leery about the wine, resveratrol is also abundant in Concord grape juice.

The Role of Antioxidants

When it comes to staving off atherosclerosis and the possibility of a heart attack, doctors often rely on the standard advice: Stop smoking, stay away from foods high in cholesterol and saturated fat, and get plenty of exercise. But beyond that, can specific antioxidants play a role in preventing a heart attack? According to Howard N. Hodis, MD, director of the atherosclerosis research unit at the University of Southern California School of Medicine in Los Angeles, the jury is still out.

"We now have sufficient data in both men and women to suggest that antioxidant vitamins, either individually, specifically vitamin E, or in combination, as with vitamins E, C, and selenium, don't have much effect on atherosclerosis or cardiovascular disease outcome," says Dr. Hodis. "The data is pretty neutral. Where there may be benefits are in those who have low levels, basically deficiency of antioxidants. [In these people] the nutrients may be effective in reducing atherosclerosis or [improving] cardiovascular outcome."

Also, adds Dr. Hodis, where studies are lacking is in those who begin taking antioxidant vitamins at a very early age. "I don't believe any studies are currently going on to see if this is helpful," he says.

Now, before you throw away all your vitamins, Dr. Hodis says that anti-oxidants can still play a role in your overall heart health. "Clearly antioxidant defenses are needed," he says. "Free radicals are the producers of almost all the biochemical reactions in our bodies. They have to be sucked up by an antioxidant. So if you don't have enough antioxidants, you are going to be at risk for all kinds of chronic diseases like cancer and heart disease."

Based on the most current research, these are the antioxidants that appear to play a role in our heart health.

The Mixed Message on Vitamin E

Few nutrients have taken us on a roller-coaster ride in recent years quite like vitamin E. Lately, a slew of studies have called the effectiveness of vitamin E at preventing heart disease into question.

Until just a few years ago, the evidence that vitamin E could prevent heart disease looked quite promising. First, vitamin E was shown to have powerful antioxidant properties. In additional studies, it appeared that this antioxidant potential could prevent the slippery slope of events that led to heart disease: oxidation of fats, platelet aggregation, and clogged arteries.

These smaller studies were soon followed by larger epidemiological stud-ies, such as the Nurses Health Study and the Health Professionals Study, both of which indicated that vitamin E caused a significant decrease in heart disease risk. In the Nurses Health Study, which involved 121,000 female nurses between ages 30 and 55, the women who took 200 IU of vitamin E a day had a 34 percent lower heart disease risk than those who took just 3 IU per day.

Recently, however, the tide has turned on vitamin E. More current ran-domized trials have shown no significant benefit of taking vitamin E supple-ments for your heart health. One prominent trial in particular, the Heart Outcomes Prevention Evaluation (HOPE), concluded that 400 IU of vitamin

E a day had no more effect on heart health than a placebo in the more than 10,000 patients studied.

So what went wrong with vitamin E? The problem, says Christopher Gardner, PhD, of the Stanford Prevention Research Center at Stanford University Medical Center, is that the whole story wasn't in before people began getting excited about it. "The original studies were very small and rather crude. Then the larger epidemiological studies didn't isolate vitamin E, so there's a good chance that those who took vitamin E were also doing a lot of other healthy stuff," he says. "As a result, people believed vitamin E was helping, when in reality it probably wasn't making a whole lot of difference."

To make things worse, in 2004 the American Heart Association concluded that those who take more than 400 IU of vitamin E a day face a greater risk of death than those who do not. These findings were based on the analysis of death rates in 14 studies of vitamin E from 1993 to 2004.

Because of this glut of new evidence against vitamin E, most of the experts we spoke with advised against vitamin E supplementation. Instead, they recommended sticking near the Daily Value of vitamin E (30 IU) through food and multivitamins. Rich food sources of vitamin E include soy, sunflower seeds, whole grains, and spinach.

Though the news for vitamin E doesn't look so good right now, Walter Willett, MD, DrPH, professor of epidemiology and nutrition at the Harvard School of Public Health, says that more research is needed before counting it out completely. In the recent Women's Health Study of almost 40,000 women, for example, overall cardiovascular deaths were 23 percent lower in the vitamin E group than the placebo group. "I think the odds are about 50-50 as to whether vitamin E has benefit for reducing heart disease in people who don't already have it," says Dr. Willett. "In such a situation, it seems reasonable to wait for further evidence before taking it."

Beta-Carotene: Preventing Heart Attacks

Although sometimes overshadowed in the lab by vitamin E, beta-carotene, the nutrient that gives carrots their color, is a champion on the dinner plate when it comes to fighting heart disease.

One study after another touts the heart-healthy benefits of beta-carotene, beginning with the Physicians' Health Study at Harvard Medical School. In this study, a group of 333 men between the ages of 40 and 84 who had severe heart disease were given 50 milligrams (83,000 IU) of beta-carotene every other day. Beta-carotene had no effect on the men's conditions during the first year. But from the second year on, the men's risk of heart attack was literally cut in half.

Researchers across the board resoundingly recommend eating five or more servings of fruits and vegetables a day, including some servings rich in carotenoids, to protect yourself against heart disease. They are less likely to recommend beta-carotene supplements.

Why would beta-carotene in the diet be better than beta-carotene in a gelcap? "One possibility is that in some of these studies, it's not just the beta-carotene that's good for you, it's also something else," says Dexter Morris, MD, PhD, clinical associate professor at the University of North Carolina at Chapel Hill School of Medicine. Beta-carotene represents only one-fifth of the most common carotenoids found in orange and yellow fruits and vegetables. So it's entirely possible that whether you get your beta-carotene from a carrot or from a gelcap full of carrot oil, these other carotenoids may contribute to some of the effect that's being credited to beta-carotene.

"A second possibility is that there may be a kind of therapeutic window for beta-carotene," Dr. Morris continues. "In other words, some is good, but too much may cause problems. There's one theory, for example, that at higher levels, beta-carotene may interfere with the protective effects of something else." Just what that might be is pure speculation, he says.

A Warning about Beta-Carotene

Despite the seeming helpfulness of beta-carotene, Dr. Hodis has an important bit of advice in regard to the nutrient. "One thing we learned in two large studies about beta-carotene is that in smokers, there was actually a worse outcome in terms of cancer, death, and cardiovascular disease," he says. "So it appears that in concert with smoking, beta-carotene becomes even a worse actor. Certainly smokers should not be taking beta-carotene."

The main concern here came from a mammoth study of 29,000 male Finnish smokers that was designed to tell whether beta-carotene and other synthetic supplements can prevent lung cancer and heart disease.

The problem is that most researchers expected to find that the supplements either reduced the chances of cancer and heart disease in the Finns or didn't do anything at all. Instead, the researchers found that male smokers who took 20 milligrams (about 33,000 IU) of synthetic beta-carotene a day actually increased their risk of both diseases.

Some researchers have attributed this finding to the fact that heavy smokers are frequently heavy drinkers, and heavy drinking destroys beta-carotene in the body. Other researchers feel that taking a high dose of beta-carotene may inhibit the absorption or effect of other antioxidants. "The mechanism is not known. It's hypothesized that beta-carotene has a pro-oxidant effect in this regard," says Dr. Hodis. "But the message is clear that if you smoke, don't take these supplements."

Vitamin C: The Antioxidant Attack Ship

Like many of the other antioxidants, the signals coming in on vitamin C and heart disease are mixed. Some real-life studies indicate that after a decade of looking good in the laboratory, vitamin C may not do as much as scientists had hoped. But other studies indicate that it clearly contributes to preventing heart disease.

When researchers at UCLA checked the amounts of vitamin C taken by more than 11,000 men and women between the ages of 25 and 74, for example, they found that people who got more than 50 milligrams of vitamin C a day, in addition to a multivitamin/mineral supplement, reduced their risk of death from cardiovascular disease by 28 percent.

Like the other antioxidants on our list, your best bet for getting your daily dose of vitamin C is from foods, such as citrus fruit, pineapple, broccoli, peppers, and strawberries. But some experts recommend taking a separate vitamin C supplement in the range of 250 to 500 milligrams a day.

Beef Up on B Vitamins

Antioxidants like vitamin C, vitamin E, and beta-carotene fight heart disease by destroying free radicals that accumulate in the bloodstream. In a similar fashion, the B vitamins (B_6, B_{12}, and folic acid) regulate homocysteine levels. Several years ago, researchers discovered that people who have elevated blood levels of homocysteine, an amino acid found in meats that can damage arterial walls and contribute to the development of atherosclerosis, frequently suffer from severe atherosclerosis and heart attacks in their twenties and thirties.

Some seem to have a genetic defect that makes their bodies unable to use homocysteine. But others seem to be suffering from deficiencies of vitamin B_6, vitamin B_{12}, or folate.

Prescriptions for Healing

Sam Sugar, MD, a physician with the Pritikin Longevity Center and Spa in Aventura, Florida, sums up the feelings of a number of our experts when it comes to heart disease and the whole foods versus supplements debate.

"There is no question in our minds here at the Pritikin Longevity Center that nutrients need to come from food," he says. "That, along with changes in lifestyle, is clearly the best way to prevent or regress heart disease."

That being said, there's no reason you can't focus your diet on the key nutrients mentioned here to equip yourself against this nation's biggest health threat. By focusing on fruits, vegetables, and whole grains that are high in vitamin E, vitamin C, beta-carotene, selenium, zinc, and magnesium, you'll be well on your way to a healthy heart. And if you feel the need for additional support, talk to your doctor about the possibilities of supplements. The experts we spoke with recommended the following dosages as being safe.

Nutrient	Daily Amount
Vitamin C	60–250 milligrams
Vitamin E	60–100 IU

In addition, there's one supplement that, while not a vitamin or mineral, all our experts recommended for your heart health.

Nutrient	Daily Amount
Omega-3 fatty acids	3–5 grams of fish oil per day, in divided doses, with meals

Researchers are still not certain what causes excess levels of homocysteine in the blood, but they're beginning to figure out how to reduce them.

"Folate prevents the buildup of homocysteine," says Frank M. Sacks, MD, professor of medicine and nutrition at Harvard School of Public Health.

In one study, researchers from Tufts University in Boston, the Clinical Research Institute of Montreal, and the Hospital Hôtel-Dieu, also in Montreal, worked with 150 men and women between ages 28 and 59 with heart disease. They found that homocysteine levels can be reduced by taking either 50 milligrams of vitamin B_6 or 5,000 micrograms of folic acid every day.

Since these amounts are between 12 and 25 times the Daily Values of

Several other nutrients also play roles in heart health. Because low levels of these nutrients seem to raise the risk of heart disease, most doctors recommend that people be sure to get the Daily Values of these nutrients through a well-balanced diet and, if necessary, a multivitamin/mineral supplement.

Nutrient	Daily Amount
Folic acid	400 micrograms
Selenium	70–100 micrograms
Zinc	15 milligrams

MEDICAL ALERT: *If you have heart disease, you should discuss vitamin and mineral supplementation with your doctor.*

The recommendations for the antioxidants vitamin C and vitamin E exceed the Daily Values of these nutrients. A wide range is recommended for each vitamin because the exact amount consumed would vary from person to person.

If you are taking anticoagulant drugs, you should not take vitamin E supplements. (Though generally a dose of up to 1,500 IU of vitamin E a day is considered safe, some recent reports suggest that taking more than 400 IU a day could be harmful to people with cardiovascular or circulatory disease or with cancer. If you have such a condition, be sure to consult your doctor before you begin supplementation.)

Selenium in doses exceeding 400 micrograms daily should be taken only under medical supervision.

these vitamins, however, the researchers opted not to recommend such high doses until further studies reveal the long-term effects. (Vitamin B$_6$ is already known to cause nerve damage in high doses.) Lower doses may be as effective, but clinical trials are ongoing, says Jacques Genest Jr., MD, director of the cardiovascular genetics laboratory at the Clinical Research Institute of Montreal, who led the study.

In the meantime, advises Dr. Sacks, "eat some spinach or take a regular multivitamin/mineral supplement." That should help you meet the Daily Value of folic acid (400 micrograms) and help keep homocysteine levels low enough to prevent a big buildup to begin with.

Meet the Fighting Trio

Aside from helping you meet your folate requirement, a well-balanced diet that emphasizes vegetables may help prevent heart disease for other reasons as well.

Researchers have found that low levels of at least three elements—selenium, zinc, and magnesium, generally found in meats, seafood, cereals, and vegetables—seem to increase your risk of heart disease.

In a study in Denmark of nearly 3,000 men between the ages of 53 and 74, researchers found that those with the lowest levels of selenium in their diets increased their risk of heart disease by 55 percent. What's more, the researchers suspected that close to 19 percent of the heart attacks among men in the study might in fact be caused by low levels of this nutrient.

The Daily Value for selenium is 70 micrograms. Most researchers agree, however, that you can take up to 400 micrograms daily without harm.

Zinc might also play a role in preventing atherosclerosis, researchers say. Laboratory studies at the University of Kentucky in Lexington indicate that zinc may be necessary to safeguard the heart's arterial walls from the damage triggered by high blood pressure, high cholesterol, and tobacco smoke, which sets the whole atherosclerotic process into motion.

Zinc is involved in repairing and fortifying any breaches in the cells lining the heart's arteries. So it's possible that zinc can help prevent atherosclerosis by keeping arterial walls in such good shape that cholesterol and fatty acids do not enter the artery walls to form artery-clogging plaque.

Zinc also has a third critical role, says Dr. Hodis. "Zinc is thought to be a necessary cation to the antioxidant vitamins," he says. "In other words, it helps them work the way they do."

The Daily Value for zinc is 15 milligrams a day.

Magnesium is of interest for its role in congestive heart failure, a secondary condition that can result from heart disease. Studies have shown that people with congestive heart failure often have deficient levels of magnesium. Interestingly enough, magnesium is also given intravenously as a treatment after a heart attack. Most people don't get the recommend 400 milligrams a day of magnesium from foods such as brown rice, spinach, oatmeal, potatoes, beans, and bananas, so it may be worth asking your doctor if magnesium supplementation is right for you.

A Word about Iron

One nutrient that has been quite a conundrum in heart disease research is iron. Although researchers once thought it was useful in preventing heart disease, it's now believed that excess iron may be a factor in actually causing heart disease in the first place.

"As time goes on, there is more and more data that indicates that iron is a platform for free radical formation," says Dr. Hodis. "So there is evidence that iron has a relationship with heart disease and cardiovascular events."

The newest research, says Dr. Hodis, is looking into the role of chelation therapy in removing excess iron from the body to see if it plays any role in reducing the risk of heart disease. Dr. Hodis says the jury is still out on this therapy, but it's worth keeping an eye on in the years ahead.

In the meantime, this doesn't mean you should completely avoid foods like beef and potatoes that are high in iron, as the mineral is necessary for preventing anemia, among other conditions.

The Daily Value for iron is 18 milligrams.

HIGH BLOOD PRESSURE

MINERAL MAGIC
CAN BRING IT DOWN

What do professional golfers and people with high blood pressure have in common?

They're both shooting for a lower score.

But while a high score could cost a pro golfer thousands of dollars, for those with high blood pressure (or hypertension) the stakes are much higher. About 50 million Americans have it, and one-third of those are completely unaware that they do. That's why it's often called "the silent killer."

If you're one of these 50 million Americans with hypertension, then the score you're shooting for is 120/80 mm Hg (which stands for millimeters of mercury). The top number, 120, refers to the systolic pressure of the heart as it's pumping, and the lower number, 80, is the diastolic pressure in arteries when the heart is at rest.

If your score jumps from the 120s to the 130s, your doctor will likely want to monitor the situation closely. Jump from the 130s to the 140s, and you may be a candidate for medication.

Medication, however, is just one way to get your blood pressure under control. A few landmark studies in recent years have shown just how powerful a healthy diet can be in reducing blood pressure to acceptable levels. The most famous of these studies were those sponsored by the National Heart, Lung, and Blood Institute that focused on the Dietary Approaches to Stop Hypertension, or DASH, diet.

"The results that came out of the DASH studies were significant," says David L. Katz, MD, MPH, director of the Yale-Griffin Prevention Research Center in Derby, Connecticut, and author of *The Way to Eat*. "In many cases, strict adherence to the diet proved to be as effective as blood pressure–lowering medications."

Furthermore, the DASH diet also provided us with more definitive information when it comes to the most controversial hypertension-related compound: salt. For more information on this and how to eat under the DASH plan, keep reading.

Now, all of this is by no means replacement for your doctor's advice if he or she recommends medication to get your blood pressure under control. But with the powerful one-two punch of diet and medication, Americans have greater hope for getting a handle on high blood pressure than ever before. So in the meantime, listen to your doctor, have your blood pressure checked often, and take a look at the following blood pressure–lowering tips.

A New Understanding of Salt

When it comes to blood pressure control, few things have caused more consternation and misunderstanding over the years than salt. For generations, doctors typically dished out just one bit of advice along with their prescriptions: Cut back on salt.

But over the years, a bevy of studies have shown that the relationship between salt and blood pressure is more complex than we initially realized. Just as important as salt, it seems, are potassium, calcium, and magnesium. In other words, if you don't get enough of these minerals, blood pressure can also spike. And when these nutrients are deficient in the body, the effects of salt are magnified.

In addition to explaining how to lower blood pressure with food (see "Food Factors" on page 304), the DASH diet studies had one other lasting legacy—proving a more definitive connection between salt and high blood pressure.

The first DASH study simply compared the diet to a standard American diet. Not surprisingly, the DASH diet significantly lowered blood pressure readings. But then researchers conducted a second study, known as DASH-Sodium. In addition to the DASH diet and a standard diet, this time researchers also looked at both DASH diets and standard diets with varying levels of salt in them.

The results were significant: Lowering the levels of sodium in the diets resulted in reduced blood pressure readings for people eating both the standard diet and the DASH diet. And the lowest blood pressure readings in the entire study were found in those eating the low-sodium DASH diet (which contained about 1,500 milligrams of sodium a day).

"Thanks to the results of the DASH diet, I think the debates about the salt–blood pressure connection can be officially laid to rest," says Dr. Katz. "The results were significant and were consistent in both men and women. There are still those that aren't salt-sensitive, but as a general rule, it's a good idea for everyone to try to limit their intake of sodium."

If the results of the DASH-Sodium study still don't convince you, then consider the INTERSALT Study, the largest epidemiological study ever conducted on the subject. INTERSALT looked at the relationship between salt and blood pressure in a mind-boggling 10,079 men and women age 20 to 59, in 32 countries.

After close analysis, the findings of INTERSALT were pretty clear: Whether young or old, male or female, hypertensive or not, level of salt intake was fairly obviously related to blood pressure. Perhaps the study's conclusion puts it best: "The INTERSALT results, which agree with findings from other diverse studies, including data from clinical observations, therapeutic interventions, randomized controlled trials, animal experiments, physiologic investigations, evolutionary biology research, anthropologic research, and epidemiologic studies, support the judgment that habitual high salt intake is one of the quantitatively important, preventable mass exposures causing the unfavorable population-wide blood pressure pattern that is a major risk factor for epidemic cardiovascular disease."

As further proof that the experts' beliefs about salt have come full circle, consider this: The Center for Science in the Public Interest (CSPI) filed a legal petition against the FDA in 2005, asking the FDA to set reasonable upper limits on the salt content of processed foods. Their reasoning? Americans' salt consumption has spiraled upward to about 4,000 milligrams a day—more than twice the recommended amount—and CSPI estimates that reducing sodium levels by half would save about 150,000 lives annually.

Food Factors

Although vitamins and minerals clearly play significant roles in preventing and perhaps treating high blood pressure, there are other dietary strategies that can also help keep your blood pressure where it belongs.

Sack the salt. Though the message has been mixed over the years, the DASH diet studies sponsored by the National Heart, Lung, and Blood Institute, among others, have pretty clearly shown the connection between high sodium intake and high blood pressure. The Daily Value of sodium is 2,400 milligrams, or a little less than a teaspoon, but most people consume around 4,000 milligrams. And the DASH diet showed the best blood pressure–lowering results at a miniscule 1,500 milligrams of sodium.

The National Heart, Lung, and Blood Institute has dozens of great tips for reducing salt intake at its Web site: www.nhlbi.nih.gov/hbp/prevent/sodium/sodium.htm. Just a handful of these include using fresh foods whenever possible, choosing low-salt options for canned or processed foods, rinsing canned foods with water to remove some of the salt, or flavoring dishes with other herbs instead of salt.

Try the DASH diet. Developed by the National Heart, Lung, and Blood Institute, this diet has proven as effective as medication in reducing high blood pressure. Its basic tenets are plentiful fruits and vegetables, lots of fiber, low-fat dairy products, and low levels of saturated fat and cholesterol. Here's a quick overview of the roughly 2,000-calorie-a-day diet:

- Grains, including whole-grain bread, rice, pasta, or cereal: 7 or 8 servings
- Vegetables, particularly raw and leafy choices: 4 or 5 servings
- Low-fat dairy products, including milk and yogurt: 2 to 3 servings
- Lean meats, such as poultry and fish: 2 or fewer servings

In addition, the following tips will help you meet the goals of the diet:

- To up your fruit and vegetable intake, try adding an extra serving at lunch and dinner.
- Cut your butter and margarine consumption by half.
- Try cutting down your portions of meat by one-third or one-half.
- Eat one or two vegetarian meals a week.
- For snacks, try nuts, raisins, yogurt, plain popcorn, and raw vegetables.

"The claims of the CSPI may be a bit extreme," says Dr. Katz, "but it shows just how serious the situation with salt has become in America."

(For some practical tips on cutting your salt consumption, see "Food Factors.")

Cut calories. Obesity is one of the biggest risk factors for high blood pressure, reports the National Heart, Lung, and Blood Institute. It can make you two to six times more likely to develop the condition than if you were at a healthier weight. That's why the institute suggests that you lose weight by cutting 500 calories a day from your diet and that you find ways to burn off even more calories by becoming more physically active.

Eat fish. Fatty fish such as herring, sardines, and salmon contain omega-3 fatty acids, a type of fat that, in large amounts, seems to reduce blood pressure. The National Heart, Lung, and Blood Institute recommends that you chow down on fatty fish as often as possible. Provided the fish is not fried, the added fat isn't a harmful addition to your total fat budget, since it would likely replace unhealthy saturated fat.

If you can't eat that much fish, try a fish oil supplement. Strive for 1 to 2 grams per day, in divided doses.

Nix the drinks. The effect of alcohol on blood pressure is so significant that some researchers believe that it accounts for up to 5 percent of all cases of high blood pressure. Researchers at Harvard Medical School found that among 3,275 nurses who were 34 to 59 years old at the start of a 4-year study, those who drank two to three alcoholic beverages daily increased their risk of high blood pressure by 40 percent. If you do drink, the National Heart, Lung, and Blood Institute suggests that you limit your intake to two or fewer drinks a day.

Cut down on sugar. "Work from my laboratory shows that sugar—the kind in your sugar bowl and in foods—raises blood pressure," says Harry Preuss, MD, professor of medicine at Georgetown University School of Medicine in Washington, DC. Researchers don't yet know how much sugar it takes to cause a problem. "But it's always a good idea to limit sugar," Dr. Preuss advises.

Think green. Some studies suggest that EGCG, an antioxidant found in green tea, may lower blood pressure. Though this is far from definitive, it certainly couldn't hurt to drink more green tea.

The Power of Potassium

While the effects of sodium have become pretty clear in recent years, it's by no means the only mineral that affects blood pressure readings. One other critical mineral is potassium.

In a 3-week study of 87 African-American men and women at the Johns Hopkins Medical Institutions in Baltimore, researchers took blood pressure measurements, divided the group in half, and gave potassium supplements of 3,120 milligrams a day to one group and placebos (inactive pills) to the other.

The result? Systolic blood pressure, the top number in a blood pressure reading, went down an average of 6.9 points in the people who received the supplements. Diastolic pressure, the bottom number, went down an average of 2.5 points. There were no blood pressure changes in the people who took the placebos.

The DASH diet also showed that potassium definitely plays a role in regulating blood pressure. This is why the diet places a strong emphasis on fruits, vegetables, and low-fat dairy products that are rich in the mineral.

Since most folks get only around 2,600 milligrams of the nutrient a day, however, most of us need to add at least three servings of potassium-rich fruits and vegetables, such as bananas and potatoes, as well as dairy products (a glass of milk has nearly as much potassium as a banana) to our diets every day. If this still doesn't do the trick, then you might want to talk to your doctor about potassium supplementation.

People who have diabetes or kidney problems or who are taking anti-inflammatory drugs, potassium-sparing diuretics (water pills), ACE inhibitors, or heart medicines such as heparin should not supplement potassium without medical supervision.

Magnesium's Magic

Along with potassium, magnesium seems to play an important role in keeping blood pressure down, particularly if you're magnesium-deficient to begin with.

In a study in Sweden of 71 people with mildly elevated blood pressure, researchers found that giving about 350 milligrams of magnesium to those who had deficiencies lowered their blood pressure readings several points.

How does it work in people with high blood pressure who may not have deficiencies?

Prescriptions for Healing

Several nutrients may play roles in keeping a lid on blood pressure. Here are the amounts that researchers recommend you get from dietary sources, if possible, or from vitamin and mineral supplements, if necessary.

Nutrient	Daily Amount
Calcium	1,000 milligrams for men ages 25 to 65, for women ages 25 to 50, and for women at menopause (ages 51 to 65) who are taking estrogen
	1,200–1,500 milligrams for women who are pregnant or nursing
	1,500 milligrams for women at menopause (ages 51 to 65) who are not taking estrogen and for men and women over age 65
Magnesium	300–400 milligrams
Potassium	3,500 milligrams

MEDICAL ALERT: *If you have been diagnosed with high blood pressure, you should be under a doctor's care.*

If you have heart or kidney problems, you should check with your doctor before taking supplemental magnesium.

Potassium supplements should not be taken by those with diabetes or kidney disease or by those using certain medications, including nonsteroidal anti-inflammatory drugs, potassium-sparing diuretics, ACE inhibitors, and heart medications such as heparin.

Some studies indicate that it won't do much of anything, although at least one indicates that it might. That study, conducted by researchers in Belgium and the Netherlands, looked at the blood pressure readings of 47 women with high blood pressure. When the women were given 485 milligrams of magnesium every day for 6 months, their systolic readings dropped an average of 2.7 points, while their diastolic readings dropped 3.4 points. A few of the women had low levels of magnesium in their blood, but most did not.

That drop doesn't sound like a lot. But to someone with borderline-high blood pressure, it can mean the difference between taking medication and eating salmon, which is rich in magnesium.

Most people should get between 300 and 400 milligrams of magnesium daily to keep their blood pressure on an even keel. (The Daily Value for this mineral is 400 milligrams.) Adult males in the United States get about 320 milligrams per day; adult women, about 230 milligrams a day. Good food sources of magnesium are green leafy vegetables, fish, whole grains, rice, legumes, and nuts.

If you have heart or kidney problems, you should check with your doctor before taking supplemental magnesium.

Calcium for Kids and Moms

Although some studies have indicated that calcium might play a role in keeping blood pressure under control, a panel of experts at the National Institutes of Health has determined that most studies indicate the mineral's role is probably minor and that a recommendation to increase calcium intake for blood pressure control is unwarranted for most people at this time.

"The two exceptions may be pregnant women who suffer from high blood pressure during their pregnancies and children who are calcium-deficient," says Matthew W. Gillman, MD, associate professor of ambulatory care and prevention at Harvard Medical School, who has investigated the relationship between calcium and blood pressure.

In a study at the University of Florida Health Science Center Jacksonville, for example, researchers found that 2,000 milligrams of calcium a day reduced the onset of high blood pressure in women during pregnancy by 54 percent.

Until scientists more clearly define whom calcium does and does not help, however, everyone should make sure to get the optimum daily intake. The National Institutes of Health recommends the following:

- Men, ages 25 to 65: 1,000 milligrams
- Women, ages 25 to 50: 1,000 milligrams
- Pregnant and nursing women: 1,200 to 1,500 milligrams
- Women at menopause (ages 51 to 65) who are taking estrogen: 1,000 milligrams
- Women at menopause (ages 51 to 65) who are not taking estrogen: 1,500 milligrams
- Men and women over age 65: 1,500 milligrams

Unfortunately, federal surveys indicate that women ages 25 to 50 get only between 685 and 778 milligrams of calcium a day through diet. Women over age 50 get between 600 and 700 milligrams daily. Adult men get closer to the mark, generally getting between 700 and 1,000 milligrams daily.

Mixed Results for Antioxidants

Though supplements of vitamins C and E have shown some mild effects in small studies, Dr. Katz says the jury is still out on these antioxidants.

"It's clear that antioxidants have some benefit for blood pressure when ingested in food," he says. "But for whatever reason, the results have not been great when these antioxidants are taken in isolation."

The best advice here, says Dr. Katz, is to try getting your antioxidants from healthy food sources like fruits, vegetables, nuts, and whole grains.

HIGH CHOLESTEROL

PROTECTING YOURSELF FROM THE BAD STUFF, GETTING ENOUGH OF THE GOOD

If you're like many Americans, you're struggling to reduce your cholesterol to a healthy level. You've probably sworn off eating eggs and liver and cut way back on your consumption of red meat. You're learning to carefully read labels to keep saturated fat and cholesterol from sneaking into your diet. And all of that vigilance is hopefully paying off with a lower level of cholesterol in your blood, plus a reduced chance of heart disease and stroke.

So with your new healthy habits in place, you can now stop worrying and get on with living. Right?

That depends. The cholesterol level in your blood is usually divided into at least three numbers. One number reflects the total amount of cholesterol circulating in your blood. Another number reflects the part of that total that contains LDL cholesterol, the "bad" stuff that gets stuck in your arteries and helps initiate the disease process that can cause a heart attack or a stroke. And the third number reflects the amount of HDL cholesterol, the "good" kind that's known to put a half nelson on the bad stuff and escort it to the liver for disposal.

Some doctors recommend that you keep your total cholesterol under 200 mg/dL, but others suggest that you aim for an even lower number, especially if you have other risk factors for heart disease. In general, the American Heart Association considers a total cholesterol level of under 200 mg/dL to be desirable. Levels between 200 and 239 mg/dL are considered borderline high risk, and a level of 240 mg/dL or over is considered high risk.

Beyond the total number, the ratio of LDL to HDL cholesterol is important. For LDL cholesterol, a level of under 100 mg/dL is considered optimal; 100 to 129 mg/dL is near optimal/above optimal; 130 to 159 mg/dL is borderline high; 160 to 189 mg/dL is high; and 190 mg/dL is considered very high. When it comes to HDL cholesterol, on the other hand, bigger is better: An HDL cholesterol level of less than 40 mg/dL, in fact, is considered too low. If your cholesterol levels fit into the at-risk categories, you should be following a diet and exercise program recommended by your doctor. As part of that program, your doctor may suggest some of the following.

Vitamin C Gives a Boost

Scientists have known for some time that keeping a close eye on your dietary fat intake and your cholesterol consumption is the key to lowering your LDL cholesterol level. The rule for cholesterol is simple: Eat less than 300 milligrams a day. The rule for fat is a little more complicated. By now we have all heard that a diet in which you get 25 to 35 percent of your calories from fat (no more than 7 to 10 percent from saturated fat) is best. But for someone with high cholesterol, that's not the case. If your LDL cholesterol is greater than 100, limit your fat intake to 25 to 35 percent of your calories, with *less than* 7 percent coming from saturated fat. While being careful not to lower your HDL is important, you should also take action to pump up your level of this good cholesterol. Researchers are just beginning to learn how you can do that.

Some studies indicate that consuming a little alcohol (one or two drinks a day), getting heart-pumping exercise most days of the week, and avoiding tobacco are three strategies that will raise HDL.

When it comes to vitamins, vitamin C has properties that seem to enable it to lower high cholesterol, but more research is required. Some studies show that taking vitamin C daily can decrease bad LDL cholesterol and increase good HDL cholesterol. It may also help to take vitamin E and vitamin C

Food Factors

Several of the most important strategies for lowering artery-damaging LDL cholesterol and raising its artery-cleaning cousin HDL cholesterol involve tinkering with your diet. Here's how experts suggest it should be done.

Watch those numbers. Cut dietary cholesterol to less than 300 milligrams a day. Most experts agree that avoiding liver, limiting eggs, reducing consumption of red meat and adding up and monitoring the cholesterol amounts listed on packaged goods are good ways to keep your cholesterol down.

Lower fat. The key strategy behind any cholesterol-lowering effort is lowering the amount of saturated fat in your diet to no more than 7 to 10 percent of calories. That's because excess saturated fat overloads the body's cholesterol-clearing system and can lead to clogged arteries.

Start lowering saturated fat by choosing fish, poultry, and very lean red meats; trimming all visible fat from meats; using low-fat dairy products; and reading labels to determine exact fat content.

Redistribute your fat. Scientists suggest that you can lower your LDL cholesterol by changing the balance of fats in your diet. What's the best mix? According to the American Heart Association, someone with high cholesterol should limit total fat intake to no more than 25 to 35 percent of total calories, limit saturated fat to no more than 7 percent of calories, and limit trans fat intake to no more than 1 percent of total calories.

Get hooked on fish. Studies measuring the effects of omega-3 fatty acids, found in fish such as tuna, mackerel, salmon, and sardines, on HDL indicate that regularly adding fatty fish to your diet at least two times a week is a good way to reduce saturated fat intake.

For instance, a recent study done at the Harvard School of Public Health reported that the death rate from heart disease was 36 percent lower among people who ate fish twice a week compared with people who ate little or no seafood.

Fill up on fiber. Another great thing you can do with respect to your diet to help lower cholesterol is up your fiber intake. "Fiber is like a resin, and it basically absorbs cholesterol in the gut," says Boyd Lyles, MD, director of the HeartHealth and Wellness Center in Dallas and medical director of L A Weight Loss. The soluble form of fiber seems to be particularly useful for lowering cholesterol. Foods high in fiber include oatmeal, beans, peas, rice bran, oat bran, barley, citrus fruits, and strawberries. The American Heart Association recommends eating at least 25 to 30 grams of dietary fiber per day.

Look for soy. Soy products, such as tofu and the texturized vegetable protein often added to ground meat, contain natural plant chemicals called isoflavones. Studies indicate that these chemicals may help flush artery-damaging cholesterol out of your body.

together because "vitamin C, together with vitamin E, helps prevent the oxidation of cholesterol, which has been implicated in atherosclerosis," says Stephen Lawson, MD, administrative officer of the Linus Pauling Institute at Oregon State University in Corvallis, Oregon.

Vitamin C seems to work by helping to protect LDL cholesterol against oxidation. It also appears to help raise good HDL cholesterol.

Despite vitamin C's healing powers, a study done at the University of Arizona in Tucson revealed that as many as 20 percent of people may not be getting the vitamin C they need. Specifically, people who were deficient reported eating less than one serving of fruits and vegetables per day. Instead, you should aim for five to nine servings, says Carol S. Johnston, PhD, RD, professor and chair of the department of nutrition at Arizona State University in Mesa. Although it may not help everyone with high cholesterol, upping your intake of vitamin C in an effort to prevent high cholesterol certainly won't *hurt*. You can take up to 3,000 milligrams of a buffered form of vitamin C divided into several doses each day. If you develop diarrhea, how-

Prescriptions for Healing

Lowering cholesterol is a key strategy in the fight against heart disease. And although scientists have not yet figured out all of the different ways that nutrients can help, studies indicate that these three vitamins can be of assistance.

Nutrient	Daily Amount
Niacin	250–2,000 milligrams (take niacin only under a doctor's supervision)
Vitamin C	500–3,000 milligrams in divided doses
Vitamin E	100–400 IU

MEDICAL ALERT: *If you have been diagnosed with high cholesterol, you should be under a doctor's care.*

If you are taking anticoagulant drugs, you should not take vitamin E supplements. (Though generally a dose of up to 1,500 IU of vitamin E a day is considered safe, some recent reports suggest that taking more than 400 IU a day could be harmful to people with cardiovascular or circulatory disease or with cancer. If you have such a condition, be sure to consult your doctor before you begin supplementation.)

ever, lower your dose and then slowly increase it until you find the dose you can tolerate.

Vitamin E: The Neutralizer

Vitamin C is a water-soluble vitamin and is found in blood and other water-containing solutions in the body. But vitamin E is a fat-soluble vitamin, which means it actually becomes part of an LDL particle in the bloodstream. Vitamin E helps prevent the LDL from oxidizing and creating what are known as "foam cells"—which clog the arteries when there is atherosclerosis or plaque buildup. With plenty of vitamin E around, the LDL particle harmlessly passes into the artery wall instead of forming plaque. Vitamin C acts as a helper by regenerating vitamin E when stores are low.

The Recommended Dietary Allowance for vitamin E is 30 IU. Up to 1,500 IU natural or 1,100 IU synthetic daily is a safe dose, according to medical experts, but you should talk to your health care professional about a specific amount for you. People with high cholesterol are advised to stay below 400 IU (180 milligrams of synthetic vitamin E or 120 milligrams of natural vitamin E) per day because studies have shown that higher levels in those at risk for heart disease, cancer, or stroke may increase the risk of death by 10 percent. People taking anticoagulants should not take vitamin E supplements.

Niacin: The Fat-Lowering B Vitamin

For lowering cholesterol, Nieca Goldberg, MD, a Manhattan-based cardiologist and author of *The Women's Healthy Heart Program*, suggests niacin. "Niacin (particularly the active nicotinic acid form) can lower bad LDL cholesterol and raise the good HDL cholesterol," she says. One of niacin's main functions is to metabolize fats, so naturally, it also lowers bad cholesterol and triglyceride levels. Begin taking 250 milligrams of niacin per day after talking with your doctor; your doctor may increase the dosage to up to 2,000 milligrams based on your individual situation. Dr. Goldberg notes that it is very important to take niacin only under medical supervision because in patients with a tendency for diabetes, niacin can raise blood sugar. Niacin also may interfere with medications to treat high blood pressure.

Keep Zinc in the Right Zone

Although it does other great things for the body, zinc—in high doses—appears to be a bit of a villain when it comes to high cholesterol. "When the mineral zinc is taken in doses of 150 milligrams or higher—more than 10 times the RDA—it has been shown to lower the good HDL cholesterol, which is bad," says Stella Volpe, PhD, RD, associate professor at the University of Pennsylvania School of Nursing in Philadelphia. "So this is one case where more is not better," she says. Talk to your doctor about the amount of zinc you are getting in your diet and/or multivitamin and how it may be affecting your cholesterol levels.

HIV

AGGRESSIVE NUTRITION PROLONGS LIFE

A nutrition specialist based in Chicago is on the phone trying to set up an appointment with someone who needs her expertise.

"Well, Wednesday I'm in Chicago, Thursday I'm in Charlotte, and Friday, I think, I'm in your area. Monday I'm in Indianapolis . . . "

Meet Cade Fields-Gardner, RD, the woman every person infected with HIV wants to see. She is the director of services for the Chicago-based Cutting Edge Consultants, a group of dietitians who use their expertise to set up and monitor HIV nutritional programs for hospitals, industries, and individuals across the country. And she is someone who is trying to make a difference in the lives of those who are infected with HIV, the virus that destroys the immune system and causes AIDS.

Fields-Gardner is hot. Physicians speak of her with respect. People who test positive for HIV speak of her with reverence. She can read lab reports the same way a Wall Street broker reads the Dow Jones. She has the information that may help people stay alive, and she is up to date on the latest research with respect to nutrition and HIV.

"At this point in the United States and most developed countries, there have been a lot of advances in care and treatment that give us confidence that we can go beyond basic survival," Fields-Gardner says. "While this is not true everywhere in the world today, we have learned a lot of lessons that have humbled us in our work about the things we did not or still do not know," she says.

One thing is for sure: Where it was practically a death sentence 25 years ago, HIV infection, when caught early enough, can now be managed with the right medications and nutrition. Today, there are many people living with HIV for years and years. "However, chronic HIV infection is still very complex, perhaps more so now than ever," Fields-Gardner says. "We better understand that the use of antiretrovirals is not a universal requirement, especially in the cases of very low viral load and adequate immune cells. We also know that there are certain interactions between antiretrovirals and other treatments, including nutrition and nutritional status," she says.

"Getting a good balance of vitamins and minerals is important to keep the immune system as strong as possible, but with HIV, especially at the end stage, at some point those vitamins and minerals aren't going to be that helpful," says Stella Volpe, PhD, RD, associate professor at the University of Pennsylvania School of Nursing in Philadelphia. Studies show that the majority of those who are HIV-positive are likely to have major deficiencies of a slew of vitamins and minerals at different stages of the disease.

"Although you certainly can't prevent HIV nutritionally, you can use vitamins and minerals to reduce the oxidative damage the virus causes," says Belinda Jenks, PhD, RD, director of scientific affairs and nutrition education at Pharmavite in Mission Hills, California.

There is no one specific nutritional regimen for people with HIV, however. An article in the *Bulletin for the Experimental Treatment of AIDS* stated that people with HIV should adopt a sensible balanced diet and consult an experienced nutrition specialist for individual recommendations.

And one thing that people with HIV should be particularly careful about is avoiding megadoses of vitamins and minerals, "because megadosing can offset the retovirus medications," Dr. Volpe says.

A Body That Can't Fight Back

Why would a well-nourished body experience almost a half-dozen nutrient deficiencies?

"Nutrition in HIV is complex," says Fields-Gardner. "In the area of nutrition, we take from both lessons we have learned in HIV care and research and lessons from a basic understanding of what infections and chronic disease do to the body. HIV is not unique—chronic inflammatory bowel disease, rheumatoid arthritis, burns, major injury or surgery, and other intermittent and chronic inflammatory conditions have taught us about the common side effects of this type of condition," she says.

HIV usually leads to malabsorption in the digestive tract, so individuals who are HIV-positive will have some gastrointestinal symptoms and some possibly will have some deficiencies, Dr. Jenks says. In some cases, the virus may indirectly injure the intestinal wall, which can make it difficult for the body to absorb nutrients. Doctors know that opportunistic infections, such as intestinal viruses and bacteria from undercooked foods, are common in people with HIV and can also affect the body's ability to absorb nutrients. Medication-induced diarrhea and malabsorption as well as metabolic changes resulting from additional liver or pancreatic disease, often seen in people with HIV, also contribute to lower blood levels of nutrients. Compounding the situation is the fact that in people with HIV, the body seems to increase the rate at which it uses nutrients. And it may actually use them differently.

All of these factors add up to malnutrition, which has three major effects on those who are HIV-positive, experts agree. It contributes to the weight loss that frequently leads to a wasting syndrome in which more than 10 percent of total body weight, mostly lean muscle, is lost. It can decrease the effectiveness of drugs designed to prolong life, or it can increase the toxicity of other drugs. And it can sabotage already compromised immune system cells, which are charged with fighting off HIV as well as any opportunistic infections and even the cancers that frequently try to gain a foothold during HIV infection.

"And any type of malnutrition can contribute to immune dysfunction," says Fields-Gardner. "The priorities for nutrition and survival are fluids, calories, protein, and only after that the micronutrients," she says. "These priorities are a matter of what you can survive without the longest. There are some recommendations that have been made to shore up micronutrient status in general, but these should always consider the patient's individual circumstances and clinical issues and whether or not the higher priorities have been satisfied."

The Beta-Carotene Lesson

Although as noted, malnutrition is common in those with HIV, there's a wide spectrum of opinion about why it exists and what should be done about it.

Food Factors

Although vitamins and minerals may play important roles in delaying or holding off the development of AIDS in those infected with HIV, medical experts say that these nutrients cannot do their jobs without three other dietary constituents. Here's what they recommend.

Stay liquid. "For those who are HIV-positive, fluids are the number-one priority, because they are the medium in which everything occurs," says HIV nutrition specialist Cade Fields-Gardner, RD, director of services for the Chicago-based Cutting Edge Consultants, a group of dietitians who use their expertise to set up and monitor HIV nutritional programs for hospitals, industries, and individuals across the country. All of the micronutrients in the world won't do you any good unless you have enough fluid in your body to process and transport them, she says. Try to get at least 8 to 10 glasses of fluids a day, preferably those that contain healthful calories (juices and nectars are good sources). Coffee and alcoholic beverages don't count, since they may cause dehydration.

Increase calories. "Calories are the number-two priority," says Fields-Gardner. They give people the sheer raw energy with which to live and to be able to use vitamins and minerals.

The nutrient-dense calories found in the basic food groups (grains, vegetables, fruits, dairy, and meats) are preferable to the empty calories in foods that are high in fat and sugar. To increase overall calories, choose higher-calorie foods such as nonfat ice cream or frozen yogurt, dried fruits, and low-fat condiments.

Level out your protein intake. Protein is the third priority for those who are HIV-positive, because most of the body is made up of protein, says Fields-Gardner. And protein is a key player in keeping the immune system on its toes.

To increase the amount of protein in your diet, try fortifying milk, soups, shakes, and other foods with nonfat dry milk. Add eggs to soups and other items that will be cooked thoroughly. You should check with your dietitian to be sure you need additional protein before adding too much, however, since excess protein may cause dehydration.

"Although it may seem obvious that any deficiency should be corrected, we don't know if there's a purpose for the deficiency, so we have to proceed cautiously," says Fields-Gardner. "We have to play detective, do trial and error, then monitor the results closely with appropriate blood tests and other tests."

Studies at Oregon Health & Science University in Portland, for example, revealed that levels of carotenoids—lutein, alpha-carotene, beta-cryptoxanthin, and the more well-known beta-carotene—are reduced early in HIV infection and that the more advanced the disease, the lower the levels of these nutrients. "In one study, HIV-infected patients, many of whom were taking the drug azidothymidine (AZT), were given either 180 milligrams (300,000 IU) per day of beta-carotene or a placebo for four weeks," says Shari Lieberman, PhD, president of the American Association for Health Freedom and author of *The Real Vitamin and Mineral Book* who runs a private nutritional practice in New York City. "Then treatments were switched, so that the beta-carotene group received placebos, and vice versa. It was found that CD4 cells and white blood cells—both of which are important for immune function—increased only during beta-carotene supplementation," she says.

Since carotenoids are known to boost levels of body chemicals that may help fight off the destructive effects of HIV, logic seems to dictate that you do everything you can to raise levels of these chemicals as high as you can, such as taking beta-carotene supplements. "Considering the immune system-enhancing effect of beta-carotene supplementation, as well as its lack of side effects, there is a possibility that the supplemented patients would not be as susceptible to opportunistic infection as would patients not receiving supplements, and that progression to AIDS would also be delayed," says Dr. Lieberman.

However, the supplement may not work for everyone. The bodies of people with a particular disease may not use nutrients in the same way that the bodies of healthy people do, explains Fields-Gardner. Healthy people, for example, will turn orange if they get more beta-carotene than their bodies can use. "But we've had reports of people who've had signs of toxicity, including high levels of triglycerides, without even turning orange first. This is worrisome in people who may have problems with the pancreas," she says. (Triglycerides are fat molecules in the blood that are markers for heart disease.)

So what should you do? Talk to your health care professional about whether or not beta-carotene supplementation is worth a try for you.

Aggressive Nutrition

Keeping in mind that supplementing various nutrients in those who are HIV-positive can have unexpected problems, HIV experts are increasingly viewing aggressive nutrition as the defining battle in the war against AIDS. "Getting adequate nutrition into the blood and body to improve nutritional status is very important because all the vitamins and minerals work in concert to improve immune system function," Dr. Jenks says. Nutrition may not be the primary therapy directed against the virus; an alphabet soup of drugs designed to slow the virus bears that standard. But many experts feel that winning the nutrition battle can at least raise the quality of life on the battlefield or even prolong the war.

A 6-year study at Johns Hopkins School of Hygiene and Public Health in Baltimore of 281 HIV-positive men, for example, found that the highest levels of thiamin, niacin, and vitamin C from both foods and supplements were associated with slower progression to AIDS. In addition, between 9,000 and 20,000 IU of vitamin A a day, two to four times the Daily Value, was associated with a 43 percent decrease in the risk of progression to AIDS, although amounts of vitamin A over that amount were associated with an increased risk. (The Daily Value for vitamin A is 5,000 IU.) Consumption of vitamins B_{12}, D, and E, plus calcium, folic acid, iron, and copper, was not associated with AIDS in one way or another. But increasing consumption of zinc was actually associated with an increased risk of AIDS. Men with higher zinc intakes were more likely to develop AIDS.

Nutrients against AIDS

But if proper nutrition can slow the progression of HIV to AIDS, won't it also slow the progression of AIDS to death? In short, won't it buy people with AIDS more time?

Alice M. Tang, PhD, associate professor in the nutrition/infection unit at Tufts University School of Medicine in Boston and lead author of the study at Johns Hopkins, had the same question more than a decade ago. She followed the survivors of the initial study for another 2 years and launched the first study in the nation to examine the relationship between nutrients and survival in people with AIDS.

The result? "There was a 40 to 50 percent increase in survival during the study among those who consumed the highest levels of certain vitamins," says Dr. Tang.

The highest consumption of thiamin, riboflavin, vitamin B_6, and niacin was associated with more than 1 year of increased survival time. Much of the protective effect appears to be from supplements rather than foods. The intake of B_6 supplements at a level more than twice the Recommended Dietary Allowance was associated with a 37 percent decrease in mortality. Similar effects were seen with thiamin and riboflavin at levels more than five times the Recommended Dietary Allowances.

"We don't know if the supplements are bringing the nutrients up to normal levels in the patients' bodies or if they're giving nutrient levels an extra boost," says Dr. Tang.

A Nutritional Surprise

Although increased levels of B vitamins seem to prolong life, more is not always better when it comes to nutrients.

"We also looked at beta-carotene and vitamin A," says Dr. Tang. Between 7,622 and 11,179 IU of beta-carotene a day was associated with a 42 percent increase in survival. But in one of those odd nutritional quirks found so often in HIV, more or less beta-carotene did not result in any improvement.

The same thing occurred with vitamin A, which is chemically related to beta-carotene. Between 9,098 and 20,762 IU a day was associated with protection.

The Recommended Dietary Allowance for vitamin A has since gone down, however, to 5,000 IU per day. "And there may be some hazards with regard to HIV infection and high doses of vitamin A supplements," notes Charles B. Stephensen, PhD, research scientist at the USDA Western Human Nutrition Research Center at the University of California, Davis. "At least one study showed an increased risk of mother to child transmission of HIV with high levels of vitamin A supplements," he says. To be safe, talk to your health care professional before supplementing with vitamin A for HIV.

Those therapeutic windows for beta-carotene and vitamin A were not the only nutritional surprises found by Dr. Tang and her colleagues. "The intake of zinc in the population we studied appeared to be harmful," she says. "Scientists have done studies in which very high levels of zinc were toxic to the immune system. But never has anybody found that ranges around the Recommended Dietary Allowance, about 15 milligrams a day, could be harmful. Yet when we looked at zinc supplements separately from food, people who were taking any zinc supplement had a 50 percent increase in their risk of mortality."

She suspects that taking zinc supplements may be like feeding HIV a spoonful of fertilizer.

Prescriptions for Healing

The body's ability to absorb and use nutrients can be affected by HIV in unexpected ways, according to experts. That's why they maintain that each individual who is HIV-positive needs a battery of blood tests to define his exact nutritional state as well as regular consultation with an HIV nutrition specialist, who can work with the individual's doctor to custom-tailor a nutritional plan. Based on evolving research, here are some recommendations for daily nutrient consumption that experts suggest you and your HIV health practitioners consider.

Nutrient	Daily Amount
Selenium	200–400 micrograms
Vitamin A	5,000 IU
Vitamin B_6	4–8 milligrams
Vitamin B_{12}	75–100 milligrams
Vitamin C	1,000 milligrams buffered vitamin C
Vitamin E	30–60 IU

MEDICAL ALERT: *If you are HIV-positive, you should be under a doctor's care.*

Do not take any vitamin, mineral, or other supplements without first consulting your doctor.

Selenium in doses exceeding 400 micrograms daily should be taken only under medical supervision.

If you are taking anticoagulant drugs, you should not take oral vitamin E supplements. (Though generally a dose of up to 1,500 IU of vitamin E a day is considered safe, some recent reports suggest that taking more than 400 IU a day could be harmful to people with cardiovascular or circulatory disease or with cancer. If you have such a condition, be sure to consult your doctor before you begin supplementation.)

"Studies have shown that the virus has something called zinc fingers," says Dr. Tang. The fingers may actually grab zinc as the virus replicates itself.

If that's true, she adds, giving the body even a milligram more zinc than it needs to carry out basic functions might be counterproductive.

"There may be a fine balance between boosting your immune system and not giving the virus too much to work with," she concludes. It should be noted that these results were found more than 10 years ago, before highly active antiretroviral treatment (HAART). "There have not been many studies published on the effects of vitamins and supplements in the HAART era," Dr. Tang says.

The Nuances of Nutrition

Given the surprises that frequently emerge in HIV nutrition, many experts are reluctant to recommend even the Daily Value of a particular vitamin or mineral.

Others say that since people with HIV are running out of time, they're willing to suggest whopping doses that may in fact prove toxic just on the chance that they might help. Nutritional intervention should consider risks and benefits to each individual person, Fields-Gardner says. "Not all patients respond the same. In fact, though there are some general problems or conditions that should be watched out for, I don't think I have seen two patients with exactly the same set of issues," she says. But anything you can do to tip the immune system in your favor seems to be a good idea. And it seems that B vitamins help do just that. A 9-year study revealed that B_{12} deficiency was an early indication of HIV progression, and that people with low levels of vitamin B_{12} developed AIDS an average of 4 years earlier than those who had sufficient levels of the vitamin. People with HIV are urged to take a vitamin B complex that provides 75 to 100 milligrams per day.

Another vitamin that appears to be effective is the antioxidant vitamin C. "The antioxidants are important in reducing the oxidative damage that happens in people with severe HIV," Dr. Jenks says. "Too much oxidative damage weakens the immune system, so having good nutritional status and antioxidants in the diet is very important," she says. Research shows that vitamin C can minimize oxidative damage in cells and lower the amount of HIV in the body. Therefore, people with HIV should take 1,000 milligrams of the buffered form of vitamin C per day. If you experience diarrhea, lower your dose and gradually increase it until you reach a level you can tolerate.

The Promise of Selenium

Scientists originally thought that HIV invaded the immune system and then laid low until some unknown trigger finally catapulted it into rabid replication.

Scientists now realize, however, that there is a "titanic struggle" going on between the immune system and the virus all the time.

In fact, the body's immune system seems to be able to mount a vigorous response and keep the virus in check for years. Eventually, however, HIV destroys more immune cells than the body can replace, and the virus spreads throughout the body, usually precipitating a drop in the immune system's CD4 cells (the fighters) and the onset of full-blown AIDS. CD4 cells are a type of white blood cell called a T-helper lymphocyte. These cells are often referred to as the conductors of the immune system because they coordinate the response of all other immune cells by using chemical messengers called cytokines. They also help other cells increase their antiviral effects.

What causes HIV to suddenly overwhelm the immune system is a matter of intense speculation in the scientific community. But one theory suggested by Gerhard N. Schrauzer, PhD, professor emeritus at the University of California, San Diego, is that HIV breaks away from its immune system hosts only after it has exhausted their available supplies of selenium. In other words, the virus is hungry. For selenium. What makes Dr. Schrauzer think this might be the case? For one thing, studies indicate that the less selenium in the body, the more advanced an HIV infection is likely to be. For another, a group of French scientists has found that adding selenium to HIV in cell cultures blocks the virus's replication. And third, an ongoing investigation by Dr. Schrauzer and a colleague in Germany seems to indicate that supplementing the diet with somewhere between 100 and 300 micrograms of selenium a day reduces symptoms and prevents life-threatening weight loss in those with AIDS.

"And there may actually be a molecular switch controlling the virus that is sensitive to selenium levels and that would be turned on when selenium levels get too low," Dr. Schrauzer says. He emphasizes that a person infected with HIV should seek a medical doctor open to all approaches of treatment and healing. "Selenium is important," he says, "but any single agent or treatment has its limitations. The best results have been obtained with comprehensive treatments." The bottom line? "Selenium should be a key complementary therapy in any AIDS program," says Dr. Schrauzer. "I recommend 200 to 400 micrograms a day." Doses of selenium in excess of 400 micrograms a day should be taken only under medical supervision.

The results of a study published in January 2007 in *Archives of Internal Medicine* back Dr. Schrauzer up: This placebo-controlled, randomized, double-blind clinical trial looked at the effects of a daily supplement providing 200 micrograms of selenium in yeast or placebo on 262 people who were

HIV-positive (average age, 40.6). In the 174 people who completed the study, the higher selenium levels were associated with decreased HIV viral load, which in turn was associated with a higher number of CD4 T-lymphocytes (the immune system cells that the virus attacks).

IMMUNITY

FORTIFYING THE TROOPS

If you wanted to learn how to wage war, you could examine the battlefield strategies of history's great generals.

Or you could study your immune system, a mind-boggling array of internal defenses designed to protect your body from the assault of disease-causing troublemakers.

Your immune system carries on a never-ending battle against a relentless horde: airborne microscopic spike-covered cold and flu viruses trying to attach themselves to your nose and throat. Cancer-causing particles sucked into your lungs. Fungus clinging to your feet after a shower at the gym. Even bacteria breeding on your unrefrigerated roast beef sandwich.

Your own standing army of immune system defenders fights a continuing battle. Is there anything you can do to help the troops fight the good fight? Yes, a great deal!

Soldiers Need Their Rations

Medical researchers have long recognized the connection between good nutrition and immune system strength. "Just about every nutrient, if it's low, will manifest as some kind of suppressed immune function," says Elizabeth Somer, RD, author of *10 Habits That Mess Up a Woman's Diet*. "Immunity is so sensitive to your nutritional status, in fact, that some researchers have recommended that we use immune tests to test for nutritional status," she says. Researchers also know that in impoverished countries, millions of children die each year of measles, pneumonia, and diarrhea because they don't get enough vitamin A to keep their immune systems up to par.

While they're usually less extreme, nutritional deficiencies present an immune system problem in the United States as well. Some experts believe that subtle vitamin and mineral deficiencies as well as enhanced nutrient requirements at different stages of life can weaken your immune system and cause it to falter in its important work.

"We know that in many older folks, for example, immune response is compromised," says Adria Sherman, PhD, professor of nutritional sciences at Rutgers University in New Brunswick, New Jersey. "It's not clear whether this is an inevitable characteristic of aging, a physiological process, years of nutritional depletion, poor eating habits, or increased needs. But in my opinion, it's probably some combination of all of these." Dr. Sherman is certainly not alone in this opinion.

"It's not that the immune systems of older people are suppressed, it's more that they are dysfunctional," says Ronald Ross Watson, PhD, professor of public health at the University of Arizona College of Medicine in Tucson. "In an older mouse, the immune cells change from a T-helper 1 type, which is more aggressive for fighting cancer, to a T-helper 2 type, which produces more inflammation," he says. In addition, older adults tend to eat less because they exercise less, which can lead to nutritional deficiencies and therefore immune system problems. The most common deficiencies are those of iron, zinc, and vitamin C. Correction of these deficiencies by following nutritional advice or by taking dietary or medicinal supplements results in a significant improvement in immunity. "For example, many seniors will be taking in 5 to

Food Factors

Eating right can help keep your immune system running strong. Besides a diet based mainly on whole grains, fruits, and vegetables, here's what the experts recommend.

Juice up your iron. Drinking a glass of vitamin C-rich orange juice while eating meat or a whole-grain food helps your body better absorb the iron in the food. But oranges need not be your only source of vitamin C. Eating broccoli, spinach, cantaloupe, or strawberries with your steak works just as well, says Adria Sherman, PhD, professor of nutritional sciences at Rutgers University in New Brunswick, New Jersey.

Avoid the sweet stuff. Medical studies have found that antibody production drops after people have as little as 18 grams of sugar, about as much as you'd find in half a can of regular soda.

7 milligrams of zinc when they should be taking 15 milligrams, which leads to a greater risk that their immune systems will become altered," says Dr. Watson.

While the whole story isn't yet in, researchers are increasingly identifying the roles that specific nutrients play in helping your immune system keep you free of disease and infection.

Vitamin A: Immune Enhancer

Vitamin A seems to be vital for a strong immune system. "Vitamin A is important to protect against pathogens," says Charles B. Stephensen, PhD, research scientist at the USDA Western Human Nutrition Research Center at the University of California, Davis.

Vitamin A deficiency causes damage to the naturally protective mucous membrane barrier of the respiratory tract, and it's thought that bacteria and viruses take advantage of that damage.

How might that affect a child's health? After a flu virus attacks, for example, the lining of a normal throat will repair itself. Not so in those who are vitamin A-deficient. "Instead, you might get that once-healthy cell replaced by an abnormal cell," says Dr. Stephensen. "That may predispose you to having a more severe episode of an infection or having another infection on top of a viral infection."

"The link between vitamin A deficiency and the severity of respiratory disease is very well established," adds Susanna Cunningham-Rundles, PhD, professor of immunology in pediatrics at Cornell University Medical Center in New York City and editor of *Nutrient Modulation of the Immune Response*.

Deficiencies such as this are common in poorer countries, where foods high in vitamin A, such as green leafy vegetables, animal foods, and fortified milk are not readily available or are not utilized. As a result, studies of vitamin A supplementation in pregnant and nursing mothers and children have shown overall benefits in the prevention of infections and reduction of death from diarrhea, measles, and acute respiratory infections.

"In my clinical expertise, I have found that vitamin A supplementation is a safe and effective immune booster," says Shari Lieberman, PhD, president of the American Association for Health Freedom and author of *The Real Vitamin and Mineral Book* who runs a private nutritional practice in New York City. "Patients who get frequent sore throats, colds, flu, sinusitis, or bronchitis have experienced a marked decrease in the frequency and severity of these respiratory infections when given optimal amounts of vitamin A," she says. "I have also found that vitamin A supplementation is effective in decreasing the symptoms associated with allergic reactions, emphysema, and asthma."

How much vitamin A is enough? The Daily Value for Vitamin A is 5,000 IU, with a minimum of 2,331 IU for women and 2,997 IU for men.

Beta-Carotene: Immune Booster

Beta-carotene is the pigment that helps turn carrots, cantaloupe, and other fruits and vegetables orange or yellow. But researchers are discovering that this nutrient does a lot more than add color to your favorite produce.

In fact, studies have shown that beta-carotene does quite a bit of immune-boosting work of its own. "There is some evidence that beta-carotene increases things like natural killer cells (immune system cells that kill abnormal or invading cells), and there is controversial evidence that it changes the number and function of T cells (immune cells that destroy invading organisms and help other cells make antibodies)," says Dr. Watson. "More specifically, beta-carotene may promote the growth of T cells," he says.

In a blinded, randomized, crossover German study published in the *Annals of Nutrition and Metabolism*, men with a diet low in beta-carotene consumed 330 milligrams per day of either tomato juice or carrot juice for 2 weeks and then consumed no juice for the following 2 weeks. The men who consumed the carrot juice experienced an increase in immune function, especially in the 2 weeks when they weren't consuming the juice, which indicates that the improvement in immunity may have a delayed response.

Riboflavin: Necessary for Robust Immunity

Some studies have shown that a deficiency in riboflavin lowers the body's ability to produce antibodies and thus fight off invaders. "Animal experiments also suggest that riboflavin deficiency may increase the susceptibility of the tissues of the esophagus to cancer," says Dr. Lieberman. The Daily Value for riboflavin is 1.7 milligrams, so try to make sure you are getting at least that much without going over the safe upper limit of 200 milligrams.

Vitamin C Gets Votes

There is general agreement in the medical community that vitamin C is vital to the production of white blood cells, the foot soldiers of your immune system.

"Vitamin C also appears to be required by the thymus gland (one of the major glands involved in immunity) and increases the mobility of the phagocytes, the type of cell that eats bacteria, viral cells, and cancer cells, as well as other harmful foreign invaders," Dr. Lieberman says. In addition, vitamin C helps keep collagen, tissue in the skin, gums, tendons, ligaments, and blood vessels, healthy. "And collagen proteins are extremely important for optimal immune system function, since those proteins help get rid of pathogens," says Carol S. Johnston, PhD, RD, professor and chair of the department of nutrition at Arizona State University in Mesa. Vitamin C also helps prevent viruses from penetrating cells. Studies show that taking 1 gram of vitamin C during cold and flu season reduces chances of getting a cold or the flu by 20 percent and can limit the duration of an illness by up to 40 percent.

Despite its powers when it comes to immunity, unfortunately, most people don't realize just how widespread is the role of vitamin C in maintaining and restoring optimum health, says Dr. Lieberman. However, no one should be deficient in vitamin C, not when so many fruits and vegetables have such high amounts. An 8-ounce glass of orange juice has 200 percent of the Daily Value, for example. And a half-cup of chopped raw red bell peppers provides 158 percent.

But is the Daily Value enough to keep your immune system functioning in tip-top form? That's the question, and most experts say "no." To boost immunity, try to take 500 milligrams of a buffered form of vitamin C up to three times per day.

Delivering Potential Benefits with Vitamin D

Vitamin D is also developing a reputation as a key player in a healthy immune system. A landmark study in the journal *Science* linked vitamin D deficiency with a susceptibility to infection. Specifically, this study revealed that certain people with vitamin D deficiency have lowered immunity and therefore are more susceptible to certain types of microbial infections, says Carol Wagner, MD, a professor in the department of pediatrics at the Medical University of South Carolina in Charleston and coauthor of the study.

One important way vitamin D seems to work is by helping to keep the immune system running smoothly. "Vitamin D is a steroid hormone and a vitamin in one, and it helps regulate the immune system," says Gerard Mullin, MD, director of integrative GI nutrition services and capsule endoscopy in the division of gastroenterology and liver disease at Johns Hopkins Hospital in Baltimore. More specifically, vitamin D helps regulate the balance of pro- and anti-inflammatory molecules that are produced by the cells in the immune system, so it helps keep everything working properly.

In addition, vitamin D seems to be able to protect against the most common type of infection in U.S. adults, which is gingivitis, Dr. Stephensen says. "And there are currently some studies investigating whether or not vitamin D deficiency may be associated with an increased risk of autoimmune diseases and juvenile-onset diabetes by affecting the immune system," he adds.

Vitamin D is found in eggs and fortified milk. You even create your own supply as a natural reaction when sunlight touches your skin.

So who wouldn't get enough? Experts say people who avoid milk to bypass stomach problems or who spend most of their time indoors, away from the sun, could be putting themselves at risk for a shortage. Vitamin D deficiency seems to be more of an issue for the elderly than young people.

Results of a study published in the *American Journal of Clinical Nutrition* estimated that 10 percent of older people were deficient in vitamin D, and 37 percent had insufficient levels. "A lot of older adults, especially those in assisted living establishments or long-term care, never get outside in the natural light," says Narinder Duggal, MD, clinical pharmacy specialist, internist, and medical director of Liberty Bay Internal Medicine in Poulsbo, Washington. It is very easy for doctors to measure vitamin D levels—which experts say should be at 50 to 60 nanograms per milliliter of 25-hydroxy vitamin D—so people of all ages should ask their doctors for this test. The Daily Value for vitamin D is 400 IU. "But some experts are saying that is too low, that it should be raised to 800 to 1,000 international units per day," Dr. Duggal says. After you have your levels tested, talk to your health care professional about how much you should aim for per day.

Vitamin E: A Well-Known Aid

The story on vitamin E and immunity is long and positive. For years, researchers have been discovering dramatic immune-enhancing effects using vitamin E supplements, including increased levels of interferon and interleukin. Both of these biochemicals are produced by the immune system to fight infection.

In one study, Tufts University researchers evaluated whether vitamin E improved the immune response in older mice and found that vitamin E indeed *significantly* improved the elderly mice's immunity.

"The work at Tufts has shown that you can boost several immune factors back up to youthful levels in seniors just by giving them vitamin E," Somer says.

Vitamin E also helps prevent oxidative damage in the body. This is a kind of damage that has been linked to lowered immune response. It seems that

Prescriptions for Healing

Good nutrition is an important key to having a healthy immune system. Experts recommend taking a multivitamin/mineral supplement that contains the Daily Values of all of the vitamins and most minerals. If the multivitamin/mineral supplement does not contain the nutrients listed below at the levels recommended, additional supplements may be needed.

Nutrient	Daily Amount
Beta-carotene	330 milligrams
Iron	18 milligrams
Riboflavin	Up to 200 milligrams
Vitamin A	5,000 IU
Vitamin C	500–1,500 milligrams
Vitamin D	400–800 IU
Vitamin E	100 IU
Zinc	15 milligrams

MEDICAL ALERT: If you are taking anticoagulant drugs, you should not take vitamin E supplements. (Though generally a dose of up to 1,500 IU of vitamin E a day is considered safe, some recent reports suggest that taking more than 400 IU a day could be harmful to people with cardiovascular or circulatory disease or with cancer. If you have such a condition, be sure to consult your doctor before you begin supplementation.)

when immune system killer cells such as macrophages do their jobs of attacking and absorbing viruses, bacteria, and other foreign invaders, dreaded free radicals are created as a by-product. Free radicals are unstable molecules that steal electrons from healthy molecules to balance themselves, weakening or damaging cells in the process. Vitamin E tames these free radicals by offering them its own electrons, therefore helping to shield healthy cells from abuse.

How much vitamin E is enough to create this immune-boosting effect? "At this point, most experts are recommending no more than about 100 international units," Somer says.

Iron: Tops for Immunity

Not only is iron an important mineral for healthy immune system functioning, but iron deficiency is fairly common, says Dr. Sherman. The deficiency can be caused by not eating enough iron-containing foods such as red meat and green leafy vegetables. Menstruating women often have low iron stores because of the monthly loss of iron-rich blood. Stomach problems such as ulcers also cause the loss of blood, as do parasitic infections and, of course, serious injuries, she says.

Stored in the liver, spleen, and bone marrow, iron is used first and foremost to produce hemoglobin in the blood. You're not considered iron-deficient until your blood hemoglobin level begins to fall, according to Dr. Sherman.

"Iron is important for immunity because it supplies oxygen to all the tissues in the body, including the tissues in the immune system," Somer says. The Daily Value for iron is 18 milligrams, which is considered enough to keep the immune system up to par. Many researchers urge caution in taking more. Getting too much can cause abdominal pain, diarrhea, and constipation.

Think Zinc

Like iron, zinc is crucial for making sure that the first wave of immune fighters, lymphocytes, has enough troops.

"When the body is exposed to a pathogen, one of the things that happens is that immune cells begin to proliferate. That is the beginning of all of the steps in killing the offender," says Dr. Sherman. "And both zinc and iron are involved in that process." Less zinc means that lymphocytes will respond more slowly to the foreign invader and that fewer will even make it to the battlefield.

Fortunately, serious zinc deficiencies are rare. Far more common, however, are moderate zinc deficiencies. Strict vegetarians are often at the greatest risk for zinc deficiency because they shun meats and seafood, the best sources of zinc.

To keep the immune system functioning properly, Dr. Watson recommends 15 milligrams of zinc per day. And getting that amount shouldn't be a problem. Just 3 ounces of any lean red meat delivers about 32 percent, while six steamed oysters provide five times the amount of zinc that you need for a healthy immune system.

Taking Some Multivitamin Insurance

There's also a good deal of research that supports the idea of taking a multivitamin/mineral supplement every day. "I like to have everyone on a multivitamin—for umbrella reasons. It can cover so many things," says Ronni Litz Julien, MS, RD, vice president of the Julien Nutrition Institute in Miami. For instance, a review done at Wake Forest University looked at nutritional interventions to treat immune dysfunctions that occur in older age and revealed that the use of a multivitamin that contains zinc, selenium, and vitamin E helped boost immunity in older adults. Why would a simple multivitamin/mineral tablet make such a difference in the performance of your immune system? It could be that older people have increased requirements or that the Recommended Dietary Allowances, or levels near the Recommended Dietary Allowances, are not adequate to support optimum immunity.

INFERTILITY

IMPROVING YOUR CHANCES

For all of the aggravation and expense that most of us go through to prevent it, you'd think that getting pregnant would be a breeze. And for most people, it is. The average couple has a 20 to 25 percent chance of conceiving each month. But according to the American Society for Reproductive Medicine, about 10 percent of the population has fertility problems. They've tried for a year or more, without luck, to produce a baby.

"A lot of the infertility issue stems from the fact that women are having their children when they are older, after they have spent a few years establishing a career," says Narinder Duggal, MD, clinical pharmacy specialist, internist, and medical director of Liberty Bay Internal Medicine in Poulsbo, Washington. "A woman is born with her full complement of eggs, so her eggs are exposed to everything she does in her lifetime," he says. The longer women go without conceiving, the older her eggs become.

Despite the shift in the average age that a woman has her first baby, infertility often results from *mechanical* problems unrelated to increasing age. A blocked fallopian tube may prevent an egg from hooking up with eager sperm. Or a varicocele, a varicose vein in a testicle, may interfere with sperm production by making blood pool in the testes, causing an increase in temperature or other changes that may decrease sperm production. Both of these conditions are usually fixed with surgery.

Sometimes, however, the problem is not so obvious and may be related to hormonal or metabolic imbalances. And here, experts say, is where it pays to do some detective work to see if your eating habits and lifestyle are jeopardizing your chances for procreation.

In both men and women, stress, smoking, and alcohol are well-known roadblocks when it comes to making babies. Exposure to toxic chemicals and drugs can also play a role, as can nutritional deficiencies or excesses.

Here's what research shows.

Vitamin C Keeps Sperm Moving

Imagine trying to move through a crowd if everyone were stuck together: No one would go anywhere. That's what seems to happen to sperm when a man's body isn't getting enough vitamin C.

A lack of vitamin C makes sperm clump together, a problem called agglutination. Vitamin C also seems to play a role in keeping sperm numerous and moving quickly. Vitamin C may be particularly effective at improving sperm quality in smokers.

In a study done at the University of Rochester Medical Center in New York, low vitamin C levels were associated with sperm DNA damage, which can contribute to infertility in men. Specifically, abnormal sperm were observed in 59 percent of the men with low levels of vitamin C compared with only 33 percent of the men with normal levels of vitamin C. In another study, infertile men with poor sperm motility and sperm count were given 1,000 milligrams of vitamin C for 2 months. At the end of the study, the average sperm count and motility (the ability to move fast) both doubled.

To get that high amount of vitamin C from foods, you'd have to eat about 25 cups of chopped rutabaga or kohlrabi, not exactly the kind of meal to get you in the mood. So doctors feel that supplements are in order to get to the 1,000-milligram mark. If you experience diarrhea, lower the dose of supplements and then increase it to the level you can tolerate. But don't forget vitamin C–rich foods, which can add some bonus C. Try citrus fruits and juices, sweet peppers, and (ahem!) passion fruit.

Check Up on Zinc

Think of it as a manly mineral.

Although zinc is essential for both men and women, it plays a particularly important role in the production of testosterone, the main male hormone. "A low zinc level leads to a reduction in the production of testosterone, which can lead to impaired fertility," explains Ananda Prasad, MD, PhD, professor of medicine at Wayne State University School of Medicine in Detroit and a leading zinc researcher.

In one study, Dr. Prasad and his colleagues found that men on a diet deliberately low in zinc had significant drops in testosterone levels and in sperm count. When the men's zinc intakes were restored to levels on a par with the Daily Value of 15 milligrams, both testosterone levels and sperm count slowly rose back to normal in 6 to 12 months.

Some experts think that low sperm counts or slow sperm can be caused by anything from too-tight shorts to lead-laden drinking water. "Two studies showed that wearing boxers instead of briefs is best because they keep the testicles away from the body, and sperm production is at its highest when the testicles are lower than the core body temperature," says Dr. Duggal.

"In my opinion, not many men in the United States are so deficient in zinc as to be infertile," says Rebecca Sokol, MD, MPH, professor of obstetrics and gynecology and medicine at the University of Southern California in Los Angeles. This is why measuring blood levels of zinc is not routinely done in infertile men, she says. However, measuring heavy metals or other chemicals in semen may provide some information about whether supplementing men with zinc or antioxidants may improve sperm function, so ask your doctor about testing for chemicals that may cause a problem with fertility,

Food Factors

Dietary changes are about as low-tech as it gets when it comes to treating infertility. "But doctors don't make money offering this sort of advice, so they don't always mention it," one doctor confides. Here's what to watch for.

Find your most fertile weight. Body fat plays an important role in hormone levels, especially for women but also, apparently, for men.

Thin women may have too little estrogen, and overweight women too much, to become pregnant, says Narinder Duggal, MD, clinical pharmacy specialist, internist, and medical director of Liberty Bay Internal Medicine in Poulsbo, Washington. "Fat is an endocrine organ, and it produces a lot of estrogen, and too much estrogen can make you infertile," he says. Similarly, thin men, such as marathon runners, may have low sperm counts, while obese men have low testosterone levels and high estrogen levels, which impede sperm production. Thin women need to gain enough weight to normalize their menstrual cycles. And while overweight women don't need to become svelte, they do need to lose enough weight to allow their periods to normalize.

Your best bet for help: a doctor who specializes in reproductive endocrinology.

Lay off the hard stuff. Experts agree that alcohol is a reproductive tract toxin for both men and women. And the more you drink, and the longer you drink, the greater the impairment of fertility may be.

How much is too much? A study by Harvard University researchers found that women who had more than seven drinks a week were 60 percent more likely to be infertile because of ovulation problems than women who did not drink. And even moderate drinkers (those having four to seven drinks a week) had a 30 percent increased risk of infertility.

One drink equals a 12-ounce beer, 4 ounces of table wine, or a shot of straight spirits.

Instead, drink green tea. "There is some evidence that green tea can increase fertility, perhaps even double it," says Dr. Duggal. So try drinking a half-cup (the amount consumed in the study Dr. Duggal is referring to) to a full cup of green tea per day.

including heavy metals, pesticides, industrial chemicals such as phthalates, and PCBs, Dr. Sokol suggests. Studies show that men generally get between 10 and 15 milligrams of zinc a day, mostly from meats and seafood. Most likely to be coming up short: vegetarians, dieters, and older people, who may be getting less than two-thirds, and in some cases less than one-half, the Daily Value.

The absolute best source of zinc is eastern oysters. Six of these succulent mollusks offer 76 milligrams of zinc (but make sure they're cooked!). Beef, veal, lamb, and crab and other seafood are also good sources, as are wheat germ, miso, and whole grains.

And zinc seems to work particularly well in infertile men when it is combined with copper, says Dr. Duggal. "We think the combination, which is 30 milligrams of zinc and 2 milligrams copper, works because of the antioxidant effect on the sperm, but we are not 100 percent sure," Dr. Duggal says. "What we do know is that zinc plays a pretty big role in the reproductive process, and the reason you should take copper is that the copper will help you absorb the zinc," he says.

Energize Sperm with Vitamin E

There is some evidence that vitamin E can boost male fertility. "A three-month study showed that men taking 800 IU of vitamin E per day—400 international units two times a day—decreased infertility," Dr. Duggal says. And another study showed that infertile *couples* who took vitamin E supplements experienced an increase in fertility. "I recommend taking 400 international units twice a day to start and then slowly decreasing the dosage," he says. Make sure you check with your doctor before taking vitamin E supplements because certain drugs, such as statins and blood thinners, can interact with vitamin E.

Speed Up Sperm with Selenium

There is some evidence that selenium may heighten sperm motility, but it doesn't seem to increase sperm count. One double-blind, placebo-controlled study showed that selenium supplements significantly helped improve sperm motility. Research has shown benefits with 100 micrograms a day for 3 months.

Bolster B Vitamins, Especially Folate

"Vitamin B complexes are very important for women who want to become pregnant because they are essential for fetal development," Dr. Duggal says. "Folic acid is crucial for neural tube development and other cellular functions and for the prevention of spina bifida," he says. "As a result, the government has put folic acid into a lot of foods and supplements, but women may still not be getting enough. I recommend 800 to 1,000 milligrams of folic acid per day," he says.

The Salt-and-Pepper Approach

Lots of other nutrients are recommended for fertility problems in both men and women. Vitamins B_6, B_{12}, and E and other nutrients are all touted now and then as being helpful.

"Many times doctors just don't know what to do. So they'll add a little salt and pepper, trying a bit of this and that without knowing for sure what's helpful and what's not," Dr. Sokol says. But when it comes to hard scientific evidence, there's no one recipe for making babies.

So use common sense, experts advise. Your best bet really is to eat a healthy balanced diet that offers at least five servings of fruits and vegetables, along with whole grains and some good-quality protein such as meats, fish, eggs, or milk.

Save Your Heart, Save Your Love Life

You can be packing millions of ready-to-go sperm. But not one of those eager swimmers is ever going to fertilize an egg if your penis can't deliver the goods. We're talking here about potency, or the ability to maintain an erection for intercourse.

Although impotence can occur for a multitude of reasons, in men ages 40 and older it's often associated with circulation problems related to atherosclerosis. The same fatty deposits that clog up the arteries to your heart can build up in the tiny arteries to your penis. The result: too little blood to pump up the spongy cylinders that cause an erection.

Drugs used to treat high blood pressure and nerve damage caused by diabetes can also cause impotence.

So to stay frisky into your fifties and sixties and even longer, stick to the same lean diet that saves your heart.

Prescriptions for Healing

Doctors agree that eating a healthy, balanced diet is the first step toward successful conception. But in some cases where conception is difficult, nutritional supplements may prove helpful. Here's what is recommended.

Nutrient	Daily Amount
For Men	
Copper	2 milligrams
Selenium	100 micrograms
Vitamin C	200–1,000 milligrams
Vitamin E	400–800 IU
Zinc	30 milligrams

Plus a multivitamin/mineral supplement containing the Daily Values of all essential vitamins and minerals

For Women	
Folic acid	800–1,000 milligrams

Plus a prenatal multivitamin/mineral supplement containing the Daily Values of all essential vitamins and minerals

MEDICAL ALERT: *More is not necessarily better. Experts say that a too-high amount of any nutrient can impair fertility.*

Some doctors recommend that women start taking prenatal supplements a few months before they stop using birth control.

Selenium in doses exceeding 400 micrograms daily should be taken only under medical supervision.

If you are taking anticoagulant drugs, you should not take vitamin E supplements. (Though generally a dose of up to 1,500 IU of vitamin E a day is considered safe, some recent reports suggest that taking more than 400 IU a day could be harmful to people with cardiovascular or circulatory disease or with cancer. If you have such a condition, be sure to consult your doctor before you begin supplementation.)

Do not take more than 15 milligrams of zinc a day unless under medical supervision.

You have to treat your body like a temple because those eggs are exposed to everything you do, from the foods you eat to the drugs you take, Dr. Duggal says. And take a multivitamin/mineral supplement (or, if you're a woman, a prenatal supplement) to cover your bases. If you're a vegetarian, make sure that you're not shortchanging yourself on zinc, vitamin B_{12}, iron, and other essential nutrients.

INSOMNIA

RESETTING THE SLEEP CLOCK

The late-night talk show hosts look more familiar than most of your relatives. You and the night cashier at the 7-Eleven are on a first-name basis. You can't remember the last time you paid full price for a long-distance call; in fact, you could use more friends in faraway time zones who would still be up when you are.

If you sometimes have trouble sleeping, you're far from alone. A National Sleep Foundation survey revealed that nearly 60 percent of adults have an occasional bad night that keeps them from functioning at their best the following day. That, by the way, is how the experts decide whether your insomnia is a problem. While an occasional bad night won't ruin your life, a whole string of them can pose some serious problems. Some of the worst industrial accidents in history have been linked to errors made by sleep-deprived workers. Insomnia is also a risk factor for depression. If you're among the 10 percent of Americans who suffer from chronic insomnia, or the one in four who experiences the occasional sleepless night, you know that lack of sleep makes a big difference in the way you feel, the way you work, and the way you relate to other people.

Sleuthing beneath the Surface

"Insomnia is a big problem in this country because we're just moving too fast," says Narinder Duggal, MD, clinical pharmacy specialist, internist, and medical director of Liberty Bay Internal Medicine in Poulsbo, Washington. "People have too much to do and no one winds down before bed," he says.

Doctors used to tell their patients that their insomnia was a symptom, not a disorder. But new evidence is suggesting that insomnia may not be a symptom of other conditions after all, but rather a condition in and of itself.

Sometimes the cause is physical, such as leg cramp or restless leg syndrome, adds Dr. Duggal. If that's the case, finding an effective treatment for those symptoms should end insomnia as well.

Sleepless nights can also be caused by environmental factors (noise), bad sleep habits (sleeping late on weekends), and circadian rhythm problems (feeling sleepy at the wrong times).

Finally, a growing body of research shows that sleep can be affected, positively or negatively, by what you put in your mouth. For instance, some medications can keep you awake. "Prozac, Zoloft, Paxil, Celebrex, bronchodilators, anti-Parkinson's drugs, Norvasc, Pravachol, thyroid hormones, and certain weight loss drugs can lead to insomnia," says Ronni Litz Julien, MS, RD, vice president of the Julien Nutrition Institute in Miami. "In addition, drinking alcohol or caffeinated drinks too close to bedtime can keep you up as well, so avoid them," she says.

Food Factors

When it comes to insomnia, what you're eating may be just as important as what you're not eating. Here's how to make sure your diet isn't sabotaging sleep.

Eliminate the usual suspects. That means coffee, tea, cola, and anything else containing caffeine. Everyone knows that too much caffeine can interfere with sleep. What we may not know is just how much is too much. Some people with insomnia are very sensitive to caffeine, and even one or two cups of coffee is too much.

Bag the nightcap. The late-night cocktail is one of the oldest sleep remedies in the book. But while a nightcap may help you become drowsy and drop off faster, it's also likely to cause you to wake up in the middle of the night.

Keep it light. Eating a heavy meal before bed can kick your digestive system into overdrive and keep you awake. Have a light but satisfying dinner, and skip any foods that tend to trigger heartburn for you.

Stop raiding the refrigerator. Try to break the habit of getting up in the night for a snack. If you often wake up hungry, have a high-protein snack before bedtime, such as yogurt or a bowl of cereal with milk. This will help prevent nocturnal hunger pangs.

"There are numerous other factors—illness, stress, depression, lifestyle— that are likely to have much stronger effects on your sleep than nutrition would," says James G. Penland, PhD, head researcher with the USDA Grand Forks Human Nutrition Research Center in North Dakota. "But once those factors have been ruled out, our research suggests that getting more or less of certain nutrients can improve the quality of sleep."

Take the Bs for Quality Zs

Most of the B vitamins seem to help with sleep in one way or another.

"If you are deficient in niacin (vitamin B_3), then the conversion of tryptophan to the neurotransmitter serotonin can't take place, which adds to poor sleep habits, and a zinc deficiency has been seen in some studies on people with insomnia," says Julien. The Daily Values for niacin and zinc are 20 milligrams and 15 milligrams, respectively, which are enough to prevent deficiency.

Another B vitamin that seems to aid in sleep is vitamin B_{12}. "In two studies, vitamin B_{12} was shown to aid in sleep problems," says Elizabeth Somer, RD, author of 10 Habits That Mess Up a Woman's Diet. "Older people become less efficient at absorbing B_{12}, and insomnia is a real problem for older people, especially menopausal women," she says. "So it wouldn't hurt to boost your intake of B_{12} to no more than 25 micrograms unless your doctor says you need more," she says.

In addition, low levels of both vitamin B_6 and thiamin have been associated with increased risk of insomnia. "If you take 2 to 5 milligrams of vitamin B_6 per day, it certainly wouldn't hurt and who knows, it might even help," Somer says. "There was also a study done at the University of California, Davis, that showed that people who supplemented with thiamin (vitamin B_1) had improved sleep patterns and a reduced need for daytime naps," she says. The Daily Value for thiamin is 1.5 milligrams, and good food sources include beef, beans, ham, oatmeal, oranges, peas, and wheat germ.

Copper Gets a Medal

A study by the USDA found that low intake of copper was associated with poor sleep quality in premenopausal women. Women on a low-copper diet of less than 1 milligram daily took longer to fall asleep and felt less rested in the

Tripping to Dreamland

Until a few years ago, the top nutritional remedy for insomnia was the amino acid tryptophan. "Tryptophan is an amino acid that helps boost levels of serotonin, a neurotransmitter that helps promote sleep," says Elizabeth Somer, RD, author of *10 Habits That Mess Up a Woman's Diet*.

Sold in health food stores, tryptophan was used successfully by thousands of people to get a better night's sleep. That changed around 1990, when several people came down with a rare blood and muscle disorder that was linked to contaminated tryptophan supplements from a Japanese manufacturer.

But while tryptophan supplements are no longer sold in the United States, some people find that eating *foods* rich in tryptophan just before bedtime seems to help them sleep, says Narinder Duggal, MD, clinical pharmacy specialist, internist, and medical director of Liberty Bay Internal Medicine in Poulsbo, Washington. It doesn't work for everyone, but it's certainly worth trying for a couple of weeks to see if it helps. Good sources of tryptophan include turkey, spinach, and milk, which may have something to do with why a cup of hot milk before bedtime became such a popular folk remedy.

morning than women who consumed the same diet but also got a 2-milligram copper supplement daily, says Dr. Penland, who directed the study.

The Daily Value for copper is 2 milligrams—a tiny amount, but more than the average American is getting. Most of us get about 1 milligram of copper a day. That is not enough of a deficiency to cause obvious symptoms, but it may be enough to affect the way we sleep. The best food sources of copper are lobster and cooked oysters. Seeds, nuts, mushrooms, and dried beans also contain copper, but you'd have to eat several servings a day to meet the Daily Value, says Dr. Penland.

Iron Makes a Difference

Another mineral that seems to have an effect on sleep quality is iron. One study by the USDA found that women who got only one-third of the Recommended Dietary Allowance for iron experienced more awakenings during the night and poorer sleep quality than those who got the full

Recommended Dietary Allowance. A number of studies, including a study done at the University of Pennsylvania School of Medicine in Philadelphia, have shown a relationship between iron deficiency and restless leg syndrome, a major cause of insomnia. And while both low-iron and low-copper diets cause total sleep time to increase, that's not necessarily a good thing, says Dr. Penland. "When people are sick, they sleep more," he says. "Greater total sleep time often indicates that the body is trying to cope with some kind of challenge, which may be the case if you're not consuming enough copper or iron." If you suspect that low copper or iron intake is affecting your sleep, a multivitamin/mineral supplement is a safe, easy way to correct the problem, says Dr. Penland. Just be sure that the supplement contains 2 milligrams of copper and the Recommended Dietary Allowance of iron, which is 18 milligrams.

Aluminum Can Foil Sleep

Another mineral that seems to have an effect on sleep quality is aluminum. Dr. Penland and his colleagues compared the sleep quality of women who consumed over 1,000 milligrams of aluminum a day with the sleep quality of women who consumed only 300 milligrams of aluminum a day. The women who consumed more aluminum reported poorer sleep quality.

We all absorb small amounts of aluminum from air and water as well as from aluminum cooking utensils and some antiperspirants, but it probably isn't enough to cause a problem, says Dr. Penland. But if you regularly take an antacid, especially a liquid, you should be aware that many brands contain as much as 200 to 250 milligrams of aluminum per teaspoon. If you take an antacid and find yourself waking up during the night, try giving it up for a few weeks to see if your sleep improves, suggests Dr. Penland. You can also try switching to tablets, which are usually aluminum-free. Check the active ingredients on the label to be sure.

Keep an Eye on Magnesium

Some research suggests that a low magnesium level can also lead to shallower sleep and more nighttime awakenings, especially in the elderly, who often experience sleeping problems. Also, some studies indicate that stress,

Prescriptions for Healing

Some doctors recommend these nutrients to send you nightly to the land of Nod.

Nutrient	Daily Amount
Copper	2 milligrams
Iron	18 milligrams
Magnesium	400 milligrams
Niacin	20 milligrams
Thiamin	1.5 milligrams
Vitamin B_6	2-5 milligrams
Vitamin B_{12}	25 micrograms
Zinc	15 milligrams

MEDICAL ALERT: *People with heart or kidney problems should consult their doctor before taking magnesium supplements.*

particularly the kind of stress that causes insomnia, may signal a magnesium deficiency. "Low magnesium status means that your magnesium intake is very low on a daily basis, probably less than 200 milligrams a day," says Dr. Penland. "It isn't uncommon, especially among people with reduced caloric intakes, such as the elderly and people on weight-loss diets."

Even if your magnesium intake is normal, certain medications can keep your body from absorbing the mineral efficiently. The most common are probably diuretics (water pills) prescribed for high blood pressure. If you're taking them, your doctor should keep an eye on your magnesium level. Just make sure your physician knows about any medications that you're taking, especially if you're being treated by more than one doctor.

The Daily Value for magnesium is 400 milligrams. If you opt for a supplement, this amount should be enough to prevent sleep problems, says Dr. Penland. If you have heart or kidney problems, be sure to consult your doctor before taking magnesium supplements.

INTERMITTENT CLAUDICATION

IMPROVING CIRCULATION

We all know the feeling of climbing multiple flights of steps—breathing gets heavier and deeper. But people with intermittent claudication experience a double whammy when they exercise; in addition to the huffing and puffing, they feel a painful cramping sensation in their legs because, due to blood flow restriction from hardening of the arteries, their limbs aren't getting the oxygen they need. In a sense, their legs are crying out for oxygen to get the job of walking up the steps done.

Clogging Up the Works

In its worst form, intermittent claudication costs someone his or her leg, but this is rare. More commonly, the condition creates mild to severe pain during exertion.

The same things that contribute to heart disease, such as smoking and too much dietary fat, also contribute to intermittent claudication. "With intermittent claudication, you get oxidative stress, which causes a buildup of lipids; on top of those lipids, you get protein deposits and then more lipids because the blood vessels are narrower and the deposits sticking out pick up more fats and minerals," says Belinda Jenks, PhD, RD, director of scientific affairs and nutrition education at Pharmavite in Mission Hills, California. When the fatty deposits build up along artery walls, they impede circulation and reduce the amount of blood that reaches the legs.

If you have this condition, at first you might find that you are able to walk long distances and suffer only minor pain. But eventually, as bloodflow continues to slow, even a short walk may cause difficulty. Skin becomes weak and susceptible to wounds from lack of proper amounts of blood, oxygen, and nutrients. Pain can develop in the hips, thighs, calves, and feet. People with advanced cases can develop sores on their toes and heels.

Because of the oxidative stress associated with intermittent claudication, antioxidants such as vitamin E and vitamin C are important for reducing

The Nutrient Catch of the Day

Think fish. What do fish have to do with improving your ability to walk farther and faster?

Some doctors recommend getting more omega-3 fatty acids, which are found in fish oil, because of their ability to help reduce both blood fat levels and the "stickiness" of blood platelet cells. Both of the benefits from these swimmers will help improve your ability to walk.

Fish oil has the ability to reverse the effects of plaqueing material. To help keep your arteries as clear as possible, take an omega-3 fish oil capsule that contains at least 1 gram of combined eicosapentaenoic acid (EPA) and docosahexaenoic acid (DHA) per day. You can also get more of these beneficial fatty acids by eating the right kinds of fish at least two times per week. A 3-ounce portion of dry-cooked Atlantic herring provides 1.82 grams of omega-3s. A similar amount of canned pink salmon provides 1.45 grams, and dry-cooked swordfish, 0.9 gram. Just avoid deep-fried fish. Deep-frying fish destroys the omega-3 fatty acids. (And if you have intermittent claudication, you should be avoiding high-fat foods.)

oxidative damage, Dr. Jenks says. A study done in the Netherlands backs this up. Researchers gave 16 patients with claudication a standard walking test before and after giving them 200 milligrams (300 IU) of vitamin E and 500 milligrams of vitamin C daily for 4 weeks. At the end of the 4 weeks, the patients showed less oxidative stress, suggesting that the vitamin C and vitamin E reduced the oxidative damage associated with the condition.

Vitamin E Helps Open Arteries

The benefits of vitamin E for claudication have long been recognized. Back in 1958, Canadian researchers divided 40 men with intermittent claudication into two groups: one that received 954 IU of vitamin E a day and one that received placebos (inactive pills). The study lasted 40 weeks.

Although only 17 men from each group completed the study, 13 of the vitamin E takers were able to walk farther without experiencing pain than the placebo takers. The researchers who conducted the study noted one finding that they considered important: "We also found that there is a considerable delay before any response can be noted, and we conclude that therapy should be continued for at least three months before being abandoned."

A long-term study in Sweden, published in 1974, gave the Canadian theory a boost. For 2 to 5 years, the Swedish researchers tracked 47 men with intermittent claudication. Half of the group took 300 IU of vitamin E a day; the other half took drugs designed to increase bloodflow to their legs.

After 4 to 6 months, 54 percent of the vitamin E takers were able to walk nearly a mile without stopping, while just 23 percent of those who took drugs were able to do the same. Arterial bloodflow also improved in the vitamin E group 12 to 18 months into the study, and by 20 to 25 months, they had a 34 percent increase in the amount of blood flowing through their legs.

Laboratory study seems to confirm the claims of those who advocate vitamin E for intermittent claudication, says Mohsen Meydani, DVM, PhD, director of the vascular biology laboratory and senior scientist at the Jean Mayer USDA Human Nutrition Research Center on Aging at Tufts University in Boston. Multiple studies have looked at vitamin E in patients with

---

Food Factors

The same dietary factors that help treat heart disease also help intermittent claudication. That's because both conditions are caused by narrowing of the arteries. Here's what doctors recommend.

Go low-fat. While high-fat foods are known to contribute to heart disease and other circulation woes, switching to an eating plan that gets less than 7 percent of its calories from saturated fat (no more than 25 to 35 percent of calories from total fat) has been shown to help prevent heart disease and claudication. You can do this by eating very little red meat and other high-fat foods and more fruits and vegetables, whole grains, low-fat dairy, poultry, and fish.

Lower salt. People with intermittent claudication often have high blood pressure, which can be controlled in part with a low-salt diet. The American Heart Association recommends limiting your total salt intake to less than 2,300 milligrams per day or less than 1,500 milligrams per day if you have high blood sugar.

Watch your blood sugar. If you have diabetes along with claudication, stay away from high-sugar and high-carbohydrate foods. "The diabetic diet includes protein at every meal with healthful, high-fiber carbohydrates and lots of fruits and vegetables," says Ronni Litz Julien, MS, RD, vice president of the Julien Nutrition Institute in Miami.

Prescriptions for Healing

Some doctors recommend the antioxidants vitamin C and vitamin E to prevent and treat intermittent claudication.

Nutrient	Daily Amount
Vitamin C	500 milligrams
Vitamin E	200 milligrams (300 IU)

MEDICAL ALERT: *If you have intermittent claudication, you should be under a doctor's care.*

It's best to check with your doctor before taking vitamin E in doses that exceed 400 IU daily. If you are taking anticoagulant drugs, you should not take vitamin E supplements. (Though generally a dose of up to 1,500 IU of vitamin E a day is considered safe, some recent reports suggest that taking more than 400 IU a day could be harmful to people with cardiovascular or circulatory disease or with cancer. If you have such a condition, be sure to consult your doctor before you begin supplementation.)

peripheral vascular disease, including intermittent claudication, and some have continued to show a benefit. Researchers at Tufts have found that when the linings of arteries are bathed in vitamin E, plaque-forming cells are less likely to stick to them than to arteries without the vitamin E treatment, he says. "It's just my clinical observation, mind you, but it makes sense that vitamin E would be useful," says Dr. Meydani.

There are at least two more reasons that vitamin E seems to help improve intermittent claudication, experts say. Even though reduced bloodflow prevents adequate oxygen from getting to muscles in the legs, vitamin E helps the muscles use what little oxygen they get more efficiently. It also helps muscles get by on less oxygen.

More important, vitamin E seems to reduce the ability of blood cells to stick together and form clots. Actually, it's a good thing that blood can form clots. This same safety mechanism causes problems, however, after fatty deposits called plaque have built up along the walls of your leg's arteries. Sensing injury at the scene of the plaque, blood cells pile on like cars at a traffic accident, clotting and further decreasing the flow of blood.

By making your blood cells less sticky, vitamin E helps prevent any further decrease in bloodflow and might even reverse some of the damage. Also, by thinning the blood, vitamin E helps blood pump more easily through your veins, thus improving circulation to the legs. The Daily Value for vitamin E is 30 IU, but higher doses, such as the 200 milligrams used in Dutch study, appear to be more effective for claudication. Talk to your health care professional about a specific dose. Also, it's best to check with your doctor before taking vitamin E in doses that exceed 400 IU daily.

KIDNEY STONES

DISSOLVING A PAINFUL PROBLEM

Take a look at a kidney stone under a microscope, and you'll understand why the pain of passing a stone is unforgettable. Most stones are spiked with razor-sharp crystals. No wonder those who've gone through the experience say the agony is equivalent to a knife in the back.

Kidney stones develop when urine concentrations of minerals and other dissolved substances get so high that the minerals can no longer remain dissolved. Stones can also form if the pH (acid-alkaline balance) of urine is too high or too low. In all cases, the minerals form insoluble crystals and precipitate, or drop out, of the urine, exactly the same way too much sugar drops to the bottom of a glass of iced tea. The crystals collect in the kidney ducts, slowly solidifying into stones.

Most doctors these days rely on both dietary measures and drugs, often diuretics (which decrease urinary calcium and increase urine flow), to keep kidney stones from coming back.

Know Your Stone

While some dietary changes seem to help prevent all kinds of kidney stones, a few work for only certain types of stones. So it's important to know the kind of stone you have formed, doctors say. The only way to do that is with laboratory analysis of a captured stone. The most common type of kidney stone, made of calcium oxalate, is found in about 70 percent of cases.

It's also important to try to find out why you're forming stones, although the answer may not always be so clear. Possible causes include a family history of stones, chronic urinary tract infections, cystic kidney disorders, and

Food Factors

Many doctors consider the following dietary adjustments proven and effective kidney stone stoppers. Here's what they recommend.

Stay well-watered. The more water you take in, the less chance that minerals in your urine will build up and form crystals that lead to stones. "Aim for at least a half-gallon of water a day or an 8-ounce glass every other waking hour," says Fred Coe, MD, professor of medicine at the University of Chicago Pritzker School of Medicine. If you care to measure, you should be producing about 2 liters of urine a day. (Large plastic soda bottles contain almost two liters, or roughly a half-gallon.) Or, your urine should be a pale straw color (not yellow, unless you recently took a vitamin or supplement). Drinking enough water helps prevent all types of stones, and it's especially important for people who live in hot, dry climates.

Shake the salt habit. Too much salt raises urine calcium levels, which ups your risk of kidney stones. The American Heart Association recommends limiting salt intake to no more than 2,300 milligrams per day. To go that low, avoid most processed foods, especially lunchmeats, soups, and frozen dinners, and toss out your saltshaker.

Don't be so sweet. "Sweet treats raise urine calcium levels at the same time they decrease urine volume, causing a very high concentration of calcium in the urine," Dr. Coe explains. If you must eat dessert, make it a small one. And avoid sweet snacks.

Don't have a cow (or a pig or a chicken). For people eating the typical American diet, high meat consumption is associated with calcium oxalate stones, studies show. Animal protein increases the concentration of both calcium and uric acid in the urine, Dr. Coe says. "Many

metabolic disorders such as hyperparathyroidism. Urine and blood tests can help identify or rule out some of these potential causes.

Check with your doctor to make sure you're selecting the best dietary changes for your specific condition before you try any of these measures.

The Calcium Conundrum

"There is a misconception that a diet high in calcium will increase kidney stones, and that's just not the case," says Elizabeth Somer, RD, author of *Nutrition for a Healthy Pregnancy* and *10 Habits That Mess Up a Woman's*

men with kidney stones are big meat eaters," he adds. "We try to get them under 10 ounces a day, and the less, the better."

Don't cut back on calcium. Cutting back on dairy products and other calcium-rich foods used to be standard advice for people with kidney stones. Because stones contain calcium, experts thought calcium may be one of the culprits. Turns out, though, that people who get more calcium in their diets are *less* likely to develop kidney stones than people who get less calcium. If you're taking calcium supplements, however, don't go above 1,000 milligrams a day without your doctor's okay, Dr. Coe says.

Go easy on C. The Daily Value for vitamin C is a mere 60 milligrams, but many people ingest much more—up to 50 times that amount—to take advantage of vitamin C's many healing benefits. It's especially important for people who've had kidney stones to not jump on the vitamin C bandwagon with too much enthusiasm. Some doctors recommend that if you are taking vitamin C supplements, you stay below 500 milligrams to help prevent stones. That's because one by-product of vitamin C metabolism may be oxalate, which makes up half of the most common kind of kidney stone, says Dr. Coe.

Scratch oxalates off your grocery list. Beans, cocoa, instant coffee, parsley, rhubarb, spinach, and black tea are all loaded with stone-causing oxalates. And ask your doctor about others. "We give our patients a list of the oxalate contents of about 200 foods," Dr. Coe says.

Don't worry about coffee or beer. Although both of these beverages up calcium excretion, they also increase urine volume, so there's no increase in calcium concentration in the urine. In fact, some people rely on beer's strong diuretic effects to flush out kidney stones, Dr. Coe says.

Diet. "It's more often other compounds in the diet, like oxalic acid and, in some cases, *low* calcium levels that are associated with increased risk of kidney stones," she says.

Stella Volpe, PhD, RD, associate professor at the University of Pennsylvania School of Nursing in Philadelphia, agrees. "People with kidney stones used to be told to decrease their milk consumption because kidney stones contain calcium, but they should do quite the opposite," she says. What happens is this: If you don't take enough calcium and your calcium level drops below normal levels, your body will try to make up for the deficit by reabsorbing calcium through the kidneys, which makes you more prone to stones, Dr. Volpe explains.

The Daily Value for calcium is 1,000 milligrams (1,200 if you are over 50), so make sure you are getting at least that much through foods and supplements. "Good sources of calcium in the diet include dairy products and other 'oxalate'-containing foods such as rhubarb, beets, collards, okra, spinach, star fruit, sweet potatoes, sesame seeds, almonds, and soy products," says Ronni Julien, MS, RD, vice president of the Julien Nutrition Institute in Miami.

Magnesium May Counterbalance Calcium

The chemistry behind kidney stone formation is complex. Some doctors believe that the ratio of calcium to magnesium, another essential mineral, in the diet is important. Magnesium seems to work by helping to break down the substances that make up kidney stones, such as calcium oxalate and calcium phosphate, the main materials that make up about 80 percent of kidney stones. Population-based studies have shown that people who live in areas where the drinking water contains a lot of magnesium have lower rates of stones.

"Magnesium inhibits formation of crystals in the urine, and most Americans' diets are low in magnesium, so upping magnesium intake a little may help," Somer says. Doctors might specifically recommend supplemental magnesium to someone whose urine is low in magnesium and high in calcium, which is a rare condition, says Fred Coe, MD, professor of medicine at the University of Chicago Pritzker School of Medicine.

To help prevent stones from forming, take 200 to 400 milligrams of magnesium in the magnesium citrate form per day with meals. If you develop diarrhea or loose stools, lower the dosage.

You can also get magnesium from foods. Good food sources of magnesium are green vegetables, nuts, beans, and whole grains.

Vitamin B$_6$ Provides Antioxalate Protection

Along with magnesium, some doctors recommend vitamin B$_6$ to people who get kidney stones.

"A vitamin B$_6$ deficiency throws up a roadblock in the body's metabolism, so more oxalic acid is made, which means that high amounts get into the urine," Dr. Coe explains. Oxalic acid then combines with calcium to form insoluble calcium oxalate, the stuff from which stones form.

In one study, conducted in India, researchers found that people with a history of kidney stones who took 40 milligrams of vitamin B$_6$ a day were

Prescriptions for Healing

Some doctors recommend these nutrients, in a range of amounts, as part of a program to prevent a recurrence of kidney stones. Check with your doctor first to determine whether these supplements might help you.

Nutrient	Daily Amount
Calcium	1,000–1,200 milligrams
Magnesium	400 milligrams
Potassium	3,500–4,500 milligrams
Vitamin B$_6$	Up to 50 milligrams (including the amount in a multivitamin/mineral supplement containing the B-complex vitamins)

MEDICAL ALERT: *No supplement program dissolves kidney stones that have already formed.*

If you have kidney or heart problems, check with your doctor before taking supplemental magnesium.

Potassium supplements should not be taken by those with diabetes or kidney disease or by those using certain medications, including nonsteroidal anti-inflammatory drugs, potassium-sparing diuretics, ACE inhibitors, and heart medications such as heparin.

Some doctors recommend taking no more than 50 milligrams of vitamin B$_6$ without medical supervision. Large doses have been associated with nerve damage. Stop taking B$_6$ if you develop numbness in your hands or feet or unsteadiness in walking.

much less likely to form stones than they were prior to beginning the vitamin. (A few people required up to 160 milligrams a day before they stopped forming stones.)

Most kidney stone specialists, however, discount the idea that people in the United States could be so shortchanged when it comes to vitamin B$_6$ that they develop kidney stones as a result. "It might be given to someone whose urine is very high in oxalic acid, but in my opinion, most stone-formers aren't B$_6$-deficient," Dr. Coe says. People with stones are seldom tested for B$_6$ deficiency or asked about their intakes of B$_6$-rich foods such as fish, bananas, and nuts. (Studies show that in the United States, both men and women get less than the Daily Value of 2 milligrams of B$_6$. Men average 1.87 milligrams a day, while women average 1.16 milligrams.)

If you're supplementing vitamin B$_6$, stick to no more than 50 milligrams a day without medical supervision, says Dr. Coe. In large doses, B$_6$ has been associated with nerve damage. Stop taking B$_6$ if you develop numbness in your hands or feet or unsteadiness in walking. Medical experts suggest that if you're taking B$_6$ supplements, make sure you're also taking a well-balanced multivitamin/mineral formula that includes the array of B-complex vitamins. (B vitamins work in harmony with each other.) But again, be sure that the two supplements combined give you no more than 50 milligrams of B$_6$ a day.

Protection with Potassium Power

Medical experts agree that eating grains, vegetables, and fruits helps avert kidney stones, and one reason for this may be that vegetarian fare offers lots of potassium. Low levels of this mineral can increase the risk of stone formation.

"People with low potassium levels, and especially those on potassium-draining diuretics such as thiazides, are likely to be prescribed potassium supplements and to be told to get more potassium in their diets," explains Lisa Ruml, MD, an internist in private practice in Wharton, New Jersey. "Low potassium can lead to low urine citrate, which is the direct reason for increased stone risk."

Doctors who recommend potassium as a preventive for kidney stones generally suggest aiming for 3,500 to 4,500 milligrams daily. You can get this amount by eating at least five servings of fruits and vegetables, including plenty of citrus fruits and juices, every day.

One form of this mineral, potassium citrate, which is available by prescription, may be helpful not only for people with low blood levels of potassium but also for many who form calcium oxalate stones, Dr. Ruml adds.

In a study done by researchers at the University of Texas Southwestern Medical Center at Dallas, people cut their chances of forming new stones to close to zero during 3 to 4 years of daily potassium citrate therapy.

"Potassium citrate changes the pH of urine, making it able to hold more calcium oxalate without forming crystals because citrate is increased," Dr. Ruml explains. "Instead of forming stones, the calcium oxalate is excreted in the urine. We use potassium citrate now in most of our patients who get calcium stones."

Potassium citrate supplements should be taken only under medical supervision, Dr. Ruml says. People taking potassium-sparing diuretics or those who have kidney disease or diabetes should not use potassium supplements of any kind without first consulting their doctor.

LEG CRAMPS

STOPPING THE SQUEEZE

There is nothing more disorienting than being awakened in the middle of the night out of a sound sleep by a gripping, knotting, painful sensation in your calf—a leg cramp. It's enough to make you want something to make the cramps stop as fast as they came on.

The Cause of the Cramp

Defining a cramp is simple enough: It's nothing more than the short, involuntary contraction of a muscle. One of your muscles literally decides to flex, and to briefly stay that way, without your permission.

Exactly what provokes this display of belligerence is a little more difficult to get a handle on. For one thing, researchers can't seem to get muscles to cramp on cue. "To have a cramp actually happen in a laboratory situation, when you're in a position to study it, can only be described as fortuitous," says Lorraine Brilla, PhD, professor of exercise physiology at Western Washington University in Bellingham.

Doctors do know that those who are more muscular seem to have more leg cramps, as are athletes, people who are ill or overweight, or people age 65 or older. They also know that pointing your toes a certain way while swimming can cause cramps. Getting your feet trapped in tight bedsheets can elicit a similar response. But bodybuilding, swimming, and playing footsie with your bedspread are among the most innocuous causes of leg cramps.

Low levels of fluids after exercise or being exposed to hot weather, or low levels of certain minerals known as electrolytes—magnesium, potassium, calcium, and sodium—have long been linked to leg cramps. (Marathon runners sweating out the miles are particularly prone to this variety.) Certain drugs, such as diuretics (substances that increase the flow of urine from the body) for the heart and for high blood pressure, have also been cited as a cause of leg cramps. Dialysis patients, who have their blood filtered by a machine because their kidneys don't work properly, often complain of leg cramps. And pregnancy, it seems, is also a factor. No matter what you think is causing your leg cramps, see your doctor to rule out more serious causes, such as circulation, nerve, hormonal, metabolic, or nutritional problems. If you get a clean bill of health, you can try some vitamins and minerals; studies have found that people with leg cramps sometimes respond to vitamin and mineral therapy.

Food Factors

These dietary tips can help you keep the nutrients that help ward off leg cramps where you need them: in your body.

Cut the cocktails. Even a single drink containing alcohol may decrease the supply of magnesium in your body.

Trim the fat. Dietary fat makes magnesium harder to absorb, increasing the chances that it will be wasted.

Cap your sweet tooth. Eating sugary foods forces your body to use magnesium just to metabolize the sweet stuff.

Can the cola. Soft drinks contain phosphates, which experts say also deplete your body of magnesium and calcium.

Stop cramps with sodium. "Sodium is a bad thing for people with high blood pressure, but it is a good thing for athletes and people with leg cramps," says Stella Volpe, PhD, RD, associate professor at the University of Pennsylvania School of Nursing in Philadelphia. "When someone comes in and tells me he or she is cramping, I tell them to be a little more liberal with salting their foods," Dr. Volpe says. "I tell people to add a little salt to their sports drinks or eat a few pretzels as a snack and see if that helps ease the cramps." If you are at risk for high blood pressure, however, make sure you do not add extra salt to your foods or drinks, and stay below 1,500 milligrams of sodium per day.

Remember old reliable: the banana. "For leg cramps, simply eating a banana each day to get some extra potassium may work," Dr. Volpe says. "Even if it doesn't help, it certainly won't hurt, so it is certainly worth a try," she says.

Put a Stop to Cramps with Potassium

As mentioned, leg cramps can result from low potassium. Potassium helps prevent leg cramps by maintaining normal fluid balance in the body and promoting muscle growth and health. It is also important for the contraction of smooth muscle tissue. So if a person is deficient in potassium, he or she is more likely to have muscles that cramp. A healthy level of potassium is 3,500 milligrams per day, and good food sources include baked potatoes with skin, beans, low-fat milk, tomatoes, broccoli, dried fruits, and bananas. "For athletes, on exercise days, I recommend that one to two potassium-rich foods be eaten," says Ronni Litz Julien, MS, RD, vice president of the Julien Nutrition Institute in Miami.

Making a Case for Magnesium

You've seen those sports drink ads on television, the ones featuring weary, sweat-soaked weekend warriors gulping bottles of fluid filled with electrolytes. Electrolytes—magnesium, potassium, calcium, and sodium—are some of the most important and most well-known nutrients in the fight against cramping. What most folks don't know, however, is that you're likely to run out of magnesium before any other electrolyte.

"The truth is, most people in this country just don't eat enough foods containing magnesium," says Robert McLean, MD, associate clinical professor of internal medicine and rheumatology at Yale University School of Medicine and an internist in New Haven, Connecticut. And even if you do eat plenty of green leafy vegetables and other foods rich in magnesium (such as nuts, figs, and pumpkin seeds), there are many things that rob your body of this important nutrient. Certain medications used to treat heart disease and high blood pressure, for example, flush magnesium from the body.

So what's the connection between magnesium and muscle cramps? Think of a key and a lock. Normally stored in muscle and bone, magnesium acts like a key that unlocks muscle cells, allowing potassium and calcium to move in and out when needed as a muscle does its job.

Without adequate levels of any of these three nutrients, the muscle becomes irritable, says Dr. McLean. "It's a crude analogy, but to keep the muscle cell adequately healthy and alive, you need to get potassium into the cell, and you need to have magnesium to open up the door to let the potassium in," he explains.

Prescriptions for Healing

Doctors recommend these nutrients to help end leg cramps.

Nutrient	Daily Amount
Magnesium	800–1,200 milligrams, taken as 2 or 3 divided doses
Potassium	3,500 milligrams

MEDICAL ALERT: *Pregnant women should not take any supplement without first discussing it with their doctor.*

If you have kidney or heart problems, don't take magnesium supplements without medical supervision. Excess magnesium can also cause diarrhea in some people.

Potassium supplements should not be taken by those with diabetes or kidney disease or by those using certain medications, including nonsteroidal anti-inflammatory drugs, potassium-sparing diuretics, ACE inhibitors, and heart medications such as heparin.

Doctors have long marveled at magnesium's powerful relaxant effect on muscles. In massive intravenous doses, this mineral is the preferred treatment for stopping premature labor contractions and a dangerous condition called preeclampsia, which causes extreme swelling and high blood pressure in pregnant women. (*Note:* Pregnant women should not take any supplement without first discussing it with their doctor.)

Before recommending magnesium supplements to ease muscle cramps, Dr. McLean does a blood test to determine an individual's blood magnesium level, to make sure that it is not unexpectedly high. If the blood level is low or even normal, then body magnesium stores may be low. Unfortunately, a normal blood level does not ensure that body magnesium stores are adequate.

Based on the results of the tests as well as the person's muscle cramp symptoms, Dr. McLean usually recommends taking one 400-milligram magnesium capsule two or three times a day. "I wouldn't go higher than that, because too much magnesium can cause you to develop diarrhea," he says. (Magnesium salt is the ingredient that makes Phillips' Milk of Magnesia, a popular bowel cleanser, do its job.)

But be careful: If you have kidney problems, taking magnesium supplements may make you accumulate the mineral too quickly, which could be toxic, says Dr. McLean. If you have kidney or heart problems, you should check with your doctor before taking magnesium supplements.

Some people taking magnesium may get relief from leg cramps right away, but a long-standing deficiency can take weeks to overcome with supplements. Some experts recommend supplementing for 4 weeks to see if it helps.

LOU GEHRIG'S DISEASE

A POTENTIALLY RADICAL SOLUTION

Theoretical astrophysicist Stephen Hawking is in his third decade of a disease that kills most people in 5 years.

He can't tell you exactly how he made it this far, but he can tell you that in the space of all of those "extra" years, he has developed the concepts of black holes, space-time and how the universe got started. And in his spare time, Hawking—who can move only a few facial muscles and a single finger on his left hand—wrote the 5.5-million-copy bestseller A Brief History of Time.

Hawking's disease is amyotrophic lateral sclerosis (ALS), the progressively degenerative condition that most of us know as Lou Gehrig's disease. It's a disease in which nerve cells of the spine and the lower part of the brain are killed off little by little. The result is a progressive muscle weakness that affects the limbs, trunk, breathing muscles, throat, and tongue. Sense of touch remains normal, as do the bladder, the bowel, and sexual function. Intellect is not affected. There are apparently two forms: one that seems to occur at random and one that may have a genetic base. Currently, there is no treatment. But there is one therapy being studied that holds out some hope for the future. And that therapy involves vitamin E and other nutrients.

"We have no idea what causes most ALS," says Gabriel Tatarian, DO, a neurologist at Thomas Jefferson University Hospital in Philadelphia.

ALS usually strikes between ages 40 and 70, and an estimated 30,000 Americans have the disease at any given time. The most information we

Food Factors

The major nutritional difficulty for those with amyotrophic lateral sclerosis (ALS), or Lou Gehrig's disease, is getting enough calories to keep their weight up. "Due to the symptoms of ALS, such as twitching, muscle weakness, [and] difficulty chewing and swallowing, getting adequate nutrition becomes an issue," says Ronni Litz Julien, RD, vice president of the Julien Nutrition Institute in Miami. To keep weight and nutrition up, Julien suggests higher-calorie nutritional liquid supplements, as well as having foods pureed or softened to match patients' level of oral functioning. "By paying attention to the texture of foods, we are able to get around some swallowing problems," she says. Foods that are sticky, crumbly, flaky, or stringy make it much more difficult to chew and swallow. In short, people should eat whatever they can.

People with ALS need to look at what they eat and how they eat in a whole new way. And because constipation can be an issue, Julien recommends people with ALS eat as many foods high in fiber as possible. Aim to get at least 25 to 30 grams of fiber per day. Check with the ALS Association for a list of clinical care facilities near you that can provide the customized nutritional advice necessary to handle this condition. You can call the association at (818) 880-9007, or log on to www.alsa.org.

have is on the hereditary form of the disease, which affects 5 to 10 percent of those with ALS. "In probably 20 percent of those cases, we've identified an abnormal gene, the copper- and zinc-dependent superoxide dismutase gene, as a problem," Dr. Tatarian says.

The gene to which Dr. Tatarian refers is one that controls the body's ability to make a natural antioxidant called superoxide dismutase, or SOD.

Antioxidants are substances that mop up the maverick molecules, sometimes called free radicals, that are set loose in the body like a bull in a china shop by normal, everyday body processes. These free radicals steal electrons from your body's healthy molecules to balance themselves. Antioxidants rein in free radicals by offering their own electrons, protecting healthy molecules from harm.

Several nutrients are antioxidants; so is SOD. "Within the body, there are several different types of SOD," says Carol Troy, MD, PhD, associate professor of pathology at Columbia University Medical Center in New York City.

"Their presumed function—and not everything is clear on this—is as a first line of defense against free radicals."

Laboratory studies indicate that excessive levels of these free radicals kill nerve cells and that when cells have chronically low levels of the antioxidant SOD, it is impossible to protect them from free radical damage.

"It's controversial as to what is going on," says Dr. Troy. "Certainly, we know that the cells have SOD for a reason. And when there are alterations in the cells, we know that there are problems, such as ALS."

To see if they could get a better handle on what happens, Dr. Troy and her colleagues set up small dishes of nerve cells in the laboratory and lowered the amount of SOD, just as it seems to occur in ALS.

And just as they did in people, the cells died.

Dr. Troy took new dishes of cells, lowered the SOD, and then added a nerve growth factor to see if it would protect the cells. Again, the cells died.

She took a third batch of cells, lowered the SOD, and then added the antioxidant vitamin E.

The cells lived.

Vitamin E Sparks New Hope

Whether or not vitamin E or any other antioxidant nutrient can prevent nerve cell death in humans with ALS is unknown. Nevertheless, that's exactly what scientists are hoping. "The results of a new study suggest that vitamin E may have some benefit in preventing ALS," says Meir Stampfer, MD, DrPH, professor of nutrition and epidemiology at Harvard School of Public Health.

Researchers at the Harvard School of Public Health compared the risk of ALS in people who regularly took vitamins C and E to the risk in those who did not take them regularly for 9 years. They found that death rates due to ALS were 62 percent lower in the people who regularly took vitamin E than in those who did not (no significant associations were found with vitamin C). The researchers concluded that because of the reduction in oxidative stress, vitamin E may help prevent ALS.

The Daily Value for vitamin E is 30 IU.

LUPUS

FIGHTING OFF AN
IMMUNE SYSTEM ATTACK

Most of the time your immune system is your best friend, fighting off invading microbes and keeping you healthy. But in certain cases—in someone with lupus, for example—the immune system gets confused about who the enemy is.

A painful and potentially life-threatening illness, lupus occurs when the immune system turns renegade and attacks the body's own tissues, causing inflammation and damage. Skin, kidneys, blood vessels, eyes, lungs, nerves, joints—just about any part of the body can be involved.

At the same time, in severe cases the immune system sometimes shirks its normal protective duties, making infections of all sorts more likely. "Symptoms of lupus include sun sensitivity, mouth ulcers, a butterfly rash across the face, and kidney issues—it is quite a global disease," says Narinder Duggal, MD, clinical pharmacy specialist, internist, and medical director of Liberty Bay Internal Medicine in Poulsbo, Washington.

No one knows what sets off the immune system in the first place, but a genetic tendency and exposure to some sort of outside trigger, perhaps a virus, may be involved. The Lupus Foundation of America estimates that approximately 1,500,000 people have some form of the disease, mostly women between puberty and menopause (ages 15 to 44) and, more frequently, African-American women. Some get the more common form of the disease, systemic lupus erythematosus, which affects the entire body. Another form of the disease, discoid lupus erythematosus, can cause disfiguring skin problems. Both conditions can flare up, then subside.

Lupus may be treated with corticosteroid drugs, such as prednisone (Deltasone), which reduce inflammation and suppress the immune response. But most people newly diagnosed with lupus don't need steroids. They may do well on nonsteroidal anti-inflammatory drugs such as aspirin or with some dietary changes. It's still important to see a doctor, preferably a rheumatologist (one who specializes in arthritis and autoimmune diseases), for assessment and long-term follow-up. One good reason: People with lupus can develop inflammation in their kidneys, connective tissues, blood vessels, and other organs but have no obvious symptoms until damage is severe. Your doctor can periodically check your kidneys with blood and urine tests.

Nutritional therapy for lupus involves correcting drug-induced deficiencies and eating a balanced diet to help prevent heart disease. Women with lupus are much more likely than normal to develop heart disease. People with kidney disease also need to follow special protein restriction guidelines.

In addition, some doctors recommend so-called antioxidant nutrients that may help reduce inflammation and protect against heart disease. There's good evidence that vitamins C and E can help prevent heart disease, and since that's such a big risk in lupus, even in these young women, it's a good idea to make sure you are getting adequate amounts of both.

Food Factors

Revamping your eating habits can go a long way toward controlling the symptoms of lupus and warding off heart problems and kidney damage, its worst side effects.

Don't chew the fat. Saturated fat, that is. "Corticosteroids are often prescribed for inflammation reduction in lupus, and corticosteroids cause weight gain," says Ronni Litz Julien, MS, RD, vice president of the Julien Nutrition Institute in Miami. So it's important to stay away from saturated fats for the sake of your waistline. Plus, evidence that saturated fat contributes to inflammation and promotes heart disease—both of which are a concern for people with lupus—is a good reason to keep the fat out of your diet as much as possible. One way to do that: Stick to small servings of lean meats and reduced-fat salad dressings and cheeses and load up on whole grains, fruits, and vegetables.

Stay away from cured meats and hot dogs. Both contain compounds that in large amounts can aggravate symptoms in people with lupus, says W. Joseph McCune, MD, professor of internal medicine at the University of Michigan Health System in Ann Arbor.

Keep the sugar down. "Occasionally with lupus, steroid-induced diabetes appears, in which case the diabetic diet can improve elevated blood sugar levels," Julien says. "To keep sugar levels under control, eat protein at every meal, fill up on healthful, high-fiber carbohydrates, and eat plenty of fruits for the antioxidants," she says.

Load up on garlic. Numerous studies show that garlic has a remarkable ability to reduce blood cholesterol levels and help prevent clotting in the arteries.

Some doctors, including Dr. Duggal, also recommend fish oil, which helps fight inflammation.

For best results, experts recommend taking a fish oil supplement that contains 1 gram of combined eicosapentaenoic acid (EPA) and docosahexaenoic acid (DHA).

In addition, people with lupus who take the drug methotrexate often become deficient in B vitamins. "So people on this drug should make sure they take extra folic acid," Dr. Duggal says.

Here are some other nutrients that may help the symptoms of this disease.

Antioxidants May Offer Protection

Inflammation produces unstable molecules called free radicals, which damage cells by grabbing electrons from healthy molecules in a cell's outer membrane. Antioxidants help stop a free radical free-for-all by generously offering up their own electrons.

There's no doubt that inflammation produces free radicals. And lupus creates inflammation, sometimes all over the body. Doctors who recommend vitamins C and E, the mineral selenium, and beta-carotene (the yellow pigment found in carrots, cantaloupe, and other orange and yellow fruits and vegetables) to people with lupus are hoping that over time, these nutrients will help reduce the inflammation by mopping up some of the free radicals.

"Selenium tends to be particularly low in people with lupus," says Dr. Duggal. To make sure your levels are up to snuff, make sure you are getting the Daily Value of 70 micrograms per day. One of the best sources of selenium is Brazil nuts—one ounce has a whopping 550 micrograms of selenium, 10 times the Daily Value! Other good sources include meat, seafood, dairy foods, wheat germ, nuts, oats, whole wheat bread, bran, brown rice, turnips, garlic, barley, and orange juice.

Studies of animals with lupus do show that the antioxidants vitamin C and vitamin E can help stop the damage from inflammation associated with lupus. A Japanese study published in the journal *Clinical Rheumatology* done on vitamin E supplementation on lupus patients revealed that patients who took 150 to 300 milligrams of vitamin E per day had a lower antibody production in response to intense sunlight than lupus patients who took a placebo, an indication that the vitamin E helped suppress the autoimmune reaction. In another study published in the *Journal of Rheumatology*, lupus

Should Fish Be Your Dish?

If you have lupus, you may have heard about the potential beneficial effects of fish oil for this condition. Doctors sometimes suggest fatty fish for several autoimmune diseases, including lupus, rheumatoid arthritis, Raynaud's phenomenon, psoriasis, and scleroderma. (Autoimmune diseases are the result of the immune system turning on the body.) These conditions involve inflammation, or pain and swelling, of the joints, skin, and vital organs. But since they don't involve infection, drugs such as antibiotics usually don't help.

"Fish oil apparently reduces inflammation by substituting for other fats when your body makes inflammation-generating biochemicals," explains William Clark, MD, professor of medicine at the University of Western Ontario in London, Ontario, and a leading researcher of lupus and fish oil.

Your body normally makes two groups of potentially inflammatory biochemicals, prostaglandins and leukotrienes, using whatever fats are available. If you eat meats and eggs, your body uses a component of the fats found in these foods, arachidonic acid, to make very potent forms of these biochemicals. (To a much lesser extent, your body can also use corn oil, safflower oil, and sunflower oil to make these biochemicals.) If fish oil is abundant, however, your body uses it to produce forms of prostaglandins and leukotrienes that are less likely to cause inflammation.

Does fish oil really help control the symptoms of lupus? Studies of mice with lupus that were fed large amounts of fish oil instead of other dietary fats show that these diets do help reduce inflammation and improve kidney function and immunity. If you have lupus and you decide that you want to try fish oil, your best bet may be to substitute fatty fish such as salmon, tuna, mackerel, or herring (broiled or poached—not fried!) for meats and eggs, experts say.

One 7-ounce serving of mackerel, Pacific salmon, or fresh albacore tuna offers 5 grams of omega-3s. (Omega-3 fatty acids are the beneficial part of the oil found in fish.) The same amount of Atlantic herring has 4.24 grams of omega-3s; canned anchovies, 4.1 grams; canned pink salmon, 3.38 grams; and bluefin tuna, about 3 grams.

Not a fish eater? A daily fish oil supplement that contains 1 gram of combined eicosapentaenoic acid (EPA) and docosahexaenoic acid (DHA) may help reduce inflammation

Some doctors worry that combining fish oil with anti-inflammatory medicines such as aspirin may prolong the amount of time it takes for blood to clot. Talk to your doctor about this potential interaction before you start eating large amounts of fish or taking fish oil.

Prescriptions for Healing

Drugs, not supplements, are standard treatment for lupus. But some experts believe that these nutrients may help ease symptoms.

Nutrient	Daily Amount
Calcium	1,000–1,200 milligrams
Selenium	55 micrograms
Vitamin C	500–1,000 milligrams
Vitamin D	400 IU
Vitamin E	400–800 IU
Zinc	15 milligrams

MEDICAL ALERT: *Anyone with lupus should be taking vitamin and mineral supplementation only after discussing it with a physician.*

Selenium in doses exceeding 400 micrograms daily should be taken only under medical supervision.

If you are taking anticoagulant drugs, you should not take vitamin E supplements. (Though generally a dose of up to 1,500 IU of vitamin E a day is considered safe, some recent reports suggest that taking more than 400 IU a day could be harmful to people with cardiovascular or circulatory disease or with cancer. If you have such a condition, be sure to consult your doctor before you begin supplementation.)

patients were given either a placebo or a combination of 500 milligrams of vitamin C and 800 IU of vitamin E. The patients receiving the vitamins C and E experienced lower levels of oxidative stress, which was probably the result of the antioxidant powers of the two vitamins.

All people with lupus should discuss any vitamin or mineral treatments they are considering taking with their doctors.

Vitamins C and E are considered safe, even in fairly large amounts. Both selenium and zinc have much smaller ranges of safety. It's best not to take more than 400 micrograms of selenium, 400 IU of vitamin E, or 15 milligrams of zinc a day without medical supervision, experts say. The cap on vitamin E is especially important if you are at risk for heart disease, stroke, or cancer. Research has shown that amounts higher than 400 IU may increase the risk of death by 10 percent.

Bone Up with Calcium and Vitamin D

Frequently, people with severe lupus need to take corticosteroid drugs such as prednisone. These drugs get inflammation under control, but at a price. One side effect is bone loss.

"If these drugs are being given to women in their twenties and thirties, a time when they should be maintaining optimum bone mass, chances are that they will begin to develop osteoporosis fairly early in life, by their forties or fifties," says W. Joseph McCune, MD, professor of internal medicine at the University of Michigan Health System in Ann Arbor. Osteoporosis, which literally means porous bones, can lead to painful, crippling fractures.

That's why doctors who treat lupus recommend that anyone taking corticosteroid drugs for the condition get at least 1,000 to 1,200 milligrams of calcium a day through foods and supplements, if necessary. "For better absorption, split the dose into half in the morning, half in the evening," says Ronni Litz Julien, MS, RD, vice president of the Julien Nutrition Institute in Miami. Experts also recommend keeping an eye on vitamin D, aiming for the Daily Value of 400 IU, to help calcium absorption. Some doctors recommend supplements; others reserve vitamin D supplements for those who are already showing signs of osteoporosis on special x-rays that measure bone density. Vitamin D can be toxic in large doses, so supplements should be taken only when approved by your doctor.

A glass of 1 percent milk, a top source of calcium, offers 300 milligrams, so you'll need to drink slightly more than 3 glasses a day to reach 1,000 milligrams. That same amount of milk provides almost 400 IU of vitamin D. Egg yolks and fatty fish such as salmon are also excellent sources of vitamin D.

MACULAR DEGENERATION

PROTECTING VISION INTO THE LATER YEARS

If you think of your eye as a camera, then the retina is the film. It's a sheet of light-sensitive cells lining the back of the eyeball. The retina captures images focused on it by the lens, converts the images to nerve impulses, and sends the impulses straight to your brain, which then has the task of figuring out whether you've set your gaze on a sock, a parking ticket, or a double-dip ice cream cone.

Smack in the middle of the retina is an area called the macula. Dense with cells that provide the brain with finely detailed, color-saturated images, the macula is the biological equivalent of Kodachrome. It doesn't get any sharper or more brilliant than this.

The macula gets the most focused light of any part of the eye. But as vital as light is to vision, it has a mean side. Focused year after year on the retina, light interacts with oxygen and may damage the retina's cells, causing the accumulation of waste material and sometimes the abnormal growth of tiny blood vessels under the retina. These blood vessels sometimes leak, swell, and cause scars that can permanently blur your sight. This whole vision-damaging process is called macular degeneration. After cataracts, it's the leading cause of blindness in people ages 50 and older.

There are two main forms of macular degeneration—wet macular degeneration and dry macular degeneration. Dry macular degeneration causes problems with seeing in dark situations or up close and a gradual decrease of vision and increase in blurriness; wet macular degeneration, on the other hand, causes visual distortions, a decrease in central vision, and a central blurry spot.

As far as a cause, "a number of genes have been shown to have a role in age-related macular degeneration, one such gene being complement factor H (or CFH)," says Ron Klein, MD, professor of ophthalmology and visual sciences at the University of Wisconsin School of Medicine and Public Health in Madison. "People with variants of the gene are at increased risk, especially when they are exposed to inflammatory stimulants in their environment, such as smoking," he says.

Fighting for Vision

Symptoms usually develop slowly. "People find it difficult or impossible to see clearly at long distances, to do close work, to see faces or objects clearly, or to distinguish different colors," says Dr. Klein. You might mistake that double-dip cone of Bing cherry vanilla for rocky road, for instance.

The current treatment options for late-stage macular degeneration are limited and include endothelial growth factor injections into the eyes to stabilize or improve vision, Dr. Klein says. So preventing macular degeneration in the first place is definitely the way to go. Avoiding smoking is one good means of prevention, Dr. Klein says. There's some evidence that retinal damage involves oxidative chemical reactions, the same reactions that make iron rust and oil turn rancid. Oxidative reactions occur when oxygen interacts with other substances, setting off a game of molecular musical chairs as unstable molecules lose electrons and then grab electrons from other molecules to balance themselves. Oxidative reactions damage cell membranes and genetic material.

There's also some evidence that certain vitamins and minerals, particularly dietary components known as antioxidants, can help prevent macular degeneration.

"There was a clinical trial a few years ago called the Age-Related Eye Disorder Study [AREDS] that showed that a combination of the antioxidants vitamin A in the form of carotene, vitamin E, vitamin C, and zinc reduced the severe loss of vision either from wet or dry macular degeneration," says Elias Reichel, MD, vice chair for research and education in the department of ophthalmology at Tufts University School of Medicine in Boston.

And a study done in the Netherlands and published in the *Journal of the American Medical Association* showed that a high dietary intake of vitamins C and E, beta-carotene, and zinc was associated with a 35 percent lower risk of macular degeneration in older people.

"The eyes contain very small microvessels and just like your large blood vessels, you have to keep them healthy—the healthier you keep the small vessels in your eyes, the lower your risk for macular degeneration," says Belinda Jenks, PhD, RD, director of scientific affairs and nutrition education at Pharmavite in Mission Hills, California. "The antioxidants vitamin A, vitamin C, vitamin E, and selenium all help keep blood vessels in the eye healthy and free of plaques," she says.

Multivitamins Get Some Votes

Several over-the-counter multivitamin/mineral products, including Icaps and Ocuvite (available in health food stores, retail stores, and pharmacies), are marketed to people with either macular degeneration or cataracts. Studies suggest that multivitamin/mineral supplements may help people with macular degeneration. Other ophthalmologists do recommend nutrients. "I'm not saying the evidence is in, either. But the facts so far seem promising enough for me to tell my patients that certain nutrients may help," says Randall

---

Food Factors

Antioxidant nutrients seem to get all of the attention when it comes to eye protection, but researchers are interested in other, less widely studied food components as well. Here's what shows promise.

Look for lycopene. "Lycopene is an antioxidant that seems particularly effective for macular degeneration," says Stella Volpe, PhD, RD, associate professor at the University of Pennsylvania School of Nursing in Philadelphia. Numerous studies have linked high intakes of lycopene with a decreased risk of macular degeneration. "So I encourage people to eat deep red fruits and vegetables rich in lycopene, such as tomatoes and tomato-based products like tomato paste and tomato sauce," she says. Other foods that contain lycopene include watermelon and pink grapefruit.

Go after glutathione. In test tube experiments, this micronutrient helped stop oxygen-induced damage to retinal tissue. (It helps form an important antioxidant enzyme called glutathione peroxidase.) Look to fresh green, yellow, and red vegetables for your supply of this nutrient. Canned and frozen vegetables lose all of their glutathione in processing.

Olson, MD, professor and chair of the department of ophthalmology at the University of Utah School of Medicine and director of the John A. Moran Eye Center, both in Salt Lake City. "Presently, the nutrients that seem to be most promising and therefore are currently being studied in the National Institutes of Health's AREDS II are the carotenoids lutein and zeaxanthin, as well as the omega-3 fatty acids in fish," Dr. Olson says. The best way to get more of these carotenoids is through foods rich in them, such as broccoli, collard greens, egg yolks, peas, romaine lettuce, yellow corn, spinach, and kale. And for omega-3 fatty acids, eat fatty fish such as tuna, mackerel, salmon, or herring at least two times per week. If you are not a fish eater or can't fit that much into your diet, take an omega-3 supplement that contains a gram of combined eicosapentaenoic acid (EPA) and docosahexaenoic acid (DHA) per day.

Orange Aid for Eyes

Need another good reason to stock up in the produce section the next time you're shopping for groceries? It turns out that vitamin C, an antioxidant that's highly concentrated in the eye, may help shield retinal cells from oxygen-generated damage.

Studies suggest that people who get plenty of vitamin C in their diets are less likely to develop macular degeneration than those whose vitamin C intakes are low. AREDS I showed that 500 milligrams of vitamin C—555 percent of the Daily Value—helped slow the progression of age-related macular degeneration in people with the condition. Therefore, doctors who recommend vitamin C to prevent or slow the progress of macular degeneration suggest 500 to 1,000 milligrams in one or two divided doses.

Vitamin E Eye Guard

Along with vitamin C and beta-carotene, vitamin E is a well-known antioxidant and therefore, as Dr. Jenks mentioned, it can help keep small vessels in the eye healthy and clear. In addition, incorporated into the fatty membranes that enclose cells, vitamin E shields cells from free radical damage. In the retina, vitamin E may help dampen the reactions between light and oxygen that may eventually cause retinal cells to malfunction.

A few studies suggest that vitamin E can be helpful in preventing macular degeneration. In a French study of 2,584 adults age 60 and older, vitamin E was shown to be protective against the condition. The adults with high intakes of vitamin E were 82 percent less likely to have macular degeneration than those with low levels of the vitamin. Doctors who do recommend vitamin E generally stay in the range of 400 IU. Even diets that include lots of vitamin E-rich foods such as wheat germ and almonds can't provide these high amounts, so supplementation may be in order. The Daily Value for vitamin E is 30 IU. (It's a good idea to talk to your doctor if you're considering taking more than 400 IU of vitamin E daily.)

Zinc May Slow Down Damage

It's well known that the retina contains high concentrations of zinc, an essential mineral. Zinc appears to play an important role in the metabolism of the retina. Zinc-deficient animals show signs of retinal breakdown, and people who are shortchanged when it comes to zinc seem to be at higher than normal risk for macular degeneration. Zinc levels gradually decrease with age, which may be one of the reasons macular degeneration sets in later in life.)

Doctors who recommend zinc to prevent or slow macular degeneration suggest amounts ranging from the Daily Value of 15 milligrams up to 80 or 90 milligrams a day. (The amount of zinc used in AREDS I was 80 milligrams.) Dr. Olson recommends 50 milligrams. "Doses higher than this may decrease heart-protective HDL cholesterol, and even this level of zinc should only be taken if you have macular changes," Dr. Olson says.

Prescriptions for Healing

Some doctors recommend these nutrients to help prevent or slow the progress of macular degeneration.

Nutrient	Daily Amount
Selenium	50–200 micrograms
Vitamin C	500–1,000 milligrams daily in 1 or 2 divided doses
Vitamin E	400 IU
Zinc	50 milligrams

Plus a multivitamin/mineral supplement containing the Daily Values of all essential vitamins and minerals

MEDICAL ALERT: If you have macular degeneration, check with your doctor before taking supplements.

Selenium in doses exceeding 400 micrograms daily should be taken only under medical supervision.

People who are taking anticoagulants should not take vitamin E supplements. (Though generally a dose of up to 1,500 IU of vitamin E a day is considered safe, some recent reports suggest that taking more than 400 IU a day could be harmful to people with cardiovascular or circulatory disease or with cancer. If you have such a condition, be sure to consult your doctor before you begin supplementation.)

Don't take more than 15 milligrams of zinc daily without medical supervision.

Selenium Adds Antioxidant Power

Because of its antioxidant properties, doctors sometimes fill out their antioxidant prescriptions with selenium, a mineral that is involved in the body's production of glutathione peroxidase, yet another protective enzyme found in the eye and in other parts of the body. Similar to zinc, selenium levels decrease in the body with age.

Doctors who recommend supplements suggest 50 to 200 micrograms a day. Doses of more than 400 micrograms daily should be taken only under medical supervision; even in small amounts, selenium can be toxic. For foods rich in selenium, try garlic, onions, mushrooms, cabbage, grains, and fish.

MEMORY LOSS

HELPING YOUR BRAIN
WORK BETTER

You've heard of the tree of knowledge? Think of your brain. Inside that 4-pound organ sitting inside your skull is a root and branch system of truly biblical proportions.

Hundreds of billions of brain cells called neurons stretch toward each other with rootlike growths called axons and dendrites.

Close as they might get, the tiny nerve endings of one axon never touch those of the dendrites branching toward it. Instead, memories and other thoughts have to hurdle what are called synaptic gaps.

Without chemicals called neurotransmitters (such as dopamine, norepinephrine, serotonin, and acetylcholine) bridging them, these tiny gaps may as well be as wide as the Grand Canyon. Information just can't get from one neuron to the other. And that means memories, though stored throughout your brain, are just out of reach.

"You know that if you have a phone, I can call you," says Manuchair Ebadi, PhD, distinguished professor of pharmacology and clinical neuroscience at the University of North Dakota in Grand Forks. "But if you don't have a phone, there's nothing I can do. That's the way it is with neurotransmitters.

In order for things to occur, you know you need transmitters. In the absence of transmitters, biological function is halted."

Turning Memories into Mush

If neurotransmitters are the stuff that helps transmit memories, then what makes neurotransmitters? Although the brain's primary fuel is glucose, experts believe that key vitamins and minerals supply the raw material for many of these neurotransmitters.

And that may be what's at the heart of many memory loss problems. Although Americans eat a lot of food, they don't always choose the right

---

Food Factors

These dietary tips can help you keep the memories flowing.

Eat berries. "When it comes to preventing memory loss, my biggest push is to tell people to eat more berries, especially blueberries, for the antioxidants," says Stella Volpe, PhD, RD, associate professor at the University of Pennsylvania School of Nursing in Philadelphia. For best results, try to eat a cup of berries a day. "Pomegranates and pomegranate juice also have a high antioxidant capacity, so if it's convenient, add this fruit to your diet as well," she says.

Put the berries on some wheat germ. Albert Szent-Györgyi, the physician who discovered vitamin C in the 1930s and won a Nobel Prize as a result, told a friend that "in order to stay young, you should eat wheat germ." That was 15 years before the discovery of coenzyme Q10, a substance found in abundance in wheat germ.

Coenzyme Q10 increases the level of memory-saving adenosine 5`-triphosphate (ATP). "As people get older, the level of ATP goes down in their brains, and that's one reason they lose their memories," says Manuchair Ebadi, PhD, distinguished professor of pharmacology and clinical neuroscience at the University of North Dakota in Grand Forks. The coenzyme Q10 in the wheat germ increases levels of ATP in the brain, which in turn helps preserve memory. "In the case of nutrition for maintaining memory, I recommend eating wheat germ daily," Dr. Ebadi says.

For best results, Dr. Ebadi recommends drizzling some honey on your wheat germ. "Honey contains acetylcholine—what I call 'the memory molecule,'" Dr. Ebadi says. "One of the best things you can do for your memory is to eat honey every day."

kinds. As a result, many of us just don't get enough brain-boosting nutrients. And even if you are among the few who are getting the Daily Values of these essential nutrients, you may not be home free as far as memory is concerned.

Some doctors wonder whether the Daily Values are set high enough to meet all of the body's needs. Not only that, but it's possible to consume all of the nutrients in all of the right amounts and still be shortchanged if your body isn't doing a good job of absorbing the nutrients. This is a situation most likely to develop among older people, precisely the population that is most likely to be beset by memory problems.

Malabsorption of vitamin B_{12}, which means that your body can't get sufficient B_{12} from foods no matter how much you eat, is thought to affect at least one in five older adults, says Sally Stabler, MD, professor of medicine and cohead of the division of hematology at the University of Colorado Health Sciences Center in Denver.

Mix already poor nutrition with improper or impaired nutrient absorption, and you have a recipe for memory loss.

Benefits of B Vitamins

It's one thing to occasionally misplace your car keys. It's another to forget where you parked your car, especially when it's in the garage, where you usually keep it. Yet that's what some research shows could happen if you don't get proper amounts of B vitamins. "The B vitamins all seem to help lower homocysteine, and elevated homocysteine levels appear to contribute to memory loss," says Elizabeth Somer, RD, author of *10 Habits That Mess Up a Woman's Diet*. One Australian study looked at the dietary intakes of vitamin B_6 and vitamin B_{12} in 1,183 middle-aged men and women and examined the association between these vitamins and self-reported cognitive function (including memory) and overall psychological well-being. Researchers found that vitamin B_6 and B_{12} were positively associated with memory function in men, meaning the more of those B vitamins they took, the better the men reported their memories to be. In the women, vitamin B_6 intakes around the Daily Value of 2 milligrams were associated with better memory.

In another study published in the *American Journal of Clinical Nutrition*, researchers looked at the cognitive function of 321 men from the Veterans Affairs Normative Aging Study, assessed their diets for 3 years, and looked at their blood levels of B vitamins and homocysteine. At the end of the study, the researchers determined that there was a significant relationship between a certain aspect of memory called special copying and low blood levels of homocysteine, vitamin B_6, vitamin B_{12}, and folate, as well as low dietary intake of the vitamins. The researchers concluded that low B vitamin and high homocysteine levels may predict a decline in overall memory and that the spatial copying mechanisms appear to be the most sensitive. There's another good reason that vitamin B_6 helps memory. Remember those all-important neurotransmitters with the long names? Vitamin B_6 apparently helps create dopamine, serotonin, and norepinephrine.

The Daily Value of 2 milligrams should be sufficient to help keep your memory in good working order. You can easily get this amount as part of a B-complex supplement that supplies the Daily Values of all B vitamins. You should never take B_6 by itself without medical supervision, as amounts above 100 milligrams can be toxic.

Boosting the Brain with B_{12}

In one study, when 39 people were treated for neurological symptoms related to vitamin B_{12} deficiency—things such as memory loss, disorientation, and fatigue—all of them improved, sometimes dramatically. "B_{12} deficiency causes problems in the nervous system, including burning pains in the feet and mental problems such as difficulty with recent memory and the ability to calculate, that sort of thing," says Dr. Stabler. A B_{12} deficiency has even been known to change brain wave activity, she says.

Up to one-third of people over age 60 can't extract the vitamin B_{12} they need from what they eat. That's because their stomachs no longer secrete enough gastric acid, the stuff that breaks down food and helps turn it into fuel for your brain and body.

The low doses of vitamin B_{12} in common supplements will not overcome the problem of malabsorption. So doctors who suspect vitamin B_{12} deficiencies in people with memory problems give them B_{12} shots, thus bypassing the faltering digestive system, or high-dose vitamin B_{12} pills that contain 1,000 to 2,000 micrograms.

Severe vitamin B_{12} deficiency caused by diet is rare when the digestive system is in good working order. That's because eating just small portions of dairy products or animal protein gives you some of this vital nutrient. Recent

---

Prescriptions for Healing

Some doctors recommend these nutrients to help avoid memory loss.

Nutrient	Daily Amount
Iron	18 milligrams
Vitamin B$_6$	2 milligrams
Vitamin B$_{12}$	6 micrograms
Vitamin E	400 IU
Zinc	15 milligrams

MEDICAL ALERT: *If you are taking anticoagulant drugs, you should not take vitamin E supplements. (Though generally a dose of up to 1,500 IU of vitamin E a day is considered safe, some recent reports suggest that taking more than 400 IU a day could be harmful to people with cardiovascular or circulatory disease or with cancer. If you have such a condition, be sure to consult your doctor before you begin supplementation.)*

---

studies are now showing that people who limit intake of animal products to only once a week may have mild deficiency. Many soy products are fortified with vitamin B$_{12}$, which may decrease the risk in vegetarians. Usually you have to adhere to such a limited diet for at least several years before a deficiency develops, says Dr. Stabler.

Virtually all animal products, such as milk, cheeses, yogurt, eggs, fish, seafood, and meats, contain vitamin B$_{12}$. The Daily Value for B$_{12}$ is 6 micrograms.

End Forgetfulness with Vitamin E

"Among vitamins, there is sufficient evidence to warrant taking vitamin E, d-alpha-tocopherol, to prevent memory loss," says Thomas Crook, PhD, president of Psychologix in Ft. Lauderdale, Florida, former chair of both the National Institute of Mental Health and the American Psychological Association Task Forces on the Diagnosis and Treatment of Age-Associated Memory Impairment, and author of *The Memory Advantage*. Vitamin E is a powerful antioxidant that can inhibit damage by free radicals to the brain, which can lead to memory problems. A study done at the National Institutes of Health looked at 815 people over the age of 65 who were part of the Chicago Health and Aging Project (CHAP). CHAP participants were free of dementia at the beginning of the project, given various antioxidants as part of the study, and followed for 3.9 years. Participants completed a questionnaire 1.7 years from the start of the project, and researchers noted that the most significant protective effect against memory problems was found among people who were in the top fifth of dietary vitamin E intake. People taking an average of 11.4 IU of vitamin E per day had a 67 percent lower risk of Alzheimer's disease than people with the lowest consumption of vitamin E (an average of 6.2 IU per day). "I personally recommend—and take—400 international units of the natural form of vitamin E, d-alpha-tocopherol (not dl-alpha-tocopherol, which is the much less active synthetic form)," Dr. Crook says.

The Lecithin-Choline Connection

Who would have thought that a food filler could help you be less forgetful? Lecithin is a common food additive; it's used in ice cream, margarine, mayonnaise, and chocolate bars to help wed the fat in these foods to water. It has healthful qualities as well, such as mildly increasing the amount of the B vitamin choline in your brain. And more choline means more acetylcholine, an important neurotransmitter that you need for your memory to function. "I call acetylcholine the memory molecule," says Dr. Ebadi.

One study showed that rats fed extra choline produced offspring that were much more adept at learning and memory than the rats whose mothers were on a normal diet. And rats deprived of choline had offspring who did relatively poorly on memory tests.

Also, several well-designed studies have shown that a form of choline called choline alfoscerate helped people who had mild to moderate Alzheimer's disease improve. To get choline, you can take lecithin or the choline itself. The recommended dose for choline is 550 milligrams for males age 14 and older and 425 milligrams for females over age 19 (400 milligrams for females age 14 to 18). Lecithin is usually taken in a dosage of two 1,200-milligram capsules two times a day. There is also a granular form of lecithin—1 teaspoon contains 19 grains or 1,200 milligrams of lecithin.

Iron and Zinc to Help You Think

While researchers have established the importance of iron and zinc in the mental development of infants, you have to dig into the scientific literature before you'll find studies showing that these minerals help make for better memories in adults as well.

Iron supports the neurotransmitters in your brain that help keep your memory sharp; if you are deficient in iron, your ability to remember where you put your car keys or when you scheduled your dentist's appointment may suffer. Women who experience heavy periods or people with poor diets are especially vulnerable to iron deficiency and, thus, memory problems. In one study, women with low iron levels missed twice as many questions on a memory test as those with sufficient iron levels. After 4 months of taking iron supplements, the women who were previously low in iron (and thus memory power) scored just as well as the best group did in the first test. If you think you may be low in iron, take a multivitamin that contains 18 milligrams of iron (8 milligrams if you are a postmenopausal woman).

For a closer look at zinc's role in helping you think, researchers at the USDA Grand Forks Human Nutrition Research Center in North Dakota fed 10 men living at the center meals containing 1, 2, 3, 4, or 10 milligrams of zinc every day for 5 weeks each.

At the end of the 25-week study, researchers noted that the week the men ate 10 milligrams of zinc a day, they were better able to remember shapes and responded faster to simple motor tasks, says James G. Penland, PhD, head researcher at the center and author of the study. "There was a very clear improvement at ten milligrams versus the other amounts, with the others being more or less the same," he says.

And how does zinc help memory? Apparently, vitamin B_6 can't do its job without zinc pitching in, says Dr. Ebadi. "In the absence of zinc, active B_6 is not formed properly in the brain, and as a result, neither are key neurotransmitters," he says. Not only that, but large amounts of zinc have been found in the brain's memory center, the hippocampus.

Some experts say that some elderly people may get less than half of the zinc that they need. (The Daily Value for zinc is 15 milligrams.)

MÉNIÈRE'S DISEASE

STOPPING THE SPINNING

If you've ever been so drunk that you feel like the room is spinning, you know exactly what someone experiencing an acute attack of Ménière's disease is going through. This disorder affects the part of the inner ear that controls balance: a tiny set of membranes and nerve endings that respond to motion. When this part of the ear is damaged, it sets off a reaction that results in stop-the-world-I-want-to-get-off vertigo that only time resolves.

"The function of the inner ear is to let your brain know where your head is relative to your body in space, so you can close your eyes and turn your body in any direction and know where your head is," says Narinder Duggal, MD, clinical pharmacy specialist, internist, and medical director of Liberty

---

Food Factors

Ear doctors and their patients agree that healthy eating can go a long way toward alleviating ear problems, for plenty of reasons. Here are the details.

Chip away at fat. A damaged inner ear is particularly sensitive to high blood levels of cholesterol. Some researchers believe that fat in the blood actually makes the blood more viscous, or thick, and impairs blood delivery through the tiny artery that leads to the inner ear.

So cut fat, especially saturated fat, from your diet. Cut saturated fat to less than 7 percent of your total daily calories. This means filling up on fresh vegetables and fruits, whole grains, beans, low-fat dairy products, fish, and lean cuts of meat. Eat only the low-fat versions of lunchmeats, mayonnaise, cheeses, frozen desserts, and baked goods.

Battle your sweet tooth. Loading up on sugar does several things. It prompts your body to pump up insulin production. (Insulin is a hormone that your body uses to get energy from sugar.) Too much sugar in your diet can also send your blood sugar levels to extremes of high and low, says Charles P. Kimmelman, MD, director of New York City Ear, Nose, and Throat Center. Your ears don't like that, he says.

It's easy enough to avoid the usual sugar-laden snacks: cookies, candy, and soda. But the sweet stuff also lurks in some unsuspected

---

Bay Internal Medicine in Poulsbo, Washington. Normally, the fluid in your inner ear is contained in two balloonlike chambers. A series of receptors in the inner ear that are sensitive to motion use the fluid to gauge the relation of your head to the rest of the world. In people with Ménière's disease, however, this mechanism is thrown off, so much so in some people that they can't walk. "Some people with Ménière's are so restricted that they cannot live independently," Dr. Duggal says. Less serious attacks leave people feeling nauseated, weak, and disoriented.

It seems that in people with Ménière's disease, something, perhaps a virus, interferes with the proper balance of fluid in the inner ear. Fluid pressure builds, eventually rupturing a tiny membrane in the inner ear. The rupture is often preceded by a feeling of fullness or ear pressure, followed by a loud, roaring noise and hearing loss that can be temporary or permanent. Other symptoms may include nausea and vomiting as well as tinnitus, in which there's persistent noise such as hissing or buzzing in the ear.

While the vertigo typically lasts for 10 to 60 minutes, the entire attack often encompasses hours. Ménière's disease can be helped by certain allergy

foods. Low-fat cookies and other snacks, fruit-flavored yogurt, flavored teas and breakfast cereals, and even some salad dressings can all pack a sugar wallop. If you're really looking to curb your sweet tooth, check labels for sugar content and enjoy these foods only in moderation.

Know your salt sources. To cut salt, nutrition experts recommend reading labels carefully and avoiding foods with more than 150 milligrams of sodium per serving (for a total of no more than 2,300 milligrams per day, 1,500 milligrams if you have high blood pressure). Either eliminate potato chips, corn chips, pickles, olives, ham, hot dogs, canned foods (soups, beans, and vegetables), hard cheeses, soy sauce, cottage cheese, tomato juice, tuna, lunchmeats, biscuits, pancakes, breads, and pizza, or use low-sodium or no-sodium versions of these foods.

You can reduce the salt in some canned foods up to 80 percent by rinsing and draining the food for 1 minute.

Try using onion powder or garlic powder as seasoning rather than salt. In fact, there's a whole world of tastes worth exploring. Try sage or savory on chicken and rosemary or marjoram on meats, and add dried mushrooms and tomatoes to casseroles.

drugs that are also ideal for relieving the symptoms of dizziness. If nausea and vomiting are major components of an extended attack, then antinausea suppositories may be used. For temporary relief, doctors frequently prescribe diuretics (water pills) to reduce fluid buildup in the ear. Some doctors also make several dietary recommendations.

Shake the Salt Habit

For most doctors, top on the list of dietary advice for people with Ménière's disease is to cut way back on sodium, an essential nutrient that's too abundant in most diets. "Some people with Ménière's seem to be extremely sensitive to salt, almost as though their ears pick up any extra salt they can," explains Michael Seidman, MD, medical director of the Center for Integrative Medicine at Henry Ford Health System in Detroit, codirector of the Tinnitus Center, and author of *Save Your Hearing Now.*

Once salt is concentrated in the fluid within the inner ear, it draws in additional fluid, increasing the pressure in the inner ear until the membrane ruptures, setting off a dizzying attack. Eventually, the membrane heals and the ear settles down. Some doctors ask their patients to make sure that they get no more than 1,000 to 2,000 milligrams of sodium per day. The higher amount is for active people living in hot climates. One study of soldiers estimated that they got about 11,000 milligrams a day! (There are 2,000 milligrams of sodium in 1 teaspoon of salt.)

Other Minerals Balance Salt

Although it's obvious that people with Ménière's disease should cut back on salt, they should be looking at other mineral needs as well. Magnesium, calcium, and potassium are other minerals that are critical to the normal functioning of the inner ear, explains Charles P. Kimmelman, MD, director of New York City Ear, Nose, and Throat Center.

Because these minerals are so important to healthy ears, some doctors tell their patients with Ménière's disease to make sure that they get at least the Daily Values.

For magnesium, that's 400 milligrams a day. Studies show that most people come up short, with men usually getting about 320 milligrams a day and

Prescriptions for Healing

Doctors recommend cutting back on salt and adding these nutrients to a healthy diet to reduce the dizziness of Ménière's disease.

Nutrient	Daily Amount
Calcium	1,000 milligrams
Magnesium	400 milligrams
Nicotinic acid	100–200 milligrams
Potassium	3,500 milligrams

Plus a multivitamin/mineral supplement containing the Daily Values of all essential vitamins and minerals

MEDICAL ALERT: *Some diuretics, which are often prescribed for people with Ménière's disease, can deplete the body of potassium and magnesium. Before taking supplements of either nutrient, however, talk to your doctor. Too much of either mineral can be harmful.*

If you have heart or kidney problems, be sure to consult your doctor before supplementing magnesium.

Potassium supplements should not be taken by those with diabetes or kidney disease or by those using certain medications, including nonsteroidal anti-inflammatory drugs, potassium-sparing diuretics, ACE inhibitors, and heart medications such as heparin.

women getting about 230 milligrams a day. Whole grains, nuts, and beans are your best magnesium sources. Green vegetables are good sources, but bananas are the only fruit that provides much magnesium.

For calcium, doctors recommend aiming for the Daily Value of 1,000 milligrams. One cup of 1 percent milk offers about 300 milligrams of calcium, 1 ounce of hard cheese (part-skim mozzarella) offers about 181 milligrams, and 8 ounces of low-fat yogurt offers about 415 milligrams.

To get a healthy amount of potassium—3,500 milligrams or more a day—load up on fresh fruits and vegetables and their juices. A cup of tomato juice, for instance, has about 537 milligrams of potassium, orange juice has 496 milligrams, and prune juice has 707 milligrams. Potatoes, yams, avocados, Swiss chard, and bananas are also good sources. Since potassium is leached out by boiling water, you'll want to stick to fresh, baked, or lightly steamed fruits and vegetables.

Note: Diuretics, pills that increase your flow of urine, are frequently prescribed for people with Ménière's disease, says Dr. Kimmelman. Some types of diuretics can deplete the body of potassium and sometimes of magnesium. If you're taking this kind of diuretic, he says, check with your doctor to make sure that you get enough supplemental potassium and magnesium to make up for the loss. Don't take potassium and magnesium supplements on your own in this situation, however. Too much of either mineral can be harmful, especially if you have heart or kidney problems or diabetes.

Open Up Your Ears with Nicotinic Acid

"Nicotinic acid has been recommended for Ménière's disease for at least 30 to 40 years," says Belinda Jenks, PhD, RD, director of scientific affairs and nutrition education at Pharmavite in Mission Hills, California. "It works by dilating the small blood vessels in the ear and improving bloodflow. For Ménière's disease, nicotinic acid has been recommended in large doses—between 100 and 200 milligrams," she says. "With nicotinic acid, you have to dose very slowly because you can get what's called 'nicotinic flush' and gastrointestinal disturbances. Start with ¼ of a dose one day with food, and then half a dose the next day and so forth," she says.

Other Vitamins May Deter Dizziness

Do any other vitamins or minerals help Ménière's disease? A number of ear doctors and other hearing specialists recommend a multivitamin/mineral supplement to their patients with Ménière's disease, but they're hard-pressed to come up with the kind of scientific proof that most doctors insist on before recommending something as being effective.

Even if you decide to take a multivitamin/mineral supplement, make sure that you follow the dietary measures recommended in "Food Factors" on page 380 as well. While nutrients can make up for some dietary indiscretions, it's unrealistic to expect them to overcome constant bad eating habits.

MENOPAUSAL PROBLEMS

REINVENTING THE
CHANGE OF LIFE

Some women have a miserable time at menopause. Others barely notice that it's happening.

Although menopause is technically defined by health care professionals as one single day, the process of menopause can last a decade or longer. Menopause results when the ovaries decrease production of the sex hormones progesterone, estrogen, and androgen and therefore stop producing eggs. A woman is said to have reached menopause when she has not had a menstrual period for 12 months. The average woman has her last period at age 51, but menopausal changes actually begin much earlier. Women often notice changes in their cycles when they're in their early forties or even before then. Periods may be shorter or longer, lighter or heavier; they may come closer together or farther apart.

The Estrogen Connection

It's during this time, known as perimenopause, that the ovaries gradually slow their production of the female hormone estrogen and that a woman begins to notice the effects this has on her body. So why do some women experience such discomfort at menopause, while others never have so much as a single hot flash?

It may be because some women experience more drastic drops in their estrogen levels than others do, says Margo Woods, DSc, associate professor in the nutrition/infection unit at Tufts University School of Medicine in Boston. Dr. Woods has done research on the effects of soy on menopausal symptoms. She found that Asian women, who have lower estrogen levels before menopause than Western women, experienced less drastic drops in estrogen, which may be one reason that they report fewer menopausal symptoms, says Dr. Woods. Many researchers feel that diet may influence menopausal symptoms.

And some lucky women, about 25 to 30 percent, don't entirely stop producing estrogen, says Susan M. Lark, MD, a physician specializing in women's health; editor of *Women's Wellness Today*; president of DrLark.com in Forrester Center, West Virginia; and author of *Menopause: Self-Help Book*. Even after their ovaries stop producing estrogen, their adrenal glands and one small area of each ovary called the stroma continue to produce small amounts of this hormone. These glands don't produce enough estrogen to promote menstruation, but they do produce enough to keep the most bothersome symptoms of menopause at bay, explains Dr. Lark.

Fighting Back with Phytoestrogens

If you're fed up with menopause, move to Japan. In the Land of the Rising Sun, hot flashes and night sweats are virtually unheard of. "Asian women and American women have reported such dramatically different experiences of menopause that it's easy to wonder if we're talking about the same thing," says Margo Woods, DSc, associate professor in the nutrition/infection unit at Tufts University School of Medicine in Boston. Of course, Japanese women don't have an easier time with menopause just because of where they live. Researchers believe that it has more to do with their traditional diet. Besides providing more vegetable protein and less animal protein than a Western diet, it's also low in fat and high in soy products such as tofu. These foods are rich in plant compounds known as phytoestrogens, which seem to mimic some of the biological activities of female hormones.

"Japanese women of all ages have higher estrogen levels than their American counterparts," says Dr. Woods. "At first we thought it was just because of their lower-fat, higher-fiber diet. Now it looks as if phytoestrogens might also play a role."

While the phytoestrogen content of soy foods varies considerably from brand to brand, one or two servings of tofu, soybeans, or soy milk a day is equivalent to the usual intake of the Asian population. It also contains approximately 35 milligrams of phytoestrogens, a reasonable goal to shoot for, says Dr. Woods.

On average, Japanese women eat from 2.5 to 3.5 ounces of tofu per day, says Dr. Woods.

"If you are having hot flashes and night sweats and don't want to take hormones, I certainly think it would be worthwhile to try it. It can't hurt," says Dr. Woods. Legumes and vegetables can be eaten without restraint and in moderation (one serving per day).

"Some women are just good estrogen producers," she says. "We don't know why."

The amount of estrogen that the body continues to produce is out of a woman's hands, adds Dr. Lark. But there are plenty of other factors that a woman can control that can reduce menopausal discomfort. "Women who avoid stress, who don't overdo caffeine, and who get regular exercise have a much easier time of it than women who don't do those things," she says.

"There isn't much hard evidence to prove it, but it has been my experience that women who have a history of premenstrual syndrome and bad menstrual cramps also have more hot flashes and other symptoms of menopause," says Dr. Lark. And here again, lifestyle factors come into play. "These women tend to have very stressful lives, poor diets, and poor coping skills," she maintains.

Finally, nutrition apparently plays an important role in determining whether your menopause will be an endurance contest or a walk in the park. Here's what experts say you can do to make the transition as comfortable as possible.

Vitamin E Snuffs Out Hot Flashes

A hot flash—that sudden, intensely hot feeling in your face and neck that makes you wish for a walk-in refrigerator—can happen any time, anywhere: at home, at work, while you're driving in traffic, or even while you're sleeping.

Caused by hormonal surges, hot flashes usually last for 3 to 5 minutes, but they can feel like an eternity. Some women get flushed, sweat profusely, and even have heart palpitations. Other women have flashes so mild that they barely notice them. About 80 percent of all women going through menopause have hot flashes at one point or another.

Studies show that thin women are more prone to hot flashes than heavier women. This is because even after the ovaries slow their hormone production, fat cells continue to produce small amounts of estrogen. So women with a lot of fat cells go through less drastic estrogen withdrawal than their leaner sisters.

While hot flashes can be relieved by hormone replacement therapy, there may be another, less drastic option: a daily vitamin E supplement.

Vitamin E can act as an estrogen substitute, explains Dr. Lark. Studies have shown that it can relieve hot flashes, night sweats, mood swings, and even vaginal dryness. "Vitamin E is really an essential part of a supplement program for women during the menopause years," she says.

If vitamin E is so effective, why hasn't your doctor recommended it? Chances are she has never heard of it, or if she has, she's waiting to see some hard scientific proof that it works. And sad to say, there isn't any. While a number of studies were done in the 1940s on vitamin E and menopause, the connection hasn't been investigated recently. A number of doctors who use nutritional therapies as part of their medical practices recommend it, however, and find that it often works.

If you get hot flashes and would like to try vitamin E, Dr. Lark recommends a fairly high dose: about 800 IU. And while vitamin E is non-toxic at this level, she says, women should get their doctors' okay before

Food Factors

Menopause is an excellent time to take stock of your eating habits and make healthy adjustments, says Susan M. Lark, MD, a physician specializing in women's health; editor of *Women's Wellness Today*; president of DrLark.com in Forrester Center, West Virginia; and author of *Menopause: Self-Help Book*. The following simple changes, she says, can make a big difference in your health during menopause and in the years to come.

Shake the salt habit. Eating too much salt can contribute to water retention, a common problem among women going through menopause, says Dr. Lark. "It's not enough to stop adding salt to your foods," she cautions. "I tell women to eliminate fast foods, salty snacks, and other highly processed foods and to use garlic and herbs instead of salt in cooking." Aim for no more than 2,300 milligrams of salt per day and no more than 1,500 milligrams if you have high blood pressure.

Switch to decaf. "A number of studies show that women who use caffeine have more hot flashes than those who don't," says Dr. Lark. A high intake of caffeine also increases anxiety, irritability, and mood swings. It depletes the body's stores of the B-complex vitamins, explains Dr. Lark, which can be a real problem for some women during menopause.

With all of these negative side effects, Dr. Lark recommends either dramatically cutting down on caffeine or eliminating it entirely. Because cutting out caffeine can cause withdrawal symptoms such as

taking this high amount, especially if they have diabetes or high blood pressure.

Reduce Bleeding with Nutrients

Many women approach menopause expecting menstrual flow to taper off and finally stop. But for a good percentage, periods during perimenopause are heavier than ever.

Besides the inconvenience—perimenopausal bleeding is often so irregular that women have to be prepared at all times—frequent heavy bleeding can seriously endanger a woman's iron stores, says Dr. Lark.

irritability and headaches, she suggests cutting back gradually. And don't forget that tea, chocolate, and cola drinks also contain caffeine, she adds.

Stay away from soda, even if it's diet. "A lot of women drink diet soda, and the phosphorus in diet soda can offset the calcium-to-phosphorus ratio," says Stella Volpe, PhD, RD, associate professor at the University of Pennsylvania School of Nursing in Philadelphia. Calcium is important to women during menopause, because osteoporosis becomes a bigger threat around this time in their lives. "A good calcium-to-phosphorus ratio is 2:1 or 1:1, and drinking a lot of soda can alter that ratio," she says. "I recommend limiting diet soda to no more than one to two cans per week. Instead, drink flavored or seltzer waters, 100 percent juice, or better yet, drink milk or soy products that are fortified with calcium," she says.

Be a teetotaler. Alcohol depletes the body's B-complex vitamins, disrupts the liver's ability to metabolize hormones, and can worsen hot flashes, says Dr. Lark. "Excessive drinking is also a risk factor for osteoporosis, which all menopausal women should be concerned about," she adds. If you can't cut out cocktails altogether, she suggests limiting yourself to no more than one or two drinks a week.

Eat more fruits and vegetables. Fresh produce is full of important vitamins and minerals, says Dr. Lark. And because they're low in fat and high in fiber, eating more fruits and vegetables can help prevent weight gain, a common problem for women of menopausal age.

Heavy bleeding can be treated effectively with nutrients, says Dr. Lark. "Some studies have shown that besides replenishing the iron lost through bleeding, a daily iron supplement may actually reduce the amount that a woman will bleed during future periods," she says.

Women with heavy bleeding also benefit from loading up on vitamin C and bioflavonoids, she says. Bioflavonoids are chemical compounds related to vitamin C; they're found in many citrus fruits and included in many supplements.

Prescriptions for Healing

While scientific studies have yet to be done, a number of doctors have found that certain nutrients may help many women avoid problems as they go through menopause. Here's what these doctors recommend.

Nutrient	Daily Amount
B-complex supplement containing . . .	
Niacin	50 milligrams
Thiamin	50 milligrams
Vitamin B$_6$	30 milligrams
Calcium citrate	1,000–1,500 milligrams (1,000 milligrams in 2 divided doses if postmenopausal and taking estrogen, 1,200 milligrams in 2 divided doses if not postmenopausal, and 1,500 milligrams in 3 divided doses if postmenopausal and not receiving estrogen therapy)
Iron	15 milligrams
Magnesium	500–750 milligrams
Vitamin C	1,000 milligrams
Vitamin E	800 IU

MEDICAL ALERT: People with heart or kidney problems should check with their doctors before taking supplemental magnesium.

If you are taking anticoagulant drugs, you should not take vitamin E supplements. (Though generally a dose of up to 1,500 IU of vitamin E a day is considered safe, some recent reports suggest that taking more than 400 IU a day could be harmful to people with cardiovascular or circulatory disease or with cancer. If you have such a condition, be sure to consult your doctor before you begin supplementation.)

"Both vitamin C and bioflavonoids reduce bleeding by strengthening the capillary walls, which are at their weakest just before and during the menstrual period," says Dr. Lark. And since bioflavonoids have many of the same chemical properties as estrogen, they can also be helpful in controlling hot flashes, night sweats, and mood swings. She recommends a daily supplement that includes at least 1,000 milligrams of vitamin C and 800 milligrams of bioflavonoids.

Because vitamin C helps the body absorb iron more efficiently, Dr. Lark recommends taking these two nutrients together. If you take a multivitamin/mineral supplement, check to make sure that it contains both vitamin C and iron. Another option is to take an iron supplement, about 15 milligrams, with a glass of orange juice. If you have a juicer, juicing the white pulp of the orange along with the rest of the fruit guarantees an abundant dose of bioflavonoids, Dr. Lark adds.

B Complex Battles the Blahs

Depression is also common around the time of menopause, though nobody knows for sure how much of it results from hormonal fluctuations and how much is triggered by the everyday stresses that women face at midlife.

Regardless of what's causing it, emotional stress can deplete the body of B vitamins, leaving a woman feeling tired, anxious, and irritable, says Dr. Lark.

"High levels of estrogen can also deplete vitamin B_6 and cause depression," says Dr. Lark. "Women who take the Pill or hormone replacement therapy sometimes have this, and some perimenopausal women go through a period of having very high estrogen levels." B_6 also plays an important role in helping the liver regulate estrogen levels, says Dr. Lark.

Vitamin B_6 should always be taken as part of the B complex, says Dr. Lark. She suggests a B-complex supplement containing 50 milligrams each of thiamin and niacin and 30 milligrams of B_6.

Coping with Surgical Menopause

While most women experience the gradual progression of natural menopause, others go through "the change" much more abruptly. Each year thousands of women undergo hysterectomy, the surgical removal of the uterus and sometimes the ovaries because of conditions as varied as pelvic infection, endometriosis, and cancer.

In most cases, the woman's ovaries are left intact; they continue to produce estrogen until the woman goes through normal menopause. But if a woman's ovaries are removed along with her uterus in what is called a complete hysterectomy, she'll experience surgical menopause, with the same symptoms as any other woman who is going through natural menopause.

Women who experience surgical menopause may actually have more severe symptoms because they go through menopause so abruptly, says Dr. Lark.

A woman who undergoes a hysterectomy can benefit from the same nutritional strategies that help women who are going through natural menopause, says Dr. Lark. "As far as your body is concerned, it's the same process," she says.

Bolster Bones with Calcium

Around menopause, women should start seriously thinking about the possibility of osteoporosis and should make sure they're getting enough calcium. "Although increased calcium intake during the first five years of menopause isn't as crucial as it is once a woman has reached postmenopause, it is a good idea to get in the habit of getting enough as soon as possible," says Stella Volpe, PhD, RD, associate professor at the University of Pennsylvania School of Nursing in Philadelphia.

Calcium is very important for maintaining bone mass and strength as women get older, and it becomes especially vital when estrogen levels decline during menopause and make women even more vulnerable to developing osteoporosis. Take 1,200 milligrams of the calcium citrate form of calcium per day in two divided doses. If you are postmenopausal and are not receiving estrogen therapy, take 1,500 milligrams of calcium citrate daily divided into three separate doses. If you are postmenopausal and taking estrogen, take 1,000 milligrams of calcium citrate per day in two divided doses.

To maximize the absorption of calcium, take a magnesium supplement to reach a ratio of magnesium to calcium of 1:2. For example, if you are taking 1,200 milligrams of calcium, take 600 milligrams of magnesium.

MENSTRUAL PROBLEMS

NUTRIENTS TO EASE
MONTHLY DISTRESS

Imagine you were moving to the North Pole for 5 years. How would you prepare for your new life? Most likely, you'd learn everything you could about coping with the cold. And if there was anything you could eat or any supplement you could take to make the experience more pleasant, of course you'd want to know about it. It's 5 years of your life, after all. You might as well be comfortable.

Maybe you never thought about it, but if you add it up—month after month, year after year—you have your period for about 5 years of your life. And if you're like most women, you'd do anything to sail through those days without feeling crampy and exhausted and swollen up like a beluga.

Why You Feel So Bad

Most women have some degree of menstrual discomfort at some point in their lives, says Susan M. Lark, MD, a physician specializing in women's health and author of the newsletter *Women's Wellness Today*. Most menstrual pain is classified as either spasmodic or congestive. Doctors know that spasmodic pain is caused by the female hormones estrogen and progesterone and by prostaglandins, hormonelike substances that control muscle tension. Women with spasmodic cramps generally have an excess of a certain type of prostaglandins called 2-series prostaglandins, which are responsible for contraction of the smooth muscles, including the uterus. Prostaglandin production increases toward the end of your cycle, resulting in cramps that are sometimes accompanied by nausea, constipation, or diarrhea.

Probably the best thing that can be said about spasmodic pain is that it tends to improve with age. It's usually most severe in women in their teens and twenties. Spasmodic pain often improves after a woman has children, says Dr. Lark.

The other type of menstrual pain is known as congestive. Women with congestive pain also tend to suffer from bloating, water retention, headaches, and breast pain. In addition, they often notice a worsening of their cramps when they eat certain foods, such as wheat and dairy products, or when they drink alcohol, says Dr. Lark. Unfortunately, congestive pain tends to get worse with age, whether or not a woman has children.

While monthly cramps aren't pleasant, they are normal, says Dr. Lark. She cautions that in some cases, the pain can be a symptom of a health problem that requires medical attention, such as endometriosis. "You should always discuss unusual menstrual symptoms with your doctor," she advises.

But most of the time, the cause of cramps is simply menstruation itself. And in such cases, some doctors maintain that a few prudent nutritional changes can do wonders to improve your quality of life during your period, says Dr. Lark. The following nutrients have been shown to help soothe menstrual symptoms.

Calcium, Magnesium, and Manganese: A One-Two-Three Punch for Painful Periods

Calcium, manganese, and magnesium all seem to ease some of the physical discomfort that so many women experience before and during their periods. "In one study, magnesium supplementation decreased lower back pain, lower abdominal pain, and lost days from work," says Shari Lieberman, PhD, president of the American Association for Health Freedom and author of *The Real Vitamin and Mineral Book* who runs a private nutritional practice in New York City. "In another, magnesium and vitamin B$_6$ together reduced the intensity and duration of menstrual cramps, and symptoms continued to improve over a four- to six-month period," she says.

And if that weren't enough, yet another study showed that 21 out of 25 women given magnesium experienced a decrease in menstrual symptoms as compared with 25 women who did not receive the supplement. "The authors of this study suggest these improvements may be due to the dramatic drop in the blood levels of certain prostaglandins as a result of the magnesium therapy, as well as magnesium's well-known ability to relax muscle spasms and dilate blood vessels," Dr. Lieberman says. To reap the same benefits, take 500 to 1,000 milligrams of magnesium per day beginning on the 15th day of your menstrual cycle and continue until your period starts. To avoid the loose stools that sometimes accompany magnesium supplementation, take the magnesium glycinate form.

Food Factors

When it comes to easing monthly discomfort, supplements are only part of the equation, says Susan M. Lark, MD, a physician specializing in women's health; editor of *Women's Wellness Today*; president of DrLark.com in Forrester Center, West Virginia; and author of *Menopause: Self-Help Book*. How you feel during your period also depends on what you eat during the rest of the month. Here's what she advises.

Beware of hidden sodium. Most women know that too much salt in the diet can aggravate monthly water retention, says Dr. Lark. But many don't know that much of the salt they're eating is hidden in seemingly healthy foods, such as canned vegetables, frozen dinners, and cheeses. Fast foods, pizza, and most snacks, such as chips and pretzels, are also heavily salted. Not to mention foods that contain soy sauce, such as Chinese food. Stop adding salt at the table and during cooking, she suggests, and get into the habit of reading food labels for sodium content. Salad dressings, prepared soups, and many condiments are loaded with sodium. Ultimately, you should aim for no more than 2,300 milligrams of sodium per day.

Focus on fiber. Constipation is a common complaint of women with menstrual cramps, says Dr. Lark. Solve the problem naturally with a fiber-rich diet that includes plenty of fruits, vegetables, legumes, and whole-grain breads and cereals. For best results, try to get at least 25 to 30 grams of fiber per day.

Try banishing wheat. Wheat can aggravate monthly symptoms in women who have food allergies, says Dr. Lark. If you suspect that you may be wheat-sensitive, she suggests substituting corn, oatmeal, brown rice, and rye bread for wheat products for a month or so to see if it helps.

Steer away from beef. A diet that contains lots of red meats such as beef, lamb, and pork may aggravate menstrual cramping, says Dr. Lark. Meat contains saturated fat, which the body uses to produce 2-series prostaglandins—chemicals that are responsible for the contraction of the smooth muscles of the uterus, which leads to cramping, she explains.

In addition, scientists at the USDA Grand Forks Human Nutrition Research Center in North Dakota have found that getting enough of certain minerals—particularly calcium and manganese—all month long can make a significant difference in how a woman feels during her period.

In one study, a group of menstruating women were fed a number of different diets over several months and questioned about how they felt at different points in their menstrual cycles. One of the diets was unusually low in calcium and manganese, a trace mineral that's found in nuts, tea, whole-grain cereals, and dried peas and beans. The same women also tried a diet that was supplemented with both minerals.

When the researchers analyzed the women's premenstrual symptoms, they noticed a clear pattern: Most women reported much less severe symptoms when they followed the diet high in both calcium and manganese.

It's interesting to note that the diet the researchers considered low in calcium, the one that produced the most uncomfortable menstrual periods, included about 587 milligrams of calcium per day. The high-calcium diet had about 1,336 milligrams of calcium, which is close to the amount experts recommend to prevent osteoporosis, the brittle bone disease.

Prescriptions for Healing

There are a few nutrients that can help make a woman's monthly cycle more comfortable. Here's what some medical experts recommend.

Nutrient	Daily Amount
Calcium	500–2,000 milligrams
Iron	15 milligrams
Magnesium	500–1,000 milligrams beginning on the 15th day of your menstrual cycle and continuing until your period starts
Manganese	2 milligrams
Niacin	25–200 milligrams, beginning 7–10 days before your period and stopping the day your period starts
Vitamin B_6	200–300 milligrams
Vitamin C	1,000 milligrams

MEDICAL ALERT: *If you have heart or kidney problems, be sure to consult your doctor before supplementing magnesium.*

Do not take niacin in doses exceeding 100 milligrams without medical supervision. Women with liver disease should use niacin only under medical supervision.

Vitamin B_6 can cause side effects when taken in doses of more than 100 milligrams daily, so it's a good idea to talk to your doctor before supplementing the amount recommended here.

Just how these minerals fend off menstrual discomfort isn't clear. Researchers know that calcium is involved in the production of prostaglandins. "It may be calcium's role in prostaglandin metabolism that's responsible for the mineral's effect on pain," says James G. Penland, PhD, head researcher at the USDA Grand Forks Human Nutrition Research Center.

Manganese's role is even more mysterious. "We do know that manganese is involved in blood clotting, and some research shows that a low intake is associated with a heavier menstrual flow," says Dr. Penland. "This is definitely an area that needs more study."

While researchers continue to try to figure out exactly how these two minerals work their magic on menstrual symptoms, a daily multivitamin/mineral supplement that includes the recommended levels of both calcium and manganese makes good sense for women who want to minimize menstrual discomfort, says Dr. Penland. The Daily Value for manganese is 2 milligrams. Because women of all ages have trouble getting enough calcium through diet, Dr. Penland recommends increasing your intake of low-fat, high-calcium foods such as low-fat yogurt and fat-free milk. If you still need more calcium, he suggests taking 500 to 1,000 milligrams of supplemental calcium a day.

If you make sure you get the calcium Dr. Penland recommends and you *still* have painful periods, up your calcium intake while you are experiencing cramps. Try taking 1,000 milligrams of calcium per day and 250 to 500 milligrams every 4 hours during painful cramping for a maximum of 2,000 milligrams per day. Calcium is best absorbed when taken with magnesium in a ratio of 2:1. For example, take 1,000 milligrams of calcium for every 500 milligrams of magnesium.

Vitamin B_6 Keeps Cramps at Bay

The whole B complex is essential for good health, but when it comes to relieving monthly symptoms, vitamin B_6 and niacin are the stars, says Dr. Lark.

Vitamin B_6 plays a key role in the production of 1-series prostaglandins, the "good" prostaglandins that relax the uterine muscles and keep cramps under control, according to Dr. Lark. But a woman's B_6 stores are easily depleted. Stress and certain medications, such as oral contraceptives, can easily cause a shortage. As a result, your body may not manufacture enough of the right kind of prostaglandins, leaving you feeling tied up in knots when your period comes. And if you're bothered by water retention or monthly weight gain, B_6 can ease those symptoms, too, Dr. Lark says.

Dr. Lark recommends taking vitamin B_6 as part of a B-complex supplement. Look for a B-complex supplement that contains no more than 200 to 300 milligrams of B_6. Large doses can be toxic, she says. It's a good idea to check with your doctor before taking doses of more than 100 milligrams daily.

Equally important in staving off cramps is niacin. "Some research shows that niacin is about 90 percent effective for relieving cramps," says Dr. Lark. To head off cramps before they start, she suggests taking between 25 and 200 milligrams of niacin a day, beginning 7 to 10 days before your period is due and stopping the day that your period starts. This treatment can be repeated every month to prevent menstrual cramps.

Because niacin can cause slight flushing in some women, start with 25 milligrams a day for the first month. "If it doesn't seem to help, you can always increase the dose the following month until you find the level that's right for you," she advises. Women with liver disease should use niacin only under medical supervision, cautions Dr. Lark.

Nutrients to Lessen Bleeding

Next to cramps, heavy bleeding is probably the most common complaint of menstruating women, says Dr. Lark. Besides being inconvenient, heavy bleeding can deplete a woman's iron stores and can even lead to anemia.

It isn't surprising, then, that doctors recommend iron supplements to women with heavy bleeding. What is surprising is that getting extra doses of this mineral doesn't just replace the iron that has been lost. It may actually reduce the amount of bleeding in the future, says Dr. Lark.

'Women need only a small amount of iron. But what they need they really need," she says. She recommends a daily supplement of about 15 milligrams.

Women with heavy bleeding also need plenty of vitamin C and bioflavonoids, says Dr. Lark. Bioflavonoids are chemical compounds related to vitamin C; they're found in many citrus fruits and included in many supplements. Both vitamin C and bioflavonoids reduce bleeding by strengthening the capillary walls, which are at their weakest just before and during the menstrual period, says Dr. Lark. She recommends a daily supplement that includes at least 1,000 milligrams of vitamin C and 800 milligrams of bioflavonoids.

Because vitamin C helps the body absorb iron more efficiently, Dr. Lark recommends taking these two nutrients together.

MIGRAINES

ENDING THE PAIN

The hammering inside your head is utterly horrendous, as if someone were using your brain for a bongo. For what it's worth, you're not the only one with a built-in percussion section: Roughly 28 to 32 million Americans reportedly suffer from migraines each year.

Although tension headaches are by far the most common types of headaches, chronic migraines are much more likely to send a desperate individual to the doctor seeking relief. Besides the agonizing pain, people who suffer from migraines often have tremendous sensitivity to light and noise. Just snapping your fingers or clapping around them can be excruciating.

The one-sided, throbbing headache known as a migraine is three times more common in women than in men. But what migraines lack in gender equality they make up for in severity. Some migraines are so extreme that they cause limb numbness, hallucinations, nausea, and vomiting.

The good news is that medical research has come up with several vitamin and mineral therapies that might prove helpful for people who have been unable to find relief elsewhere.

"B" Headache-Free

Fifty-two quarts of chocolate syrup. Nine hundred bowls of cornflakes. These might prevent a migraine—if they weren't guaranteed to give you a stomachache first. They add up to a super high dose of riboflavin, which research hints may ward off the someone's-put-a-soccer-ball-in-my-head pain.

In a study done at Kaiser Permanente in California and published in the journal *Headache*, participants took a daily dose of a combination of 400 milligrams of riboflavin, 300 milligrams of magnesium, and 100 milligrams of feverfew or 25 milligrams of riboflavin for 3 months. At the end of the study, researchers found no difference in reduction of migraines—the people taking 25 milligrams of riboflavin had the same results as those taking the combination, indicating that 25 milligrams of riboflavin may be just as effective for preventing migraines as a combination of higher doses of riboflavin, feverfew, and magnesium.

Food Factors

A host of foods contain chemicals that can cause severe headaches. Here's what nutrition experts say to avoid.

Say no to MSG. A flavor enhancer used in restaurants and in prepared foods such as soups, salad dressings, and lunchmeats, monosodium glutamate (MSG), even in small amounts, can provoke severe headaches as well as flushing and tingling in headache-prone people, says Seymour Diamond, MD, director and founder of the Diamond Headache Clinic and director of the inpatient headache unit at Saint Joseph Hospital in Chicago. In fact, one study showed that roughly 30 percent of those who eat Chinese food suffer these same symptoms. Although more research needs to be done, MSG seems to act as a vasodilator, which means it opens and then closes the blood vessels in the head. This process is exactly what happens in a migraine. Because of these negative effects, a lot of Chinese restaurants have eliminated MSG from their cooking, but to be sure, ask when you order whether or not the food is MSG-free.

When it comes to food you eat at home, however, because of all of the bad press, spotting MSG on food labels is harder than ever. "Natural flavor" and "hydrolyzed vegetable protein," for example, substitute for MSG in everything from frozen dinners, potato chips, and sauces to canned meats.

Nix the nitrites. Commonly used as a preservative in hot dogs, salami, bacon, and other cured meats, nitrites have been known to provoke migraines, says Dr. Diamond.

Corral the caffeine. The experts are divided here. Coffee, cola, and tea all contain caffeine, which can act as a vasoconstrictor and, as a result, limit bloodflow through the blood vessels in your head.

"A little bit of caffeine may help a headache, but you get either withdrawal or a rebound phenomenon from having too much," says Dr. Dia-

Why would something like riboflavin work? Researchers have noticed a deficit in certain energy generators in the brain cells of some people with migraines. They suspect that flooding the system with riboflavin could indirectly help regenerate this flagging energy system and somehow short-circuit migraine pain.

What's attractive about riboflavin, if rigorous scientific studies support these preliminary findings, is that it's likely to have fewer side effects than current headache preventives (although no one knows for sure what the long-term effects of this much riboflavin might be).

mond. Still, even 2 cups of a caffeine-containing beverage per day removes precious magnesium from your system, he says.

The bottom line: If you're having a problem with migraines, avoid caffeine for a month or so and see if it helps.

Consider cutting down on aspartame. Although few studies show a direct link between this artificial sweetener and headaches, some people do report problems with it, especially when they ingest a lot, says Dr. Diamond. "My advice to people is that it probably won't bother you, but if you can relate a headache to it, you should not use it," he says.

To test whether this or any other food is causing your headaches, keep a diary of your meals as well as any headaches for a month. If you see a pattern and it looks like one of the foods you're eating is causing the problem, cut the food out of your diet and see if it helps, advises Dr. Diamond.

Keep track of tyramine. A whopping 30 percent of migraine sufferers seem to have sensitivity to an amino acid called tyramine. Found in stronger aged cheeses, pickled herring, chicken livers, canned figs, fresh-baked goods made with yeast, lima beans, Italian beans, lentils, snow peas, navy beans, pinto beans, peanuts, sunflower seeds, pumpkin seeds, and sesame seeds, tyramine means migraine pain for many, says Dr. Diamond. Try eliminating these tyramine-containing foods and see if it helps, he suggests.

Cut your Kisses. Chocolate contains a chemical called phenylethylamine that, like tyramine, can cause headaches, says Dr. Diamond.

Ban the booze. The alcohol in drinks can dilate the blood vessels in your brain and cause a headache, warns Dr. Diamond. Also, chemicals known as congeners as well as impurities in Scotch and other hard liquors have the same effect, he says. And if that weren't enough, the dehydration caused by drinking alcohol can also make your head pound.

Although riboflavin generally is quite harmless, it's a good idea to check with your doctor before supplementing with such a high amount.

Making the Magnesium-Migraine Link

An increasing number of doctors believe that a fairly large percentage of the most severe cases of migraines may actually be caused by an imbalance of key minerals such as magnesium and calcium.

"Magnesium is probably one of the strongest vascular protective minerals available, and many people are deficient in it," says Narinder Duggal, MD, clinical pharmacy specialist, internist, and medical director of Liberty Bay Internal Medicine in Poulsbo, Washington. "Most of the data shows that if you take magnesium, it improves migraine headaches," he says.

Many studies have shown intravenous magnesium's effectiveness for easing migraines, and some preliminary studies have shown that magnesium taken orally is effective as well. And still other studies have shown that women who are deficient in magnesium have a higher rate of menstrual migraines than women who have adequate levels. To understand why magnesium might do the trick, it helps to take a look at how migraines happen.

Migraines are thought to be caused by vascular changes, or changes in the blood vessels, that reduce blood or oxygen flow in the scalp and brain. What causes these vascular changes? Things such as muscle contractions during times of stress and biochemicals called catecholamines and serotonin, which are circulating in the blood. Too much serotonin can cause bloodflow to slow; too little can cause blood to move through too rapidly.

While mainstream researchers have long known that changes in serotonin and catecholamine levels cause migraine pain, stopping these changes has been a hit-or-miss proposition. Aspirin, for example, temporarily inhibits the effects of serotonin but does nothing to prevent a migraine from coming back.

Among its many important roles in the body, magnesium helps regulate blood vessel diameter and, therefore, the availability of serotonin. It's very likely that magnesium deficiency is a widespread cause of migraines, maintains Dr. Duggal. In fact, an estimated 50 percent of migraine sufferers have a magnesium deficiency. Studies show that many people don't even come close to getting the Daily Value of magnesium, which is 400 milligrams. What's more, several different things, from the caffeine in just 2 cups of coffee a day to the chemicals in most asthma medications, remove some magnesium from your system. "Research indicates that dietary intake by many people in developed countries, including the United States, is less than the recommended level," says Karen Kubena, PhD, professor of nutrition at Texas A&M University in College Station. "Furthermore, many medications, including a number of those used by patients with cardiovascular disease, and alcohol increase the loss of magnesium from the body. People with diabetes who have continual elevated blood sugar excrete more magnesium in the urine and, as a result, may develop a magnesium deficiency," she says. Even stress, a frequent cause of migraines, can remove magnesium from your system.

Prescriptions for Healing

While vitamin and mineral supplements are by no means the first line of treatment for migraines, there are a couple of therapies that just might work when all else fails. Here's what some experts recommend.

Nutrient	Daily Amount
Magnesium	600 milligrams in 2-3 divided doses
Riboflavin	25-400 milligrams

MEDICAL ALERT: Doses for these two therapies are extremely high. If you wish to try these supplements to treat migraines, you should discuss it with your doctor.

People who have kidney or heart problems should supplement magnesium only under medical supervision.

So can getting more than your share of magnesium every day prevent migraines? Studies evaluating magnesium supplements for migraines have had mixed results. One study done on patients with menstrual migraine showed that headaches improved with magnesium supplements. Another German study showed a modest improvement in migraines in people taking magnesium, but the follow-up study didn't show the same results. And a small study done by headache expert Alexander Mauskop, MD, of the New York Headache Center showed that people with cluster migraine headaches improved after taking magnesium. So it certainly can't hurt to try to get adequate magnesium—especially through your diet. Foods rich in magnesium include almonds, cashews, soybeans, dark green leafy vegetables, seafood, bananas, and milk. Unfortunately, some foods abundant in magnesium are also headache triggers, such as nuts, beans, and fresh bread. If you are sensitive to these triggers, you may need to take magnesium supplements rather than trying to get the mineral from foods.

For people with migraines, experts who suggest magnesium supplements recommend taking 600 milligrams divided into two or three doses. Large doses of magnesium can cause diarrhea. In people who experience diarrhea, the magnesium glycinate form of the supplement may work better.

In other people with migraines, magnesium gluconate—the more biologically active form—may be more effective. "The active form of magnesium is ionized magnesium. When a substance is chemically bound, it's sort of neutralized, if you want to use a *Star Trek* term. When it's ionized, it is available to do what it is supposed to do, which in this case is possibly prevent constriction of blood vessels in your brain and scalp," explains Dr. Kubena.

The Calcium Connection

Even if you monitor your magnesium level like a maniac, you're still at risk for migraines if your calcium level is out of whack. The reason: Magnesium and calcium interact with each other.

It seems that higher than normal blood levels of calcium cause the body to excrete the rest, which in turn triggers a loss of magnesium.

"Let's say you have just enough magnesium and too much calcium in your blood. If calcium is excreted, the magnesium goes with it. All of a sudden, you could be low in magnesium," says Dr. Kubena.

In fact, people who have low magnesium and elevated calcium levels are among those who are most successfully treated with magnesium.

MITRAL VALVE PROLAPSE

EASING SYMPTOMS
OF A TROUBLED HEART

Normally, the valves that regulate bloodflow through the heart close neatly, snapping shut with the *lub-dub* sound that we recognize as a heartbeat.

In mitral valve prolapse, however, an additional click—*lub-dit-dub*—is added to the heartbeat. The extra sound occurs because the valve between the two left chambers of the heart is pushed out of shape by high blood pressure in the compressing heart. The valve pops upward, almost like a parachute being snapped in the wind. The condition happens when one of the fibrous cords that hold the valve in place stretches out too far or when either of the two leaflets that make up the valve is elongated, thickened, or floppy. If the valve does not seal perfectly, blood may leak backward, causing the swishing noise that's known as a heart murmur.

"Mitral valve prolapse syndrome is considered a hereditary disorder," explains Kristine Scordo, PhD, RN, CNP, professor at Wright State University in Dayton, Ohio, and author of *Taking Control: Living with the Mitral Valve Prolapse Syndrome*. "People with the disorder—and there are three times as many women as men—are often tall and slender, with long arms and fingers and thin chests."

Although mitral valve prolapse usually causes no life-threatening problems, it has been associated with an array of disturbing symptoms, including heart palpitations, chest pain, shortness of breath, dizziness, fatigue, anxiety, headaches, and mood swings. Doctors refer to these collectively as mitral valve prolapse syndrome. "These symptoms aren't caused by the valve itself," Dr. Scordo says. "But they are often part of the package."

These symptoms seem to be caused by disturbances in the body's autonomic nervous system. That's the nervous system that works without conscious control and governs the glands, the heart muscle, and the tone of smooth muscles, such as those of the digestive system, the respiratory system, and the skin.

People with mitral valve prolapse often have overreactive autonomic nervous systems. Their bodies have a hard time adjusting to changes in the environment. They may be sensitive to light and noise, for instance.

"The symptoms are believed to be caused by a number of physiological changes and can often be helped by lifestyle changes such as cardiovascular exercise and dietary changes such as increasing fluid intake and avoiding caffeine. In fact, dietary changes are often all that's needed to alleviate symptoms," Dr. Scordo says. Here's what is recommended.

Magnesium Plays a Role

There's no doubt that minerals play important roles in a properly beating heart. Both the nerves that coordinate the heartbeat and the muscles that contract to move blood through the heart need magnesium in order to do their jobs.

One mineral that has gotten some attention when it comes to mitral valve prolapse is magnesium. "There's evidence that magnesium deficiency may play a role in [mitral valve prolapse syndrome] symptoms," Dr. Scordo says. Several studies have found that a high percentage of people with mitral valve prolapse have lower than normal magnesium levels. And one study by researchers at Lund University in Sweden found that people with mitral valve prolapse had significantly lower levels of magnesium in their white blood cells than healthy people, suggesting that a magnesium deficiency may play a role in the condition.

Another study done at the University of Alabama School of Medicine in Birmingham looked at 94 people with mitral valve prolapse and found that 62 percent of them had low red blood cell levels of magnesium. Those people were also more likely to have additional symptoms: muscle cramps, migraines, and a condition called orthostatic hypotension, in which their

---

Food Factors

The following dietary adjustments won't correct a faulty mitral valve. "But they will help relieve many of the symptoms associated with the disorder," explains Kristine Scordo, PhD, RN, professor at Wright State University in Dayton, Ohio, and author of *Taking Control: Living with the Mitral Valve Prolapse Syndrome*.

These dietary changes are just as important as any vitamin or mineral supplement that you take, experts say. In fact, two dietary recommendations, less caffeine and less sugar, help your body retain the magnesium it needs.

Junk the java. Some of the most bothersome symptoms of mitral valve prolapse—anxiety, chest pain, and shortness of breath—worsen when people consume too much caffeine. "Caffeine is a stimulant and has an adrenaline-like effect, which exaggerates the problems of mitral valve prolapse," Dr. Scordo says. "We tell people to avoid coffee, cola, tea, and chocolate altogether, if they can."

Ditch the sweets. That sugar high you've heard of is for real, Dr. Scordo says. Foods that contain sugar that's quickly absorbed, such as candy, cookies, soda, and the like, make your body pour out insulin. That greatly increases the activity of the sympathetic nervous system, the body's "accelerator," making symptoms worse.

Go for eight a day. Glasses of water, that is. This is to maintain normal blood pressure. "Even slight dehydration can aggravate symptoms of light-headedness and dizziness," Dr. Scordo says. "Most people can alleviate these symptoms in about two weeks just by getting enough fluids and salt."

Diet with care. Crash diets and fad diets aren't just ineffective in the long run; most of the initial weight loss that's achieved is through water loss, just the opposite of what someone with mitral valve prolapse symptoms needs. If you do need to lose weight, doctors suggest going for no more than a 1-pound weight loss per week.

blood pressure dropped when they first stood up, making them light-headed.

Fifty of the 94 people took 250 to 1,000 milligrams of magnesium daily, in addition to their regular treatment, for 4 months to 4 years. Overall, there was a 90 percent decrease in muscle cramps, a 47 percent decrease in chest pain and a definite decrease in blood vessel spasms in the people taking magnesium, reports the study's main researcher, Cecil Coghlan, MD, clinical professor of medicine at the University of Alabama School of Medicine. Palpitations also were markedly less, and a certain kind of heart arrhythmia called premature ventricular contraction was reduced by 27 percent. People taking magnesium also reported fewer migraines and less fatigue.

Magnesium deficiency can be induced by the very drugs meant to help heart problems, such as digitalis and some types of diuretics (water pills). These drugs cause the body to excrete both magnesium and potassium, leaving people in short supply of these nutrients.

Others most likely to come up short on magnesium, in Dr. Scordo's opinion, are those who drink a lot of soft drinks or alcohol, those under stress, and anyone eating a poor diet with lots of calories from sugar or fat.

"Therefore, changing their diets along with magnesium supplements often helps relieve symptoms," Dr. Scordo says. In addition, people with mitral valve prolapse syndrome should avoid foods that inhibit the absorption of magnesium, such as dietary fats. "Dietary phosphates—very high in certain sodas—also may inhibit reabsorption of magnesium," Dr. Scordo says. "And refined foods, especially white sugar and grains, cause large losses of magnesium. One half-cup of brown sugar contains 20 milligrams of magnesium and white sugar has none, so substitute brown sugar for white in cooking and baking," she says. "And steam vegetables instead of boiling them to preserve magnesium."

In addition to eating a balanced diet, Dr. Scordo recommends 420 milligrams of supplemental magnesium for men and 360 milligrams for women (slightly above the Daily Value). Although magnesium is considered to be a fairly safe mineral, even in high doses, people with heart problems or kidney problems should take supplements only under medical supervision. Too much magnesium could cause a dangerous buildup of the mineral in the blood.

"So don't take supplements without first consulting your doctor," Dr. Scordo says.

Note that people can have normal blood levels of magnesium and still have inadequate supplies in their tissues. If you are severely deficient, you may benefit by initially getting intravenous magnesium or high oral doses. This treatment, of course, would have to be administered by your doctor.

Prescriptions for Healing

Only one nutrient, magnesium, is thought to be helpful for symptoms related to mitral valve prolapse. But vitamins that work in conjunction with magnesium, especially vitamin B$_6$, also are often recommended by some experts.

Nutrient	Daily Amount
Calcium	1,000–1,200 milligrams
Magnesium	420 milligrams for men; 360 milligrams for women
Vitamin B$_6$	Up to 100 milligrams

MEDICAL ALERT: *If you have been diagnosed with mitral valve prolapse, you should be under a doctor's care.*

People with heart or kidney problems should take magnesium only under medical supervision.

Meats are a good source of magnesium, but if you want heart-healthy sources, try steamed or broiled halibut and mackerel, rice bran, nuts, seeds, tofu, green leafy vegetables such as spinach and Swiss chard, and fruits such as apples, apricots, and bananas.

And since the magnesium that's found in plants depends on the amount of magnesium in the soil, consider buying organically grown produce, which contains a better balance of minerals than produce grown with potassium-rich inorganic fertilizers.

Calcium May Help Contraction

In addition to magnesium, another mineral that may help with the symptoms of mitral valve prolapse is calcium. "Calcium helps with muscle contraction—what we call blood vessel patency," says Stella Volpe, PhD, RD, associate professor at the University of Pennsylvania School of Nursing in Philadelphia. "So it may help ease some of the symptoms of mitral valve prolapse," she says. Aim for a minimum of 1,000 milligrams of calcium per day, 1,200 milligrams if you are over 50.

MORNING SICKNESS

TAMING THE TURBULENT TUMMY

You can be tickled pink at the idea of impending motherhood but still roll out of bed every morning, head straight to the bathroom, and heave. Studies show that morning sickness hits 50 to 90 percent of pregnant women. Luckily, some experts believe there is a safe and effective vitamin therapy to reduce stomach-churning symptoms.

Vitamin B_6 to the Rescue

Several studies done back in the 1940s suggested that vitamin B_6 is an effective treatment for morning sickness. More recently, two studies have confirmed this vitamin's effectiveness. Researchers at the University of Iowa College of Medicine in Iowa City found that pregnant women who took 25 milligrams of B_6 every 8 hours had significantly less vomiting and nausea than women who took placebos (inactive pills). And in a study that included almost 350 moms-to-be, researchers in Thailand found that 10 milligrams every 8 hours reduced symptoms as well.

"This is something more and more obstetricians are hearing about, and it's definitely worth trying," says Jennifer Niebyl, MD, professor and head of obstetrics and gynecology at the University of Iowa College of Medicine. "It's safe, with no risk of side effects or birth defects at 25 milligrams, and it works for at least half of the women who try it." Both studies found that the vitamin worked best in women with moderate to severe nausea.

No one really knows why pregnant women get nauseated or how vitamin B_6 works, Dr. Niebyl says. "It probably has to do with high hormone levels, but we don't know which hormones cause nausea or how B_6 affects nausea," she says.

She recommends taking vitamin B_6 first thing in the morning, even before getting out of bed, then in midafternoon and before bed. Stick to no more than 75 milligrams of B_6 a day—three doses of 25 milligrams—to be on the safe side, Dr. Niebyl recommends. Amounts higher than 100 milligrams a day have been associated with nerve problems.

If vitamin B_6 is going to help your symptoms, you should feel relief after the first few doses, Dr. Niebyl says. If it hasn't worked by then, you may need to ask your doctor about other forms of treatment.

Beyond vitamins, if you have morning sickness, you should try to eat whatever you can keep down or do whatever it takes to ease the nausea, says Elizabeth Somer, RD, author of 10 Habits That Mess Up a Woman's Diet. "I have had clients who have sniffed a lemon and it calmed their stomachs,"

Food Factors

What goes down the hatch can make a big difference when it comes to whether or not it comes back up. Some doctors recommend trying these dietary measures the next time you need to steady a pitching stomach.

Eat gingerly. There's good scientific proof that ginger, the popular peppery spice used to flavor cookies, cakes, and Asian foods, can calm even supersensitive stomachs.

In one study, 940 milligrams of ginger (about a half-teaspoon) worked as well as the standard dose of Dramamine, a common over-the-counter remedy, in relieving motion sickness. A similar dose kept Danish sailors from turning green during a 4-hour jaunt on the high seas.

British researchers found that ginger worked as well as drugs, and without side effects, in relieving the nausea and vomiting common after surgery that involved general anesthesia. And Danish doctors report that one-eighth teaspoon of powdered ginger, given four times a day, relieved morning sickness in pregnant women so seriously stricken that they were hospitalized.

Ginger apparently works directly in the gastrointestinal tract to interfere with so-called feedback mechanisms that send "time to throw up" messages to the chemoreceptor trigger zone in your brain, says Narinder Duggal, MD, clinical pharmacy specialist, internist, and medical director of Liberty Bay Internal Medicine in Poulsbo, Washington. Although ginger ale or ginger tea may calm your tummy, the powdered stuff packs the most punch, says Jennifer Niebyl, MD, professor and head of obstetrics and gynecology at the University of Iowa College of Medicine in Iowa City. "The usual dosage is about a half-teaspoon," she says. Ginger has no known adverse side effects, she adds.

Graze and pick. "Eating frequent light meals that are rich in carbohydrates and low in fat may help your nausea, so it's worth a try," says Dr. Niebyl. "The idea is to always have some easy-to-digest food in your stomach, but not to have a full stomach." That's why eating a few crackers before you get out of bed in the morning helps, she adds.

Prescriptions for Healing

Here's what some doctors recommend for nausea associated with pregnancy.

Nutrient	Daily Amount
Vitamin B$_6$	75 milligrams, taken as 3 divided doses (every 8 hours)

MEDICAL ALERT: *As a general rule, pregnant women should get a doctor's okay before taking any supplements. More than 100 milligrams of vitamin B$_6$ a day has been associated with nerve damage.*

she says. "Others dip carrots into vinegar because they crave the crunchy/sour combination. The good news is that once you pass your first trimester, you are usually fine, and morning sickness does not have any long-term effects on the baby," she says. As a general rule, pregnant women should never take any drugs or supplements without first discussing it with their physician.

MULTIPLE SCLEROSIS

SLOWING A NERVE-RACKING DISEASE

Just as electrical wires are covered with an insulation that keeps them running smoothly and safely separates them from surrounding walls, your nerves are covered with an insulating barrier that keeps their conduction strong and separates them from surrounding tissues; this nerve insulation is called a myelin sheath. In people with multiple sclerosis, their immune system attacks the fatty insulating myelin sheath, which leaves nerves vulnerable and slows down their conduction.

The breakdown occurs mostly in the brain and spinal cord. Once the fatty sheath starts to go, messages traveling to and from the brain are blocked. A message from the brain to "shake a leg," for instance, may simply dead-end while it's still in the brain, never reaching the muscles in the leg that could perform the task.

"Multiple sclerosis is very difficult to diagnose because we still don't know the exact cause," says Narinder Duggal, MD, clinical pharmacy specialist, internist, and medical director of Liberty Bay Internal Medicine in Poulsbo, Washington. "It is like a two-strike disease where you have some genetic predisposition and then you get a virus or trigger," he says.

Luckily, there are ways to make life with MS easier. The first drug that helps treat relapsing-remitting MS, called Betaseron, was approved in 1993. Two other drugs—Avonex and Copaxone—were approved in 1996. Together, these three drugs, known as "ABC drugs," do not stop MS, but they do reduce frequency and intensity of attacks and appear to slow the progression of the damage the disease causes.

Fending Off the Immune System

"No one knows for sure what sets off the immune system to attack nerves," says Timothy Vollmer, MD, director of the neuroimmunology program at Barrow Neurological Institute in Phoenix. "There are good data to suggest that genetics plays a role in determining risk and that other risk factors include some sort of outside trigger, possibly exposure to a virus, that apparently sets off immune system changes."

MS is in a class of diseases called autoimmune diseases, where the immune system attacks a person's own body—in this case, the myelin sheath. "When you look at an MRI, you see pockets of no myelin sheaths and nothing to insulate the wires, so to speak, so nerve conduction is lower in that area," Dr. Duggal says.

Depending on which nerves lose their fatty sheaths, symptoms may include blurred or double vision, numbness, loss of bladder control, and fatigue or tremors in the arms or legs. Fatigue so extreme that it has been called paralyzing also strikes some. Most symptoms wax and wane, with problematic conditions and remissions occurring over the years.

Dr. Vollmer believes most doctors think that nutrition has little, if anything, to do with the development or progression of MS and that no dietary measure can repair damaged nerve cells.

"Many of us do, however, think that a healthy, well-balanced diet high in fruits and vegetables is important to maximize function and to decrease the disability that occurs in MS," Dr. Vollmer says. "We want to avoid

Food Factors

Dietary changes are not the mainstay of traditional treatment for multiple sclerosis (MS). Still, some say dietary changes can make a difference in the course of the disease, says Mary Dan Eades, MD, author of *Protein Power* and *The Doctor's Complete Guide to Vitamins and Minerals*.

Try fatty acids. Increasing intake of two essential fatty acids, gamma-linolenic acid (GLA) and eicosapentaenoic acid (EPA), can help people with MS, says Dr. Eades. Some reports also suggest that elimination of all grains containing gluten may benefit MS sufferers, as some research indicates that similarities in the chemical composition of gluten may trigger an autoimmune reaction against the nerve sheath in susceptible people, she says. Gluten is found not only in wheat, but in oats, barley, and spelt. Nongluten grains include rice, amaranth, and buckwheat.

Eat more fiber. To coax the sluggish bowel associated with MS, get plenty of fiber every day, urges Timothy Vollmer, MD, director of the neuroimmunology program at Barrow Neurological Institute in Phoenix. Whole grains, fruits, vegetables, and beans can all help keep you regular.

Drink plenty of water. Getting lots of water relieves constipation, too. And it can ward off the bladder infections that can plague people with MS, Dr. Vollmer says. (Try cranberry juice for extra infection-fighting power.)

Find your food foes. The idea that food allergies or intolerances can contribute to symptoms of MS remains entirely unproven. Still, some doctors believe that for some people, certain foods can trigger or worsen symptoms.

Two Dutch doctors cite several reports of people whose symptoms worsened after chocolate binges, which suggests that chemicals in cocoa, coffee, and cola can be toxic to nerve cells in large amounts. (It's true that large amounts of chocolate can be toxic to some animals. For instance, a dog that gobbles up a box of chocolates might develop twitching and muscle and heart weakness and lose control of bowel and urinary functions, the same symptoms associated with MS.)

One case report implicates fresh pineapple as the cause of a woman's muscle weakness and loss of vision. And in the United States and 21 other countries, the incidence of MS correlates most strikingly with milk consumption, according to one survey.

While most doctors pooh-pooh these possible connections, common sense suggests that if your symptoms seem to worsen after eating a particular food, drop that food from your diet for a least a few weeks to see if you notice improvement.

nutritional deficiencies and keep our patients as healthy as possible so that they don't develop some additional chronic ailment such as heart disease or diabetes, which can magnify the symptoms of MS." Even an infection that raises body temperature as little as 1°F can worsen symptoms of MS, Dr. Vollmer says.

Here's what nutritional research suggests may play a role in controlling the symptoms of MS. Keep in mind that even the doctors who recommend nutritional therapy use it along with other medical care, including physical therapy. Dr. Vollmer suggests that you enlist your doctor to work with you in devising a treatment plan that is best for your particular case.

Antioxidant Nutrients May Help

There's some evidence that the MS-associated damage to a nerve's fatty sheath is caused by what is known as oxidative injury. That damage, also called lipid (fat) peroxidation, occurs because unstable molecules called free radicals steal electrons from the healthy molecules in this fatty covering, causing breakdown and scarring that eventually destroys the nerve. Free radicals can be generated by attacking immune cells. They also occur when the body is exposed to certain toxic chemicals.

Some doctors recommend that their patients with MS take the array of so-called antioxidant nutrients, which neutralize free radicals by offering up their own electrons, protecting your body's healthy molecules from harm. These nutrients include vitamins C and E, beta-carotene, and the mineral selenium. Amounts recommended can vary widely.

"I recommend taking at least 500 milligrams of vitamin C two or three times a day and 100 micrograms of selenium and 400 to 800 international units of vitamin E once a day," says Mary Dan Eades, MD, author of *Protein Power* and *The Doctor's Complete Guide to Vitamins and Minerals*. It's a good idea to check with your doctor before taking more than 400 IU of vitamin E a day. Vitamin C in doses exceeding 1,200 milligrams a day can cause diarrhea in some people.

Check Out Vitamin B$_{12}$

Most doctors in the United States say there is no proof that a vitamin B$_{12}$ deficiency contributes to the development of MS or that taking B$_{12}$ helps

Prescriptions for Healing

Drugs are the mainstay of treatment for multiple sclerosis. There are, however, a few nutrients that may prove helpful. Here's what some doctors recommend.

Nutrient	Daily Amount
Selenium	100 micrograms
Vitamin B$_{12}$	6 micrograms (talk to your doctor about higher levels)
Vitamin C	1,000–2,000 milligrams, taken as 2–4 divided doses
Vitamin D	400 IU
Vitamin E	400–800 IU

Plus a multivitamin/mineral supplement containing the Daily Values of all essential vitamins and minerals

MEDICAL ALERT: *If you have been diagnosed with multiple sclerosis, you should be under a doctor's care.*

Selenium in doses exceeding 400 micrograms daily should be taken only under medical supervision.

Injections of vitamin B$_{12}$ are required for people who have problems absorbing this nutrient.

Vitamin C in doses exceeding 1,200 milligrams a day can cause diarrhea in some people.

If you are taking anticoagulant drugs, you should not take vitamin E supplements. (Though generally a dose of up to 1,500 IU of vitamin E a day is considered safe, some recent reports suggest that taking more than 400 IU a day could be harmful to people with cardiovascular or circulatory disease or with cancer. If you have such a condition, be sure to consult your doctor before you begin supplementation.)

reduce symptoms. Nevertheless, there appear to be some potential links between the nutrient, which is so essential for proper nerve function, and this debilitating disease. For instance, vitamin B$_{12}$ deficiency can mimic some of the symptoms of MS, such as numbness and tingling in the arms and legs, loss of balance, and fatigue. Therefore, a B$_{12}$ deficiency may aggravate the symptoms or make treatment more difficult. Some studies show that B$_{12}$ deficiency may contribute to early onset of MS (before age 18). In addition, people with MS who are being treated with intravenous steroids may also be low in vitamin B_{12}. To find out if you are deficient in B_{12}, consult your doctor. The Daily Value for vitamin B_{12} is 6 micrograms. To return deficient levels to normal, some people receive vitamin B_{12} through an injection, and others do better on the sublingual (under the tongue) form of the vitamin.

Defend against MS with Vitamin D

The latest studies on vitamins and multiple sclerosis point to a vitamin D deficiency as a potential risk factor for the disease. "While the research is preliminary in humans, there is clear evidence that those people who live farthest from the equator (and therefore get low amounts of sunlight and make low levels of vitamin D) are at the highest risk for MS, suggesting a vitamin D deficiency as the cause," says Elizabeth Somer, RD, author of *10 Habits That Mess Up a Woman's Diet*. "When researchers study MS in mice, they inject myelin into the animals who then develop the antibodies to destroy myelin in much the same mechanism that's seen in MS," Somer explains. "But none of this damage occurs if the animals are first given vitamin D," she says.

In addition, a Harvard study published in the *Journal of the American Medical Association* showed that as circulating levels of vitamin D increased in a group of military personnel, the risk of multiple sclerosis decreased. "And at the same time, a review of 27 clinical trials on vitamin D done by researchers at the Council for Responsible Nutrition came together and concluded that vitamin D is nowhere near as toxic as we once thought. They concluded that the safe upper limit should be increased five-fold," Somer says. The current Daily Value for vitamin D is 400 IU. Until the safe upper limit is officially raised, talk to your health care professionals about how much vitamin D you should take to prevent MS and other conditions.

NIGHT BLINDNESS

EYES NEED VITAMIN A

Night blindness is a complex subject. Doctors now know that it can result from nutritional factors, genetics, uncorrected nearsightedness, or an eye disease such as cataracts, macular degeneration, or retinitis pigmentosa. And anything that affects vitamin A metabolism, such as liver disease, intestinal surgery, malabsorption, or alcoholism, can also cause the problem. Vitamin A is absolutely connected to the retina, so a decrease in vitamin A could make the condition worse, says Stella Volpe, PhD, RD, associate professor at the University of Pennsylvania School of Nursing in Philadelphia. Some forms of night blindness can be corrected with a pair of new glasses. Other forms require surgery. Still other forms of night blindness respond to something as simple as vitamin A.

The Vitamin Connection

What does vitamin A have to do with vision?

The answer is complex, says Elias Reichel, MD, vice chair for research and education in the department of ophthalmology at Tufts University School of Medicine in Boston. But it involves the part of the eye called the retina.

"The retina is that part of the eye that acts like the film in a camera," he explains. "It's used to perceive light." On the retina there are structures called rods and cones. These house four kinds of pigments, one of which binds to an eye-friendly form of vitamin A. When you enter a sunny room and light enters your eye, the pigment transforms. Instantly, the vitamin A in your eye changes shape and, in that process, excites nerve endings to start transmitting electrical impulses to your brain to let it know what's going on—that you've entered a sunny room.

When you enter a dark room, the vitamin A changes shape again and helps your eyes realize that you've entered a dark room.

But nothing is ever completely light or completely dark. That's why you have 120 rods and 7 million cones in each eye that make the minute adjustments necessary to perceive light and dark. And they're all dependent on vitamin A to do their jobs.

Despite this heavy demand for vitamin A, it still is pretty hard to develop a deficiency of this nutrient in the United States, where the foods in which it is contained are plentiful. Common staples such as milk and margarine are fortified with vitamin A, and orange and yellow foods such as sweet potatoes and carrots are rich sources of beta-carotene. (Beta-carotene is a precursor of vitamin A and converts to vitamin A in the body.) We need to depend on outside sources for vitamin A because the body can't make its own. Besides, since a healthy liver is usually able to store up to a year's supply of vitamin A, you'd have to be chronically deprived of vitamin A food sources for quite a while for it to affect your sight, as is the case with millions of children in developing nations.

"Night blindness resulting from vitamin A deficiency is very, very, very, very rare in individuals who live in America," says Dr. Reichel. And even if it does develop, it can frequently be reversed within an hour by injections of vitamin A.

Most people with night blindness have eyes that mobilize vitamin A so slowly that it takes a while to adjust to the dark, says Dr. Reichel. People notice it most often when they're going into theaters or driving at night.

Slowing Genetic Damage

Not only is vitamin A an effective treatment for deficiency-induced night blindness, but it may also slow night blindness that is induced by several hereditary conditions, usually grouped under the name retinitis pigmentosa.

Retinitis pigmentosa is considered rare in the United States, occurring in an estimated one in 4,000 people. But it is the most common inherited cause of blindness in people between the ages of 20 and 60, striking those who have a genetic mutation that slowly destroys the light-sensing structures in their eyes. The mutation is inherited from a parent, who frequently is unaware that he or she carries a gene that can imperil the child's vision.

Unfortunately, it does. People with retinitis pigmentosa usually begin to develop a loss of daytime side (peripheral) vision in young adulthood that progresses to tunnel vision and eventually to loss of vision in midlife. Without treatment, most people with retinitis pigmentosa will have significantly reduced day vision between the ages of 50 and 80.

Fortunately, research has shown that vitamin A can slow the retinal damage that can cause night blindness in adults with retinitis pigmentosa. In a study of 208 people with retinitis pigmentosa between the ages of 18 and 55, researchers at the Berman-Gund Laboratory for the Study of Retinal

Prescriptions for Healing

Night blindness caused by deficiency of vitamin A can be reversed by adding vitamin A to the diet or by taking vitamin A supplements, according to medical experts. The genetic eye disease known as retinitis pigmentosa is associated with night blindness as well as with the loss of day vision. This condition can be slowed with vitamin A supplements or by eating foods rich in vitamin A and beta-carotene. "This doesn't mean you have to eat 100 carrots a day, but try to increase your consumption of fruits and vegetables that contain vitamin A or beta-carotene," says Stella Volpe, PhD, RD, associate professor at the University of Pennsylvania School of Nursing in Philadelphia. Foods rich in vitamin A and beta-carotene include apricots, broccoli, carrots, cantaloupe, dark green leafy vegetables, mangos, peaches, pumpkin, and sweet potatoes.

Nutrient	Daily Amount
Vitamin A	15,000 IU (vitamin A palmitate)

MEDICAL ALERT: *If you have symptoms of night blindness, you should see your doctor for proper diagnosis and treatment.*

People taking high doses of vitamin A may be at risk for toxicity and side effects such as diarrhea, hair loss, dry skin and lips, headache, muscle and joint pain, and fatigue. The therapeutic dose of 15,000 IU greatly exceeds the Recommended Dietary Allowance of vitamin A, which is about 3,000 IU for males and 2,310 IU for females. If you'd like to try this therapy, discuss it with your doctor first, especially if you are a woman of childbearing age. Women who are pregnant should not use this therapy.

Degenerations at Harvard Medical School reported that 1,200 milligrams of docosahexaenoic acid (DHA) plus 15,000 IU of vitamin A given as retinyl palmitate could slow the progression of retinal degeneration that can cause night blindness as a result of retinitis pigmentosa by at least 2 years.

"The study suggests that if you are starting vitamin A, if you start DHA at the same time, it will be more beneficial than the vitamin A alone," Dr. Reichel says. "And in patients who were already on vitamin A palmitate, it was observed that those patients who had a diet higher in omega-3 fatty acids—from tuna, herring, mackerel, or sardines—had a lower risk of loss of visual field than the patients with a lower intake of omega-3," he says.

But not all types of vitamin A will do the job. Although there are several forms of vitamin A, they all have different functions in the body and cannot be used interchangeably. The form used in the study was vitamin A palmitate.

There are no reports of otherwise healthy adults with retinitis pigmentosa becoming ill from 15,000 IU of vitamin A palmitate daily. But that doesn't mean that it's okay to take more than this amount or that more is better. People taking high doses of vitamin A may be at risk for toxicity and side effects such as diarrhea, hair loss, dry skin and lips, headache, muscle and joint pain, and fatigue. The therapeutic dose of 15,000 IU greatly exceeds the Recommended Dietary Allowance of vitamin A, which is about 3,000 IU for males and 2,310 IU for females. If you'd like to try this therapy, discuss it with your doctor first, especially if you are a woman of childbearing age. Women who are pregnant should not use this therapy.

Vitamin E May Protect Eyes . . . In Small Doses

Vitamin E seems to be one vitamin that can help sharpen eyesight when given with other antioxidants and in small doses. In a study done at Johns Hopkins University School of Medicine in Baltimore, researchers gave some mice daily injections of vitamin E (alpha-tocopherol at 200 milligrams) and vitamin C (250 milligrams), together with a few other antioxidant chemicals. They found that the mice treated with the antioxidant mixture had less cone cell death, indicating that the antioxidants may provide protection against retinitis pigmentosa. In high doses, however, there is some evidence that vitamin E can destroy light-sensing cells by inhibiting the transport of vitamin A in the retina.

In a study published in the *Archives of Ophthalmology*, people with retinitis pigmentosa who took 400 IU of vitamin E every day appeared to lose their vision faster than those taking a trace amount of vitamin E. The researchers noted that they had no evidence to suggest that small amounts of vitamin E, such as those found in multivitamin/mineral supplements, affect those with retinitis pigmentosa.

OSTEOARTHRITIS

SLOWING JOINT WEAR AND TEAR

Check out a chicken drumstick the next time you bake a bird. You'll note that the knobby end of the thighbone is covered with a tough, rubbery coating. That's cartilage, a tissue designed to cushion joints and ensure smooth motion.

In osteoarthritis, cartilage breaks down. It becomes frayed, thin, perhaps even completely worn away in areas. The underlying bone disintegrates, while painful bone spurs may grow around the edges of the joint. A formerly smooth, quiet joint may feel like it's grinding. It might even sound rough, like crinkling cellophane, when it's moved.

No one really knows why cartilage breaks down. Heavy use of a joint is sometimes a contributing factor. Also, a joint injured in the past tends to develop osteoarthritis sooner than a normal joint, perhaps because misalignment causes cartilage wear.

Osteoarthritis usually develops slowly, over many years. Some people never have more than a mild ache. Others develop crippling pain, and a few even end up trading in a creaky old hip or knee for a shiny new titanium-alloy model.

Many doctors who treat osteoarthritis consider it pretty much an unavoidable part of growing older. In fact, more than half of people ages 65 and older can expect to have at least a touch of osteoarthritis. Those same doctors think there's not a whole lot that can be done for this disease, except to nurse aching joints with mild painkillers such as acetaminophen or aspirin, heat, and a careful balance of exercise and rest.

The relatively few doctors who treat osteoarthritis with nutritional therapy take a different stance, however. They contend that osteoarthritis is a metabolic disorder, a breakdown in the body's ability to regenerate bone and cartilage. Although they concede that the breakdown is partly the result of old age, they also believe that providing the proper nutrients, in proper amounts, can help stop the process of deterioration and reduce pain and swelling.

Unfortunately, while there is some sketchy evidence that certain nutrients can help osteoarthritis, the kind of large scientific studies that would confirm these benefits have yet to be done.

Until then, here's what doctors say may be helpful.

B$_{12}$ and Folate Give Bones a Boost

Vitamin B$_{12}$ is best known for its role in maintaining a healthy blood supply. In the bone marrow, B$_{12}$ stimulates stem cells, a certain type of bone cell, to make red blood cells. When B$_{12}$ levels are low, people develop anemia.

But that's not the only role vitamin B$_{12}$ plays in bone. A few years ago, researchers at the University of Southern California School of Medicine in Los Angeles discovered that B$_{12}$ also stimulates osteoblasts, another type of bone cell that generates not red blood cells but bone. That could be important to people with osteoarthritis, because underneath degenerating cartilage, bone also deteriorates, causing additional pain and further cartilage erosion.

This finding about vitamin B$_{12}$ led researchers at the University of Missouri-Columbia to try giving B$_{12}$ to people with osteoarthritis in their hands. They found that people who took 20 micrograms of B$_{12}$ (3.3 times the Daily Value of 6 micrograms) and 6,400 micrograms of folic acid, another B vitamin that works in concert with B$_{12}$, for 2 months had fewer tender joints and better hand strength and took less medicine for pain than people not getting this B vitamin combo. (This amount of folic acid is 16 times the Daily Value and should be taken only under medical supervision, as excess folic acid can actually mask signs of B$_{12}$ deficiency.)

Food Factors

Taming osteoarthritis may well be a matter of adding nutrients while subtracting calories.

Drop some pounds. Research shows that people who maintain their proper weight or stay close to it are much less likely to develop osteoarthritis in certain joints than people who are overweight.

Staying slim spares weight-bearing joints such as the knees and hips. Joints can be so compressed by excess body weight that the fluid-filled space normally found between the cartilage-covered surfaces of bone ends becomes obliterated, says Robert McLean, MD, associate clinical professor of internal medicine and rheumatology at Yale University School of Medicine and an internist in New Haven, Connecticut. "If you already have osteoarthritis, losing some weight can help decrease stress on some of the joints and thereby reduce pain," Dr. McLean says. Your doctor can recommend specific exercises, designed to strengthen the muscles supporting the joints (especially around the knees), to help reduce the pain of osteoarthritis, he adds.

Accost Osteoarthritis with Omega-3s

Omega-3 fatty acids have been used in veterinary medicine for racehorses, dogs, and other animals with joint problems. And recent studies show that omega-3 fatty acids help *people* with inflammatory disorders such as osteoarthritis as well. Several laboratory studies of cartilage-containing cells have shown that omega-3 fatty acids help reduce inflammation and decrease activity of enzymes that break down cartilage.

"So it certainly won't hurt to try a fish oil supplement," says Elizabeth Somer, RD, author of *10 Habits That Mess Up a Woman's Diet*.

Ronni Litz Julien, MS, RD, vice president of the Julien Nutrition Institute in Miami, agrees: "Fish is the number one anti-inflammatory food," she says. "I suggest four to five servings of fatty fish such as white albacore tuna, shark, kingfish, and mackerel [per week]." Not a fish eater or don't feel you can fit that much into your diet? Take a daily fish oil supplement that provides 1 gram of combined eicosapentaenoic acid (EPA) and docosahexaenoic acid (DHA).

Vitamin E Eases Painful Joints

Joints damaged by osteoarthritis don't get as hot and swollen as joints hit with rheumatoid arthritis, but they are somewhat inflamed. That's one reason doctors sometimes recommend vitamin E for osteoarthritis. Vitamin E fights inflammation by neutralizing the biochemicals that are produced during inflammation. These biochemicals, released by immune cells, contain free radicals, unstable molecules that grab electrons from your body's healthy molecules, damaging cells in the process. Vitamin E offers up its own electrons, protecting cells from damage.

In a study by Israeli researchers, people with osteoarthritis who took 600 IU of vitamin E every day for 10 days had significant reductions in pain compared with when they were not taking vitamin E. "Vitamin E also apparently stimulates the body's deposit of cartilage-building proteins called proteoglycans," says Joseph Pizzorno Jr., ND, adjunct professor of naturopathic medicine, president emeritus, and co-founder of Bastyr University in Seattle.

Doctors recommend 400 to 600 IU of vitamin E, amounts that are considered safe. These large amounts are available only by supplementation and should only be taken after you clear it with your health care professional. To get some vitamin E from foods, try sunflower oil, almond oil, and wheat germ. Most people get about 10 IU a day.

Selenium, a mineral that increases the effectiveness of vitamin E, is often added to the osteoarthritis formula in amounts of about 200 micrograms a day. That amount is considered safe, but you won't want to take more than 400 micrograms a day without medical supervision.

Prescriptions for Healing

Many doctors do not make dietary recommendations for the treatment of osteoarthritis beyond maintaining normal weight. Some nutrition-oriented doctors, however, recommend an array of nutrients, including these.

Nutrient	Daily Amount
Folic acid	6,400 micrograms
Niacinamide	500 milligrams
Selenium	200 micrograms
Vitamin B$_{12}$	20 micrograms
Vitamin D	400–600 IU
Vitamin E	400–600 IU

Plus a multivitamin/mineral supplement containing the Daily Values of all essential vitamins and minerals

MEDICAL ALERT: *If you have symptoms of osteoarthritis, you should see your doctor for proper diagnosis and treatment.*

This amount of folic acid should be taken only under medical supervision, as excess folic acid can actually mask signs of vitamin B$_{12}$ deficiency.

Large amounts of niacinamide can cause liver problems. Doses significantly above 100 milligrams a day require careful medical supervision. If you have liver disease, you should not use this treatment.

The amount of selenium recommended here exceeds the Daily Value for this mineral. Selenium in doses exceeding 400 micrograms daily should be taken only under medical supervision.

If you are taking anticoagulant drugs, you should not take vitamin E supplements. (Though generally a dose of up to 1,500 IU of vitamin E a day is considered safe, some recent reports suggest that taking more than 400 IU a day could be harmful to people with cardiovascular or circulatory disease or with cancer. If you have such a condition, be sure to consult your doctor before you begin supplementation.)

According to a study done at the University of North Carolina at Chapel Hill's Thurston Arthritis Research Center, selenium deficiency itself may contribute to osteoarthritis. Researchers compared x-ray evidence of osteoarthritis in 940 people according to how much selenium they had in their systems. The people with less than normal amounts of the mineral had a higher risk of osteoarthritis in one or both knees. Good food sources of selenium include Brazil nuts (1 ounce has 550 micrograms!), meat, seafood, oats, turnips, garlic, and orange juice.

Vitamin C Stimulates Cartilage Repair

Most of us know vitamin C as an infection fighter and an immunity builder. But vitamin C is also used throughout the body to manufacture a variety of tissues, including collagen. Collagen forms a network of protein fibers that lay down the structural foundation for many tissues, including cartilage, bone, tendons, and muscles, all necessary to keep joints strong and operating smoothly.

"It's well known that animals deficient in vitamin C develop an array of health problems associated with collagen breakdown, including joint pain and cartilage breakdown," Dr. Pizzorno says.

Guinea pigs, one of the few animals besides humans that can't make vitamin C in their bodies, show the classic symptoms of osteoarthritis—cartilage erosion and inflammation—when put on a diet containing only a small amount of vitamin C.

And one study suggests that large amounts of vitamin C encourage the growth of cartilage cells (chondrocytes) by stimulating synthesis of these cells' genetic material, report researchers at the State University of New York at Stony Brook.

"Although there are no human studies confirming a benefit, there's enough evidence out there, I think, to include vitamin C in a program to slow osteoarthritis," Dr. Pizzorno says. And there's some evidence that vitamins C and E work together to protect cartilage from breakdown. You can get sufficient vitamin C for this purpose in a multivitamin/mineral supplement, he says.

Prevent Joint Problems with Vitamin D

"Vitamin D may play a role in the prevention of osteoarthritis," says Boyd Lyles, MD, director of the HeartHealth and Wellness Center in Dallas and medical director of L A Weight Loss. Vitamin D deficiency is relatively common in people with osteoarthritis, and therefore maintaining healthy levels of vitamin D can help conserve bones and prevent the breakdown of cartilage. Ask your health care professional to test your levels of vitamin D to make sure you don't have a deficiency. For vitamin D boosting and maintenance, you can get some vitamin D from foods and supplements, but your body also makes it through exposure to bright sunlight. Take 400 to 600 IU of vitamin D per day, and aim for 15 to 30 minutes of bright sun per day.

Niacinamide Could Be Worth a Try

You may not have heard of niacinamide. It's a form of niacin, one of the B-complex vitamins. Studies show that niacinamide may decrease the inflammation that goes along with osteoarthritis. No one really knows why niacinamide seems to help osteoarthritis. The vitamin is thought to somehow improve the metabolism of joint cartilage. One study on niacinamide and osteoarthritis showed that people with the condition were able to reduce their intake of nonsteroidal anti-inflammatory drugs when they took daily niacinamide tablets. To aim for the same results, take 500 milligrams of niacinamide per day. Do not take niacinamide without checking with your health care professional—at high doses, it can lead to organ toxicity.

Adding a Bit of Insurance

Doctors who treat osteoarthritis make an additional recommendation that's designed to cover all bases. They recommend a multivitamin/mineral supplement that provides the Daily Values of all of the essential vitamins and minerals.

That recommendation might not be such a bad bit of advice. There's a scattering of evidence that a host of nutrients—pantothenic acid, vitamin B_6, zinc and copper, and other trace minerals—may play roles in maintaining healthy bones and cartilage.

OSTEOPOROSIS

WALKING TALL INTO YOUR GOLDEN YEARS

Imagine a bank that never let you know how much (or how little) money you have in your account. Unless you were a diligent bookkeeper, chances are that sooner or later, you'd start bouncing checks. Well, your bones are that bank, only instead of money, you're withdrawing calcium.

Essentially, that's what happens when people get osteoporosis, a disease causing porous bones: Their skeletons become bankrupt. Their bodies have withdrawn more calcium from the bones than has been deposited over the years, and all that's left is a fragile shell.

Osteoporosis is responsible for 1.5 million fractures each year, most notably fractures of the vertebrae (these cause the hunched appearance often seen in elderly women), forearms, wrists, and hips (these are often crippling and sometimes fatal). By the time they reach age 90, one in three women and one in six men will experience a hip fracture, which can lead to permanent disabilities.

That's the bad news. The good news is that osteoporosis is both preventable and treatable.

"There is no reason this disease should exist. It's preventable just through nutrition and exercise, if a woman starts young enough," says Ruth S. Jacobowitz, former vice president of Mount Sinai Medical Center in Cleveland, a member of the National Council on Women's Health, and author of *150 Most-Asked Questions about Osteoporosis*. "It is never too early and never too late to build bone. Even very elderly women can still build some amount of bone density."

Making Deposits into the Bone Bank

The first step in building bone is understanding how bones work. Even after we've stopped growing, our bones undergo constant remodeling. Remodeling is the actual term that doctors use to describe the body's ongoing process of removing old bone and forming new bone. Generally, the formation of new bone stays ahead of, or even with, the removal of old bone during the first 20 to 30 years of our lives.

Sometime after age 30, our bones begin operating in the red, and both men and women lose slightly more bone than they form—that is, until women hit menopause and stop producing estrogen, one of the hormones that regulate remodeling. Then they lose significantly more bone than men, up to 2 to 5 percent a year during the first 5 to 7 years after menopause. For this reason, 80 percent of people affected by osteoporosis are women, though it does occur in elderly men.

That is why it's particularly important for women to build and maintain peak bone mass, the maximum amount of bone you can form during your lifetime. And you form peak bone mass by taking in calcium and getting plenty of exercise, explains Clifford Rosen, MD, director of the Maine Center for Osteoporosis Research and Education at St. Joseph's Hospital in Bangor. The earlier you start, the better, because the majority of peak bone mass is achieved by your mid-twenties, though some researchers believe you can build bone until age 35.

Does that mean you're doomed if you're already past age 30 and just learning what peak bone mass is? "Absolutely not," says Dr. Rosen. Calcium and exercise can prevent the bone loss that occurs in your thirties and forties. "And slowing bone loss is enough to keep you from having osteoporosis, no matter how low your peak bone mass," he says.

One of the most effective ways of preventing bone loss and osteoporotic fractures is hormone replacement therapy. Unfortunately, HRT has been found to carry some major risks. Recent research has found that taking hormones may increase the risk of heart disease in women, which is pushing many women and doctors to look for alternative treatments. While HRT at one time was considered a mainstay of osteoporosis treatment, it's now a second line of treatment among many doctors.

And medical experts agree that for both women and men, a healthy diet plays an important role in preventing and treating osteoporosis.

In addition to calcium, the nutrients shown by research to have the best bone-building potential include vitamin D, boron, magnesium, fluoride, manganese, copper, zinc, and vitamin K. Here's what we know so far.

Straight from the Cow

Mom always said "Drink your milk, or you won't have strong teeth and bones." As usual, she was right.

Calcium, a mineral abundant in milk, is essential for strong, healthy bones. In fact, 99 percent of the body's calcium is stored in the skeleton. But you also need a stable level of serum calcium (calcium in your blood) for normal heartbeat, nerve and muscle function, and blood coagulation. It's your bones that suffer when there isn't enough to go around.

Maintaining enough calcium in the blood is the body's ultimate priority, explains Dr. Rosen. "If it doesn't have enough, it goes to the reservoir and takes it," he says. The reservoir, in this case, is your bones.

Unfortunately, Americans aren't building up enough of a reservoir. One survey found that 88 percent of women and 63 percent of men don't get enough calcium from food.

According to researchers at the University of California, San Diego, every little bit of calcium counts. Of the 581 60- to 79-year-old women they studied, those who had drunk one or more glasses of milk daily as adolescents and young adults had significantly higher bone mineral density at the mid-forearm (3 to 4 percent), spine (5 percent), and hip than those who had not. The effect of drinking milk on bone mineral density was even greater at the hip (4 percent) and spine (7 percent) for adults ages 20 to 50.

Calcium can also be helpful in treating osteoporosis once the disease has developed. Investigators at Winthrop-University Hospital in Mineola, New York, studied 118 women past the age of menopause. Over a 3-year period, they gave the women 1,700 milligrams of calcium, 1,700 milligrams of calcium plus the female hormones estrogen and progesterone, or placebos (medically ineffective pills). Though the calcium-hormone mix was most effective, calcium alone significantly slowed bone mineral loss. Researchers measured bone mineral loss in the upper thighbone, noting a 0.8 percent decline a year in the women taking calcium versus a 2 percent decline a year in those taking the placebos.

When it comes to getting enough calcium, however, drinking more milk is by no means the final word. Calcium from dairy products can be difficult to absorb, and many people have difficulty digesting dairy products, says Neal Barnard, MD, president of the Physicians Committee for Responsible Medicine in Washington, DC, and author of Eat Right, Live Longer. He recommends foods such as beans, broccoli, and fortified orange juice as calcium sources instead. Other calcium-rich foods include collard greens, kale, mustard greens, butternut squash, tofu, and sweet potatoes.

The Daily Value for calcium is 1,000 milligrams. And the National Institutes of Health recommends the following intakes.

- Men, ages 19 to 50: 1,000 milligrams
- Women, ages 19 to 50: 1,000 milligrams
- Pregnant and nursing women: 1,000 milligrams
- Men and women ages 51 and over: 1,200 milligrams

Because calcium is abundant in food, you can get enough from your diet if you eat three servings of high-calcium foods a day, such as milk, yogurt, cheese, or calcium-fortified juice and cereal, says Felicia Cosman, MD, clinical director for the National Osteoporosis Foundation.

Food Factors

There is an abundance of vitamins and minerals that build and maintain a healthy skeleton, but there are also plenty of everyday foods that are nothing less than bad to the bone. Here are some to avoid.

Drink a little less java. Though controversy still brews on how much caffeine is too much, experts agree that caffeine consumption increases the urinary excretion of calcium.

The Rancho Bernardo Study, a 3-year study of 980 women past the age of menopause, found that coffee drinkers had less bone. The study noted a significant decrease in hip and spinal bone mass associated with lifetime caffeine intake equivalent to only 2 cups of coffee per day among women who did not drink milk on a daily basis.

Although drinking at least 1 glass of milk per day offset the bone loss in this study, it's wise to limit caffeine, since most women are not taking in enough calcium to begin with, says Ruth S. Jacobowitz, former vice president of Mount Sinai Medical Center in Cleveland, a member of the National Council on Women's Health, and author of *150 Most-Asked Questions about Osteoporosis*.

Can the cola. Cola definitely has a negative effect on bones, but researchers aren't yet sure which chemical is the culprit. In the past, researchers thought phosphorous blocked calcium absorption, but more recent research has found that it's not phosphorous or caffeine that's affecting bone, says Felicia Cosman, MD, clinical director for the National Osteoporosis Foundation. "It's probably something else in the cola that is specifically causing problems at the bone cellular level," she says.

One thing researchers do know, however, is that drinking cola seven times a week has detrimental effects on your bones.

Researchers at Tufts University in Boston measured the bone density of more than 1,500 men and women in the Framingham Osteoporosis Study and found that women who drank cola every day had a significantly lower bone mineral density than those who drank less than one serving of cola a month. (Researchers didn't see a similar connection among men.)

If you can't cut the cola from your diet completely, it's a good idea to restrict it to less than seven cans a week, or try to switch to a noncola soda, which wasn't associated with low bone density in the Tufts study.

However, the average American gets only one serving a day. In that case, supplement 300 milligrams for every serving that's missing from your diet. If you get only one serving a day, take 600 milligrams, Dr. Cosman says. If you get two servings, supplement 300 milligrams.

Power up with protein. Protein helps build the scaffolding that bones form around, so it's important to get the recommended 46 to 56 grams a day from foods like cottage cheese, ground turkey, and tofu.

Think greens and beans. While protein is an important part of your diet for both bone formation and overall health, it's important not to get too much from meats and other animal products because they may increase calcium loss and thereby weaken bones, says Neal Barnard, MD, president of the Physicians Committee for Responsible Medicine in Washington, DC, and author of *Eat Right, Live Longer*.

"The majority of the problem with osteoporosis in this country is the result of calcium loss," Dr. Barnard says. He advocates getting protein from grains, beans, and vegetables and getting calcium from greens such as broccoli, kale, collards, and beans to avoid the animal protein found in milk (1 gram per fluid ounce).

Stay strong with potassium. Getting potassium in your diet will help even out your body's acid levels and keep your bones strong. Good sources include orange juice, raisins, fish, and fat-free milk.

Pass on the salt. High salt intake increases urinary excretion of calcium, says Dr. Barnard. "It is well-documented that cutting your daily sodium intake to 1,000 to 2,000 milligrams can save 160 milligrams of calcium per day," he says. That means keeping your salt intake to a teaspoon or less a day.

Go easy on the spirits. Researchers have found reduced bone mass and increased osteoporotic fractures in a significant percentage of men with chronic alcoholism. Moderate drinking, however, is fine, Dr. Cosman says.

Nix the aluminum. Although more research is needed, there is evidence that too much aluminum may also cause bone loss, says Jacobowitz. She notes that aluminum not only can bind with phosphorus and calcium, drawing them into the urine, but also deposits on bones, causing osteomalacia (soft bones).

"It's a bad idea to use aluminum-based antacids for calcium supplementation. Not only will it do you no good, it could do you harm. Read labels," she warns.

When you buy calcium supplements, your best bet is to choose calcium citrate. Experts think it's more easily absorbed by the body, particularly among people with a lower amount of stomach acid. Calcium carbonate is less expensive, but it may not be as effective at preventing osteoporosis.

Also, keep in mind that your body absorbs calcium best in doses of 500 milligrams or less at a time. If you want to get 1,000 milligrams of calcium a day, it's a good idea to take 500 milligrams twice a day.

Play in the Sunshine for Vitamin D

Often referred to as the sunshine vitamin, vitamin D is a must if you want all of that calcium to do any good. Vitamin D, which your skin makes whenever it's exposed to sunlight (except during the winter at northern latitudes), helps your body absorb calcium and build good bones. Studies have shown that using both calcium and vitamin D together is important in protecting your bones, but experts believe that about half of all Americans don't get enough vitamin D.

"In my experience with patients, people tend to overdo the calcium and they don't get enough vitamin D," Dr. Cosman says. But vitamin D is required for calcium absorption and aids in bone mineralization.

Research has shown that vitamin D plays a major role in preventing fractures. In 2005, researchers looked at studies involving vitamin D and fractures over a 45-year period and found that taking 700 to 800 IU of vitamin D a day lowered the risk of hip and nonvertebral fractures by about 25 percent. The same benefits weren't seen in doses of only 400 IU a day. In the majority of cases, those study participants who saw a lower risk of fractures also consumed more than 700 milligrams of dietary calcium a day.

Doctors believe that vitamin D not only helps prevent bone loss but also increases muscle strength and balance, making it less likely that older people will fall.

"Research here in Boston and in Europe has found that up to 40 percent of elderly men and women with hip fractures are vitamin D-deficient," says Michael F. Holick, MD, PhD, professor of medicine, physiology, and biophysics in the section of endocrinology, diabetes, and metabolism and director of the General Clinical Research Center at Boston University Medical Center.

Unfortunately, your skin's ability to manufacture vitamin D decreases with age, says Dr. Holick. Matters are even worse for those living where the days are short and the winters are long. You can't make any vitamin D in the wintertime at northern latitudes such as Boston. "During the months from November through February in Boston, even if you exposed your entire body to sunlight from sunrise to sunset, you would not be able to make enough vitamin D to satisfy your body's requirement," Dr. Holick says. And the closer your abode to the polar ice caps, the longer that stretch.

"This problem is compounded by the use of sunscreen in the summer," adds Dr. Holick. "Sunscreen with an SPF of eight is enough to markedly diminish your ability to make vitamin D. Clothing completely prevents it."

Although it's okay to drink fortified milk, you shouldn't count on it as your primary source of vitamin D, notes Dr. Holick. "There's great variability in the vitamin D content of milk, and our research has shown that only 30 percent of milk samples contain the amount of vitamin D shown on the label. That percentage is even lower in skim milk samples."

That makes it rather difficult to get adequate amounts of vitamin D from your diet alone. Fortunately, the answer to the vitamin D dilemma is as close as your local drugstore, especially if you walk there on a sunny day.

The Daily Value for vitamin D is 400 IU, but there's mounting evidence that those recommendations need to be higher, Dr. Cosman says. The National Osteoporosis Foundation recommends that most adult individuals take a vitamin D supplement of 1,000 IU a day. Choose a supplement that contains vitamin D_3, which is the form of vitamin D your skin makes.

Vitamin D can be toxic in large doses, although research has shown that you can take up to 10,000 IU a day for up to 6 months without adverse effects. Dr. Holick recommends taking 1,000 to 2,000 IU a day. Many multivitamin/mineral formulas contain 400 IU of vitamin D, so adding an extra 1,000 IU in single supplements would put you in the right range. "We also recommend that people, particularly the elderly, go outside for five to ten minutes, two or three times a week, during the spring, summer, and fall for sun exposure on their hands, faces, and arms.," Dr. Holick says. "It is casual exposure to sunlight that provides us with more vitamin D."

Take Magnesium to Regulate Calcium

Magnesium, an essential mineral used to treat almost everything from depression to heart attack, is also crucial to bone health. Magnesium helps calcium get into the bones and also converts vitamin D to its active form in the body. Nearly half of the body's magnesium is found in the skeleton.

Magnesium may also help in the treatment of osteoporosis. Researchers in Israel studied 31 women with osteoporosis who were past the age of menopause. They gave the women daily magnesium supplements of 250 to 750 milligrams for 6 months and then 250 milligrams for 18 months. At the end of that period, 22 women increased their bone density by 1 to 8 percent, and 5 women experienced decreases in their rates of bone loss. Conversely, bone density decreased markedly in 23 women who did not receive magnesium supplements during the same period.

Here in the United States, the USDA continues to study magnesium's role in osteoporosis, says Forrest H. Nielsen, PhD, center director for the USDA Grand Forks Human Nutrition Research Center in North Dakota. "Based on what we know about magnesium regulating calcium, we can say that an adequate magnesium diet is necessary to maintain healthy bones," he says.

The Daily Value for magnesium is 400 milligrams. You'll find magnesium in oat bran, wheat germ, sunflower seeds, pumpkin seeds, nuts, brown rice, seafood, dairy products, and green leafy vegetables. But since many Americans lack sufficient magnesium in their diets, doctors who recommend magnesium supplements advise taking 200 to 400 milligrams daily. (If you have heart or kidney problems or if you're taking hypertension medication, you should talk to your doctor before taking magnesium supplements. Certain types of hypertension medications can make people retain magnesium, Dr. Nielsen says.)

Boron Plugs the Calcium Leak

Researchers have speculated that boron, a trace mineral may reduce urinary excretion of both calcium and magnesium and therefore help prevent osteoporosis.

According to preliminary research, boron may play a role in the body's absorption of key players in bone health: calcium, magnesium, and vitamin D. Research also suggests that boron may help reduce the amount of calcium lost in urine.

Research biologist Curtiss Hunt, PhD, at the Grand Forks Human Nutrition Research Center in North Dakota has discovered that boron in the diet affects mineral metabolism and improves bone structure. Diets low in boron allow a small amount of calcium and magnesium to escape the body in urine.

Boron is found in fruits, vegetables, and legumes, particularly peanuts. You can get 0.5 milligram of boron just by eating one good-size apple.

Something in the Water Could Help

Fluoride, the electrically charged form of fluorine, has long been touted for its cavity-fighting ability. Now some researchers believe it can build bones as well.

"The women in our study had a 70 percent reduction in spinal fractures over a 30-month period and close to a 5 percent increase in spinal bone density every year for almost three years," says Khashayar Sakhaee, MD, professor of internal medicine at the Center for Mineral Metabolism and Clinical Research at the University of Texas Southwestern Medical Center at Dallas.

In the study, Dr. Sakhaee gave 48 women who were past menopause 25 milligrams of slow-release fluoride and 800 milligrams of calcium (as calcium citrate) twice a day for three 12-month cycles, with a 2-month break from fluoride between cycles. With this method of delivery, Dr. Sakhaee says, fluoride treatment is safe and effective.

"Other researchers used to use a rapid-release fluoride that went right to the skeleton, and the patients were getting toxic levels," says Dr. Sakhaee. The rapid-release formula did create dense bones, he explains, but the bone material it formed was brittle and weak. The new slow-release formula is creating strong bones. The slow-release formula is being used in European countries, but the FDA hasn't approved it for the treatment of osteoporosis in the United States, Dr. Sakhaee says.

Researchers remain leery about rapid-release sodium fluoride. Very high doses of fluoride, from 2,500 to 5,000 milligrams, can be fatal, though amounts needed for bone health are nowhere near that level, says Dr. Sakhaee.

"People really aren't getting enough fluoride to do their bones any good," says Dr. Sakhaee. He notes that soil and well water are rich in fluoride, but in towns and cities where the water is fluoridated, government standards prohibit more than 1 milligram of fluoride per liter of water. And many communities don't have fluoridated water at all.

Fluoride supplements are available only with a doctor's prescription. If you want to try fluoride, you'll have to discuss these supplements with your doctor. If your water isn't fluoridated, good food sources of fluoride include tea, mackerel, and canned salmon with bones. Daily intake of up to 10 milligrams of fluoride from foods and water is considered safe for adults.

Zinc, Copper, and Manganese: Working Together for Stronger Bones

For years, researchers have looked for connections between osteoporosis and the minerals zinc, copper, and manganese. While it's well-documented that deficiency of any one of these nutrients has a negative impact on bone health, research shows that they may work best together.

Recognizing the importance of each of these minerals, investigators at the University of California, San Diego, studied the effects of zinc, copper, and manganese when taken together. During a 2-year study of 59 women past the age of menopause, the researchers found that 1,000 milligrams of calcium slowed spinal bone mineral loss. Adding a "mineral cocktail" of 15 milligrams of zinc, 2.5 milligrams of copper, and 5 milligrams of manganese, however, actually stopped bone mineral loss in these women.

It's particularly important for the elderly to consider the balance of minerals they're getting because they may be lacking in some essential nutrients. In a study conducted at the University of Michigan School of Public Health, researchers found that study participants—all between ages 65 and 90—consumed just 70 percent of the recommended amount of zinc and 79 percent of the recommended amount of magnesium in their diets. Compounding the problem, some medications that are common among the elderly may affect the absorption of minerals in the body.

Nobody knows just how important any of these minerals are in osteoporosis prevention, Dr. Cosman says, but they have been implicated in one or two different studies as being important for bone health. Her recommendation is to follow a good, balanced diet with lots of fruits and vegetables and take a multivitamin. "We're not recommending that people take these specific supplements," she says.

The Daily Value for zinc is 15 milligrams; for both copper and manganese, it's 2 milligrams. Since too much zinc can block the absorption of copper, it is important to keep them in balance.

Prescriptions for Healing

Doctors agree that good nutrition is essential for bone health. Experts recommend these nutrients to help prevent osteoporosis or slow its progression.

Nutrient	Daily Amount
Boron	3 milligrams from food
Calcium	1,000–1,200 milligrams
Copper	2 milligrams
Fluoride	Up to 10 milligrams from food and water
Magnesium	200–400 milligrams
Manganese	2 milligrams
Vitamin D	1,000 IU
Vitamin K	80 micrograms
Zinc	15 milligrams

Plus a multivitamin/mineral supplement containing the Daily Values of all essential vitamins and minerals

MEDICAL ALERT: *If you have been diagnosed with osteoporosis, you should be under a doctor's care.*

If you have heart or kidney problems, you should talk to your doctor before taking magnesium supplements.

Vitamin K: The Unsung Hero

If you were to tell someone to get vitamin K, their response would probably be "Vitamin what?" Yet vitamin K, abundant in the food chain and produced by intestinal bacteria, plays a key role in bone formation. And vitamin K deficiency, which was previously thought to be very rare, may be a factor in osteoporosis. After following more than 72,000 women for 10 years, investigators for the Nurses' Health Study found that women with the lowest intake of vitamin K were at 30 percent higher risk for suffering a bone fracture than women with the highest intake. Meanwhile, the Framingham Heart Study found that getting 250 micrograms of vitamin K a day, which is about a half-cup of broccoli or mixed greens, lowered the risk of hip fractures in elderly men and women.

The Daily Value for vitamin K is 80 micrograms, and it's easy to get this vitamin in your diet. Just getting one serving a day of dark greens—such as spinach, kale, or broccoli—and eating a fair amount of fruits and vegetables will give you the vitamin K you need, says Jay Kenney, PhD, director of nutritional education for the Pritikin Longevity Center and Spa in Aventura, Florida. Vitamin K is found in all fruits and vegetables, but leafy vegetables tend to be the richest sources.

The Grab Bag

In addition to these vitamins and minerals, some doctors have suggested the possible benefits of vitamin C, vitamin B_6, and folic acid. Researchers don't recommend individual supplements of these nutrients for osteoporosis, but they don't hesitate to recommend a little multivitamin/mineral insurance.

OVERWEIGHT

NOURISHING YOURSELF THIN

Shakes, puddings, powders, and grapefruit: Name the diet, and you've tried it, each time hoping it would be the one that works. Then you watched that dreaded needle on that dreadful scale drift right back up to where you started.

Despite sage advice against dieting from physicians and national experts, we're still doing it. According to a 2006 survey of more than 2,000 adults in the United States, two-thirds had tried a diet at least once in the previous 5 years. Among those who dieted, 65 percent said the attempt failed. Regardless of all that calorie counting, our national waistline continues to expand at an alarming rate. According to the National Center for Health Statistics, about 66 percent of Americans are overweight or obese.

Could it finally be time to throw in the towel and pick up the fork? "No," says Judy Dodd, RD, assistant professor at the University of Pittsburgh and past president of the American Dietetic Association. "We just have to be sensible about our diets. Even people who are genetically predisposed to putting on weight do not have to be overweight. There are steps you can take to beat it, such as exercise and nutrition."

Multivitamins May Lend a Hand

And what about vitamins and minerals? What role do they play in a sensible no-diet weight-loss plan? Although the topic is controversial, some doctors believe that multivitamin/mineral supplements, combined with a healthy food and exercise plan, can help. They find that the struggles of overweight people are often brought on by a combination of poor general nutrition and dieting that leaves them feeling fatigued and craving food.

There's no doubt that nutrient deficiency makes it difficult to manage your weight, says Carol Forman Helerstein, PhD, a licensed clinical nutritionist in private practice on Long Island in New York. It's particularly true when it comes to B vitamins—such as folate, B_6, and B_{12}—because they're involved in energy production. When you're deficient in vitamin Bs, you may lack energy, crave food, and feel anxious. When you get enough of the vitamins, you're more likely to have the energy you need and feel calm, Dr. Helerstein says.

"It's kind of like a dog chasing its tail," Dr. Helerstein says. "You're depleted in the micronutrients that on a cellular level make everything work."

And it's not hard to be deficient in B vitamins. "In America today, we're all deficient because the foods we eat are so processed that we simply don't get what we need," she says. The solution: a multivitamin. When you get all of the micronutrients your body needs, you'll have fewer cravings and more energy. Scientists at the Fred Hutchinson Cancer Research Center surveyed 15,000 people with cancer and found that those who had taken a multivitamin, vitamin B_6, vitamin B_{12}, and chromium for 10 years had gained less weight—up to 14 fewer pounds—than those who hadn't taken vitamins.

Following fad diets may also have a huge effect on your nutrition. "Some of the old fad diets, such as the high-protein diet, are popular again, and people tend to skimp on important dietary elements such as fruits, vegetables, and dairy," Dodd says.

According to diet research, the most popular diets—those emphasizing high or low levels of protein, carbohydrates, and fat—all lead to deficiencies in important vitamins and minerals, particularly vitamins A and C, thiamin, iron, and calcium. And low-calorie diets, even those that are well balanced, typically lack folate, vitamin B_6, magnesium, and zinc.

Whether you're following a fad diet or not, simply eating less will make it harder to get all of the micronutrients you need from food. "Nutrition is a problem when people restrict calories," says Dodd. "I encourage people to get their vitamins and minerals from natural food sources, but if they go below 1,200 calories, they should consider a multivitamin/mineral supplement with 100 percent of the Daily Values."

Aside from multivitamin/mineral supplements, here are some of the nutrients that many experts believe can help you stay healthier and feel better and may even promote weight loss.

Nutrients to Build Immunity

As if the well-documented health risks associated with overweight, such as heart disease and diabetes, weren't bad enough, some researchers now believe that overweight people have lowered immunity, perhaps because of deficiencies of vitamins and minerals, especially the antioxidants.

Antioxidants such as vitamins C and E are important because they protect our bodies against free radicals, unstable oxygen molecules that damage the body's cells by stealing electrons from healthy molecules. Antioxidants offer their own electrons, neutralizing free radicals and protecting cells. Vitamin A arms your immune system by making white blood cells that attack bacteria and viruses and prevent infections. And if you don't exercise enough, the antioxidant vitamin E may mimic exercise's effect on free radicals in your body, protecting cells from damage. Although exercise should always be in your daily routine, taking extra vitamin E will help make up for any shortfall.

"Antioxidants are very, very necessary," Dr. Helerstein says. We create free radicals simply by living, such as when we digest food or breathe in pollution. Antioxidants protect us from those free radicals.

According to a study done in Poland, overweight people may not be reaping antioxidant benefits. Researchers at the National Institute of Food and Nutrition in Warsaw studied 102 overweight women and found that the women had significantly lower levels of the antioxidant vitamins C and E, as well as of vitamin A, and a higher prevalence of overall vitamin deficiency compared with women of normal weight.

These deficiencies are at least partially responsible for depressing immunity in overweight individuals, leaving them more susceptible to cancer and infectious illness, say some researchers.

Because of abnormal hormone activity, overweight people may also have greater need for antioxidants than people who are not overweight. Studies show that the excess fat in people who are very overweight drives estrogen production up and testosterone down, a deadly combination that scientists believe could be a major factor in certain female reproductive cancers.

Dr. Helerstein recommends getting a multivitamin that includes more than 100 percent of the Daily Value of the antioxidant vitamins C and E. Current recommendations from the government are set only to help prevent diseases that result from deficiencies. For instance, the Daily Value of 60 milligrams for vitamin C will keep you from getting scurvy but won't give you enough antioxidant protection.

If you'd like to take a separate supplement from your multivitamin, aim for 1,000 milligrams of vitamin C and 400 to 800 IU of vitamin E a day, Dr. Helerstein says.

But when it comes to vitamin A, don't get more than the Daily Value of 5,000 IU. Research has found that taking 10,000 IU of vitamin A daily in early pregnancy can cause birth defects. For this reason, more than the Daily Value should be taken only under medical supervision, especially if you are a woman of childbearing age. And pregnant women should talk to their doctor about taking supplements.

To get more antioxidants through your diet, reach for fruits and vegetables. Those with bright orange coloring, such as sweet potatoes, carrots, and cantaloupe, are rich in beta-carotene (a precursor of vitamin A); broccoli, brussels sprouts, and citrus fruits will give you a burst of vitamin C; and wheat germ and kale are good sources of vitamin E.

Calcium May Curb Fat

This mineral may traditionally be thought of as an aid in osteoporosis prevention, but there's mounting evidence that a diet high in calcium helps break down fat and leads to weight loss. Experts also believe that calcium from food and supplements may bind to fat in the digestive tract and carry it out of the body.

In one study, 32 adults who were obese were split into three groups. One group ate a diet that included 400 to 500 milligrams of calcium, another ate a standard diet and added a calcium supplement of 800 milligrams, and the third ate a diet that included 1,200 to 1,300 milligrams of calcium a day. Each group cut 500 calories from their diet over 24 weeks. The group getting up to 1,300 milligrams of calcium a day lost the most weight.

It's not just the calcium in food that's beneficial. You may lose more

Food Factors

When it comes to weight loss, selecting your foods can be a real balancing act. You have to lose some of what you've grown accustomed to and add some items that may be new to you. Here's what experts recommend to promote weight loss.

Reduce fat. With regard to fat, the research is clear: Diets too high in fat promote overweight. You should strive to consume no more than 25 percent of your calories from fat.

The good news is that there are plenty of low-fat options these days. Good choices for reduced-calorie snacks include a low-fat cheese stick or a cup of low-fat yogurt with fruit. Indulging in a cup of halved strawberries is not only a good nonfat snack option, it also provides 90 milligrams of vitamin C.

Go mini. Eating minimeals every 3 or 4 hours will help you become leaner. Research has found that women who eat small meals and two or three small snacks a day weigh less than women who eat two or three big meals, even when it's the same number of calories. Grazing on small amounts of food throughout the day keeps your metabolism running.

To make your meals smaller, cut 100 calories by skipping croutons on your salad and using one fewer tablespoon of butter on your bread.

Don't be so sweet. Numerous studies have linked table sugar to increased calorie consumption. While sugar doesn't do as much dietary damage as fat, you'll find that when you eat sweets, you simply want to eat more . . . of everything. Not only that, but sugar also makes your body excrete chromium, and chromium is a mineral that helps your body build calorie-burning lean tissue.

A major source of sugar may be in your beverage. Americans have been drinking more and more soda over the past 40 years, and that's adding up to a significant amount of calories. Eighteen ounces of a sweetened drink adds 225 calories to your diet, which adds up to almost 7,000 extra calories a month, or a gain of 2 pounds.

Drink up. "If people want to keep their nutrients in balance, they need to drink plenty of plain, unflavored water every day," says Judy

weight if you take calcium supplements. After reviewing 10 years' worth of data from more than 5,000 women between ages 53 and 57, researchers at the University of Washington found that those who got 1,100 milligrams of calcium or more in their diet gained 2 pounds less than women who got less. The women who reached their calcium level with a supplement lost a pound more than the women who consumed calcium through their diet.

Some studies have contradicted the ones that show a benefit from

Dodd, RD, assistant professor at the University of Pittsburgh and past president of the American Dietetic Association. Water not only acts as a solvent for many vitamins and minerals but also is responsible for carrying nutrients into and wastes out of cells, so the body functions properly. As a rule of thumb, you should drink a half ounce of water for every pound of body weight daily, unless you're very active, in which case you should increase your water intake to two-thirds of an ounce per pound of body weight daily.

Fill up on fiber. You can curb your hunger by increasing your intake of dietary fiber, which is filling, so you feel full but eat less. Research shows that women who regularly eat high-fiber diets have a lower risk of obesity and heart disease. Experts recommend eating more fruits, vegetables, and whole-grain cereals. Broth-based soups with raw veggies are a great way to fill up on fiber. People who eat soup regularly lose more weight than people who don't.

Get treatment for food allergies. Some researchers believe that overweight is the result of people craving foods that they are allergic to. For these people, weight loss is extremely difficult until they figure out what those trigger foods are and eliminate them from their diets.

When you're intolerant to certain foods, it causes inflammation in your body, and that puts your immune system into high gear. When your immune system remains chronically active, your body reacts by storing fat, says Roger Davis Deutsch, author of *Your Hidden Food Allergies Are Making You Fat* and founder and chief executive officer of ALCAT Worldwide, a company that tests for allergies.

Experts also theorize, although it hasn't been shown yet in research, that irritable bowel syndrome may lead to lower levels of serotonin, which make people crave high-glycemic foods that lead to weight gain.

Getting tested for food allergies will help. "When we test somebody for food intolerance and we change their diet accordingly, they lose their cravings for sugar," Deutsch says.

calcium, but calcium is so important for a variety of reasons that it can't hurt to ensure you're getting enough of the mineral every day. And considering 88 percent of women and 63 percent of men in the United States don't get enough calcium from their food, a supplement may be a good idea. Another advantage to supplements: They don't add extra calories.

There's another reason to get calcium: Your bones may suffer if you're cutting calories. Rutgers University scientists have found that people who are trying to lose weight show up to a 3 percent loss of bone after 6 months of dieting. They found that eating less shifts hormones in your body and makes it harder to absorb calcium from food and supplements.

If you're dieting, make sure you're getting 1,000 to 1,200 milligrams of calcium a day. If you're over 50, increase your goal to 1,500 milligrams a day to make up for lower absorption.

Also, vitamin D is just as important for your bones. Although the Daily Value for vitamin D is 400 IU, many experts recommend aiming for 1,000 IU a day.

Chromium Can Help

It might not be the waist-whittling miracle mineral that some advertisements tout it as, but according to some research, chromium picolinate (a supplemental form of chromium) may indeed help build lean tissue and reduce fat in adults who exercise.

In one study of 59 college-age students at Louisiana State University in Baton Rouge, researchers found that women taking 200 micrograms of chromium picolinate a day gained almost twice as much lean body mass as those who did not take the supplements, an effect that could result in long-term reductions in body fat, since lean body mass burns more calories than fat.

"What makes the effectiveness of chromium more and more believable is that the results we see in humans are so well-documented in animal studies," says Richard Anderson, PhD, research chemist in the nutrient requirements and functions laboratory at the USDA Beltsville Human Nutrition Research Center in Maryland and a leading chromium researcher. And although chromium will benefit only those who are deficient, Dr. Anderson reports that most people in Westernized countries receive only 25 percent of the Daily Value of 120 micrograms. So a lot of people are deficient.

Chromium also improves the effectiveness of insulin, the hormone that allows cells to pick up glucose (a simple sugar that your body uses for fuel) from the bloodstream. For this reason, chromium may also be helpful in preventing diabetes, which is common in people who are overweight. People

Prescriptions for Healing

Some nutrition experts find that overweight people have special vitamin and mineral needs, especially if they're trying to lose weight. Here's what these experts recommend.

Nutrient	Daily Amount
Calcium	1,000–1,200 milligrams; 1,500 milligrams if you're over 50
Chromium	50–200 micrograms (chromium picolinate)
Copper	1.5–3 milligrams (1 milligram for every 10 milligrams of zinc)
Iron	15 milligrams
Magnesium	250–500 milligrams
Vitamin A	5,000 IU
Vitamin C	1,000 milligrams
Vitamin D	1,000 milligrams
Vitamin E	400–800 IU
Zinc	15–30 milligrams

Plus a multivitamin/mineral supplement containing the Daily Values of all essential vitamins and minerals

MEDICAL ALERT: *People with diabetes who take chromium should be under medical supervision, since their insulin dosage may need to be reduced as their blood sugar levels drop.*

Do not take more than 3 milligrams of copper per day without medical supervision.

If you have heart or kidney problems, you should talk to your doctor before taking magnesium supplements.

Vitamin A in the amount recommended here should be taken only under medical supervision, especially if you are a woman of child-bearing age. Women who are pregnant should not use this therapy.

If you are taking anticoagulants, you should not take vitamin E supplements. (Though generally a dose of up to 1,500 IU of vitamin E a day is considered safe, some recent reports suggest that taking more than 400 IU a day could be harmful to people with cardiovascular or circulatory disease or with cancer. If you have such a condition, be sure to consult your doctor before you begin supplementation.)

Doses of zinc in excess of 15 milligrams daily should be taken only under medical supervision.

with diabetes who take chromium should be under medical supervision, since their insulin dosage may need to be reduced as their blood sugar levels drop.

Dr. Helerstein recommends going to a health food store and looking for a supplement under the category of weight loss or blood sugar level control or balance. Those supplements will include chromium and other agents that help control blood sugar and help with weight management, such as cinnamon, green tea extract, and fenugreek.

The National Institutes of Health warn, however, that the studies that show a link between chromium and weight loss have included a small number of participants and were short in duration. Also, a 2003 review of 24 studies that used from 200 to 1,000 micrograms of chromium a day failed to find an impact on body mass.

Doctors who recommend chromium picolinate supplements suggest daily doses ranging from 50 to 200 micrograms. If you'd like to increase chromium through your diet, try whole-grain cereals, black pepper, cheeses, and brewer's yeast.

Think Zinc

It's well documented that zinc, a mineral found in wheat germ, seafood, and whole grains, frequently gets left by the wayside when calorie intake dips below 1,200.

Most experts do not recommend such low-calorie regimens. If you're among those who keep a too-tight daily calorie tally anyway, you should know that zinc deficiency not only depresses the immune system but also can be a barber's nightmare, causing brittle, dry hair and hair loss.

Experts usually recommend between 15 and 30 milligrams of zinc daily. Since zinc competes with other metals in the body, however, daily doses of more than the Daily Value of 15 milligrams warrant medical supervision. For the best results, you should take 1 milligram of copper for every 10 milligrams of zinc.

Minerals Make a Difference

Magnesium and iron are the major minerals that doctors find deficient in people who are overweight, particularly in those who are trying to slim down.

Magnesium is essential for every major biological function, including your heartbeat. According to research, even marginal magnesium deficiency is not to be taken lightly, especially when you are dieting and losing weight, as it can lead to potentially fatal heart abnormalities.

Doctors who recommend magnesium supplements call for between 250 and 500 milligrams daily, which is right around the Daily Value of 400 milligrams. (If you have heart or kidney problems, you should check with your doctor before taking magnesium supplements.) Good dietary sources of magnesium include seafood, green vegetables, and low-fat dairy products.

Iron is another frequent victim of low-calorie dieting. The most common complication arising from a lack of iron is iron-deficiency anemia, which can cause headaches, shortness of breath, weakness, heart palpitations, and fatigue.

Doctors who recommend supplementing iron suggest 15 milligrams a day, particularly for adults who are following a low-calorie diet to lose weight. To pump some iron into your diet, try steamed clams, Cream of Wheat cereal, tofu, and soybeans.

PARKINSON'S DISEASE

SMOOTHING OUT THE TREMORS

Dr. Alex MacGregor's life was about control. As a bariatric surgeon, he relied on fine motor control every day to do his job. And then around age 59 his hands took on a will of their own. While he was sitting at his desk, his right hand began to flop around, utterly out of his control.

When medication couldn't control the tremors anymore, he was forced to lay down his scalpel forever. Up until then he had been diagnosed and treated for tremors, but several months later he was diagnosed with Parkinson's disease. Parkinson's had stripped his brain of the power to signal his muscles into action or inaction. In church, he had to sit on his left hand to restrain it. When his knees began to shake, he had to hold them down with his right hand, the only one that was free.

Eleven years later, Dr. MacGregor couldn't walk, dress himself, or control the muscles in his face. He and his family lived with the fear that he would choke on his food. In the meantime, his ability to communicate began fading away as his voice became softer and softer.

Dr. MacGregor has regained some of his function from deep brain stimulation, a procedure in which wires are implanted into portions of his brain and are stimulated by a small engine placed in his chest. The stimulation takes away his tremors and allows him to work part-time reviewing scientific papers for the American Society for Bariatric Surgery. But unfortunately, Parkinson's has taken away his ability to drive, show facial expression, and speak in anything but a very soft voice.

Dr. MacGregor and his wife Christine live with the knowledge that he isn't going to get better, but they work on maintaining the abilities he has right now.

A key factor in maintaining his health is nutrition. Treating Parkinson's means looking after the whole person, Christine says. Dr. MacGregor eats nutritionally optimal meals every day, along with orange juice and plenty of liquids. The orange juice provides the antioxidant vitamin C and helps his body absorb his medications, Christine says. And if he doesn't stay hydrated with plenty of liquids, he becomes confused.

He doesn't need supplements because his diet provides everything he needs, Christine says. Other than the Parkinson's disease, he's in very good health, thanks to a lifetime of eating well and getting exercise. Dr. MacGregor played all types of sports and even was a gymnast at a younger age. Today he works out at a gym three times a week.

Parkinson's disease is characterized by damage to brain cells in the substantia nigra, an area deep in the center of the brain that helps coordinate muscle movement, as well as to brain cells in other areas that influence certain aspects of cognition, emotion, and autonomic function. These cells produce a chemical called dopamine, a neurotransmitter that's essential for the brain to send messages to the muscles. As the cells die and dopamine levels drop, muscle control suffers.

Nobody knows for sure why the cells die, but a combination of exposure to environmental toxins and genetic susceptibility, along with normal wear and tear, seems to be the most likely reason, says Caroline M. Tanner, MD, PhD, director of clinical research at the Parkinson's Institute in Sunnyvale, California. "Certain chemicals can cause symptoms similar to Parkinson's in both animals and humans," Dr. Tanner says. An estimated 1.5 million Americans suffer from the disease.

Getting the Rust Out

One aspect of nutritional therapy for Parkinson's is directly related to the disease's probable causes, says J. William Langston, MD, founder and chief executive officer of the Parkinson's Institute.

"Both normal aging and possible exposure of this part of the brain to toxins may cause oxidative chemical reactions that allow the release of free radicals, molecular particles that steal electrons from other molecules, setting off a chain reaction of cell damage," Dr. Langston explains.

Even dopamine, the neurotransmitter highly concentrated in this part of the brain, is oxidized as part of the message-sending process, Dr. Langston explains. "It's as if dopamine were too hot to handle, and over many years, as it's oxidized, it may eventually kill the very same cells that make it and use it to cause normal motor function," he says.

Vitamin E and sometimes vitamin C have been recommended for people with Parkinson's because these two nutrients act as antioxidants. They stop the chain reaction of free radicals by offering their own electrons, sparing healthy molecules from harm. Most attention has been on vitamin E, since it acts in the fatty parts of cells (brain and nerve tissues contain lots of fatty membranes). Here's what research shows.

Vitamin E: Promise and Disappointment

"The theory behind giving vitamin E for Parkinson's disease is that this nutrient is a free radical scavenger and therefore can protect against free radical damage to the brain," Dr. Langston says. "If you have excessive production of all of these potentially damaging, reactive chemicals over time, and if you put in something like a sponge, something that can soak up or block their effects, you might protect against further damage to the brain."

That's the theory, anyway. In practice, research results have been mostly disappointing.

There were times when antioxidant supplements looked promising for Parkinson's patients. One study found that people with early Parkinson's disease who took vitamins E and C were able to postpone taking medication for symptoms for 2½ years longer than people not getting these vitamins. (The vitamin takers gradually increased to 3,200 IU of vitamin E and 3,000 milligrams of vitamin C daily, taken in four divided doses.)

But a large nationwide study that followed, the DATATOP study, found that 2,000 IU of vitamin E, taken for up to 2 years, offered no apparent benefit to people with Parkinson's.

All in all, there's no evidence-based medicine that points to vitamin E as a factor in slowing the progression of Parkinson's disease, says Lily Jung, MD, interim medical director at the Swedish Neuroscience Institute in Seattle. The best studies—the ones that are randomized—fail to find a connection.

The problem isn't that the antioxidants don't work, it's that there's a barrier between the blood and the brain, Dr. Langston says. "It's very hard to get drugs into the brain."

Food Factors

If you're taking the drug levodopa to relieve the tremors, stiffness, and poor muscle control of Parkinson's disease, you know that the way you eat can have a major impact on your symptoms. Here are the dietary changes that doctors are most likely to recommend.

Take your medicine on an empty stomach. Levodopa is absorbed in the small intestine, not the stomach, so it's a drug you can take on an empty stomach, says J. William Langston, MD, founder and chief executive officer of the Parkinson's Institute in Sunnyvale, California. If you take the medication with food, the stomach will hold onto your meal to start the digestive process and the drug won't be able to be absorbed for an hour or two. Because of this delay in the action of the drug, it's better to take it on an empty stomach, Dr. Langston says.

Save protein for dinner. Protein is made up of amino acids, and the amino acids in foods interfere with levodopa getting into the brain. (Levodopa is also an amino acid.)

Although you shouldn't go below the minimum daily requirement of protein that your doctor determines is right for you, you may want to hold off on eating protein until dinner. Because your Parkinson's symptoms will likely become worse after eating protein, save it for the evening so you can stay home afterward, Dr. Langston says.

Beware the fava bean. This flat, tan bean, used in Mediterranean and Middle Eastern dishes, contains dopamine. Eating it with your daily dose of levodopa can cause symptoms of dopamine overdose, including agitation and extra involuntary movements. Dr. Langston recommends avoiding fava beans all together.

Dr. Langston spent time looking at "prescription antioxidants," chemically engineered varieties not found in nature that get into the brain more easily than vitamin E, but he says the research hasn't been fruitful. "Antioxidants don't look very promising in spite of very strong scientific theory that they should be," he says.

Although vitamin E doesn't seem to help once a patient has been diagnosed with the disease, studies show that dietary intakes of vitamin E may protect against developing Parkinson's disease. A 2002 Harvard University study looked at more than 76,000 women and 47,000 men and found that those who had the highest dietary intake of vitamin E had a significantly lower risk of Parkinson's disease.

Good sources of vitamin E are wheat germ oil, almonds; sunflower seeds; hazelnuts; peanut butter; spinach; broccoli; kiwi; mango; and sunflower, safflower, and soybean oils.

Promising New Research

Although vitamin E has been disappointing, there are two supplements that are giving researchers hope: coenzyme Q10 and creatine.

Our bodies make coenzyme Q10, which serves as a link in the chain of chemical reactions that produce cell energy, called mitochondrial function.

As a supplement, "coenzyme Q10 seems to improve the energy packets in each cell where energy is made," Dr. Langston says. Parkinson's patients have lower levels of coenzyme Q10 in their mitochondria, and animal studies show that coenzyme Q10 can protect the part of the brain that's damaged in Parkinson's patients.

The compound also acts as an antioxidant, destroying potentially hazardous chemicals that are created during metabolism.

A preliminary study of 80 patients in the early stages of Parkinson's disease found that coenzyme Q10 might slow the progression of the disease. The study participants were split into four groups, with one group receiving 300 milligrams a day of coenzyme Q10, a second group receiving 600 milligrams a day, a third group receiving 1,200 milligrams a day, and a fourth group receiving a placebo. All four groups also took vitamin E.

After 16 months, the group getting the largest dose saw the slowest decline in mental and motor functions. The groups taking up to 600 milligrams of coenzyme Q10 had better results than the placebo group but didn't see the same effects as the group getting 1,200 milligrams.

In addition, the groups that took coenzyme Q10 had more of the compound in their blood and experienced a significant rise in energy-producing reactions within their mitochondria.

"We think there's enough evidence to go on and do a much larger study," Dr. Langston says.

Another compound showing promise is creatine, the supplement that's commonly associated with improving the performance of athletes. Creatine works in the same way coenzyme Q10 does, by boosting the production of energy inside cells and acting as an antioxidant.

In research done on mice, creatine was able to prevent the loss of cells that are typically affected by Parkinson's disease. Creatine also passed a "futility trial," in which researchers test a drug—in this case, 10 grams of creatine—to see if it is ineffective at slowing down a disease, Dr. Langston says. As a result, the National Institutes of Health is launching a trial involving 1,720 patients to look at creatine's effect on Parkinson's symptoms.

More research is needed before Dr. Langston will begin to recommend coenzyme Q10 or creatine supplements to patients, but patients may decide on their own to take them. "They're very safe," he says, but warns that they're expensive. To match the doses used in the studies, you'll have to pay hundreds of dollars a month.

Talk to your doctor if you plan to take coenzyme Q10 and you're taking

---

Prescriptions for Healing

Drugs, not vitamins and minerals, are the mainstay of treatment for Parkinson's disease. Doctors who also offer nutritional guidance are most likely to make these recommendations.

Nutrient	Daily Amount
Coenzyme Q10	1,200 milligrams
Creatine	10 grams

Plus a multivitamin/mineral supplement containing the Daily Values of all essential vitamins and minerals, including the trace minerals

MEDICAL ALERT: If you have Parkinson's disease, take supplements only under the supervision of your doctor.

the blood-thinning medication warfarin. Coenzyme Q10 may decrease warfarin's effects.

Add a Little Insurance

Some experts recommend that Parkinson's patients take a multivitamin/mineral tablet that includes the Daily Values of all of the essential vitamins and minerals, including the trace minerals. There's a bit of evidence that selenium, a mineral with antioxidant properties, may play a role in Parkinson's. In people with this disease, the part of the brain that's involved, the substantia nigra, is low in a selenium-based antioxidant called glutathione peroxidase. Some experts speculate that low levels of this substance may help set the stage for cell damage.

PELLAGRA

DECODING A TURN-OF-THE-CENTURY MYSTERY

Offer someone sow bellies and cornmeal grits for dinner tonight, and you'll probably find yourself eating alone. But in the Deep South about 100 years ago, these foods were the staple diet that's thought to have caused an outbreak of a niacin-deficiency disease called pellagra.

Characterized by a progressive decline that often starts with itchy, red skin, moves on to diarrhea and depression, and ends in death, pellagra was called the disease of the four Ds: dermatitis, diarrhea, dementia, and death. Spanish peasants were thought to have had it in 1735, and there are reports in the United States from the 1820s that point to pellagra.

It became a real problem in the United States in the early 20th century after the advent of the roller mill, which changed the way corn was processed, says Michael Flannery, head of historical collections at the University of Alabama at Birmingham. The new process depleted the cornmeal of niacin.

By 1912, South Carolina had 30,000 cases of the disease, which had a mortality rate of 40 percent. And by 1940, about 3 million people had suffered from pellagra in the United States and 100,000 had died.

In 1914, the U.S. Congress called on the Surgeon General to do something about the problem. Dr. Joseph Goldberger led the investigation and soon disproved what medical experts had assumed about pellagra all along: that it was an infectious disease. While examining the afflicted in orphanages, mental hospitals, and cotton mill towns, Dr. Goldberger noticed that the staff never contracted the disease and insisted the cause of the symptoms was the result of a dietary disorder, although he didn't know that lack of niacin was the culprit.

An experiment involving orphans in Jackson, Mississippi, who had pellagra gave him clues to the mystery. Just a few days after doctors added milk, meats, and eggs to the corn grit diet of the children, their pellagra disappeared.

To confirm dietary deficiency as a cause, another study was conducted, this time involving convicts. When pellagra-free prisoners agreed to eat nothing but sow bellies, corn grits, gravy, and fried mush for 5 months, nearly all developed pellagra.

To eliminate lingering doubts that pellagra might be an infectious disease, still another study was launched involving convicts. The prisoners, and the experimenters themselves, were injected with blood from people with pellagra or were exposed to their nasal or throat excretions. When the subjects didn't come down with the disease, researchers realized that pellagra could not possibly be infectious.

But throughout his experiments, Dr. Goldberger received harsh criticism from the medical community, who refused to believe that pellagra developed because of a nutritional deficiency. To prove his point, Dr. Goldberger even injected himself and his assistant with blood from pellagra patients, and neither contracted pellagra.

True Grits Not Enough

It wasn't until 1937 that researchers pinpointed the exact source of the problem. When the selective service began rejecting an alarming number of soldiers because of nutritional deficiencies and other diseases, the U.S. government mandated the enrichment of food, which conquered the disease, Flannery says.

The problem was that corn not only contains a form of niacin, a B vitamin, that the body cannot easily use but also can create an amino acid imbalance. Amino acids are the building blocks of protein, the stuff of which the body is made. Eating corn as part of a well-balanced diet is not a problem, but a diet that consists almost exclusively of corn and corn products is devastating. As a result of the fortification of flours and cereals with niacin, pellagra is now rare except in developing countries where nutrition is poor. Malawi, in Southern Africa, experienced a pellagra epidemic in 1990.

A few people still get pellagra, however, for reasons that have nothing to do with eating corn. Alcoholics and individuals with severe gastrointestinal problems often have difficulty getting enough niacin. Even then, diagnosing pellagra is not easy. The early symptoms, such as reddening of the skin, cracked lips, weight loss, tiredness, confusion, and mild diarrhea, can be subtle.

Niacin to the Rescue

Fortunately, the effects of early-stage pellagra are easily reversed. Patients are given niacin supplements along with a high-protein diet that includes milk, meats, peanuts, green leafy vegetables, whole and enriched grains, and brewers' dry yeast, which can enhance the intake of niacin.

Within 24 hours of being treated, patients see dramatic results. They become mentally clear, swelling and redness of the tongue subside, and nausea, vomiting, and diarrhea go away.

Supplements of either nicotinic acid or niacinamide will correct the

---

Prescriptions for Healing

These days, pellagra is rare. Once this niacin-deficiency disease is diagnosed, doctors recommend niacinamide, a form of niacin that is known to have few side effects.

Nutrient	Daily Amount
Niacinamide	50 to 500 milligrams, sometimes taken in 2 or 3 doses

MEDICAL ALERT: If you have symptoms of pellagra, you should see your doctor for proper diagnosis and treatment.

This amount of niacinamide is prescribed for severe cases of pellagra and should be taken only under medical supervision.

deficiency, says Doug Heimburger, MD, professor of nutrition sciences at the University of Alabama at Birmingham. Nicotinic acid also works to lower cholesterol levels.

The amount prescribed probably has to do with the condition of the patient as much as it has to do with the physician. Some physicians will prescribe very high doses, and others will be more conservative and give the patient a minimal amount, Dr. Heimburger says. It should take only one "substantial" dose to cure pellagra: 50 to 500 milligrams of nicotinic acid or niacinamide, administered orally or intravenously. Some doctors may divide the amount into two or three doses.

Since high amounts of niacin can be toxic, this amount should be taken only under the supervision of a physician.

Of course, the key is to make sure the patient continues to maintain niacin levels to avoid another deficiency. Some of the best food sources of niacin are chicken breast, turkey, beef, salmon, nuts, tuna, and fortified cereal. The Daily Value for niacin is 20 milligrams.

PHLEBITIS

STAYING OUT OF DEEP TROUBLE

You might think you've been kicked in the leg or you've pulled a muscle, but you can't for the life of you remember just when or where or how it happened. That's because it didn't happen. That painful knot you feel in your calf isn't a bruise or a muscle injury. It's phlebitis, a swollen, inflamed vein that can be caused by anything from staying put too long to birth control pills.

Phlebitis is not uncommon. And it's not necessarily serious when it occurs in a superficial vein, since these veins are numerous enough to permit your body to rechannel the flow of blood, bypassing the inflamed vein.

Phlebitis that occurs in deep veins, called thrombophlebitis, is a serious matter. It usually involves formation of a blood clot in the vein, and it can lead to life-threatening circulation problems. The clot could break free, travel to the lungs, and block a pulmonary artery, which could lead to death. That's why doctors advise getting up and taking short walks every hour when you're on an airplane or pulling over for a short walk during long car rides. If you can't get up, doctors advise flexing your ankles at least 10 times an hour.

Thrombophlebitis doesn't always have clear symptoms, but it can be detected with ultrasound. It must be treated promptly with blood-thinning medication. Superficial phlebitis, which is most likely to occur in varicose veins, responds to a judicious combination of exercise and resting with your feet elevated. Smoking is also a risk factor, so quitting can go a long way to preventing the problem. These nutritional approaches may also help prevent phlebitis and its worst consequences.

B Vitamins May Help Stop Clots

Several years ago researchers discovered that people with high blood levels of an amino acid called homocysteine had a high risk of developing damage to endothelial cells, the cells lining artery walls. Once these cells are damaged, cholesterol deposits can build up fast. These people frequently suffered from severe heart disease, experiencing heart attacks in their twenties and thirties.

Dutch researchers discovered a second problem connected with homocysteine. They found elevated blood levels of this substance in people who had recurring blood clots in their veins. As the blood levels of homocysteine increased, so did people's risk of forming clots. Even moderately elevated levels of homocysteine were linked to two to three times the normal risk of recurrent blood clots.

What do B vitamins have to do with all of this? Three B vitamins—folate (the naturally occurring form of folic acid), vitamin B_6, and vitamin B_{12}—have been found to help break down and clear homocysteine from the blood. For a while, that led doctors to recommend supplements of these vitamins to prevent a stroke or cardiovascular disease. But more recent clinical trials have contradicted that advice.

In a 2006 study of more than 5,500 patients who were age 55 or older and had vascular disease or diabetes, researchers found that those who took folic acid, vitamin B_6, and vitamin B_{12} didn't have a significantly lower risk of death from heart disease, although none of the patients who took the supplements had a stroke. Another study of more than 3,700 men and women who had had a recent heart attack found that taking B vitamins didn't lower the risk of cardiovascular disease after a heart attack.

Does this mean B vitamins should be ignored when it comes to preventing

---

Food Factors

Your diet can help prevent the blood clots that lead to phlebitis. Here's what research has shown.

Indulge in a little chocolate. If you smoke, you're at a higher risk for blood clots, but the flavonoids in chocolate may help. Swiss researchers gave 10 male smokers 1.4 ounces of dark chocolate, which is rich in flavonoids, and another 10 smokers white chocolate, which doesn't contain flavonoids. After 2 hours, an ultrasound showed that those who ate the dark chocolate had 36 percent less clot-forming activity and 59 percent greater artery flexibility.

Enjoy kiwifruit. Researchers at the University of Oslo in Norway found that study participants who ate two or three kiwifruit daily for 28 days significantly lowered their chances of forming a blood clot.

---

blood clots, stroke, and heart disease? No, says J. David Spence, MD, professor of neurology and clinical pharmacology at the University of Western Ontario, director of the Stroke Prevention and Atherosclerosis Research Centre at Robarts Research Institute in London, Canada, and author of *How to Prevent Your Stroke*. He argues that the studies didn't use a high enough dose of vitamin B_{12} to see improvement.

"Elevated levels of total homocysteine do increase clotting of blood, and since stroke is more dependent on blood clotting and on emboli (clots that form elsewhere and then travel through the arteries to the brain) than are heart attacks, vitamin therapy probably does reduce the risk of stroke, if not yet shown to reduce the risk of heart attacks," he says.

That doesn't mean everyone should take all three vitamins as a supplement. Grains are fortified with folate in North America, so it's not necessary to get extra, Dr. Spence says. Getting enough vitamin B_6 also isn't an issue. What people should be paying attention to is vitamin B_{12}, Dr. Spence says, especially after age 50. That's because people lose the ability to absorb vitamin B_{12} from food as they get older. Under age 50, only about 12 percent of people have a vitamin B_{12} deficiency, but it goes up to 30 percent for people over age 71. There are also hereditary reasons why some people don't absorb vitamin B_{12}, he says.

But here's a major problem: most doctors don't understand that people have trouble absorbing vitamin B_{12} as they get older. Making matters worse, a standard blood test will come back normal even in people who actually are deficient in vitamin B_{12}, Dr. Spence says. A test that measures methylmalonic acid is a better way to look for deficiency because adequate levels of vitamin B_{12} suppress methylmalonic acid.

Because the main source of vitamin B_{12} is meat, it's not something people should eat more of when they're trying to lower the risk of stroke and a heart attack. That's where supplements come in. Dr. Spence recommends that people who have a severe deficiency take 1,200 micrograms of vitamin B_{12} twice a day either through a weekly injection or in pills. People who have a less severe deficiency should take 1,000 micrograms of vitamin B_{12} a day, he says. One thing to keep in mind: If you're getting vitamin B_{12} through injections, you need them once a week because the vitamin is water-soluble and injections elevate levels for only about a week.

Prescriptions for Healing

These nutrients won't cure a raging case of phlebitis. But some medical experts feel that they might help prevent a recurrence.

Nutrient	Daily Amount
Folic acid	2,500 micrograms
Vitamin B_6	25 milligrams
Vitamin B_{12}	1,200 micrograms twice a day for severe deficiency; 1,000 micrograms a day for less severe deficiency
Vitamin E	200–600 IU

MEDICAL ALERT: *If you have phlebitis, you should be under a doctor's care.*

Consult your doctor before supplementing your diet with these B vitamins. Blood tests need to be done to determine your exact deficiencies before a doctor can prescribe the best combination and amounts. In addition, folic acid in doses exceeding 400 micrograms daily can mask symptoms of vitamin B_{12} deficiency.

If you are taking anticoagulant drugs, you should not take vitamin E supplements. (Though generally a dose of up to 1,500 IU of vitamin E a day is considered safe, some recent reports suggest that taking more than 400 IU a day could be harmful to people with cardiovascular or circulatory disease or with cancer. If you have such a condition, be sure to consult your doctor before you begin supplementation.)

Vitamin E May Improve the Flow

Evidence is mounting that vitamin E helps protect against cardiovascular disease by helping to block the chemical processes that lead to atherosclerosis, or hardening of the arteries.

Vitamin E plays an additional role, one that's particularly important to people with phlebitis. Several studies indicate that vitamin E can help protect against potentially life-threatening blood clots. Specifically, vitamin E helps prevent platelets, components involved in blood clotting, from sticking to each other and to blood vessel walls.

"Sticky platelets can cause blood clots to build up fast," explains Joseph Pizzorno Jr., ND, president emeritus of Bastyr University in Seattle. Studies suggest that reducing platelet stickiness with vitamin E could have a role in the treatment of "thromboembolic events," or traveling blood clots, especially in people with type 1 (insulin-dependent) diabetes, who are at particularly high risk for blood-clotting problems.

If you're going to take vitamin E, Dr. Pizzorno suggests that 200 to 600 IU daily should do the trick. Some research suggests that 200 IU is enough to reduce platelet adhesion.

People taking anticoagulants (sometimes called blood thinners or heart medicine) should not take vitamin E supplements.

PREMENSTRUAL SYNDROME

PUTTING AN END TO MONTHLY DISCOMFORT

Ask 10 women what premenstrual syndrome feels like, and you'll probably get 10 different answers.

A few of those answers will be pretty predictable: bloated, sore, tired, headachy. Other women feel okay physically but ride an emotional roller coaster of anxiety and depression.

And—something you probably don't want to hear if you have premenstrual syndrome—some women don't experience any premenstrual symptoms at all.

Experts estimate that at least 85 percent of menstruating women in the United States have some degree of premenstrual syndrome, or PMS. Whether you're one of them depends on a variety of factors, including your genetic inheritance, how much stress you're under, whether you drink alcohol or caffeine, and how much you exercise. Age is also a factor: Women in their thirties and forties are more likely to get PMS than younger women.

And finally, some researchers believe that nutrition exerts a powerful influence on how a woman feels both before and during her period. It's the reason that women tend to have PMS in their thirties after they've been pregnant, says Carol Forman Helerstein, PhD, a licensed clinical nutritionist in private practice on Long Island in New York. Because pregnancy depletes the body of nutrients, women are more likely to be deficient in B vitamins and magnesium after pregnancy.

According to Dr. Helerstein, a key aspect to preventing PMS symptoms is avoiding refined sugar and high-fat foods. "There's a lot of science that shows that when you eat a high-fat, high-sugar diet, you're going to have more PMS than someone who eats a well-balanced diet," she says.

But it may not be so easy to eat well when you're having PMS. The hormone changes your body goes through before your period are a stressor on the body, and as a result your body releases the stress hormone cortisol, which initiates insulin and causes cravings, Dr. Helerstein says.

Vitamins and minerals can help put an end to PMS discomfort. Here's what researchers have learned about the nutrition connection.

Calcium: Woman's Best Friend

If you've picked up a health book or magazine lately, you know all about calcium's role in preventing osteoporosis, the brittle-bone disease that incapacitates thousands of women (and men) each year. But if scientific studies are any indication, there may be another, more immediate reason to add a calcium supplement to your medicine chest: It may relieve PMS.

In one study, researchers studied the diet of more than 3,000 women over 10 years and found that those who consumed 1,200 milligrams of calcium and 400 IU of vitamin D a day through food had up to a 40 percent less chance of experiencing PMS. And it appears that choosing the low-fat

Food Factors

How you feel in the days before your period depends at least in part on what you eat and drink all month long.

Don't turn to the bottle. Resist the temptation to unwind with a cocktail. While it has been said that severe PMS drives some women to drink, research suggests that drinking is more than a reaction to monthly discomfort. Studies show that women who consume 10 drinks or more per week over the course of a month are more likely to have premenstrual symptoms than lighter drinkers or teetotalers.

Don't be so refined. If you experience PMS every month like clockwork, it's possible you're just too refined, at least as far as your diet is concerned. Some studies show that women who get PMS eat more refined sugar and carbohydrates, such as breads, cakes, pastas, and other starchy foods made of white flour.

In general, these types of foods are low in vitamins, minerals, and fiber, says Carol Forman Helerstein, PhD, a licensed clinical nutritionist in private practice on Long Island in New York. Getting most of your calories from them means you're losing out on essential nutrients. Replacing refined foods with their heartier cousins, such as whole-grain breads and cereals and naturally sweet fresh fruits, will result in a more nutrient-dense diet and possibly fewer premenstrual symptoms, she says.

Kick the can. The cola can, that is. While the caffeine in your coffee, tea, or soda doesn't cause PMS, it can aggravate symptoms in some women, Dr. Helerstein says.

Go easy on sugar and salt. This can be difficult when you're craving chocolate and potato chips, but giving in to your cravings can create a vicious cycle, Dr. Helerstein says. Sugar affects the way your body uses the hormone insulin, and any excess can create sharp fluctuations in your blood sugar levels. These fluctuations can lead to increased appetite, fatigue, dizziness, and more cravings. And both sugary and salty foods can aggravate monthly water retention, according to Dr. Helerstein.

Love those veggies. Studies have found that women in the United States have more PMS than women in Asia. Some doctors believe it's because Asian women eat a smaller amount of animal protein and more vegetable protein than American women. But Dr. Helerstein says that women in the United States may have more PMS because the meat supply has hormones and other unhealthy additives that change body chemistry. "Animal protein in and of itself may not be the culprit," she says.

You may find relief from PMS by limiting the meats and other animal products that you eat or by eliminating these foods altogether. Women who eat a vegetarian diet tend to have milder or no PMS symptoms, Dr. Helerstein says.

versions of high-calcium foods made a difference. Women who drank 2 percent milk or lower had fewer symptoms than women who drank whole milk.

This study didn't find a benefit from calcium supplements, but another study by researchers at Columbia University in New York City did. They found that women who supplemented 1,200 milligrams of calcium a day reported a 48 percent decline in PMS symptoms.

It isn't clear exactly why calcium relieves PMS, but researchers suspect that it eases the muscular contractions that lead to cramping.

And those aren't the only studies to find a connection between calcium and PMS. A small study at the USDA Grand Forks Human Nutrition Research Center in North Dakota found an intriguing connection between a diet low in both calcium and the trace mineral manganese and PMS. Women who experienced PMS on a low-calcium, low-manganese diet had fewer symptoms when their diet was supplemented with the two minerals.

What's interesting is that the diet that produced the worst premenstrual symptoms is actually closest to the way most American women eat. Studies show that most women get about 587 milligrams of calcium a day, nowhere near the 1,000 milligrams they're supposed to get to build healthy bones and prevent osteoporosis.

Manganese intake among American women is only about 2.2 milligrams a day. That's a little more than the Daily Value for this mineral.

While researchers continue studying the connection between calcium and manganese and PMS, a daily supplement that includes both minerals can't hurt and might help if you're prone to PMS. Check to see if your multivitamin/mineral formula provides 2 to 5 milligrams of manganese. As for calcium, doctors recommend getting at least 1,000 milligrams from three to four servings of calcium-rich foods such as low-fat yogurt and milk. If that is difficult, consider taking 500 to 1,000 milligrams of supplemental calcium a day.

Mellow Out with Magnesium

Magnesium is another mineral that seems to have a beneficial effect on women with PMS. A few studies have found lower magnesium levels in women with PMS than in women without symptoms. Other studies suggest that increasing magnesium levels might reduce or eliminate premenstrual discomfort, especially emotional symptoms such as tension and anxiety.

Magnesium deficiency causes a shortage of dopamine, a chemical found in the brain that regulates mood, according to Dr. Helerstein. This shortage may have something to do with the premenstrual tension and irritability that many women experience.

In one study, researchers gave women 250 milligrams of magnesium for 3 months and scored their PMS symptoms. The women reported a 35 percent drop in PMS symptoms after taking the magnesium.

The Daily Value for magnesium is 400 milligrams. The best sources of magnesium are nuts, legumes, whole grains, and green vegetables, all of the staples of a low-fat, high-fiber diet. But if your diet leans more toward white bread, white rice, meats, and dairy products, your body is probably coming up short on magnesium.

To help even things up, you may want to consider taking a magnesium supplement of 300 to 400 milligrams, Dr. Helerstein says. Taking too much can cause diarrhea, however, so you may need to adjust your dose according to how well your bowel tolerates it. If you have heart or kidney problems, be sure to talk to your doctor before taking magnesium supplements.

A daily supplement of 400 milligrams of magnesium a day may also help you retain less water and feel less bloated, and it may relieve some breast tenderness, according to the Mayo Clinic.

Vitamin E Smoothes Out Rough Edges

Doctors recommend vitamin E for PMS because it interferes with the production of hormonelike substances called prostaglandins, which cause cramps and tender breasts.

In two separate studies, a team of Baltimore scientists examined the effect of vitamin E supplements on women prone to PMS. The women received vitamin E in the form of d-alpha-tocopherol every day for two consecutive menstrual cycles. The supplement made a substantial difference in premenstrual symptoms such as mood swings, cravings, bloating, and depression.

It isn't clear why vitamin E has an effect on PMS. Some experts have suggested that it works by slowing the production of prostaglandins.

Because vitamin E is fat soluble and stays in the liver for a long time,

Prescriptions for Healing

Getting the right nutrients can make a big difference in whether you suffer monthly symptoms of premenstrual syndrome. Here's what some experts recommend.

Nutrient	Daily Amount
Calcium	500–1,000 milligrams
DIM	100–200 milligrams
Magnesium	300–400 milligrams
Manganese	2–5 milligrams
Vitamin B₆	150–200 milligrams
Vitamin E	400 IU (d-alpha-tocopherol)

MEDICAL ALERT: If you have heart or kidney problems, you should talk to your doctor before taking magnesium supplements.

High doses of vitamin B₆ can cause side effects and should be used only under the supervision of your doctor.

If you are taking anticoagulant drugs, you should not take vitamin E supplements. (Though generally a dose of up to 1,500 IU of vitamin E a day is considered safe, some recent reports suggest that taking more than 400 IU a day could be harmful to people with cardiovascular or circulatory disease or with cancer. If you have such a condition, be sure to consult your doctor before you begin supplementation.)

there's been some concern by researchers about whether or not taking a vitamin E supplement is safe. But as long as you don't take too much, vitamin E is a "superb antioxidant," Dr. Helerstein says. "Vitamin E influences inflammatory pathways, stops oxidative stress, and decreases DNA damage," she says. "It's a very, very important nutrient." The upper tolerable intake level for vitamin E, set by the Institute of Medicine, is 1,500 IU.

If you'd like to try vitamin E for PMS, experts generally advise a dosage of 400 IU daily. The d-alpha-tocopherol form of vitamin E used in the study is readily available; just check the label before you buy. (Other forms of the vitamin haven't been studied for PMS.)

Beat PMS with B₆

Finally, if you're bothered by premenstrual weight gain and emotional symptoms, vitamin B_6 can help control them. In a study of 25 women with PMS, a high-dose supplement of B_6 reduced premenstrual weight gain and lessened the severity of other premenstrual symptoms.

The women in the study were given high doses of vitamin B_6: 500 milligrams a day for 3 months. (The Daily Value is only 2 milligrams.) B_6 at this level eases PMS by changing blood levels of two female hormones, estrogen and progesterone. But high doses of the vitamin can be dangerous and may even cause neuropathy, so high-dose supplementation should be used only under the supervision of your doctor.

If you'd like to try vitamin B_6 for premenstrual symptoms, Dr. Helerstein recommends taking it as part of a B-complex supplement. It's important to balance it with other B vitamins because it may cause deficiencies of other nutrients.

And if you're taking B_6, also make sure you're getting enough magnesium. A good guideline is to take twice as much magnesium as vitamin B_6, Dr. Helerstein says. So if you're taking 150 to 200 milligrams of B_6, take 300 to 400 milligrams of magnesium.

The Best Vegetables in a Pill

Cruciferous vegetables such as broccoli, cauliflower, and cabbage contain a compound called diindolylmethane, or DIM, that works on the liver to promote a positive effect on the metabolism of estrogen.

Taking DIM as a supplement every day helps to detoxify the bad estrogens in your body and lessen symptoms of PMS, such as breast tenderness, Dr. Helerstein says.

Cruciferous vegetables are also touted for their ability to help prevent breast, cervical, prostate, and uterine cancers. They contain compounds that kill carcinogens before they can damage DNA and prevent cells from turning cancerous. Some products in the vegetables work specifically on estrogen to prevent hormone-sensitive cancer. The National Cancer Institute recommends five to nine servings of vegetables a day to help prevent cancer, but it hasn't put a recommendation on cruciferous vegetables.

If, like most Americans, you're not getting enough servings of vegetables a day, you may want to consider taking a DIM supplement. "DIM is very protective and very helpful for all women," Dr. Helerstein says. If you'd like to take a DIM supplement for PMS symptoms, the recommended dose is 100 to 200 milligrams a day.

PROSTATE PROBLEMS

DEALING WITH A COMMON CONDITION

For most men, it seems as inevitable as gray hair and wrinkles. At first you notice a little hesitancy when trying to start the flow of urine. Your urine stream may be weak or intermittent. You find yourself getting up at night to urinate, or you feel like your bladder is still partly full after you've gone. These are all signs of benign prostatic hyperplasia (BPH), an enlargement of the prostate gland.

Statistics suggest that BPH is hard to avoid. More than half of all men over age 50 have significant prostate enlargement, and the rest have at least some. Simply getting older seems to be the main risk factor.

"The vast majority of men have some degree of prostate involvement as they age," says Sam Sugar, MD, a physician at the Pritikin Longevity Center and Spa in Aventura, Florida. "It's a consequence of aging that's almost unique to the human species."

Enlargement does not inevitably lead to drugs or surgery, however. The best way to attack the problem early is by getting routine prostate exams every year after age 55, Dr. Sugar says. And some doctors contend that it's possible to slow enlargement enough to avoid surgery and drugs, especially if you take the right steps at the first signs of problems. The steps they recommend include dietary changes, herbs, and nutritional therapy.

Small Gland, Big Problems

While most men may think of the prostate as nothing but trouble, the truth is that this chestnut-size gland does serve a useful purpose. Located just below the bladder, the prostate encircles the urethra, the tube that passes urine from the bladder to outside the body. The prostate produces semen and secretes it into the urethra, providing the liquid medium that sperm cells need for nourishment as well as to exit the body.

Prostate enlargement problems occur when the cells in the inner core of the gland, surrounding the urethra, grow to form fibrous nodules, eventually squeezing in on the urethra and blocking the flow of urine. The cells apparently grow in response to hormones, especially testosterone, and the growth seen in older men may be related to alterations in hormone balance associated with aging, experts say.

Nutritional intervention for BPH includes a healthy low-fat, high-fiber diet, weight loss if necessary, vitamin and mineral supplements, and, in some cases, essential fatty acids such as flaxseed oil. Some doctors also consider the herb saw palmetto an essential part of treatment.

Research findings are disappointingly slim when it comes to nutrition and BPH, however. Here's what studies show.

Food Factors

More than any vitamin or mineral, fat may influence prostate health, say the experts. Here are some dietary changes that they recommend.

Lose that gut. Men with 43-inch waists or greater are 50 percent more likely than normal-weight men to report symptoms of prostate enlargement or to have surgery for this condition, Harvard University researchers report. Losing about 7 inches of waistline, about 35 pounds in most cases, could be a method of treating and preventing prostate enlargement, they say.

The best way to shake this stubborn fat? Eliminate alcohol and cut way back on sugar and dietary fat. At the same time, burn calories by walking, biking, swimming, or running.

Trim the fat. A lean diet may be the best way yet to slash your risk of prostate cancer, experts say. Avoid saturated and hydrogenated fats (hard at room temperature) and stick to monounsaturated fats (olive oil or canola oil) for cooking.

Sam Sugar, MD, a physician at the Pritikin Longevity Center and Spa in Aventura, Florida, recommends minimizing red meat in your diet as much as you can. "We prefer that it's not present at all," he says. Instead, eat fish, chicken, and vegetable protein.

Flush it. Drinking plenty of fluids—2 to 3 quarts of water every day— helps prevent the bladder infections, cystitis, and kidney problems sometimes associated with an enlarged prostate, doctors say.

Zinc May Shrink Enlarged Gland

Zinc is highly concentrated in the prostate gland, but many doctors think zinc deficiency has little, if anything, to do with prostate enlargement. Some doctors, however, do recommend zinc for BPH, and with some apparent success. And there is a bit of scientific evidence supporting its use.

One doctor, Irving Bush, MD, professor of urology at the University of Health Sciences/Chicago Medical School; senior consultant at the Center for Study of Genitourinary Diseases in West Dundee, Illinois; and former chair of FDA panels on gastroenterology, urology, and dialysis, did a small study of the use of zinc in treating BPH. The men in the study took 150 milligrams of zinc sulfate every day for 2 months, followed by 50 to 100 milligrams a day as a maintenance dose. Dr. Bush found that 14 of the 19 men experienced shrinkage of the prostate.

And researchers at the University of Edinburgh Medical School in Scotland found that in test tube experiments using prostate tissue, high doses

Fiber up. A high-fiber diet helps reduce your risk of prostate cancer by slightly lowering your body's levels of reproductive hormones. In population studies, men who eat the most fiber from beans, whole grains, fruits, and vegetables are least likely to develop prostate cancer.

Go fishing. Adding omega-3 fatty acids to your diet may help you reduce your risk of prostate cancer. Studies have found that men who eat fish more than three times a week have a lower risk, and a population-based study of more than 6,000 men over 30 years found that not making fish a part of your diet increases your risk of prostate cancer by two or three times.

Get the right fats from flaxseed. The plant source of omega-3 fatty acids, flaxseed oil, is also a healthy addition to your diet. Flaxseed oil contains lignans, which are naturally occurring plant hormones that come from the hull of flaxseeds, Dr. Sugar says. In theory, the estrogenic effects of the lignans oppose the action of testosterone and keep the prostate healthy. "It's hard to measure the results, but it's a wonderful thing to take anyway," he says, since flaxseed oil is good for your health in many ways, including reducing constipation.

Experts recommend taking 1 tablespoon of flaxseed oil a day. Make sure you buy freshly ground flaxseeds because the lignans will oxidize and become worthless over time, Dr. Sugar says.

of zinc inhibited the activity of 5-alpha-reductase, the enzyme that converts testosterone to its more powerful cousin, dihydrotestosterone.

"Stimulation of the prostate gland by dihydrotestosterone contributes to its growth, so reducing levels of this hormone should lead to a reduction of prostate size," says Fouad Habib, PhD, a cell biologist at the University of Edinburgh Medical School.

Other studies have shown that the high levels of zinc in pumpkin seeds help shrink an enlarged prostate.

Unfortunately, zinc hasn't been tested in men with BPH in any large scientific studies, and until it is, most doctors will remain skeptical.

It's important to work with a doctor knowledgeable in nutrition if you want to try zinc for prostate problems, experts say. Normal amounts of zinc, up to 20 milligrams a day, have no effect on prostate enlargement, Dr. Habib says.

On the other hand, too much zinc is just plain toxic. Researchers are finding that more than 100 milligrams of zinc a day can lead to prostate cancer. In a study of 47,000 men, the National Cancer Institute found that those taking more than 100 milligrams of zinc a day had double the risk of developing advanced prostate cancer, compared with men who didn't take zinc. And other experts suggest not taking more than 15 milligrams daily without medical supervision. Too much zinc can cause anemia and immunity problems.

Lycopene Lends Protection

Scientists have known about the link between lycopene, a powerful antioxidant found in red tomatoes and watermelon, and lower risk of prostate cancer for years. Epidemiological studies show the higher the lycopene intake, the lower the risk for prostate cancer, says Omer Kucuk, MD, professor of oncology and medicine at the Karmanos Cancer Institute and Wayne State University, both located in Detroit, and a leading researcher on prostate cancer.

Nobody knows exactly how lycopene affects the prostate, but lycopene works as an antioxidant in our blood, fighting oxidative stress and free radicals. "We need [antioxidants] to block damaging effects of oxidative stress," Dr. Kucuk says. "Lycopene is a potent antioxidant—better than vitamin E."

Research shows that the best protection against prostate cancer comes from eating food high in lycopene, such as fresh tomatoes, tomato juice, tomato paste, and watermelon. When researchers used a lycopene compound alone to inhibit cancer cell growth, they saw weaker results than if they combined the lycopene with another compound found in tomatoes, such as beta-carotene, Dr. Kucuk says. That's because when you eat a tomato, you're

Prescriptions for Healing

Some doctors recommend a veritable smorgasbord of nutrients to treat benign prostatic hyperplasia (BPH). Solid scientific evidence that these nutrients help is sadly lacking, but some doctors say that they see a difference in men who take them. Here's what is often recommended.

Nutrient	Daily Amount
Flaxseed oil	1 tablespoon a day
Saw palmetto	320 milligrams, twice a day
Zinc	150 milligrams for 2 months under a doctor's supervision

MEDICAL ALERT: *If you have symptoms of BPH, you should see your doctor for proper diagnosis and treatment.*

Zinc in doses exceeding 15 milligrams daily should be taken only under medical supervision.

ingesting many other compounds that have positive effects on your health, such as carotenoids, vitamin C, and others.

Unfortunately, the intake of lycopene in the United States pales in comparison to other places in the world, such as the Mediterranean. Researchers haven't pinpointed exactly how much lycopene men should eat to get the benefits, but Dr. Kucuk says aiming for five servings of fruits and vegetables a day is a good rule of thumb to live by.

An Herb That Helps

Saw palmetto may be one of the most important supplements for prostate health, Dr. Sugar says. Studies have shown that it's as effective as the prescription drug finasteride in treating BPH, but without the side effects, such as decreased sexual function.

German researchers saw an improvement in nighttime urination, one of the most common symptoms of an enlarged prostate, and better urinary flow when they gave patients saw palmetto over 3 years. However, studies have been mixed. Another study in the *New England Journal of Medicine* failed to confirm these results.

A standardized extract of the herb appears to be more effective than a tea or tincture. Doctors recommend taking 320 milligrams of saw palmetto twice a day from an extract standardized to contain 80 to 90 percent fatty acids.

Other Nutrients Round Out the Program

Zinc isn't the only nutrient that doctors use to treat BPH. Some doctors use a smorgasbord of supplements that include vitamin A, beta-carotene, vitamin E, vitamin C, and selenium. All of these have been associated with reduced risk of cancer. Other supplements that are sometimes prescribed are magnesium and vitamin B_6.

If you would like to try a nutritional program along these lines, you should discuss it with your doctor.

PSORIASIS

PRESCRIPTION VITAMIN D DELIVERS HOPE

For years, experts and people with psoriasis scratched their heads (not to mention other body parts) in despair over medical science's inability to fight this troubling skin disease. Then groundbreaking research by Michael F. Holick, MD, PhD, professor in the section of endocrinology, diabetes, nutrition, and weight management and director of the General Clinical Research Center at Boston University Medical Center, unleashed the dramatic healing power of vitamin D and revealed just how to make it work against psoriasis.

A Plague Called Plaques

Vibrant, healthy skin seems to just happen for some people. Like clockwork, they shed skin cells in the form of minute, invisible flakes while new cells push to the surface in a 15-stage cycle that is as natural as it is uneventful. And every 28 to 30 days, they're clad in a completely new suit of skin.

Not so for people with psoriasis. It's as if parts of the skin-renewing cycle were put on fast-forward—really fast-forward. Within 4 to 5 days, the affected patches of skin, called plaques, undergo just five changes before they pile up like the Sunday paper. The result: red, itchy, scaly plaques that often cover the knees, elbows, and scalp.

Nor does psoriasis stop at the surface. "It ranges from localized mild patches on the skin to a totally disabling total body disease," says Joel Schlessinger, MD, a dermatologist in private practice in Omaha, Nebraska, and president of the American Society of Cosmetic Dermatology and Aesthetic Surgery. About 25 percent of the 4 to 5 million psoriasis cases in the United States are so bad that people are completely disabled, often with a crippling form of arthritis.

While experts say that such prolific skin shedding is caused by some as-yet-unknown genetic problem, things such as stress, infections, cuts, scrapes, certain medications (quinine, beta-blockers, and lithium, among others), and alcohol can also spark flare-ups. "While psoriasis is an inherited disease, a whole series of other events can bring out the disease in a person who is genetically predisposed," says Dr. Schlessinger.

Defeating Psoriasis with Vitamin D

Added to milk and other dairy products, vitamin D has long been known as the cure for rickets, a disease that causes bone deformity and stunted growth in children.

Special receptors in your skin also make use of sunlight-produced vitamin D, a fact that has led some to try tanning in an attempt to end their psoriasis. In fact, nude sunbathing at the Dead Sea in Israel has become such a popular treatment for psoriasis that the *Wall Street Journal* suggested the influx (about 10,000 visitors a year and growing!) is creating a modern mecca for psoriasis treatment. It's the host to psoriasis treatment centers, and studies have found that about 80 to 90 percent of psoriasis patients who visit the Dead Sea clear or significantly improve their symptoms. However, results take about 4 weeks.

Why the Dead Sea? At 1,200 feet below sea level, the Dead Sea is the lowest point on the earth's surface. The location's low elevation prevents the sun's harshest rays from reaching sunbathers, allowing them to stay out longer without burning, experts say. The Dead Sea's mineral-rich water, so salty that plants and fish can't survive, is also thought to help psoriasis.

Researchers exploring the role of vitamin D receptors in the skin have found a way to help people with psoriasis. Dr. Holick discovered that skin cells have receptors for what is called activated vitamin D, essentially the hormone that prevents skin cells from growing and shedding too rapidly.

The next step was to develop a superpotent yet nontoxic form of activated vitamin D, strong enough to slow the growth of psoriatic skin cells. "We wanted to take advantage of the observation that we had made, using a high enough concentration to alter the growth of the skin cells without harm," Dr. Holick explains. The result was a product called Dovonex, which is widely

Fishing for a Cure

Some experts think that there's something fishy about treating psoriasis with fish oil. Only one in four controlled studies find a benefit of omega-3 fatty acids for psoriasis compared with a placebo (an inactive pill). But at least one study, done several years ago, showed that the fatty acids found in fish may be beneficial after all.

In a Finnish study, 80 people with psoriasis took two capsules containing fatty acids from fish three times a day for 8 weeks. At the end of the study, seven people were completely healed, and 13 reported 75 percent healing. Those who showed the best results in the study had the least severe cases, the researchers noted.

"It's neither the best treatment for psoriasis nor the only treatment that people should use, but it may be of some benefit," says Dr. Holick.

Thirty-four of the people included in this Finnish study also had psoriatic arthritis, a form of arthritis related to psoriasis. All 34 reported less severe joint pain after taking the capsules. Fatty acids from fish apparently act as an anti-inflammatory, and that action is particularly effective in some cases of psoriatic arthritis that involve considerable inflammation, says Dr. Holick.

A study in The Lancet found that when psoriasis patients took 10 fish oil capsules every day for 8 weeks, they saw a significant improvement in symptoms such as itching, redness, and scaling. Those in the placebo group, who took the same amount of olive oil capsules, didn't see an improvement.

Fish oil seems to work because it alters the reaction of the immune system, and psoriasis is an autoimmune response. MaxEPA fish oil supplements, which are sold over the counter, were the supplements used in the Lancet study that showed benefits, according to the National Psoriasis Foundation.

Atlantic herring and pink salmon are among the fish highest in helpful fatty acids. Unfortunately, you'd have to eat between 1 and 2 pounds a day to get close to the dose of fish oil that the volunteers took during the study. So you might want to ask your doctor about taking fish oil capsules to help combat psoriasis.

Food Factors

These dietary tips may help you keep your psoriasis at bay.

Ban the booze. Alcohol and psoriasis apparently go together like martinis and olives. Researchers looked at 818 psoriasis patients in Italy and found that drinking 2 or more glasses of alcohol a day made the study participants twice as likely to have more severe psoriasis.

Give acid the slip. One small study showed a reduction of psoriasis symptoms among people who avoided acidic foods such as coffee, tomatoes, soda, and pineapple. If you discover that certain foods cause you problems, listen to your body and avoid them, says Michael F. Holick, MD, PhD, professor in the section of endocrinology, diabetes, nutrition, and weight management and director of the General Clinical Research Center at Boston University Medical Center.

Bring on the veggies. Could eating less protein help tame your psoriasis? Some reports have suggested improvement in symptoms when people with psoriasis ate a vegetarian diet low in protein for several weeks.

used as a first-line treatment for psoriasis and is available only by prescription.

Applied to the skin as an ointment, Dovonex not only slows skin cell growth to levels much closer to normal but also reduces itching and inflammation, says Dr. Holick. "Among those who use Dovonex topically, upward of 50 to 60 percent have seen significant improvement," he says. Such improvement usually begins to appear in 2 to 3 weeks. However, there are people who have developed a resistance to Dovonex and need a topical steroid along with the drug, which helps rejuvenate and maintain steroid-damaged skin.

Wouldn't megadoses of over-the-counter vitamin D have the same positive effect on psoriasis? Not at all, says Dr. Holick. "The reason is that the body is very particular about the amount of vitamin D that it takes in. It will not make any more activated vitamin D (1,25-dihydroxy vitamin D_3), regardless of how much of the vitamin you take. You can become vitamin D-intoxicated, but you won't be able to treat your psoriasis," says Dr. Holick.

Virtues of Vitamin A

Although it's reserved for more severe cases, a superpotent form of vitamin A called acetretin (Soriatane) is also available for the treatment of psoriasis, but only by prescription.

Prescriptions for Healing

Ask your doctor about Dovonex, a prescription topical form of superpotent vitamin D, and etretinate (Tegison), a prescription oral form of superpotent vitamin A.

Many doctors also recommend a multivitamin/mineral supplement containing the Daily Values of folic acid and iron.

Taken orally, activated vitamin A helps skin cells grow to maturity before shedding. Unfortunately, it also has some severe side effects, including serious birth defects in women who are pregnant, dry mouth, and hair loss. Women shouldn't take the drug if there's a possibility they could be pregnant or could become pregnant.

In some cases, Dr. Schlessinger uses both acetretin and 6 grams of omega-3 fatty acids, which are found in fish oil, to limit any side effects. "We take blood tests when we have people on these drugs, but it's usually okay to combine them," he says.

Unfortunately, taking a regular form of vitamin A won't help psoriasis at all, Dr. Schlessinger says. Don't take vitamin A with acetretin or accutane (another drug prescribed for psoriasis patients) because it can lead to dangerously high vitamin A levels.

The Case for a Multivitamin

Although no one suggests that any vitamin or mineral taken orally can cure psoriasis, there is some evidence that psoriasis itself can cause certain vitamin and mineral deficiencies.

In a study of 50 people hospitalized with psoriasis, researchers found that some were low in protein, iron, and folate (the naturally occurring form of folic acid), according to Janet Prystowsky, MD, PhD, a dermatologist in private practice in New York City.

Rapid skin cell growth and shedding deplete stores of protein, iron, and folate because psoriatic skin seems to take precedence over other parts of the body, she says. "While nutritional supplementation is not a remedy for psoriasis, it could improve the general health of a person with the disease," according to Dr. Prystowsky.

RAYNAUD'S PHENOMENON

DEFROSTING FRIGID DIGITS

Is it possible that Moses had Raynaud's phenomenon?

The Bible tells of how the Hebrew leader, high on a mountaintop, watched his hand turn snow white after he touched a rod that God had commanded him to pick up. There's no doubt that Moses was a little anxious at the time. After all, God was asking him to do something pretty scary, since the rod he picked up had been a snake only moments earlier. God then ordered Moses to stick his hand inside his shirt, where it promptly regained its normal color.

People with Raynaud's don't need to be in such a chilly and frightening situation to experience this disease's finger-blanching symptoms. Just a bit of cold or nervousness can often set them off.

Chilled to the Bone

Raynaud's is actually an extreme exaggeration of a normal response. When our hands are exposed to cold, the tiny arteries in our fingertips constrict, shunting blood to the interior of the body, where it can stay warm. When our hands sense warmth, the arteries relax, allowing normal blood flow to the fingers to resume.

In Raynaud's, however, arteries clamp down and stay clamped for the slightest reason. The muscles in the wall of the blood vessels close off blood-flow, says Edwin Smith, MD, professor of medicine at the Medical University of South Carolina in Charleston. Taking a tray of ice cubes from the refrigerator or getting tense may bring on symptoms. Fingers turn first white as blood drains out, then blue as poorly oxygenated blood pools in them. Then they flush red as oxygenated blood returns. An entire episode may take less than a minute or go on for hours. It happens to 5 to 10 percent of the population, Dr. Smith says.

The primary form of the disease comes on for no reason and tends to have a bigger effect on women between ages 15 and 40. It's also more common in areas with colder temperatures.

The secondary form of Raynaud's is a symptom of an autoimmune disease such as scleroderma, lupus, rheumatoid arthritis, cryoglobulinemia, and several other conditions, Dr. Smith says. (An autoimmune disease results when the immune system attacks the body itself rather than going after viruses and bacteria.)

Certain medications, including beta-blockers (used to treat high blood pressure) and ergot (used to treat migraines), can cause Raynaud's, Dr. Smith says. So can certain blood-clotting abnormalities. Also, an underlying condition may cause both Raynaud's and carpal tunnel syndrome, he says. So it's smart to see your doctor to figure out what is causing your symptoms. If you have Raynaud's phenomenon and you take birth control pills, your pills may make you more prone to attacks.

In the United States, nutritional therapy generally isn't used much for this disorder. Two nutrients, niacin and vitamin E, are sometimes recommended to help relieve symptoms, however. Here's how they work.

Food Factors

You'd be hard-pressed to find an Eskimo with Raynaud's phenomenon. But if you can't find whale blubber at your local supermarket, try this fishy alternative.

Have a sardine sandwich. A study by researchers at Albany Medical College in New York found that the omega-3 fatty acids concentrated in fatty fish such as salmon, mackerel, tuna, and, yes, sardines seemed to help keep blood vessels open in some people with Raynaud's phenomenon.

The same study found that symptoms stopped altogether in 5 of 11 people taking 12 fish oil capsules (a total of 3.96 grams in the form of eicosapentaenoic acid and 2.64 grams in the form of docosahexaenoic acid) daily for 2 consecutive 6-week periods. The other 6 people extended the time that they could keep their hands submerged in cold water before bloodflow to their fingers shut down from 31 to 47 minutes, an increase of 50 percent.

In a comparison group of nine people with Raynaud's taking olive oil, only one person showed any significant improvement.

Edwin Smith, MD, professor of medicine at the Medical University of South Carolina in Charleston, recommends taking 6 grams of fish oil a day, but doing so under a doctor's care.

Niacin Keeps Blood Vessels Open

One of the B-complex vitamins, niacin is well known for its talents in dilating blood vessels. Take enough of this nutrient, and you'll experience the "niacin flush," a burning, itching, reddening, tingling sensation, usually in the face, neck, arms, and upper chest, that may persist for a half hour or even longer. In fact, a slow-release form of niacin called inositol nicotinate is available overseas as a drug called Hexopal and is prescribed precisely for Raynaud's phenomenon.

Inositol nicotinate is available in this country in health food stores but can be obtained from some doctors who commonly use nutritional therapies in their practices. Look for inositol hexaniacinate, a form of inositol nicotinate that is less likely to cause flushing. (One brand name is Flush-Free Hexa-Niacin from Enzymatic Therapy.) In a number of studies, people who took this drug had fewer and shorter finger-freezing attacks.

"If you try inositol nicotinate, take 500 to 1,000 milligrams three or four times a day," suggests Mary Dan Eades, MD, author of *The Doctor's Complete Guide to Vitamins and Minerals.* "The inositol combination slows the release of the niacin."

Or you can take nicotinic acid, although it also causes flushing. Depending on your sensitivity, flushing may occur at doses as low as 50 milligrams. Dr. Eades recommends taking the lowest dose that relieves your symptoms and taking no more than 100 milligrams a day without medical supervision.

Regardless of the form in which it's taken, niacin has been known to cause liver damage in high doses. If you have liver disease, Dr. Eades feels that it's best to take no more than the Daily Value of niacin, 20 milligrams, without medical supervision.

Niacin can thaw your icy fingers, but not all doctors recommend it because of its side effects. In addition to itching and flushing, niacin may cause nausea, headaches, and intestinal cramps.

Vitamin E May Improve Bloodflow

Most doctors consider so-called case reports, in which a physician reports his or her observations of a patient who has a particular disease or is undergoing a particular treatment, a less reliable means of assessing a treatment than scientific studies. In fact, there are no studies to show the potential benefits of vitamin E for Raynaud's phenomenon. But several case reports attest to its benefits,

Prescriptions for Healing

Nutrients that preserve circulation in the tiny capillaries of the fingers are most helpful for Raynaud's phenomenon. Many doctors suggest these.

Nutrient	Daily Amount
Inositol nicotinate	1,500–4,000 milligrams, taken as 3 or 4 divided doses
Or	
Nicotinic acid	Take the lowest dose that relieves symptoms, but no more than 100 milligrams per day
Vitamin E	800 IU, taken as 2 divided doses

MEDICAL ALERT: Both inositol nicotinate and nicotinic acid are forms of niacin. Niacin has been known to cause liver damage in high doses. If you have liver disease, it's best to take no more than the Daily Value of niacin, 20 milligrams, without medical supervision.

Depending on your sensitivity, nicotinic acid may cause flushing at doses as low as 50 to 75 milligrams. Doctors recommend staying at the lowest dose that relieves your symptoms and going no higher than 100 milligrams a day without medical supervision.

If you are taking anticoagulant drugs, you should not take vitamin E supplements. (Though generally a dose of up to 1,500 IU of vitamin E a day is considered safe, some recent reports suggest that taking more than 400 IU a day could be harmful to people with cardiovascular or circulatory disease or with cancer. If you have such a condition, be sure to consult your doctor before you begin supplementation.)

and one report in particular stands out because of the dramatic results obtained.

The report, by Samuel Ayres Jr., MD, a Los Angeles dermatologist, told of a 45-year-old man who for 6 months had had worsening ulcers and gangrene on the tips of his fingers. Dr. Ayres prescribed 400 IU of vitamin E twice a day, along with vitamin E applied to the fingertips. Within 8 weeks, the man's fingers had completely healed, and they remained healed 1 year later on a maintenance dose of vitamin E. Dr. Ayres says that he has treated an additional 20 people in his practice who had circulation problems in their hands, the majority of whom have benefited from taking vitamin E supplements.

"Vitamin E could be helpful for a number of reasons," Dr. Eades says. "It may improve blood flow through tiny capillaries by reducing the tendency for cells to stick to the sides of blood vessel walls and to each other. Plus it may speed the healing of and reduce the scarring from ulcers, which are sometimes associated with Raynaud's disease."

Check with your doctor before taking more than 400 IU of vitamin E daily, as high doses can cause side effects in some people.

RESTLESS LEGS SYNDROME

WHEN YOUR LEGS HAVE A LIFE OF THEIR OWN

What happens when you want to sit still but your legs want to move? Diane Dobry had that feeling for years without knowing what caused it. One day she mentioned the feeling to her mother, and her mother said it sounded like restless legs syndrome. That got her interested, and she began reading about it on the Internet.

"Everything I read was exactly how I felt," Diane says. She describes it as a feeling of having electricity in her legs that makes her want to move them. Sometimes she needs to stand up and walk, run, or stomp her feet. "It feels like there's energy circulating in my calves and shins," she says. Sometimes her legs kick involuntarily. It can be a problem when she takes the train to her job as communications director for the Teacher's College at Columbia University in New York City. Sometimes on the train she stands up just to move her legs around a little bit, and there have been occasions when she runs home after getting off the train to get the energy out of her legs.

She was kicking all night long, too, but she didn't know it until she participated in a study at Columbia in which she was monitored while she slept. "They had it on video that my legs were kicking throughout the night," she says. It could explain why she woke up feeling tired in the mornings.

Something that may have made RLS worse for Diane was L-tyrosine, a supplement she was taking for depression to affect dopamine levels in the brain. Dopamine levels in the brain seem to have a connection with RLS, doctors say. But then when Diane cut back and eventually stopped taking L-tyrosine, the sensation in her legs calmed down.

Another thing that has helped: A few mornings a week Diane walks about 2 miles. It seems to help her RLS throughout the day, she says, including during the train ride to and from work.

She also noticed there's a difference in her RLS when she gets all of the nutrients she needs in her diet. When she plugged the food she was eating into an online nutrient tracker, it showed her that her diet was low in folate, something doctors believe may be related to RLS. Ever since then, she's been getting enough folate by eating Romaine lettuce, peanuts, Cheerios, Special K, and chicken broth, and her symptoms have improved. She also has noticed that her legs get an intense urge to move when she drinks alcohol.

Finding the Answers

Unfortunately, people like Diane haven't always been taken seriously when they tell others about their symptoms.

"Drug companies have been known to create diseases to sell drugs," says Mark Mahowald, MD, director of the Regional Sleep Disorders Clinic in Minneapolis. But any doctor who has patients with RLS knows that it's a very real problem. It's the most common cause of severe insomnia, he says.

And for any lingering skeptics, in 2007 researchers in Iceland identified a gene variant related to RLS.

Restless legs syndrome was previously thought to affect only 2 to 5 percent of people, but recent surveys have found that about 25 percent of the adult population report uncomfortable feelings in their legs, such as the creepy, crawling sensation associated with RLS, at least a couple of times a month. Many

---

Food Factors

Other than helping to offset iron or folate deficiency, foods don't seem to play much of a role in the development of restless legs syndrome. Pay heed, however, if you're a coffee fan.

Junk the java. In a study of 62 people with restless legs, researchers at St. Mary's Hospital in Passaic, New Jersey, found that the elimination of caffeine and other related compounds in tea, chocolate, and cola caused improvement in restless legs symptoms.

Incidentally, caffeine and other components of coffee and tea as well as sugar can rob your body of iron, folate, magnesium, and other nutrients that play roles in restless legs syndrome.

times, it goes undiagnosed. In 2005, researchers conducted a survey of more than 15,000 people in the United States and Europe. Among the 416 people who met the diagnostic criteria for RLS, 81 percent had told their doctor about their symptoms, but only 6 percent had received a diagnosis of RLS.

The Swedish neurologist Karl A. Ekbom named the condition in the 1940s (that's why RLS is sometimes called Ekbom syndrome). Although it can affect people at any age—even as infants—those with the most severe symptoms tend to be around age 50 or older. In about two-thirds of the people who have RLS, the symptoms progress over time.

No one really knows what causes restless legs. It does tend to run in families, however, and may appear as "growing pains" in children or as pregnancy-related "leg cramps." And it tends to get worse as people get older, experts say.

The disorder seems to have something to do with dopamine, a neurotransmitter in the brain that is involved in movement. Most people with RLS respond to the drug levodopa, which contains dopamine, but doctors aren't sure why. RLS doesn't seem to be related to a dopamine deficiency, Dr. Mahowald says.

But in some cases, at least two nutritional deficiencies may be related to RLS: iron and folate.

Iron Weighs In as a Factor

It was in the 1960s that Dr. Ekbom noted that about one of four people with restless legs syndrome had iron-deficiency anemia and that when these people were treated with iron for their anemia, their legs calmed down, too.

Although case reports of iron's benefits continued in the intervening decades, little research was done that would confirm these findings until researchers at Royal Liverpool University Hospital in England delved into the matter again.

They gave 35 older people with restless legs 200 milligrams of iron (ferrous sulfate) three times a day for 2 months, without telling the people that it might help their restless legs. When the people were later quizzed on their symptoms, about one-third reported substantial reductions in severity.

Those obtaining the most relief from iron supplements were people with low blood levels of ferritin, an iron-protein complex that is the main storage form of iron in the body.

Autopsies of the brains of people with restless legs syndrome clearly show a deficiency of iron in the brain. In 2003, scientists performed autopsies on the brains of seven people who had suffered from restless legs syndrome and

Prescriptions for Healing

Nutrients play roles in some cases of restless legs syndrome. Here's what experts say might help.

Nutrient	Daily Amount
Folic acid	5,000–20,000 micrograms
Iron	18 milligrams
Magnesium	400 milligrams
Vitamin E	100–400 IU

MEDICAL ALERT: *The Daily Value for folic acid is 400 micrograms. Higher doses may hide important symptoms of pernicious anemia, a vitamin B_{12} deficiency disease, so be sure to talk to your doctor before starting supplementation.*

The amount of iron recommended here is the Daily Value. Your doctor, however, should prescribe your iron dosage based on the results of a blood test that measures your blood level of ferritin.

If you have heart or kidney problems, be sure to consult your doctor before starting magnesium supplementation.

If you are taking anticoagulant drugs, you should not take vitamin E supplements. (Though generally a dose of up to 1,500 IU of vitamin E a day is considered safe, some recent reports suggest that taking more than 400 IU a day could be harmful to people with cardiovascular or circulatory disease or with cancer. If you have such a condition, be sure to consult your doctor before you begin supplementation.)

compared them with the brains of five people who hadn't had neurological problems. They found that the substantia nigra regions of the brains from the restless legs patients lacked iron, which may have made those brain cells malfunction and cause the symptoms.

That doesn't mean everyone with restless legs syndrome is deficient in iron, the study authors said. Rather, iron isn't effectively getting into the brains of people with restless legs syndrome.

If you have been diagnosed with restless legs syndrome, you should have your doctor check your blood level of ferritin. If it is low or borderline, you may benefit from iron supplements.

Experts don't know how low iron stores can lead to restless legs syndrome, but taking iron supplements may improve symptoms. The dose depends on your current iron level and could be a few hundred milligrams of ferrous sulfate a day.

Your doctor will monitor your dosage by periodically checking your blood ferritin level. Once your level is well within the normal range, a maintenance dosage can be established, or you may be able to get enough iron from iron-rich foods such as clams and fortified cereals.

Note that it's important to determine the cause of your iron deficiency and to correct it. The Daily Value for iron is 18 milligrams. Since daily intake of high amounts of iron can be harmful, don't take more than the Daily Value in supplements unless your doctor confirms the need with a blood test.

Folic Acid May Aid Some

While you're having your blood checked for iron deficiency, it might be worthwhile to have your doctor check your blood level of another nutrient: folate, a B vitamin that is essential for normal nerve function. Deficiency of this nutrient appears to be associated with restless legs problems in a small percentage of people.

Some studies have found that women who are pregnant and deficient in folic acid will develop restless legs syndrome, while increasing their intake of folic acid eases their pain and discomfort. It's also particularly important for pregnant women to make sure they're getting enough folic acid because too little may increase the risk for neural tube defects.

Your doctor can determine if you're coming up short in this essential nutrient by measuring folate levels in your red blood cells, which is a more accurate way to determine your real status than simply measuring blood levels.

There is no established dosage of folic acid to treat restless legs, so your doctor is likely to prescribe an amount that corrects your deficiency. Some doctors have given up to 20,000 micrograms a day, but most stick to 5,000 to 7,000 micrograms a day.

Since the Daily Value for folic acid is only 400 micrograms, you should talk to your doctor before taking a higher amount. High doses of folic acid can mask the symptoms of pernicious anemia, a condition caused by a deficiency of vitamin B_{12}. For this reason, your doctor should also check your blood for B_{12} deficiency and provide a supplement if necessary.

Vitamin E: Popular but Unproven

Although there are a few reports from doctors that vitamin E in doses of 100 to 400 IU daily has helped this condition, no large studies have been done to confirm its effectiveness. A small study of nine people did find that vitamin E helped to ease symptoms, but doctors who treat this condition don't tend to recommend vitamin E.

If you decide to take vitamin E supplements, don't neglect other, possibly more helpful treatments for this condition.

A Case of Mistaken Identity

It's possible that what you and your doctor think is restless legs is instead severe leg cramps. While leg cramps are muscle contractions, the striking feature of RLS is that patients have a difficult time describing the discomfort they're feeling, Dr. Mahowald says. They rarely say it's painful, he says. Rather, people say they have "fidgety legs" or they feel a crawling sensation in their legs, particularly when they lie down to sleep. The feeling goes away as soon as they get up and walk around but comes back once they get back into bed.

If you think you are experiencing leg cramps, it might be helpful for you to make sure that you are getting the Daily Values of calcium, magnesium, and potassium (and sodium, too, if you've been on a very restrictive diet). These minerals all play roles in muscle contraction and relaxation. Deficiency of any one can lead to muscle cramps. (If you have heart or kidney problems or diabetes, be sure to check with your doctor before taking magnesium or potassium supplements.) For the full details on using nutrients to deal with leg cramps, see page 355.

One study, from Romania, suggests that magnesium supplements can also help bona fide restless legs. So it might be worth your while to make sure you're getting the Daily Value of this mineral, which is 400 milligrams. Most people fall short of that amount.

RHEUMATOID ARTHRITIS

COOLING DOWN THE
INFLAMMATION

Even though there are doctors who specialize in the disease (they're called rheumatologists), rheumatoid arthritis remains something of a medical mystery. No one knows exactly what causes it, and no one knows why the disease seems to come and go. No one knows why some people get it so badly that they are permanently crippled or why a few lucky people have a single flare-up and never again have symptoms.

"There's a lot we still have to learn about this disease," admits Robert McLean, MD, associate clinical professor of medicine at the Yale University School of Medicine and an internist in New Haven, Connecticut.

In a person with rheumatoid arthritis, the body's own infection-fighting immune cells attack joint tissue and cause inflammation, with pain, redness, heat, and swelling. The inflammation doesn't always confine itself to joints; sometimes other organs, such as the skin, heart, and lungs, can be affected.

Rheumatoid arthritis is usually treated by simply suppressing symptoms. Doctors prescribe anti-inflammatory drugs such as aspirin or ibuprofen. For severe cases, they may recommend steroid drugs, which dampen the body's immune response and so reduce inflammation. They may recommend other medications that modulate the immune system in different ways, including cancer chemotherapy drugs such as methotrexate (Folex), azathioprine (Imuran), and cyclophosphamide (Cytoxan).

These drugs do reduce pain and swelling, but at a price. Most have side effects, from stomach upset to bone loss and reduced resistance to infection.

Medications are the first line of defense among doctors to treat rheumatoid arthritis, but studies show that nutrition does appear to have an impact on symptoms. The Arthritis Foundation admits that food sensitivities may trigger symptoms and that your overall health, which is highly dependent on diet, may affect how your body handles symptoms.

Food Factors

The strongest evidence to date that diet has anything to do with rheumatoid arthritis comes from studies of omega-3 fatty acids.

Make fish your dish. Mackerel, salmon, and tuna all contain omega-3 fatty acids, which are known to be anti-inflammatory. At least six studies have shown that diets rich in these fatty acids help reduce the pain and stiffness of rheumatoid arthritis and the biochemical signs of inflammation.

Evidence so far suggests that about 6 grams of these fatty acids a day seems to have an anti-inflammatory effect. If you're not taking fish oil capsules, try eating two or three meals of fatty fish each week. It might be up to 4 months before you notice any improvement in your condition.

Some doctors recommend plain old cod liver oil, in doses of up to 3 tablespoons (9 teaspoons) a day. In fact, there's some evidence that it reduces pain and swelling.

Even though cod liver oil has been used over the years with apparent safety, it is possible to get too much of a good thing. That's because unlike omega-3 fatty acids, cod liver oil contains hefty amounts of vitamins A and D. Although it's important to get the Daily Values of both of these nutrients, more than 15,000 IU of vitamin A (three times the Daily Value) or 2,000 IU of vitamin D (more than three times the Daily Value) can be toxic if taken over a long period of time, even if taken in foods. In addition, research has found that vitamin A can cause birth defects when taken in doses of 10,000 IU during early pregnancy.

So don't mix cod liver oil with supplements, even in modest doses, without knowledgeable medical supervision, especially if you are a woman who is pregnant or of childbearing age. And stop your regimen if you develop headaches, nausea, or vomiting.

Cut back on other fats. Doctors who prescribe fish oil say that this oil works better to relieve pain and stiffness when it's used along with a diet low in animal fats.

That makes sense, since fats compete with each other for use in the body's production of biochemicals called prostaglandins. When the body selects fish oil, as it does when fish oil molecules are abundant, the prostaglandins produced are anti-inflammatory. When the body chooses arachidonic acid from animal fats, the prostaglandins produced are pro-inflammatory.

Cut back on fats by going easy on meats (especially lunchmeats), whole-fat dairy products (such as ice cream, cheeses, and butter), mayonnaise, baked goods, and salad dressings.

Pinpoint possible trouble foods. Most doctors believe that only a small percentage of people with inflammatory arthritis have symptoms that are aggravated by foods. But many nutrition-oriented doctors believe that more people than previously suspected have food-related arthritis symptoms and that everyone with arthritis should at least try an elimination diet to detect trouble foods.

"Research is looking at the possibility that some people develop antibodies (a normally protective immune system reaction to invasion) against proteins they eat and that those antibodies then go on to attack similar proteins in the body," says Robert McLean, MD, associate clinical professor of medicine at Yale University School of Medicine and an internist in New Haven, Connecticut. "So the idea of food-related arthritis is not so far out as it once seemed."

You may want to keep a food diary for a few weeks to see if certain foods seem to be contributing to your symptoms. "One quick way to figure out if foods are part of your problem is to put yourself on a weeklong program of eating foods that you don't normally eat or to go on a juice fast," says Jonathan Wright, MD, medical director of the Tahoma Clinic in Renton, Washington, and author of *Dr. Wright's Guide to Healing with Nutrition.* If you improve during this time, then you'll need to slowly reintroduce foods to see if your symptoms flare.

Almost any food may cause problems, but milk, wheat, sugar, corn, and soy appear to be common triggers. Some people also seem to have trouble with tomatoes, potatoes, eggplant, paprika, green and red bell peppers, and chili peppers, all members of the nightshade family.

However, there are no good scientific studies that implicate any particular food substance or family as more or less likely to contribute to an aggravation of any autoimmune-mediated arthritis, including rheumatoid arthritis. "For that reason, I do not suggest that my patients go on an extensive elimination diet looking for the magical culprit, when it is very unlikely to exist," Dr. McLean says.

Cut back on caffeine. Four or more cups of coffee a day may increase your risk of developing rheumatoid arthritis, so keep caffeine intake to a minimum.

Nutritional Backup for Treatment

Doctors who prescribe nutritional therapy take these tactics: They eliminate foods from the diet that may aggravate rheumatoid arthritis; they add anti-inflammatory fats such as fish oil; and they provide optimum amounts of nutrients, including those nutrients thought to help reduce inflammation and other vitamins and minerals needed for general good health. It's an approach based on the simple premise that people who have a chronic disease such as this need extra amounts of certain nutrients to help their bodies fight the disease.

People with rheumatoid arthritis have been found to be low in a number of nutrients. One study by Finnish researchers, for instance, found that people with low blood levels of vitamin E, beta-carotene, and selenium (a mineral with anti-inflammatory properties) had more than eight times the risk of developing rheumatoid arthritis compared with people with high levels of these nutrients.

In another study, researchers compared the diets of people with rheumatoid arthritis against people without the disease and found that those with arthritis consumed significantly lower amounts of vitamin A and beta-carotene in their diets.

Doctors who specialize in nutritional therapy use an array of nutrients to fight rheumatoid arthritis.

"I find that a broad approach is best," says Joseph Pizzorno Jr., ND, president emeritus of Bastyr University in Seattle. "People won't necessarily be cured of their arthritis, but they will get enough relief to be able to cut back on their medications, and they are often willing to put up with a bit of discomfort in exchange for fewer side effects from drugs."

Here, then, is what doctors who practice nutritional therapy recommend.

Quench the Flames with Vitamin C

When it comes to rheumatoid arthritis or other conditions that involve inflammation, nutrition-oriented doctors almost always include vitamin C in their prescriptions. Because inflammation is mediated by free radicals, if you get rid of free radicals with antioxidants like vitamin C, you can get rid of the inflammation.

Free radicals are molecular bad guys that grab electrons from your body's healthy molecules. This electron stealing harms cells. Free radicals congregate in gangs in rheumatic joints because immune cells generate free radicals in their attack on joint tissue. Vitamin C and other antioxidants disarm free radicals by offering their own electrons and so spare cells.

In 2004, researchers studied the diets of 23,000 people who entered a large cancer study in the United Kingdom. Between 1993 and 2001, 73 people in the study developed polyarthritis, which means they experienced rheumatoid arthritis in two or more joints for at least 4 weeks. After examining their diet, the researchers discovered that patients who had developed rheumatoid arthritis had lower intakes of fruits and vegetables, particularly vitamin C. In fact, patients who had the lowest amount of vitamin C had three times the risk of developing rheumatoid arthritis in two or more joints, the study found.

Doctors recommend different amounts of vitamin C, but most call for at least 600 milligrams a day. Some suggest taking as much ascorbic acid (another name for vitamin C) as an individual can tolerate without developing diarrhea and gas. That may be up to 60,000 milligrams a day, which is well above the Daily Value of 60 milligrams.

Drinking a solution of powdered ascorbic acid mixed with water is the most economical way to take vitamin C. Just be sure to drink the mixture through a straw because ascorbic acid can erode tooth enamel. Powdered ascorbic acid is available in health food stores and through vitamin supply houses.

Vitamin C is considered safe, even in large amounts, because any extra is eliminated in the urine. If you want to take large amounts of vitamin C—more than 1,200 milligrams a day—it's still a good idea to discuss it with your doctor.

Selenium May Help Stop Inflammation

Selenium is essential to the body in small amounts. It is thought to be helpful for rheumatoid arthritis because it, too, fights inflammation. Selenium is used in the body for the production of glutathione peroxidase, an enzyme that works inside joints to round up free radicals.

In one study done in Belgium, 15 women with rheumatoid arthritis who took 160 micrograms of selenium or 200 micrograms of selenium-enriched yeast every day for 4 months experienced significant improvement in joint movement and strength compared with women receiving placebos (inactive pills).

Doctors who recommend selenium for people with rheumatoid arthritis prescribe 200 to 300 micrograms a day. In large amounts, selenium can be toxic, so experts say that it's probably best not to take more than 400 micrograms a day without medical supervision.

Studies show that people generally get about 108 micrograms of selenium a day in their diets. Top food sources include seafood, meats, and whole grains.

Vitamin E Adds Anti-Inflammatory Power

Doctors add vitamin E to their rheumatoid arthritis prescriptions because it, too, cleans up free radicals and may fight joint inflammation.

In one study, Japanese researchers looked at laboratory animals deficient in vitamin E as well as at those given large doses of vitamin E. When both groups were given toxins that cause joint damage similar to that caused by rheumatoid arthritis, those deficient in vitamin E had many more of the biochemical markers of inflammation in their blood.

In another study by researchers at the University of Buffalo in New York, vitamin E and fish oil lowered the number of proteins that caused joint swelling in mice. Fish oil and vitamin E both help establish a balance between proteins called cytokines that either increase or decrease inflammation. The study authors said the supplements won't prevent rheumatoid arthritis, but they may delay symptoms.

Vitamin E has even been shown to be as effective as the drug diclofenac in treating rheumatoid arthritis, according to a German study.

Doctors who recommend vitamin E generally call for amounts far beyond the Daily Value of 30 IU. "I recommend 400 international units a day," Dr. Pizzorno says. Since foods contain relatively little vitamin E, that amount is available only in supplements.

Beta-Carotene May Reduce Swelling

People with rheumatoid arthritis who become vegetarians often report that their symptoms of pain and swelling are relieved.

Such a diet may be helpful in several ways. In particular, a veggie-dense diet is likely to include more than the normal slim pickings of foods that contain beta-carotene, the yellow pigment found in carrots, winter squash, cantaloupe, and other orange and yellow fruits and vegetables.

Like vitamins C and E and selenium, beta-carotene rounds up free radicals. In one study done in Switzerland using laboratory animals, beta-carotene

Prescriptions for Healing

Most doctors who treat rheumatoid arthritis do not make dietary recommendations beyond that of eating a balanced diet.

Those who do provide nutritional therapy make sure that a person is getting at least the Daily Value of every essential vitamin and mineral. They might recommend larger doses initially, if necessary, to restore normal blood levels of these nutrients. These doctors also recommend continuing to take large doses of some of the nutrients known to play roles in regulating inflammation in the body. Here's their daily prescription.

Nutrient	Daily Amount
Beta-carotene	25,000 IU
Copper	2 milligrams (Daily Value) or 3 milligrams (1 milligram for every 10 milligrams of zinc)
Selenium	200–300 micrograms
Vitamin C	600–60,000 milligrams
Vitamin E	400 IU
Zinc	30 milligrams (zinc picolinate or zinc citrate)

MEDICAL ALERT: If you have rheumatoid arthritis, you should be using vitamin and mineral supplementation only after discussing it with your physician.

Do not take more than 3 milligrams of copper per day without medical supervision.

Doses of selenium that exceed 400 micrograms daily should be taken only under medical supervision.

If you want to take more than 1,200 milligrams of vitamin C daily, discuss it with your doctor, as large doses can cause diarrhea in some people. If you're taking vitamin C in the form of powdered ascorbic acid, be sure to drink the mixture through a straw, since ascorbic acid can erode tooth enamel.

If you are taking anticoagulant drugs, you should not take vitamin E supplements. (Though generally a dose of up to 1,500 IU of vitamin E a day is considered safe, some recent reports suggest that taking more than 400 IU a day could be harmful to people with cardiovascular or circulatory disease or with cancer. If you have such a condition, be sure to consult your doctor before you begin supplementation.)

Doses of zinc that exceed 15 milligrams daily should be taken only under medical supervision.

helped stop symptoms of a type of experimentally induced arthritis similar to rheumatoid arthritis.

Doctors who include beta-carotene in their anti-arthritis formulas recommend about 25,000 IU a day. That amount is considered safe.

Zinc Zeros In on Pain

Think zinc belongs only on your galvanized trash can? Think again.

Another mineral that fights inflammation, zinc is an important component of the nutritional package for rheumatoid arthritis. Several studies have shown that people who have rheumatoid arthritis have low blood levels of zinc, often associated with high levels of inflammatory biochemicals in the blood.

"Our bodies use zinc, along with copper, to make an inflammation-fighting enzyme called superoxide dismutase. This enzyme is found in inflamed joints, where it neutralizes free radicals," says Jonathan Wright, MD, medical director of the Tahoma Clinic in Renton, Washington, and author of *Dr. Wright's Guide to Healing with Nutrition*. Zinc also functions as a building block for 200 or so other enzymes that play essential roles throughout the body, including repairing joints and helping the immune system to do its job.

In one study by researchers at the University of Washington in Seattle, people with rheumatoid arthritis who took 50 milligrams of zinc three times a day for 3 months experienced significant improvement in joint swelling, morning stiffness, and walking time compared with when they were not taking zinc.

In another study, people with psoriatic arthritis, an inflammatory condition that is a combination of arthritis and the skin disease psoriasis, improved while taking 250 milligrams of zinc three times a day. In this study, relief of symptoms reached its peak after about 4 months of zinc supplementation and continued for several months after participants stopped taking zinc supplements.

"I recommend taking no more than 30 milligrams of zinc picolinate or zinc citrate without medical supervision," says Dr. Wright. Some doctors start their patients at amounts of up to 150 milligrams a day, then cut back as blood levels of zinc rise to normal. But prolonged high doses of zinc can cause problems, Dr. Wright warns. That's why most experts feel that it's a good idea not to take more than 15 milligrams (the Daily Value) of zinc daily without medical supervision.

Most people get 10 to 15 milligrams of zinc a day through foods, although older people may get only half of that amount. Whole grains, wheat bran, wheat germ, beef, lamb, oysters, eggs, nuts, and yogurt all contain good amounts of zinc. (*Note:* Because bacteria in raw oysters can cause serious illness in people with certain health conditions, make sure oysters are fully cooked before you eat them.)

The Copper Connection

For years, doctors have been fascinated—and stumped—by copper's possible link to rheumatoid arthritis. Blood levels of copper are often elevated in people with rheumatoid arthritis, which leads some researchers to believe that copper is being drawn out of body tissue stores and transported by the blood to fight inflamed joints.

What is known is that copper, like zinc and selenium, is used to form anti-inflammatory compounds in the body, including superoxide dismutase and ceruloplasmin, a protein found in the blood. Both of these biochemicals are known to help counteract the inflammation that occurs with rheumatoid arthritis.

Copper is also essential for the body's manufacture of connective tissue, the ligaments, tendons, and such that wrap around a joint like rubber bands and keep it stable.

And in the body, copper combines with salicylate, a compound found in aspirin, and improves the drug's pain-relieving ability, Dr. Wright says. "People who take copper supplements often find that they can get by with less aspirin or other nonsteroidal anti-inflammatories," he says.

Doctors who recommend copper supplements say that people should make sure they are getting either the Daily Value of 2 milligrams or 1 milligram of copper for every 10 milligrams of zinc that they take. The body works on a delicate balance of zinc and copper; too much zinc interferes with copper absorption and can lead to copper deficiency. Higher amounts of copper should be used only under medical supervision. Even in small amounts, copper can be toxic.

Studies show that generally, women get about 1 milligram a day and men get 1.6 milligrams a day in their diets. For food sources, try shellfish, nuts, seeds, fruits, cooked oysters, and beans.

Copper bracelets have commonly been promoted as a remedy for the aches and pains of arthritis. The Arthritis Foundation states that "there is no scientific evidence" that copper bracelets have any benefit for arthritis. If you want to get copper into your system, you'll have to take it orally.

RICKETS

BUILDING STRONG BONES

Was Tiny Tim, the lovable crippled child in Charles Dickens's classic *A Christmas Carol*, suffering from the vitamin D-deficiency bone disease called rickets?

One expert argues that it's likely, since 19th-century London was, as he puts it, "miserable." Any sunlight capable of piercing the English gloom was almost certainly trapped by industrial smog back then.

Sunlight is not the only potential source of rickets-preventing vitamin D, of course. But the Cratchit family's meager diet was hardly healthful enough to prevent a case of the infamous disease that crippled so many 19th-century children.

Bah, humbug, retort other experts. The Cratchit child clearly had some other crippling disease.

That the experts amuse themselves by debating Tiny Tim's condition says a lot about the frequency of rickets today. Aside from cases in which people avoid certain foods or the sun for dietary or religious reasons, this condition, called common rickets in children and osteomalacia in adults, is more a medical curiosity than an ongoing concern.

Almost Gone, but Not Forgotten

Rickets was a major problem in the 1930s in the United States, but fortifying milk with vitamin D nearly eliminated the disorder completely. Vitamin D-fortified milk contains about 400 IU per quart, so drinking 1 cup gives you half of the recommended amount for most adults.

However, cases of rickets still occur. Children who have diseases such as cystic fibrosis have a problem absorbing nutrients and are at risk for rickets, says Doug Heimburger, MD, professor of nutrition sciences at the University of Alabama at Birmingham.

And there's another group at risk: infants and children with milk allergies. Parents aren't advised to take their babies out into the sun, which would allow their bodies to convert the sun's ultraviolet rays into vitamin D. And if they're not getting vitamin D from milk products or a multivitamin, they'll become deficient.

In one case described in the *Annals of Allergy, Asthma and Immunology*, a 2-year-old boy with an allergy to cow's milk showed delayed growth and suffered from asthma and dermatitis, among other conditions. But once he was treated for a deficiency of vitamin D, he made a full recovery.

Awareness and supplementation are key when children have a milk allergy, the authors of the article say.

Children from certain cultures are also at higher risk for vitamin D deficiency. In the early 1990s, a few cases of rickets among Ethiopian and African-American Muslim children who were breastfed made the news. The dark skin of the mothers and their tendency to leave the house heavily clothed didn't allow them to make enough vitamin D to pass on to their babies. These were rare cases, as babies who are breastfed usually get plenty of vitamin D from their mothers' milk, according to La Leche League International.

Today cases of rickets are still emerging. In 2003, 21 cases of rickets were reported in Memphis, Tennessee, 20 of which involved African Americans. Researchers think that rickets is more common among immigrants from Asia, Africa, and Middle Eastern countries because they're more likely to wear clothes that cover much of their dark skin, which is already less efficient at converting the sun's rays to vitamin D.

Without sunlight or dairy products, both sources of vitamin D, young, growing bones are unable to perform a task known as mineralization, which is the process that adds minerals needed for bone development. Dark skin, colder climates, abundant clothing, and industrial pollution are all potential barriers to vitamin D production by the skin.

Boning Up on Vitamin D

Bone is a dynamic organ that is constantly being formed and reformed. Vitamin D is essential for bone formation and mineralization. It also ensures that there are proper amounts of calcium and phosphorus on hand for bone growth. It does this in three ways: first, by making certain that these minerals are absorbed in the intestines; second, by bringing calcium from bones into the blood; and third, by aiding the reabsorption of calcium and phosphorus by the kidneys.

A child with rickets will have ankles and wrists that flare, with noticeable knobby bumps, and weakened leg bones that bow under the child's own

---

Prescriptions for Healing

Because vitamin D is so readily available from sunshine and fortified milk products, rickets, a vitamin D deficiency disease, is relatively rare in the United States. Here's what doctors recommend for both prevention and treatment in children.

Nutrient	Daily Amount
Prevention	
Vitamin D	400 IU for children and adults
Treatment	
Vitamin D	1,000 IU for children; for adults, 50,000 IU per week until levels return to normal

MEDICAL ALERT: *Doses of more than 600 IU of vitamin D a day can be toxic. Symptoms may include high blood pressure, kidney failure, and coma. Vitamin D in such high daily doses should be taken only under the supervision of your doctor.*

---

weight. Other symptoms include a lack of muscle tone, a disproportionately large head and forehead, and delayed infant milestones such as sitting up, standing, and the appearance of teeth.

Prevention of rickets and osteomalacia is as simple as including good sources of vitamin D, such as fish (especially sardines and salmon) and fortified milk, in the diet. For infants who are breastfed, the National Institutes of Health recommends that they receive 200 IU of vitamin D a day to be sure they're getting enough of this essential vitamin. Two cups of vitamin D-fortified formula daily will cover their needs. Infants who are mainly fed formula already get all of the nutrients they need.

Of course, once a child stops taking formula, vitamin D-fortified whole milk is important. Because of fortification, an 8-ounce glass of milk provides about 100 IU of vitamin D. The Daily Value is 400 IU, but experts say that it's safe to take up to 2,000 IU a day.

For confirmed rickets cases, doctors will give the patient oral supplements of vitamin D. "A child with absorption problems would need much higher doses as opposed to a child without absorption problems," Dr. Heimburger says.

The recommended dose for rickets is 1,000 IU of vitamin D daily by mouth, while adults with osteomalacia are given 50,000 IU of vitamin D a week, Dr. Heimburger says. What's most important is to continue to test the patient's blood levels to make sure the dose is in the correct range, he says.

In addition to getting vitamin D from foods, a multivitamin for children or infants will also help prevent future cases of rickets.

SCLERODERMA

SOFTENING ROCK-HARD SKIN

Talk about being a prisoner in your own body. People with scleroderma—literally, hard skin—can become encased in thick scar tissue. The disease can turn a formerly animated face into an expressionless mask and stiffen hands into claws. About one in three people with the disease may also have problems with the intestines, kidneys, heart, or lungs.

Scleroderma, like lupus and rheumatoid arthritis, is an autoimmune disease. This means that the immune system, the white blood cells that normally protect against bacteria, viruses, and other foreign invaders, turns renegade and attacks the body's own tissues. In this case, the attack is on connective tissue called collagen. Collagen is found throughout the body, including in the skin, the muscles, and the organs.

The immune system attack first produces inflammation that can make the joints hurt and cause the hands to become puffy. Ultimately, scar tissue forms and makes the skin thick, hard, and shiny. Muscles can become weak. And almost everyone with scleroderma also has Raynaud's phenomenon, an extreme sensitivity to cold in the hands and feet. Raynaud's phenomenon causes blood vessels to constrict and fingers and toes to turn white, resulting in stinging pain and discomfort.

The most aggressive form of scleroderma is systemic and affects your skin, blood vessels, and major organs. The systemic form is very rare, says Joel Schlessinger, MD, a dermatologist in private practice in Omaha, Nebraska. Localized scleroderma, on the other hand, is limited to the skin and deep tissues underneath the skin.

Dermatologists treat the skin symptoms that result from both forms of scleroderma, while rheumatologists treat the systemic form of the disease.

Battling Toxic Exposure

Just what causes most cases of this relatively rare disease is not known, says David Pisetsky, MD, PhD, chief of the division of rheumatology, allergy and clinical immunology at Duke University. A clue to the cause is provided by the occurrence of similar problems in people who have been exposed to environmental chemicals such as polyvinyl chloride (found in soft plastics) and trichloroethylene (a grease dissolver used in manufacturing and dry cleaning). Coal miners may develop scleroderma after years of work, and outbreaks of similar connective tissue diseases have been associated, in Spain, with contaminated cooking oil and, in the United States, with contaminated tryptophan, an amino acid supplement used to treat insomnia.

Food Factors

Doctors agree: If you have scleroderma, healthy eating habits can help you function better. Here's what they recommend.

Subtract fat. Chances are you've heard this advice a few times before, as prevention for heart disease and cancer. In the case of a chronic inflammatory condition such as scleroderma, you'll want to cut back on the fat in your diet, especially saturated fat, because fat helps fuel the fire of inflammation. High-fat meals are also harder to absorb than low-fat meals. To do this, stick to low-fat dairy products, lean meats, and reduced-fat salad dressings.

Fill in with fish. The oil in fatty fish such as mackerel, salmon, and tuna actually has a mild anti-inflammatory effect. Some people take fish oil capsules, but since you want to stay low-fat, a better tactic may be to replace high-fat dishes such as macaroni and cheese with broiled fish.

Use yogurt to your advantage. Although antibiotics may be essential to knock out harmful bacteria in your digestive system, these powerful medications also destroy helpful bacteria. Eating plenty of yogurt or taking acidophilus tablets restores these friendly bacteria to the bowel, which helps protect it from a new bout of harmful overgrowth. Research has found that people who ate two servings of yogurt a day while taking an antibiotic had a lower chance of experiencing diarrhea.

Doctors also are looking into a drug that was used in the past for magnetic resonance imaging (MRI). When doctors want to look at a patient's organs or blood vessels, they inject a contrasting agent to distinguish the organ or blood vessels they're studying from other tissue. Some research has suggested that high doses of the contrasting agents used in MRIs may have led to the development of a condition called nephrogenic fibrosing dermopathy, which causes skin tightening in certain areas of the body that's similar to scleroderma. The connection has been made only in patients who had moderate to end-stage kidney disease when they were given the MRIs.

The medical community has stopped using this contrasting agent, Dr. Schlessinger says. There's hope that learning more about the connection between the agent and nephrogenic fibrosing dermopathy could lead to clues about the causes of scleroderma, but it's still too early to tell, he says.

Doctors treat scleroderma with drugs that suppress the immune system and reduce inflammation. They may also recommend medications that help the heart and kidneys function better. Antibiotics and drugs that stimulate gut motility, or the movement of food from one end of the digestive tract to the other, can combat the bacterial overgrowth and absorption problems that sometimes accompany scleroderma.

Nutrition isn't thought to play much of a role in the development or progression of scleroderma, and unfortunately doctors haven't found much—nutritionally or otherwise—that gets to the root of the problem. Rather, the drugs doctors prescribe for scleroderma treat the symptoms, Dr. Schlessinger says.

"Vitamins hold a very beneficial role in the treatment and potential improvement of many medical conditions," he says. "But with scleroderma, nothing has been proven to be helpful—vitamins or medical therapies."

That doesn't mean you shouldn't aim for optimal nutrition in your diet. When you take care of yourself and eat a healthy diet, you're giving your body the chance to function as optimally as possible, despite the disease, Dr. Schlessinger says.

Inflammation Fighters

Doctors agree: Scleroderma starts with inflammation, and its progress depends on how much inflammation continues to occur in the body. As a result, a few doctors may recommend that patients with any sort of

Prescriptions for Healing

Although most doctors do not recommend supplements to people with scleroderma, some doctors say they've found that certain supplements may help the two biggest problems that people with scleroderma face: malabsorption and inflammation.

If you have scleroderma and wish to take supplements, you should discuss it with your doctor, especially if you have kidney damage or high blood pressure.

If you are taking anticoagulant drugs, you should not take oral vitamin E supplements. Though generally a dose of up to 1,500 IU of vitamin E a day is considered safe, some recent reports suggest that taking more than 400 IU a day could be harmful to people with cardiovascular or circulatory disease or with cancer. If you have such a condition, be sure to consult your doctor before you begin supplementation.

inflammatory disease—rheumatoid arthritis, lupus, or scleroderma—get optimum amounts of antioxidants, such as vitamin E, selenium, and beta-carotene, a yellow pigment found in dark green leafy vegetables and in orange and yellow fruits and vegetables.

These nutrients are thought to help to dampen inflammation by neutralizing some of the biochemicals associated with the process.

Inflammation produces unstable molecules called free radicals, which damage a cell by grabbing electrons from healthy molecules in the cell's outer membrane. Antioxidants offer free radicals their own electrons, disarming the free radicals and saving cells from harm.

As yet, as Dr. Schlessinger pointed out, there hasn't been much in the way of actual scientific study of the use of supplemental antioxidants to treat scleroderma. In one study using laboratory animals, supplemental vitamin E helped prevent calcium deposits in soft tissues, which can be a problem for people with scleroderma. In another study, three people with scleroderma who took 800 to 1,200 IU of vitamin E daily had reductions in the stiffness and hardness of their hands, reductions in calcium deposits in soft tissues, and, in two of the three, healing of ulcerated fingertips.

It's difficult to study the effects of anti-inflammatory treatments on conditions such as scleroderma because there are usually several other health issues affecting the patient, Dr. Schlessinger says.

Also, patients may be taking several medications when they have scleroderma, and taking vitamin supplements on top of the medications may interfere with the actions of the drugs in the body, he says.

For these reasons, you shouldn't take any supplements unless your doctor recommends them. That also applies to a multivitamin, Dr. Schlessinger says.

And take special precaution with vitamin C. Vitamin C promotes the body's production of collagen, and scleroderma involves the overproduction of collagen. In fact, one study attempted to treat scleroderma by putting people on a diet very low in vitamin C, but the results were inconclusive. Although doctors generally don't tell scleroderma patients to avoid eating vitamin C-rich foods such as citrus fruits, talk to your doctor before you take a vitamin C supplement.

Fighting Absorption Problems

Perhaps the biggest nutritional problem that people with scleroderma face is malabsorption. Their intestines absorb less than normal amounts of nutrients from foods because of scarring and bacterial overgrowth. Doctors often recommend treatment with antibiotics to knock out the bad bugs and help restore some absorption. But some people also require liquid nutritional supplements or, in some cases, intravenous nutrition.

SCURVY

SOLVED WITH VITAMIN C

Chances are the last time you heard someone mention scurvy, an Errol Flynn type was being forced to walk the plank at swordpoint in a bad old pirate movie: "We'll make shark bait outta ya, ya scurvy dog!"

The name given to a set of symptoms that develop during a severe long-term shortage of vitamin C, scurvy is rare these days. But make no mistake: At one time, scurvy was a plague of epic proportions. In fact, one expert maintains that after famine, scurvy is "probably the nutritional deficiency disease that has caused the most suffering in recorded history."

Source of Sailors' Suffering

Once called the scourge of the navy, scurvy killed or incapacitated countless sailors during the age of naval exploration. Often, long sea voyages, even aboard grand sailing ships led by legendary explorers such as Ferdinand Magellan and Vasco da Gama, literally became death trips for the crew. In fact, da Gama lost 100 of 160 men to scurvy during one 10-month voyage.

Soldiers bogged down on long winter campaigns often suffered the same fate: wounds that wouldn't heal, muscle pain, bleeding gums, lost teeth, fatigue, kidney failure, pneumonia, and, finally, death.

Between 1556 and 1857, more than 100 scurvy epidemics occurred throughout Europe, including Ireland's infamous Great Potato Famine (potatoes were that country's main source of vitamin C).

Many early medical experts thought that scurvy was contagious, and no one had any idea what caused the disease. Finally, James Lind, a young Scottish physician in the British navy, theorized that sailors' diets, which often consisted of nothing more than biscuits and salted meats such as beef and pork, lacked "acidic principles."

To test his theory, Dr. Lind divided some sick sailors into groups. A few sailors ate oranges in addition to the ship's rations; others ate lemons. Still others were given vinegar. One group even drank seawater!

Within 6 days, the sailors who ate the oranges and lemons were healthy enough to be reassigned to active duty. And for his part, Dr. Lind had shown that this devastating illness could be cured with the right nutrients. In 1754, Dr. Lind published "A Treatise on Scurvy," describing the study and his recommendations for treatment.

Dr. Lind's observations weren't widely accepted for another 50 years. But they had impact, and not just on health. Soon British sailors were known as limeys, a nickname that poked fun at the lime juice they drank while at sea.

Scurvy Still Exists

Healthier diets featuring lots of foods rich in vitamin C have come close to ending scurvy in the United States.

In general, Americans get more than the recommended amounts of vitamin C a day (75 milligrams for women and 90 milligrams for men). But surveys show there still are parts of the population—as much as 18 percent—who are deficient. The UDSA's survey of food intakes from 1994 to 1996 found

Prescriptions for Healing

Although scurvy is extremely rare, doctors still see an occasional case. What's more common is a condition known as subscurvy. Here's how the experts treat both.

Nutrient	Daily Amount
For Scurvy	
Vitamin C	500–1,000 milligrams for 1 week, then 100 milligrams for 1 month, then 60 milligrams thereafter
For Subscurvy	
Vitamin C	200 milligrams

MEDICAL ALERT: Anyone with scurvy should be under medical care and should receive a vitamin prescription from a doctor.

that 14 percent of teenage boys and 20 percent of teenage girls got less than 30 milligrams of vitamin C.

People 65 and older had the lowest rate of vitamin C deficiency compared with other adults because seniors are more likely to take supplements, according to the USDA findings. Supplements of vitamin C are among the most popular in the United States.

However, the elderly, particularly those who are institutionalized, have special needs and may need more vitamin C than most.

It's a serious problem because deficiency can have a snowball effect. People who have scurvy lose their appetite, which makes it hard to overcome the disease with dietary changes. Also, painful gums can discourage eating.

Who's at Risk

While few doctors ever see full-blown cases of scurvy, nutrition experts warn that a potentially large number of older folks teeter on the brink of a condition known as subscurvy. Living alone or in nursing homes, they might eat just enough fruits and vegetables to get the daily amount needed of vitamin C.

But this amount might not be enough for some older people, according to Tapan K. Basu, PhD, professor emeritus of agriculture, food, and nutritional science at the University of Alberta in Edmonton and coauthor of

Vitamin C in Health and Disease. Many older folks take aspirin or other analgesics daily to manage arthritis pain, and that can reduce the amount of vitamin C in the body by as much as 50 percent, he explains. "You get a combination effect of aspirin impeding vitamin C absorption in the gastrointestinal tract as well as damaging the vitamin C itself," he says.

People with ulcers are also at risk for subscurvy. Avoiding acidic foods to help keep pain at bay often means cutting back on solid sources of vitamin C such as oranges and lemons, says Dr. Basu.

Smoking a pack of cigarettes a day has also been found to cut the amount of vitamin C in your body by 50 percent. According to the new dietary reference intake guidelines, smokers should be getting an additional 35 milligrams of vitamin C daily.

Combine all three—prolonged low vitamin C intake, smoking, and daily aspirin use—and you're well on your way to subscurvy. Symptoms include delayed wound healing, small red spots that show up particularly when pressure is applied to the arms, severe fatigue, and bleeding gums.

Treating Deficiency

How much vitamin C does it take to overcome the symptoms of scurvy and subscurvy? The amount pretty much depends on how severe the deficiency is in the first place, says Dr. Basu.

To begin with, a person with full-blown scurvy should be under a doctor's care. During the first week of treatment, between 500 and 1,000 milligrams of vitamin C a day is usually enough to replenish depleted reserves and help end symptoms such as bleeding gums and those purplish red spots, says Dr. Basu. During the second week, he reduces the daily dose to 100 milligrams and then prescribes that level for the next month. After that, the Daily Value (60 milligrams) is usually enough to avoid a recurrence, he says.

But how much vitamin C should you take if you think you're at risk for subscurvy? Generally, 200 milligrams a day, says Dr. Basu.

For those who use aspirin frequently, Dr. Basu suggests waiting 3 hours after taking your aspirin to take vitamin C, giving your body enough time to absorb the aspirin without harming the vitamin C. Taking vitamin C soon after a meal and not on an empty stomach is the answer for people with ulcers. You could also try ester-C, a calcium-based version of vitamin C, to prevent acid-related pain, he advises. This form of vitamin C is available in health food stores, he says.

SHINGLES

CHICKENPOX REVISITED

Childhood chickenpox is usually no big deal. A rash of itchy blisters, a touch of fever, a couple of days in bed, and a few bowls of ice cream, and you're better. You might not even remember having had it.

But the virus that causes chickenpox remains in your body in nerves at the base of your spine, and it may reactivate years later as a searing case of shingles, or herpes zoster, its medical name.

When the virus flares, it moves out along the pathway of whatever nerve is involved, usually on the trunk, neck, or face. The nerve becomes inflamed and extremely sensitive to touch. The area where the nerve reaches the skin burns and stings, then erupts in a splay of painful blisters that may last for up to a week or longer.

Shingles isn't something that you can just shrug off. And you shouldn't ignore it, even if you could. Doctors consider it a "pain emergency" and can offer some relief. Some studies also suggest that postherpetic neuralgia, the lingering pain that sometimes follows an attack of shingles, is less likely to occur if you are treated within 72 hours of the onset of blisters with high doses of drugs that stop the virus from multiplying.

People with infections such as HIV and those taking chemotherapy drugs for cancer or immunity-suppressing drugs to protect organ transplants are at highest risk for a shingles episode. And your risk goes up simply as you get older. Among people who have had chickenpox, 1 in 10 will develop shingles as adults, usually after age 50.

"Most doctors use drugs to treat shingles, and a few drugs now in the pipeline may provide more help than ever," says Stephen Tyring, MD, PhD, professor at the University of Texas Graduate School of Biomedical Sciences at Houston.

Vaccines are also helping prevent the disease. The FDA approved the varicella virus vaccine in 1995 to prevent chickenpox in children. And another vaccine, Zostavax, has been approved to help prevent shingles in people age 60 and older.

Still, some doctors add nutritional therapy to their treatments, hoping to reduce inflammation, protect nerves, and restore strong immunity. Here's what they recommend.

Vitamin B₁₂ May Aid Recovering Nerves

It's considered an old-fashioned remedy, and apparently, it doesn't work for everyone. But some doctors give injections of vitamin B_{12} to their patients with shingles. They say it helps make shingles less painful and may help people recover more quickly.

A study by Indian researchers reported that 21 people with shingles showed "dramatic response," as judged by relief of pain and the speed with which blisters disappeared, starting the second or third day of treatment with vitamin B_{12} injections. What's more, none developed the lingering pain of postherpetic neuralgia.

Vitamin B_{12} is known to play an important role in nerve function. Vitamin B_{12} helps the nervous system by protecting the fatty membranes called the myelin sheath around the nerves.

Injections of vitamin B_{12} are absorbed more efficiently by the body than supplements. If you're interested in B_{12} injections, you'll need to enlist the aid of your doctor. Doses vary. One study in the journal *Geriatrics* recommended an injection of 1 milligram of vitamin B_{12} a day for 6 days or weekly for 6 weeks.

It's impossible to get this large amount of vitamin B_{12} from foods, and absorption from supplements isn't as beneficial as injections. This amount of B_{12} is extremely high (the Daily Value is only 6 micrograms) and should be taken only under a doctor's supervision, but high amounts of vitamin B_{12} are thought to be safe by doctors.

Along with vitamin B_{12}, some doctors give injections of folic acid and the rest of the B-complex: thiamin, riboflavin, niacin, vitamin B_6, and the like.

Vitamin C May Dry Up Blisters

It's not exactly what you would call recent research. But two studies, one from 1949 and another from 1950, suggest that people having shingles outbreaks get substantial relief from intravenous doses of large amounts of vitamin C.

In one of the studies, by researchers in North Carolina, seven of eight people with shingles reported relief from pain within 2 hours of the first dose, drying of blisters within 1 day, and complete clearing in 3 days. In the other study, French researchers reported that they were able to cure all 327 people with shingles with 3 days of intravenous vitamin C.

More recently, the Spring 2006 issue of the *Journal of American Physicians and Surgeons* described two cases in which vitamin C was used to treat shingles. In one case, an 84-year-old man had shingles blisters on the side of his scalp and was injected with vitamin C. Within just a few hours, his pain went down considerably. The other case involved a 40-year-old woman with severe blisters on her chest. After four injections of vitamin C spaced 12 hours apart, her pain nearly disappeared. In both cases, the patients also took vitamin C orally.

Doctors think vitamin C bolsters immunity. Additionally, studies show that in large doses, vitamin C can inhibit replication of certain types of viruses, including those in the herpes family, and impair the ability of certain viruses to cause infection.

By virtue of its antioxidant ability, vitamin C can also neutralize inflammation-causing biochemicals that are produced by immune cells as they do battle. That talent may help spare nearby cells that would otherwise be damaged by the battle between immune cells and viruses.

Many of the doctors who prescribe vitamin C for viral infections use it

Food Factors

The shingles virus, herpes zoster, responds to the same dietary changes used for herpes simplex, the virus that causes cold sores and genital herpes. Here are the details.

Pay attention to amino acids. Research indicates that large doses of lysine, an essential amino acid, inhibit replication of the virus responsible for shingles.

"I recommend 2,000 to 3,000 milligrams of lysine a day during a shingles outbreak, more in stubborn cases," says Robert Cathcart, MD, a physician in private practice in Los Altos, California, who specializes in nutritional therapy. Although lysine is commonly found in foods such as beef, pork, eggs, and tofu, it may be necessary to take a supplement in order to get this high amount. The amino acid appears to have no side effects, since it's taken in high doses for only a short period of time, Dr. Cathcart adds. Lysine supplements are available in health food stores.

Ax arginine-rich foods. These include chocolate, nuts, and seeds. Lysine seems to work best when people cut back on arginine, another amino acid, says Dr. Cathcart. That's because lysine may work by blocking the virus's ability to absorb arginine.

both intravenously, as neutralized sodium ascorbate, and in the largest oral dose that can be tolerated without causing diarrhea, says Robert Cathcart, MD, a doctor in private practice in Los Altos, California, who specializes in nutritional therapy. "We literally flood the body with vitamin C," he says. This large amount helps keep both blood levels and levels inside cells high enough to dampen inflammation, he explains. He usually gives daily intravenous doses for 3 to 5 days, by which time the blisters are gone. "I've never had a case that goes on to postherpetic neuralgia or neuritis," he says. "This handles it very nicely."

Large amounts of vitamin C can cause diarrhea. For this reason, Dr.

Prescriptions for Healing

The main treatment for shingles consists of drug therapy. There are, however, a few nutrients that some doctors recommend.

Nutrient	Daily Amount
Vitamin B$_{12}$	1,000–2,000 micrograms
Vitamin C	Largest dose tolerated without diarrhea, as prescribed by your doctor
Vitamin E	400 IU

MEDICAL ALERT: *If you have shingles, you should be under a doctor's care.*

The amount of vitamin B$_{12}$ recommended here is many times the Daily Value and should be taken only under medical supervision. Depending on the severity of your condition, your doctor may choose to administer B$_{12}$ by injection.

Before prescribing a high dose of vitamin C, your doctor should determine how much of this nutrient you can tolerate. Some people experience diarrhea with amounts of more than 1,200 milligrams daily. For this reason, it's important that you discuss this therapy with your doctor.

If you are taking anticoagulant drugs, you should not take vitamin E supplements. (Though generally a dose of up to 1,500 IU of vitamin E a day is considered safe, some recent reports suggest that taking more than 400 IU a day could be harmful to people with cardiovascular or circulatory disease or with cancer. If you have such a condition, be sure to consult your doctor before you begin supplementation.)

Cathcart explains, a doctor should determine how much vitamin C can be tolerated without diarrhea before a high dose is prescribed. If you'd like to try this therapy for shingles, you should discuss it with your doctor.

While it's impossible to get a high enough dosage of vitamin C from foods, many doctors suggest that you'd still do well to include citrus fruits in your daily diet. That's because the white rinds and membranes of citrus fruits contain bioflavonoids, chemical compounds related to vitamin C that are also potential immunity boosters and inflammation fighters.

Vitamin E May Ease Long-Irritated Nerves

One of the worst potential consequences of a shingles attack is pain that just won't quit, caused by chronic nerve inflammation. Although it hasn't been studied recently, several older research reports suggest that high doses of vitamin E can help resolve this persistent pain.

One report, published in 1973 by Los Angeles dermatologists Samuel Ayres, MD, and Richard Mihan, MD, found "highly gratifying results" with vitamin E used orally and topically. Of 13 people treated, 9 experienced complete or almost complete relief from pain, 2 were moderately improved, and 2 were slightly improved. Two of those who experienced complete or almost complete relief from pain had had postshingles pain the longest: one for 13 years, the other for 19 years.

Vitamin E is incorporated into the fatty membranes of all cells, including nerve cells, which are protected by the myelin sheath, the thick wrapping of fatty membranes mentioned earlier. There, vitamin E helps shield cells from the damage that occurs during a viral attack. Vitamin E can neutralize harmful biochemicals that are produced by immune cells as they ward off viruses. It may help stop the damage that can lead to lingering inflammation.

Dr. Ayres and Dr. Mihan used high doses of vitamin E in their study: 1,200 to 1,600 IU daily. Consider medical supervision for doses of more than 400 IU daily.

Order the Complete Package

Vitamin E, along with other nutrients, stimulates immunity in other ways that may be helpful to people with shingles, especially those who seem to have weakened immunity, says Dr. Cathcart. "Many of my patients with herpes zoster have low immunity, so I work with an array of nutrients to rebuild their systems," he explains. These nutrients include vitamin A, the B-complex vitamins, zinc, selenium, and others. (For the full story on boosting your immune system, see page 324.)

SMOG EXPOSURE

PROTECTION FROM POLLUTION

From campfires to jet engine exhaust, where there's civilization, there's smog, a combination of noxious chemicals, light-as-air particles, and moisture that hangs in a yellowish gray haze over cities. Smog not only makes your eyes sting and lungs twitch but can even nibble the nose off a marble statue of Ulysses S. Grant.

Smog contains a long lineup of chemical nasties, including ozone, nitrogen dioxide, sulfur dioxide, and tiny particles of everything from asbestos to soot, that can settle deep in the lungs and cause general havoc. "Smog is a soup that contains a lot of stuff, and people inhale everything that's in it, a whole bunch of toxic chemicals," says Daniel Menzel, PhD, professor emeritus of community and environmental medicine at the University of California, Irvine. "They're a significant threat to people's health."

A high concentration of or long exposure to any one of these chemicals can cause shortness of breath, wheezing, coughing, bronchitis, pneumonia, headaches, inability to concentrate, chest pain, and, in some cases, lung cancer.

Smog Hurts

Breathing smog changes the way that lung cells do business, Dr. Menzel explains. In some people, the lungs become supersensitive, reacting to smog exposure with inflammation, bronchial spasms, coughing, asthma attacks, or increased production of mucus.

Smog can also make lung cells vulnerable to attack by bacteria and viruses that are always in the air. Smog can kill cells, making the lungs less efficient at doing their job of gas exchange (absorbing oxygen and releasing carbon dioxide). And some of the chemicals in smog can cause genetic mutations in cells that lead to cancer in the lungs or nasal passages.

Many of the harmful interactions between the noxious substances in smog and lung cells happen during a chemical process known as oxidation. This is the same process that causes butter to turn rancid and iron to rust. Oxidation, as you might guess, is a chemical reaction that requires oxygen in order to take place, and there's plenty of oxygen in the lungs. During oxidation, free radicals, which are unstable molecules of harmful chemicals, snatch electrons from the healthy molecules that compose the cells in order to balance themselves. This starts a chain reaction of electron stealing. The end result: serious damage to cells.

The best way to deal with smog, of course, is to avoid it as much as possible. Don't run along heavily trafficked roads. Aerobic exercise makes you breathe deeply, so you draw pollutants deep into your lungs. And don't smoke cigarettes. Smoking exposes your lungs to some of the same toxins found in smog, plus it makes your lungs more sensitive to smog's effects.

If you can't avoid smog entirely, you may want to protect yourself by

Food Factors

Antioxidant nutrients are your surest protection against damage from chemical exposure. But these additional dietary adjustments may help, experts say.

Scratch the saturated fat. Researchers at the National Cancer Institute in Rockville, Maryland, reported a strong association between saturated fat intake and adenocarcinoma, a type of lung cancer that is most common in nonsmokers. They found that women who consumed the greatest amounts of fat, typically from hamburgers, cheeseburgers, meat loaf, cheeses and cheese spreads, hot dogs, ice cream, and sausage, had six times the risk of lung cancer of those who ate the least fat.

Think raw. Researchers at Yale University found that the risk of lung cancer among men and women eating lots of salad greens and other raw vegetables, along with fresh fruits, was almost half of the risk seen among people not putting these foods on their plates.

taking nutrients that provide a measure of internal pollution protection: vitamins A, C, and E; beta-carotene; and selenium.

Vitamin E Equals Protection

Vitamin E, found in wheat germ, certain vegetables, nuts, seeds, and vegetable oils, is well known both for its ability to enhance the immune system and as an antioxidant. Antioxidants offer their own electrons to free radicals, disarming those renegade molecules and protecting healthy molecules from damage.

"Vitamin E is the strongest antioxidant found in the body," Dr. Menzel explains. "It gets incorporated into cell membranes, where it shields cells from harm. It helps stop the chain reaction that starts with exposure to smog and so is very effective at limiting the amount of damage done to cells."

However, vitamin E has lost some of its appeal in recent years. In the past, researchers thought vitamin E could significantly reduce the risk of nonsmokers developing lung cancer. But research in the last 10 years tells a different story. Randomized trials haven't shown that vitamin E helps reduce the risk of lung cancer and even shows that vitamin E can be harmful in high doses, says Susan Taylor Mayne, PhD, professor in the division of chronic disease epidemiology at Yale School of Public Health.

Researchers at the Johns Hopkins School of Medicine studied 19 clinical trials involving vitamin E supplements in 2005 and found that taking more than 400 IU of vitamin E a day increased risk of mortality. However, the authors noted that the trials that included high doses of vitamin E were small and involved patients with chronic diseases, rather than healthy adults. Doctors who recommend vitamin E suggest that you take 400 IU a day. This amount is considered safe, but it's more than you can get from even the best food sources. Research indicates that the Daily Value of vitamin E, 30 IU, is not enough to offer optimum smog protection, Dr. Menzel says.

Breathe Easier with Vitamin D

Vitamin D does everything from protecting your bones from osteoporosis to lowering your risk of hypertension. Researchers now believe it's also good for your lungs.

Researchers from the University at Auckland in New Zealand examined more than 14,000 people ages 20 and older and found that those with higher concentrations of vitamin D showed significantly better lung function. However, the researchers didn't know if the benefits from vitamin D were a result of dietary intake or supplements.

The Daily Value of vitamin D is 400 IU. You'll find vitamin D in salmon; sardines; mackerel; and fortified milk, orange juice, and cereals. Of course, most of our vitamin D comes from the sun. Our bodies convert the sun's ultraviolet rays into vitamin D. Many experts recommend supplementing vitamin D if you live in a northern state where the suns rays are weak in the wintertime or if you have a job that requires long hours indoors.

Prescriptions for Healing

For healthy lungs, avoid smog-filled areas and supplement your diet with these nutrients, which some doctors recommend as protection against air pollution.

Nutrient	Daily Amount
Beta-carotene	25,000 IU
Selenium	50–200 micrograms
Vitamin A	5,000 IU
Vitamin C	1,200 milligrams
Vitamin D	400 IU
Vitamin E	400 IU

MEDICAL ALERT: *Selenium in doses exceeding 400 micrograms daily can be toxic and should be taken only under medical supervision.*

If you are taking anticoagulant drugs, you should not take vitamin E supplements. (Though generally a dose of up to 1,500 IU of vitamin E a day is considered safe, some recent reports suggest that taking more than 400 IU a day could be harmful to people with cardiovascular or circulatory disease or with cancer. If you have such a condition, be sure to consult your doctor before you begin supplementation.)

Orange Aid for Air Pollution

Vitamin C is another well-known antioxidant. Like vitamin E, it helps stop free radical chain reactions.

Vitamin C helps maintain healthy lung function both in the general population and in people with asthma, say researchers at Harvard Medical School. They found that people who were getting at least 200 milligrams of vitamin C (about three oranges' worth) a day did best on tests that measured their lungs' capacity to expand and draw in oxygen.

Here again, usual dietary amounts may not be adequate protection, Dr. Menzel says. Researchers who recommend nutritional therapy to offset the effects of smog exposure suggest that you get about 1,200 milligrams of vitamin C a day. That amount is considered to be within the safe range, but it does require taking supplements.

Vitamins C and E work together in the lungs, and Yale University researchers have shown that a combination of the two helps keep lung tissue healthy. In one study, people who took daily supplements of 1,500 milligrams of vitamin C and 1,200 IU of vitamin E built up levels of a protective protein that prevents enzymes released during inflammation from destroying the lung's elastic properties. This lack of elasticity can be harmful: People with emphysema, for instance, who've lost lung elasticity from years of cigarette smoking, struggle for every breath.

Treat Your Lungs to a Carrot

The research evidence that's piling up about the protective effects of beta-carotene looks more and more like a cornucopia of fruits and vegetables. Those that contain beta-carotene, the yellow pigment found in carrots, cantaloupe, and other orange and yellow fruits and vegetables, apparently help shield lungs from air pollution. "In population studies, foods rich in beta-carotene seem to offer protection against lung cancer, even among nonsmokers," says Dr. Mayne.

Unfortunately, a highly publicized 1994 study of male Finnish smokers found that 20 milligrams (about 33,000 IU) of supplemental beta-carotene a day did not reduce the incidence of lung cancer. Does that mean you shouldn't take beta-carotene to help protect your lungs from smog?

Some researchers feel that this study tested amounts of beta-carotene that were too little and given too late. They believe that there are still plenty of good reasons to get enough of this nutrient, Dr. Menzel says. Both beta-carotene and vitamin A (beta-carotene is converted to vitamin A in the body) help keep cells on track as they grow and divide and so help prevent genetic mutations that can lead to cancer, he explains.

Most experts recommend getting beta-carotene from foods rather than supplements, as foods contain many other substances that may also be important for cancer prevention. Dr. Menzel suggests that people get about 25,000 IU of beta-carotene a day from foods or supplements. That's roughly the amount found in 1 cup of chopped cooked spinach, 1¼ large carrots, or 2½ large sweet potatoes. Some doctors also recommend taking the Daily Value of vitamin A, which is 5,000 IU.

Selenium Shields Cells

Medical researchers round out their antipollution prescriptions with the mineral selenium. "Selenium is needed in the body to activate glutathione peroxidase, an important antioxidant enzyme that helps keep lung tissue elastic," Dr. Menzel explains.

Doctors recommend getting from 50 to 200 micrograms of selenium daily from foods and supplements. Studies show that most people get about 108 micrograms a day from foods. (Rich sources of selenium include grains, seeds, and fish.) So it's probably not necessary to take a supplement. If you do take a supplement, don't exceed 400 micrograms daily without medical supervision. In high amounts, selenium can be toxic.

SMOKING

CONTROLLING DAMAGE
WHILE KICKING THE HABIT

Unless you live on another planet, you know the evils of smoking. And if you're a smoker, you've likely tried to quit more than once. And you plan to try again. That's good.

While kicking the habit is your number one priority, there are measures you can take nutritionally to block smoking's path of destruction while you work on "butting out" once and for all. For a little motivation, it helps to first understand how cigarette smoke damages your body.

A Radical Habit

Though all of the harmful reactions caused by smoking are not completely understood, researchers agree that the lion's share of smokers' ailments are the result of free radicals. Free radicals are unstable molecules that are missing electrons. They pillage your body's healthy molecules for replacement electrons, leaving more free radicals and damaged cells and tissues in their wake. This process is called oxidation, and it's what makes iron rust and fruit turn brown. And scientists are beginning to believe that oxidation is what makes people age.

Though free radicals are formed during everyday functions such as breathing, environmental stress factors such as smoking dramatically accelerate their production. In fact, each puff on a cigarette generates millions of free radicals, making smokers much more susceptible than nonsmokers to the ravages of oxidative tissue damage.

To fight this free radical onslaught, you need a strong defense. And according to research, one of the best defenses consists of nutrients known as antioxidants, most notably vitamins C and E and beta-carotene. Antioxidants act as your body's kamikaze fighters, protecting your body's healthy molecules by sacrificing their own electrons to neutralize hostile free radical invaders.

Though antioxidants aren't miracle cures and certainly shouldn't lure you into a false sense of security about smoking, these nutrients can help stave off smoking-related damage while you're kicking the habit. Here's what experts recommend.

E Is Essential for Smokers

When it comes to protecting your body from smoking's nasty side effects, vitamin E, an antioxidant found in sunflower seeds, sweet potatoes, and kale, is a top performer.

Food Factors

When it comes to smoking, the health advice is clear: Don't do it. But if you're still lighting up, one of the best ways to help protect yourself is by improving your diet. Here's how.

Eat fruits and veggies. There's no arguing that people who eat lots of fruits and vegetables have a higher protection from cancer than people who don't.

In fact, in a study in Japan, where cigarette consumption per capita is among the highest in the world and the incidence of lung cancer is among the lowest, researchers evaluated the effects of eating raw vegetables, green vegetables (especially lettuce and cabbage), and fruits in 282 smokers. They found that the relative risk of lung cancer was markedly decreased in those who included fruits and raw vegetables in their daily fare.

Experts recommend that for optimum protection, smokers eat seven half-cup servings of fruits and vegetables every day. Remember to reach for orange, red, and dark green vegetables for the benefits of beta-carotene.

Go easy on acids. If you're trying to quit via a nicotine replacement product such as nicotine gum or a nicotine patch, then steer clear of orange juice, grapefruit juice, and other acidic beverages, says Thomas M. Cooper, DDS, professor emeritus at the University of Kentucky. "By making your urine more acidic, you clear your body of nicotine faster, which is what you don't want if you're trying to minimize withdrawal with a nicotine replacement product," he explains.

This differs from the advice smokers received when going cold turkey was the only method available. At the time, smokers were urged to use lots of orange juice, grapefruit juice, and other acidic beverages to speed the elimination of nicotine from the body. Today, however, Dr. Cooper recommends eating more vegetables if you're on nicotine replacement therapy. They'll make your urine more alkaline, which will slow the elimination of nicotine from the body, and therefore minimize withdrawal symptoms.

Nix the alcohol. Smoking and heavy drinking each have devastating effects on the pancreas, which, combined, can put you at higher risk for diabetes. Alcoholism can cause inflammation of the pancreas, which hinders the organ's ability to secrete insulin. In the meantime, smoking increases blood sugar levels and makes it harder for your body to use insulin. Also, the chemicals in tobacco may damage blood vessels, muscles, and organs, which can lead to diabetes.

One of vitamin E's most important functions for smokers is slowing the progression of atherosclerosis, a condition in which the coronary arteries harden from deposits of cholesterol, calcium, and scar tissue, gradually restricting bloodflow and leading to heart disease. Studies show that before atherosclerosis can occur, LDL cholesterol, the "bad" kind, has to undergo oxidation-related changes that allow it to deposit on artery walls. Vitamin E helps prevent those changes.

Additionally, investigators believe that vitamin E's ability to scavenge free radicals can protect tissues from smoke irritation and discourage the cell mutation that marks cancer and other tobacco-associated chronic diseases.

If you smoke, getting enough vitamin E is important. Research has found that the levels of several antioxidants are lower in smokers than in nonsmokers, even when both are getting the same amount in their diet. Smoking produces so many free radicals that antioxidants are used up quickly to fight them. The problem is that smokers, in general, don't eat as well as nonsmokers.

For optimum effects, experts recommend getting 100 to 200 IU of vitamin E a day. Since you would have to eat between 10 and 20 cups of foods such as chopped kale and diced sweet potatoes to reach that amount, supplements are generally called for.

Beta-Carotene Protection

Ever notice how Popeye is able to puff away on that pipe, yet never suffer from the smoking-related ailments typically seen in a man his age? That may be the result of his penchant for spinach, a vegetable rich in beta-carotene, which appears to have protective, immunity-building effects against cancer.

But before you start popping beta-carotene, you should know that although supplementation is considered okay by most experts, doctors say it's even better to eat beta-carotene-rich foods such as spinach and other dark green leafy vegetables, as well as cantaloupe, carrots, and other orange and yellow fruits and vegetables. Why? Because studies show that beta-carotene is good, but it's probably not the whole story.

On the one hand, myriad small studies have found positive results from beta-carotene supplementation in smokers. Canadian researchers, for example, found that 25 smokers experienced significant reductions in oxidation-related damage after receiving 20 milligrams (about 33,000 IU) of beta-carotene daily for just 4 weeks.

But in one large study from Finland of 29,133 male heavy smokers between 50 and 69 years of age, those who received the same amount of beta-carotene for 5 to 8 years not only didn't reap any benefits but actually experienced a higher incidence of lung cancer.

Which study should we believe? Both, says Jeffrey Blumberg, PhD, director of the antioxidants research laboratory at the Jean Mayer USDA Human Nutrition Research Center on Aging at Tufts University in Boston. Dr. Blumberg contends that the Finnish study represents what we already know: "You can't undo a lifetime of damage by taking a vitamin pill for five years."

"That population was at extraordinarily high risk," says Dr. Blumberg. "They smoked an average of a pack a day for 30 years. Most of them were overweight. They had high cholesterol. They had moderate to high alcohol consumption. It would have been a public health nightmare if the study had worked, because it would have said 'Smoke and drink and eat all you want. This pill can turn around all of the damage.'"

Actually, the group in the Finnish study that did not receive supplements also taught us something, says Dr. Blumberg. "Among the people who weren't supplemented, those who had the highest blood levels of beta-carotene had the lower risk of lung cancer," he says.

The bottom line? Dr. Blumberg doesn't recommend separate beta-carotene supplements, but says it's okay to get small amounts in a multivitamin.

Finally, it's as important to remember that beta-carotene is just one of many related substances called carotenoids that protect the body from cell damage. It's best to strive for getting as much of your beta-carotene intake as possible from foods. Foods rich in beta-carotene include carrots, pumpkin, cantaloupe, apricots, sweet potatoes, mangos, collard greens, broccoli, kale, spinach, and other orange, red, and dark green fruits and vegetables. If you're having trouble meeting your needs in this way, then talk to your doctor about supplementation.

Vitamin C for Healthy Cells and Sperm

It's a joke among male smokers that they don't feel as bad about smoking when they buy packs with the "Do not smoke while pregnant" warning on the side panel. Well, according to researchers, it may be time for male smokers to get a warning of their own.

Studies have found a connection linking smoking, low levels of ascorbic acid (vitamin C), and sperm abnormalities. These abnormalities could play roles not only in infertility in men but also in birth defects and childhood cancer in their offspring, the studies show.

"We've known that many gene mutations come through the male line, but since women carry the babies, most of the birth defect studies are done on women," says Bruce Ames, PhD, professor of biochemistry and molecular biology at the University of California, Berkeley, and senior scientist at Children's Hospital Oakland Research Institute. "We're looking into the effects of paternal smoking on sperm damage, and the effects of antioxidant depletion are significant."

Smokers must ingest two to three times the daily intake of vitamin C recommended for nonsmokers, or about 180 milligrams, just to maintain comparable levels of ascorbic acid, says Dr. Ames. He has also found that as a group, smokers tend to make their deficiencies worse by not eating enough vitamin C-rich foods.

While studying the vitamin C consumption of 22 smokers and 27 nonsmokers, Dr. Ames and his colleagues found that the smokers consumed less vitamin C than the nonsmokers. In addition, the level of oxidative damage in the sperm was 52 percent higher in the smokers than in the nonsmokers.

Of course, sperm are not alone in their need for vitamin C. The rest of your body, whether you're male or female, needs it, too. Vitamin C maintains your tissues, promotes healing, and boosts immunity. And because smokers have too little vitamin C in their bodies and need more vitamin C to fight free radical damage, experts suggest that they take much more than nonsmokers: up to 2,000 milligrams a day, if they are older and smoke heavily. Researchers say that smoking produces so much oxidative damage that smokers need large amounts of vitamin C to combat it. Just keep in mind that the Daily Value for vitamin C is only 60 milligrams. Higher amounts are considered safe but may cause diarrhea in some people.

Calcium May Help Prevent Bone Loss

Research shows that people who smoke, especially women, accelerate the bone loss that occurs naturally with age, putting them at greater risk for osteoporosis, a condition of brittle, easily fractured bones.

In fact, a study done at the University of Melbourne in Australia looked

Prescriptions for Healing

Let's say it again: If you smoke, the only way to truly prevent smoking-related diseases is to quit. In the meantime, however, some doctors recommend these nutrients to help preserve your health.

Nutrient	Daily Amount
B-complex supplement containing . . .	
Biotin	300 micrograms
Folic acid	400 micrograms
Niacin	20 milligrams
Pantothenic acid	10 milligrams
Riboflavin	1.7 milligrams
Thiamin	1.5 milligrams
Vitamin B$_6$	2 milligrams
Vitamin B$_{12}$	6 micrograms
Calcium	1,500 milligrams
Vitamin C	180–2,000 milligrams
Vitamin E	100–200 IU

Plus a multivitamin/mineral supplement containing the Daily Values of all essential vitamins and minerals

MEDICAL ALERT: *Some people may experience diarrhea when taking vitamin C in doses that exceed 1,200 milligrams daily.*

If you are taking anticoagulant drugs, you should not take vitamin E supplements. (Though generally a dose of up to 1,500 IU of vitamin E a day is considered safe, some recent reports suggest that taking more than 400 IU a day could be harmful to people with cardiovascular or circulatory disease or with cancer. If you have such a condition, be sure to consult your doctor before you begin supplementation.)

at 41 pairs of female twins between 27 and 73 years of age in which one of the twins smoked and the other did not. The researchers reported that by the time the women reach menopause, those who smoked a pack a day throughout adulthood had an average bone density deficit of 5 to 10 percent compared with those who were smoke-free.

Though the only surefire way to stem this bone deterioration is to snuff your cigarette habit, some doctors recommend stepping up your calcium intake in the meantime to nourish your bones. And while it will help to increase your intake of calcium-filled foods, including low-fat dairy products and certain vegetables such as broccoli, the best way to get the 1,500 milligrams that experts recommend is through supplements.

Better Body Function with B Complex

Because the B vitamins are essential for maintaining physical and mental fitness and healthy skin, eyes, nerves, and tissues—things that are deteriorated by smoking—many experts also recommend taking supplements of the B-complex vitamins.

Especially important, say researchers, is folic acid, a nutrient that is often deficient in smokers and one that your lungs love. Studies have shown that increased folic acid intake can lessen symptoms of bronchitis as well as reduce the number of abnormal or precancerous bronchial cells in smokers. Plus inadequate folic acid intake has been linked to increased susceptibility to cancerous changes in the lungs of smokers.

Some doctors recommend taking a B-complex supplement that contains the Daily Values of all of the B vitamins.

Finish Off with a Multivitamin

Smoking depletes the body of all vitamins, and a multivitamin/mineral supplements will help restore some of what's lost.

SUNBURN

PROTECTING YOURSELF
FROM HARMFUL RAYS

You're all ready for a day at the beach. You have a blanket, a radio, and a big bottle of baby oil . . . oops. Nix the oil. You've heard the warnings about ultraviolet rays and skin cancer, so it's on with the sunscreen instead, right?

Right. But somehow, whether it's from snoozing too long in the midday warmth or forgetting to reapply your lotion after a dip in the ocean, you, like most people, probably still manage an occasional burn. Maybe not one of the Maine lobster scorches that you got as a kid, but a fairly vivid shade of pink nonetheless. Worse yet, studies show that even if you never forget your sunscreen, unless you block out 100 percent of the ultraviolet rays, lolling in the sun will damage your skin whether you burn or not.

What's a sun worshiper to do—carry a parasol? That certainly helps, say the experts. Limiting your time in the sun, especially during midday hours, is absolutely essential. And if you want some extra protection, take your vitamins and minerals. According to research, oral supplements of vitamin E and selenium, as well as topical applications of vitamins C and E, can give your sunscreen a boost by partially preventing the skin damage that occurs once you've been exposed.

How Sunburn Does Damage

To understand how vitamins and minerals can help shield you from sun damage, it helps to know how that damage comes about in the first place.

Sunlight exposes skin to two types of ultraviolet rays: UVA and UVB. UVB rays are high-intensity rays absorbed by the surface of the skin. They are the primary cause of sunburn and immediate skin damage. UVA rays are of lower intensity, but they penetrate below the skin's surface, causing long-term damage such as premature wrinkles.

Both types do significant damage by forming free radicals, unstable molecules that steal electrons from your body's healthy molecules to stabilize themselves. Though some free radicals are formed during everyday functions

Food Factors

Although there are no foods that you can eat to protect your skin from the sun, there are a few that can add fuel to the fire. Here's what you might want to avoid before a day at the shore.

Don't be a silly rabbit. While you certainly shouldn't stop eating carrots, these vegetables, along with celery, parsley, parsnips, and limes, contain psoralens, chemicals that may make you unusually sensitive to the sun.

"Though most people would have to eat huge amounts of these foods before they would have problems, some people are really sensitive to these chemicals. For them, the effects can be quite nasty," says Douglas Darr, PhD, a biotechnology industry consultant in Research Triangle Park, North Carolina.

And even if you're not psoralen-sensitive, you should wash your hands after handling these fruits and vegetables, because anyone's skin can be more susceptible to burning after direct contact with the chemical.

Eat the whole orange. According to one study, eating the peel of oranges and other citrus fruits may lower your chances of developing squamous-cell carcinoma. Biting into the peel is the key, the study found. Drinking the juices isn't enough. An alternative would be to grate the zest on top of salads or into homemade salad dressings.

such as breathing, environmental stress factors such as sun exposure create additional droves of them.

Although you have natural defenses against free radicals generated by sun exposure, they often aren't enough. Sunscreen does a good job of protecting you, but many brands still block predominantly UVB rays. Even those that block both UVB and UVA rays generally allow some exposure. Look for a sunscreen labeled "broad-spectrum coverage," suggests Douglas Darr, PhD, a biotechnology industry consultant in Research Triangle Park, North Carolina. And look for the ingredients oxybenzone and methoxycinnamate, which absorb some UVA rays. Remember that only clothing and zinc oxide totally block UVB and UVA rays.

Fortunately for your skin and your body, there are chemical substances that mop up free radicals by offering them electrons, sparing healthy molecules from harm. These substances, known as antioxidants, include vitamins C and E and the mineral selenium. Sun exposure, however, quickly depletes your skin's supply of these antioxidants.

Although you can get some protection through oral supplementation of these nutrients, researchers agree that the best protection generally comes from topical application.

In the past, you had to apply a cream with antioxidants separately from your sunscreen, but today you can buy sunscreen with antioxidant vitamins C and E built right in.

"No one is proposing that vitamins will ever replace sunscreen, but they can make sunscreen better. It would also be nice to replace some of the chemicals in sunscreen with vitamins," says Dr. Darr. "Right now we're soaking in all of these chemicals that are photodecomposing into unknown compounds. And because there are no lifetime studies, we can't make the blanket statement that they are completely safe."

Here's what the research says about adding vitamins and minerals to your sun protection regimen.

The Vitamin C Solution

Vitamin C is well known for its role as a collagen (skin tissue) builder when used topically. It's also a pretty impressive sun protectant, say the experts. But don't get it confused with sunscreen, says John C. Murray, MD, professor of medicine at Duke University School of Medicine. Vitamin C creams can't absorb ultraviolet rays.

"Sunscreen is a chemical that acts as a shield and absorbs ultraviolet light, so you're not as red," he explains. "Vitamin C is a photoprotectant. It possibly works by scavenging the free radicals caused by sun exposure."

Also, unlike sunscreen, you can't wash off vitamin C, says Dr. Murray. "Once you put it on, it's soaked into your skin," he says. "You can't rub it off."

To measure vitamin C's effectiveness, researchers at Duke University Medical Center studied ten fair-skinned individuals. They found that when the volunteers applied a 10 percent vitamin C solution, the amount of ultraviolet light needed for them to burn increased by an average of 22 percent for nine of them. And once they did burn, half of the volunteers experienced much less severe burns than they would have without the solution.

In another study, topical vitamin C decreased the amount of sunburned cells and began to repair damaged skin when it was applied 30 to 60 minutes after the skin was exposed to ultraviolet rays.

But if you plan on trying vitamin C, don't try spraying your skin with orange juice; you'll just make yourself sticky, says Dr. Murray. "Vitamin C is very unstable," he says. "It needs to be in a special preparation to stay effective."

Extra Protection with Vitamin E

Like vitamin C, vitamin E is a free radical scavenger. But unlike vitamin C, vitamin E is being recommended by researchers for after-sun use, rather than presun use, to soothe your skin and prevent a burn after exposure.

In fact, it's even effective if you apply it a half day later, say researchers at the University of Western Ontario in London, Ontario, but it's better to do it as soon as possible. In studies using laboratory animals, the researchers found that vitamin E acetate, which converts to vitamin E in the body, prevented inflammation, skin sensitivity, and skin damage when applied up to 8 hours following UVB exposure.

Vitamin E can also work from the inside out. As an oral supplement, it can significantly reduce the inflammation and skin damage caused by sun exposure, says Karen E. Burke, MD, Ph.D., a dermatologic surgeon and dermatologist in private practice in New York City. If you are inadvertently exposed to sun, take a lot of natural vitamin E (d-alpha-tocopherol, d-alpha-tocopheryl acetate, or d-alpha-tocopheryl succinate): five capsules of 400 IU each for 1 to 2 days, says Dr. Burke. For optimum protection, Dr. Burke recommends taking daily supplements of 400 IU of vitamin E in the form of d-alpha-tocopherol. (It's okay to take oral vitamin E before you go out in the sun.)

Another reason to take vitamin E: Along with vitamins C and A, it's been shown in animal studies and human epidemiological research to lower the risk of basal cell carcinoma. According to a study done in France, 25 volunteers who took daily doses of various antioxidants (including vitamin E, selenium, beta-carotene, and lycopene) for 7 weeks were lees likely to get sunburned.

To boost your intake of vitamin E, try cooking with sunflower oil or safflower oil and adding more nuts, whole grains, and wheat germ to your daily fare. Although vitamin E oil and vitamin E-fortified creams can be bought over the counter in drugstores, these products almost always contain only the low concentrations of the inactive ester forms (also a mixture of 32 synthetic molecular forms, not the natural vitamin E d-alpha-tocopherol), which can cause allergies, and they're not very effective in reducing sun damage, says Dr. Burke.

Prescriptions for Healing

Unlike the usual prescriptions, wearing your nutrients is often better than taking them when it comes to sunburn. Here are the doses that some doctors say work best against sun damage.

Nutrient	Daily Amount/Application
Oral	
Selenium	50–200 micrograms (l-selenomethionine)
Vitamin E	400 IU (d-alpha-tocopherol), taken before sun exposure
	2,000 IU, taken as 5 divided doses of 400 IU each, for 1 or 2 days after sun exposure
Topical	
Vitamin C	10% lotion
Vitamin E	5%–100% cream or oil, applied after sun exposure
Zinc oxide	As an ointment

MEDICAL ALERT: Selenium can be toxic in high amounts. For this reason, doctors recommend that doses exceeding 400 micrograms daily be taken only under medical supervision.

If you are taking anticoagulant drugs, you should not take oral vitamin E supplements. (Though generally a dose of up to 1,500 IU of vitamin E a day is considered safe, some recent reports suggest that taking more than 400 IU a day could be harmful to people with cardiovascular or circulatory disease or with cancer. If you have such a condition, be sure to consult your doctor before you begin supplementation.)

Vitamin E creams and oils contain the ester form of the nutrient, which can cause allergic reactions in some people.

Antioxidant Cocktails

While using vitamins C and E separately will go a long way toward giving you extra protection from the sun, the latest research shows that combining antioxidants within one topical application actually works better than any single antioxidant can.

A new serum developed by Sheldon Pinnell, MD, distinguished professor emeritus of dermatology at Duke University and a consultant for SkinCeuticals, called C E Ferulic, combines vitamin C, vitamin E, and the plant antioxidant ferulic acid in one topical application. It helps prevent skin damage and premature aging from the sun, enhances collagen production, and helps prevent DNA mutations related to skin cancer. It also reduces sunburn cells.

During his research, Dr. Pinnell discovered that adding ferulic acid to the serum doubled the photoprotection of the serum, compared to a topical formula that used only vitamins C and E.

Since sunscreen doesn't give you 100 percent protection from the sun's rays and studies have shown that people tend to apply one-fourth to one-fifth the amount of sunscreen required to give them optimum protection, turning to antioxidants will help fill in the gaps.

But don't skip your sunscreen when you take C E Ferulic. The serum should be used along with a broad-spectrum sunscreen because the products work in different ways. Sunscreen literally blocks the sun's rays and absorbs energy in the UVAs/UVBs, Dr. Pinnell says. Antioxidants, on the other hand, get into the skin and neutralize oxidative stress.

You apply the serum by placing about six to eight drops on your face and a few drops on your hands and rubbing them in. C E Ferulic is produced by SkinCeuticals and is found at spas and doctor's offices. To find a dealer near you, go to www.skinceuticals.com and click on Products/Find a Dealer.

Selenium Also Shines

Like vitamins C and E, the mineral selenium can quench free radicals at the cellular level, says Dr. Burke, thereby reducing the inflammation and skin damage associated with too much sun.

Although she's hoping that a cream will soon be available that can be used as an adjunct to sunscreen, Dr. Burke says that in the meantime, you can get some of the benefits by taking selenium supplements.

For best results, she suggests taking 50 to 200 micrograms of selenium in the form of l-selenomethionine, depending on where you live and your family history of cancer. Superior food sources of selenium include fish, such as tuna and salmon, as well as cabbage. Selenium can be toxic in very high doses, so you should take no more than 400 micrograms daily; such higher amounts should be taken only under medical supervision. Children shouldn't take selenium supplements until they have their adult teeth.

Zinc Oxide: The Lifeguard's Standby

You know the white stuff that lifeguards wear on their noses? It's zinc oxide, and it may look funny, but it's a great skin protectant.

"In this case, the zinc is acting not as a micronutrient but as a physical blocker of ultraviolet light," explains Norman Levine, MD, a retired professor in the dermatology unit at the University of Arizona College of Medicine in Tucson. "And it does a terrific job."

If you don't like the white, zinc oxide is now being broken down into nearly invisible particles and put into sunblocks. It's also available in designer colors, for those who like their zinc on the wild side.

And remember, since zinc works as a topical barrier, upping your dietary zinc may make you healthier, but it won't protect your skin.

SURGERY

MINDING YOUR MENDING

No doubt about it: Surgery is a major insult to your body. Even though it's done with the best of intentions and in a clean environment, your body needs to put out extra effort to mend from even minor surgery. And while you're recuperating, you're more vulnerable than usual to pneumonia, bed-sores, urinary tract infections, and other kinds of infections.

That's why good nutrition is vital both before and after surgery. "It gives your body the building blocks to fight off infection, replenish lost blood, and mend tissues, all things that can help you heal as quickly as possible with the least pain and discomfort," explains Ray C. Wunderlich Jr., MD, PhD, a doctor in St. Petersburg, Florida, who practices nutritional/preventive medicine and health promotion and author of *Natural Alternatives to Antibiotics*.

Medical experts are well aware that every single nutrient your body normally needs is also needed when you're facing surgery, including everything from calories and protein to copper and vitamin B_6. "Keep in mind that every person's condition when undergoing surgery is different, so the types of vitamins and minerals that your doctor prescribes for you, if any, will depend on your own particular case," says Joanne Curran-Celentano, PhD, professor

Taking Your Supplements to the Hospital

You may not think twice about packing up your supplements when you're heading to the hospital, but don't be surprised if they're confiscated once you get there.

Vitamins are considered drugs and may contain chemicals that interact with the medications your doctor prescribes in the hospital, says Linda LaRue, RN, a former head nurse at the Pritikin Longevity Center in Santa Monica, California, and a Los Angeles-based athletic trainer for her own mind-body company called reZeneration, Inc. Some supplements can interfere with the narcotic drugs you may be given to relieve pain.

That doesn't mean you're forbidden from continuing your supplements while you're in the hospital, but you do need to talk with your doctor in the days leading up to your surgery about the vitamins and minerals you take. If they won't interfere with the drugs you're given during your hospital stay, your doctor is likely to give you clearance to bring them with you.

In some cases, the nurses will take your supplements and dispense them to you so they can keep a record of just how much you're taking. There's good reason for this, LaRue says. "People don't make the best decisions when they're being medicated and they're in pain," she says. A nurse will ensure that you don't end up taking too much.

of nutritional sciences at the University of New Hampshire in Durham. "Because of the wide range of problems and conditions surrounding surgery, it is recommended that anyone who is about to undergo surgery check with his doctor before taking any kind of supplementation." Although many nutrients are essential to proper healing, just as many can interfere with the medications and dosages your doctor may prescribe, she says. That's why it's important to always tell your doctor about all of the vitamin and herbal supplements you take before surgery.

Not all doctors have the same approach to nutritional therapy and surgery. If you are facing surgery and want to pay special attention to nutrients that might be helpful, you'll have to find a doctor who uses methods that you feel most comfortable with.

Here are a few key nutrients that some doctors believe are important for getting your body on the high road to healing.

Vitamin C Speeds Healing

Doctors know that any kind of trauma, including surgery, can pull the plug on your vitamin C stores. After surgery, blood levels of vitamin C drop rapidly. And it's no secret that a vitamin C deficiency makes wounds heal slower. Delayed healing was noted hundreds of years ago in sailors with scurvy, a mystery disease at the time that turned out to be nothing more than severe vitamin C deficiency. "Today, it's more likely that people simply won't be getting enough vitamin C for optimum healing," Dr. Wunderlich says.

Many studies have shown that vitamin C is essential for the body to produce wound-healing collagen, which provides the basic structure for many tissues, including skin, bone, and blood vessels. Vitamin C is also needed for the skin to produce elastin, a tissue that lets wounds stretch without breaking.

Vitamin C also helps maintain a healthy immune system, vital for anyone who's undergoing surgery, Dr. Wunderlich says.

Finding Healthy Hospital Fare

You're going to the hospital, so the last thing you may be thinking about is the food you're going to be served. But, as you know, nutrition is an important part of the healing process. With this in mind, many hospitals are transforming mushy green beans, limp salad, and processed meats into food you'd get in a five-star restaurant. Even better, you choose what you want from a three-page menu and it's made fresh and delivered to your room in 30 minutes.

About 30 percent of hospitals in the United States are offering this type of hotel room service, says chef/dietitian Don Miller, the owner of a San Diego company that helps hospitals transform their food service operations. "Hospitals are in the middle of a huge revolution," he says.

Even food that follows diabetic, low-salt, or low-calorie diets—meals that typically are considered lacking in flavor—are now tasty and appealing. "Health care professionals have come to the realization that if the food tastes bad, the patient won't eat it," Miller says. "And having a patient who doesn't eat can do harm to the healing and recovery process."

You'll even find the transformation in hospital cafeterias. Tuscan-style cafés are pushing out the traditional cafeterias, and you're more likely to find ethnic foods from around the world being served.

Food Factors

Major surgery with general anesthesia requires a delicate approach to eating. Anesthesia anesthetizes your entire body, including your gastrointestinal tract.

"Until it wakes up, it's not moving," says Linda LaRue, RN, a former head nurse at the Pritikin Longevity Center in Santa Monica, California, and a Los Angeles-based athletic trainer for her own mind-body company called reZeneration, Inc. Eating too much too soon after surgery may cause some people to vomit. If they've had abdominal surgery, the vomiting can cause a rip in their incision, so that's why it's important to take it slow.

Sip clear liquids. Within hours after surgery you'll be given clear liquids, such as apple juice, and soft foods, such as gelatin or pudding. Start with small sips to prevent vomiting, LaRue says. You'll be on liquids and soft foods for about 6 to 8 hours after surgery.

Intravenous therapy will keep you hydrated and give you nutrients and electrolytes. Once you're taken off an IV, continue to drink 6 to 8 eight-ounce glasses of fluids a day. It's key to staying hydrated and flushing out the bladder, which is prone to infection if you've had a urinary catheter.

Eat light. Once the nurse hears a gurgling sound or audible bowel sounds in your GI tract with a stethoscope, you'll be able to eat a light meal of 300 calories or less, LaRue says. Again, it's important to take it slow because your GI system is just starting to get moving again.

Find a friend in fiber. An important part of your first meals after surgery is fiber, because your next step is to have a bowel movement, LaRue says. Many people turn to prunes, prune juice, fruits, vegetables, legumes, whole grains, or the kind of fiber that will help prevent constipation. Often you won't be released from the hospital until you have a bowel movement or at least pass gas, she says. Once that happens, you're ready for a regular meal.

Pick up some protein. Once you're eating normally again, make sure you're getting good amounts of protein, such as chicken, tuna, and turkey. "Major injuries call for increased protein," says Thomas K. Hunt, MD, professor emeritus of surgery and director of the wound healing laboratory at the University of California, San Francisco. But don't increase your calorie intake, which could cause an insulin response in your body. "It is now clear that high blood sugar impedes resistance to infection," Dr. Hunt says.

One study, by Russian researchers, found that people who had gallbladder surgery who received 200 to 250 milligrams of supplemental vitamin C a day were able to leave the hospital 1 or 2 days earlier than people who simply got their vitamin C from foods.

In another study, doctors gave patients in a surgical intensive care unit 1,000 milligrams of vitamin C intravenously and 1,000 IU of vitamin E by mouth for 28 days or less, depending on when they were discharged from intensive care. Among the 595 patients who received the antioxidants, 57 percent had a significantly lower incidence of multiple organ failure compared with the control group. The group receiving the antioxidants also was discharged from the intensive care unit 17 percent faster than patients who didn't receive the antioxidants. At most hospitals, you're expected to get your vitamin C from foods such as citrus juices and fruits. Eight ounces of orange juice, for instance, offers about 124 milligrams, while one orange has about 70 milligrams.

Some doctors, however, recommend amounts of vitamin C that are much higher than you normally obtain from foods alone. Dr. Wunderlich believes this to be especially important when you're recovering from surgery.

He tells his patients that "if you can take 1,000 milligrams of buffered or esterified vitamin C every eight hours for two weeks before and several weeks after surgery, you'll most likely be able to keep the vitamin C in your blood at a level that promotes optimum healing." Some people experience diarrhea and other digestive discomforts from such high levels of vitamin C. Buffered vitamin C and esterified vitamin C (a slow-release form) are easier on the stomach, says Dr. Wunderlich. Vitamin C can interfere with the results of certain diagnostic blood and urine tests, however, so it's important that you discuss supplementation with your doctor.

Dr. Wunderlich also recommends 1,000 milligrams of bioflavonoids a day to some of his patients. These chemical compounds are related to vitamin C and are often found in the same foods as the vitamin, especially citrus fruits. Dr. Wunderlich maintains that bioflavonoids can help maintain blood vessel strength and control inflammation.

Vitamin A Mends Skin

Vitamin A has been called the skin vitamin, and with good reason. At burn centers such as Shriners Burns Institute in Cincinnati, large amounts of vitamin A are added to liquid formulas designed to help prevent infection and promote the growth of new skin.

In studies with laboratory animals, vitamin A enhances healing that has been retarded by steroid drugs, immune suppression, diabetes, or radiation, reports Thomas K. Hunt, MD, professor emeritus of surgery and director of the wound healing laboratory at the University of California, San Francisco.

"Vitamin A works in many different ways," Dr. Hunt says. "It's required for cell growth and differentiation, or the ability of a cell to mature into its final form. This is important for the generation of new tissues." Vitamin A also seems to activate the production of connective tissue, including collagen, and to promote the growth of new blood vessels, he explains. That's important for nourishing newly forming tissues.

"Adequate vitamin A really is essential for anyone undergoing surgery," Dr. Wunderlich agrees. He recommends up to 25,000 IU of water-soluble vitamin A (available in health food stores) for certain patients undergoing surgery. Vitamin A can be toxic in doses exceeding 15,000 IU daily and has been found to cause birth defects in doses of 10,000 IU daily when taken during early pregnancy. For this reason, the dosage of vitamin A recommended here should be taken only under medical supervision, especially if you are a woman of childbearing age. And you should not use this therapy if you are pregnant.

Studies show that most people get about 5,000 IU of vitamin A per day from foods such as carrots, eggs, and vitamin A-fortified milk.

Zinc Zeros In on Tissue Repair

Medical research shows that in people who are low in zinc, supplements can dramatically speed up the healing of surgical incisions. In a study by researchers at Wright-Patterson Air Force Base in Ohio, people taking 220 milligrams of zinc sulfate three times a day were completely healed in roughly 46 days, while a group taking no zinc required about 80 days to heal.

Zinc, like vitamins A and C, is needed in the body for many things, Dr. Wunderlich says. It's necessary for the production of collagen, the connective tissue that allows scars to form. It interacts with vitamin A, making the vitamin available for use. And it plays a vital role in immune function.

Diarrhea can lead to loss of zinc, and people who have had gastrointestinal surgery or digestive disorders are at risk for being deficient in zinc, according to the National Institutes of Health. There isn't a test that can tell doctors if patients are losing zinc, but signs of a deficiency include hair loss, appetite loss, weight loss, delayed healing, and taste problems.

Dr. Wunderlich recommends 15 milligrams of zinc citrate (an easily absorbed form) twice daily to a number of his patients undergoing surgery. It's best to take this much zinc only under your doctor's care, as amounts exceeding 15 milligrams daily can be toxic.

Vitamin E: For Healing Hearts

Some doctors add vitamin E to their on-the-mend menus, especially for people who've had heart surgery. There's some evidence that vitamin E helps stop the process of atherosclerosis, or the buildup of fatty deposits in arteries. And one study, by researchers at the University of Toronto, suggests that it can also help limit tissue damage during coronary bypass surgery.

In this study, half of a group of people undergoing bypass surgery took vitamin E before their operations. The other half took placebos (inactive pills). After the surgery, the people taking 300 IU of vitamin E for 2 weeks prior to surgery had "small but significant" improvement in heart function compared with the people taking the placebos.

Heart cells can be damaged when their blood supply is cut off and then restarted, a condition called reperfusion injury. When oxygenated blood circulates through the oxygen-deprived heart, free radicals can form and can injure the heart cells. (Free radicals are unstable molecules that steal electrons from your body's healthy molecules to balance themselves.)

Vitamin E is known as an antioxidant. In the right place at the right time, it neutralizes harmful free radicals by giving up its own electrons, sparing healthy molecules from harm.

The University of Toronto study suggests that for people at high risk—those with unstable angina, for instance—treatment with vitamin E prior to bypass surgery may be of benefit. (For people who require immediate surgery, a water-soluble form of vitamin E can be given intravenously just prior to or during surgery.)

Prescriptions for Healing

Every nutrient is important when it comes to bouncing back from surgery. The problem is that nutrient needs vary widely depending upon your current nutritional status and the kind of procedure that you'll be having. Your best bet is to have a frank discussion about nutrition with your doctor well before your surgery. Many doctors recommend that their patients take multivitamin/mineral supplements both before and after surgery. Some suggest additional supplements as well. You should let your doctor know what you are currently taking and ask whether any changes are in order.

Doctors who recommend vitamin E to their surgery patients often prescribe about 400 IU of vitamin E daily. Don't take more than 400 IU without your doctor's okay, especially if you've had a stroke or bleeding problems in the past. "In large amounts, I'd say more than 800 international units, vitamin E can enhance bleeding problems," Dr. Wunderlich says. If you're taking anticoagulants, it's best not to take vitamin E supplements.

In fact, when you're going into surgery, it's a good idea to be aware of any and all nutritional therapy you are taking that might interfere with blood clotting, Dr. Wunderlich advises. "Some of my heart patients take garlic for their conditions, and since garlic can cause bleeding problems, I recommend stopping the garlic for a few weeks prior to surgery," he says.

"Remember, taking any kind of supplementation may interfere with your surgical procedure and recovery," says Dr. Curran-Celentano. "To be safe, take supplements only under medical supervision." A few weeks prior to surgery, you might want to discuss any supplements you've been taking with your doctor.

The most commonly offered bit of advice, from doctors and dietitians alike? Ask your doctor about taking a multivitamin/mineral supplement that provides the Daily Value of every essential nutrient. And if necessary, get enough protein and calories by adding nutritional liquids to your menu.

TASTE AND SMELL PROBLEMS

SENSE-SATIONAL NUTRITION

Imagine being unable to smell a bank of honeysuckle blooming along a country road or to savor the sweetness of a freshly picked raspberry. Most of us would feel seriously deprived if we were denied these simple pleasures.

Unfortunately, that's what happens to people with taste and smell problems. (The two senses are so closely linked that people who can't smell often complain that they can't taste anything, either.)

For some people, these two vital senses may tend to decrease with age, for no apparent reason. For others, taste and smell drop off quickly, the result of a viral infection, a head injury, or cancer therapy or as a side effect of certain prescription drugs.

People may also develop disturbing sensory changes, such as a metallic, bitter, or salty taste that can occur by itself or be triggered by foods (citrus is a common culprit). In some cases, senses recover after a time, although they may never be as sharp as they once were.

Although most physicians are unfamiliar with these problems, it's still best to seek medical attention if something seems to be wrong with your

---

Prescriptions for Healing

Doctors who recognize the role that nutrition can play agree that most taste and smell disorders are not caused by zinc deficiency alone but that deficiency may be a factor. Here's what these doctors recommend.

Nutrient	Daily Amount
Zinc	30 milligrams (zinc acetate or zinc gluconate)

MEDICAL ALERT: Doses of zinc exceeding 15 milligrams daily should be taken only under medical supervision, as high amounts of this mineral can be toxic.

---

sense of taste or smell. See your family doctor or an ear, nose, and throat specialist, or call the nearest university hospital to find out if there's a taste and smell clinic nearby. Such centers draw on a variety of specialists to troubleshoot the problem.

While there are any number of treatments that your doctor may consider, you should be aware that one nutrient has definitely been linked to taste and smell disorders: zinc, an essential mineral, according to researcher Robert Henkin, MD, PhD, director of the Taste and Smell Clinic of the Center for Molecular Nutrition and Sensory Disorders in Washington, DC. Here's the latest thinking—and controversy—on this connection.

Zinc May Account for Good Taste

There's no doubt that people with severe zinc deficiencies, which are rare in the United States, often lose their sense of taste. But there's one thing that many of the doctors who treat taste and smell disorders apparently do not know (or believe, for some reason): Even a relatively mild zinc deficiency can cause problems, says leading zinc researcher Ananda Prasad, MD, PhD, professor of medicine at Wayne State University School of Medicine in Detroit.

"Years ago in Iran, we found aberrations in taste in young boys who were zinc-deficient. Their growth and sexual maturity were retarded, and they ate clay," he explains. (Eating clay is a strange deficiency symptom known as geophagia.) "More recently, we found that volunteers made mildly zinc-deficient also lost some of their taste acuity."

The volunteers, all healthy young men, weren't being seriously deprived of zinc, Dr. Prasad says. They ate what might be considered a fairly typical vegetarian diet, getting about 5 milligrams of zinc a day, one-third of the Daily Value. And they ate soy as their main source of protein. "Soy and grains contain phytates, compounds that interfere with the absorption of a variety of nutrients, including zinc," Dr. Prasad explains. The volunteers' sense of taste diminished after 6 months on the diet. (They also developed problems adapting their eyes to darkness.)

When these people were supplemented with 30 milligrams of zinc a day, their ability to taste returned in about 2 to 3 months.

Both taste buds and olfactory (smell) cells, which are found high in the nose, are specialized cells. They depend on zinc, along with other nutrients, for their growth and maintenance, Dr. Prasad explains.

Taste buds are especially dependent on zinc, says Dr. Henkin. He found that cells in the salivary glands make gustin, a zinc-dependent protein that is secreted in saliva. "Gustin is important in maintaining the sensation of taste," Dr. Henkin says. "It acts on the stem cells that are in the taste buds, causing these cells to differentiate and develop into new taste bud cells."

Gustin directly stimulates the stem cells of the taste bud to grow and mature into the multiple cells of the bud, which turn over rapidly through the program provided by the stem cell. In people who have taste problems, the growth of these stem cells is inhibited.

The same system holds true for the nose and a sense of smell. Gustin is secreted in nasal mucus and stimulates stem cells in the olfactory epithelium in the same way it stimulates stem cells in the taste bud, Dr. Henkin says. When the growth of your stem cells is inhibited, you'll have trouble smelling.

In the past, Dr. Henkin believed that about 20 to 25 percent of taste and smell problems were related to zinc deficiencies, but today he and other experts believe it's less common than previously thought. The problems don't necessarily occur because people are zinc-deficient but because their bodies are unable to use zinc properly. "About half of these people benefit from additional zinc, but others don't improve no matter how much zinc they get," he says. He believes that these people have problems making gustin.

Supplementing zinc when a deficiency is the problem will do more than simply replace the nutrient, Dr. Henkin says. Zinc acts as a drug by stimulating the secretion of gustin and correcting the defect. It also acts to prevent the death of cells.

However, gustin is just one member of a family of enzymes that stimulate stem cells, and all of these growth factors are necessary in preserving normal taste and smell. "There is an elegant push-pull in these systems as there are in most systems for both growth and death of cells, which lead to normal sensory function," Dr. Henkin says.

If you believe that your taste or smell problem may be linked to low zinc intake, discuss it with your doctor. And if your doctor recommends blood tests, keep in mind that the most commonly done tests, blood plasma and serum zinc levels, detect only severe deficiency, not mild to moderate deficiency, Dr. Prasad says. He measures the zinc content of lymphocytes (white blood cells), a much more sensitive test performed in only a few laboratories nationwide. Dr. Henkin, on the other hand, uses a measurement of zinc in saliva, which reflects the activity of the zinc-dependent enzyme that stimulates taste bud cells to grow and develop, and in nasal mucus, which reflects the activity of the zinc-dependent enzyme that stimulates olfactory receptor cells to grow and develop. These tests, however, are not readily available.

Dr. Prasad believes most people can safely get up to 30 milligrams of zinc a day from foods and supplements. "More than that amount of zinc may interfere with copper absorption and so requires supplementation of 1 to 2 milligrams of copper daily, along with regular blood tests to check for anemia," he cautions. In addition, it's best to consult your doctor before taking more than 50 milligrams of elemental zinc a day, since this may induce copper deficiency.

Seafood and meats provide the most easily absorbed form of zinc. Eastern oysters are far and away the best source, with six cooked medium-size oysters providing about 76 milligrams of zinc. Three ounces of beef, veal, lamb, crab, or pork provide about 7 milligrams of zinc. If you're taking supplements, zinc acetate and zinc gluconate deliver the goods with less stomach upset than zinc sulfate, Dr. Prasad says.

If zinc is going to improve your taste, it should begin to do so within 3 months, Dr. Prasad says. If you don't notice an improvement by then, it's likely that zinc is not going to help you. You should then cut back to the Daily Value, 15 milligrams, and consider some other cause of your problem, he advises.

Zinc-related sensory abnormalities, including decreased taste and smell acuity and problems adjusting your eyes in the dark, have been associated with a number of conditions, Dr. Prasad reports: liver disease, kidney disease, Crohn's disease, cystic fibrosis, Parkinson's disease, thyroid problems, multiple sclerosis, serious burns, type 2 (non-insulin-dependent) diabetes, flulike infections, sickle-cell anemia, and anorexia. These abnormalities have also been noted in people taking penicillamine, a rheumatoid arthritis drug. Dr. Prasad also believes that vegetarians and older people who don't eat much food, including meats, are often shortchanged on zinc. "Mild deficiency is much more common than most people realize," he says.

TINNITUS

SILENCING THE RING

Most of us have noticed that our ears can play their own tune for a time after being blasted by loud music or machinery, firecrackers, or gunshots. Usually, the sound is barely noticeable, lasting anywhere from a few minutes to a couple of days.

For people with a condition called tinnitus, though, the ringing, hissing, chirping, roaring, or buzzing becomes a persistent presence. Tinnitus, which in Latin means "tinkling like a bell," has been reported to reach volumes as high as 70 decibels. That's equivalent to having a vacuum cleaner in your head.

More than 50 million Americans have had some degree of tinnitus, but about 12 million have had severe cases that require a trip to the doctor. In about 2 million people, the ringing is so severe that they can't function normally.

Tinnitus is often caused by loud noises, such as a jet engine or a rock concert, so it's not surprising that in 90 percent of cases, people with tinnitus

Food Factors

It's hard to believe that what you put in your mouth will have much of an impact on what you hear in your ears, but the food you eat may make the ringing worse.

Avoid additives. You may find that eating sugary foods makes your tinnitus seem louder. Although some people are more susceptible to foods and additives than others, salt, caffeine, simple sugars such as candy and candy bars, monosodium glutamate (MSG), aspartame, food colorings, and alcohol may all have an effect on the ringing in your ears, says Michael Seidman, MD, medical director of the Center for Integrative Medicine at Henry Ford Health System in Detroit, codirector of the Tinnitus Center, and author of *Save Your Hearing Now*.

It's a good idea to pay attention to how your tinnitus responds to the food you eat. Adjusting your diet may give you some relief from the ringing.

Go for ginkgo. Dr. Seidman's patients report that their tinnitus gets better when they take a pure form of ginkgo. In fact, research has found that ginkgo increases bloodflow to the brain, which may mean a better blood supply to the inner ear and an improvement in tinnitus.

But the kind of ginkgo you buy is important. "I found that some people went to the local drugstore and picked up a cheap brand that led to a stomachache and had no effect on their tinnitus," Dr. Seidman says. His other patients who went to a health food store and bought a better-quality brand complained of a headache for the first few days but found that their tinnitus improved.

Now Dr. Seidman recommends that his patients buy Arches Tinnitus Relief formula because it's highly purified and it includes garlic and zinc, which also help with tinnitus. (Dr. Seidman's company, Body Language Vitamin, sells this brand. For more information, visit the company Web site at www.bodylanguagevitamin.com.)

experience hearing loss. If your ears are particularly sensitive, it may take just one blast of a loud noise to set off a ringing or buzzing that doesn't go away. Tinnitus occurs when nerve cells in the cochlea, the tiny, snail-shell-shaped inner ear, are damaged, explains Michael Seidman, MD, medical director of the Center for Integrative Medicine at Henry Ford Health System in Detroit, codirector of the Tinnitus Center, and author of *Save Your Hearing Now*. These nerves project hairlike endings into the cochlea, which is filled with fluid that moves in waves in response to sounds traveling through the ear. When a sound sends waves through the cochlea, the hairlike endings send a signal to the brain that gets interpreted as sound. When the sounds are too loud and the waves through the cochlea are too intense, the tiny nerve endings become damaged and may send abnormal signals that can cause hissing or buzzing.

Noise-induced spasms of the tiny arteries feeding the inner ears can also damage the tiny hairlike cells by cutting off their blood supply. The nerve cells can also be damaged by viruses, high blood pressure, and high blood cholesterol and high insulin levels as well as by drugs, particularly aspirin, some narcotics such as acetaminophen and hydrocodone, and the "-mycin" antibiotics. Aminoglycosides such as gentamicin, which are often used to treat pneumonia, are a top offender, says Dr. Seidman. Tinnitus is often one symptom of Ménière's disease, a condition that is believed to be caused by excess fluid pressure in the inner ear.

Finally, degeneration of the aging ear, usually because of poor circulation, accounts for a large percentage of cases.

If you develop tinnitus, it's important to see a doctor to make sure that you don't have a tumor on an ear nerve or a damaged ear membrane, Dr. Seidman says. Both are treatable conditions.

While most doctors don't yet use nutrition to treat tinnitus, there is some intriguing new research, mostly from Israel, that holds promise for some people with this condition. Here's what doctors say may help.

Vitamin B_{12} Sheathes Ear Nerves

When it comes to nerves, vitamin B_{12} plays a special role. The body needs this nutrient to manufacture myelin, the fatty sheath that wraps around nerve fibers, insulating them and allowing them to conduct their electrical impulses normally.

A vitamin B_{12} deficiency can raise blood levels of homocysteine, an amino acid that is thought to be toxic to nerves. Low levels of B_{12} have been

Prescriptions for Healing

Tinnitus is one of those conditions that often resist treatment. Most ear specialists do not recommend nutrients to prevent or treat tinnitus. Some doctors, however, feel that certain nutrients can be helpful for some people. Here's what they recommend trying.

Nutrient	Daily Amount
Beta-carotene	100,000 IU, taken as two divided doses
Copper	1.5 milligrams (1 milligram for every 10 milligrams of zinc)
Magnesium	400 mg
Selenium	50–200 micrograms
Vitamin B_{12}	1,000 micrograms
Vitamin C	500 milligrams, taken as 2 divided doses
Vitamin E	400 IU
Zinc	15 milligrams

Plus a multivitamin/mineral supplement containing the Daily Values of all essential vitamins and minerals

MEDICAL ALERT: *If you have heart or kidney problems, be sure to talk to your doctor before beginning magnesium supplementation.*

Doses of selenium exceeding 400 micrograms daily can be toxic and should be taken only under medical supervision.

If you are taking anticoagulant drugs, you should not take vitamin E supplements. (Though generally a dose of up to 1,500 IU of vitamin E a day is considered safe, some recent reports suggest that taking more than 400 IU a day could be harmful to people with cardiovascular or circulatory disease or with cancer. If you have such a condition, be sure to consult your doctor before you begin supplementation.)

linked to a number of nervous system disorders, including memory loss, decreased reflexes, impaired touch or pain perception—and, apparently, tinnitus and noise-induced hearing loss. Experts think about 10 to 15 percent of people over 60 are deficient in vitamin B_{12}.

Researchers from the Institute for Noise Hazards Research and Evoked Potentials Laboratory at Chaim-Sheba Medical Center in Ramat Gan and from Tel Aviv University, both in Israel, looked at a group of 385 people with tinnitus and found that 36 to 47 percent suffered from vitamin B_{12} deficiency. All of the people low in B_{12} received injections of 1,000 micrograms weekly for 4 to 6 months. At the end of that time, their hearing and tinnitus were evaluated. Fifty-four percent reported improvement in their tinnitus, and approximately 25 percent reported reductions in the measured loudness of their tinnitus.

In another Israeli study of 113 people who were exposed to occupational noise, researchers found that those with low blood levels of vitamin B_{12} had a significantly higher chance of having tinnitus. When 12 of those patients were given vitamin B_{12}, they saw some improvement in their symptoms.

If you have tinnitus, and especially if you also have memory problems, ask your doctor to check your blood level of vitamin B_{12}.

Although most people get enough vitamin B_{12} from foods, absorption problems can cause shortages, especially in older people. Strict vegetarians, who eat no meats, dairy products, or eggs, are also at risk for deficiency, since B_{12} comes only from animal foods.

If your doctor determines that you have absorption problems, you'll need vitamin B_{12} shots for the rest of your life. If you don't have absorption problems, experts say that it's safe to take about 1,000 micrograms of B_{12} a day.

Magnesium May Shield Sensitive Ears

Experts know from studying lab animals that magnesium deficiency combined with loud noises can lead to damage in the nerve cells of the ear. Low magnesium levels can also cause blood vessels, including the tiny arteries going to the inner ears, to constrict. (Remember, noise-induced vasospasm is thought to play a role in tinnitus.)

Human ears, even young, healthy, normal-hearing ones, can benefit from extra magnesium. Research has found that Israeli soldiers who got an additional 167 milligrams of supplemental magnesium daily had less inner ear damage than soldiers getting placebos (inactive pills). A study has also shown that supplemental intake has this same protective effect against long-term noise exposure.

If you're faced with a noisy environment, you'll want to make sure that you're getting the Daily Value of magnesium, which is 400 milligrams. Most people fall short in that regard, with men getting about 320 milligrams a day and women averaging 230 milligrams a day. Green vegetables, whole grains, nuts, and beans are packed with magnesium. (If you're considering taking magnesium supplements, be sure to talk to your doctor first if you have heart or kidney problems.)

If your tinnitus includes a sensation of fullness in your ear and balance problems, experts recommend that you get adequate amounts of calcium and potassium as well. These additional symptoms could be a sign of Ménière's disease. (For the full details on treating Ménière's with nutrients, see page 380.)

Antioxidants May Help Save Ears

Tinnitus is sometimes caused by impaired bloodflow to the ears, which can happen in two ways, Dr. Seidman says. First, the tiny artery leading to the inner ear can get clogged with cholesterol, causing a kind of stroke in the ear, he explains. Second, loud noises can send this artery into spasm, reducing blood supply to the cochlea. In either case, an interrupted blood supply can lead to hearing problems.

That's where the antioxidant nutrients—vitamin C, vitamin E, beta-carotene, and others—come in. "Antioxidants work by helping to prevent oxygen-caused damage to cell membranes," Dr. Seidman explains. Antioxidants also help keep arteries open and free of plaque buildup, experts say.

In a study by Italian researchers, 31 patients with tinnitus were given phospholipids and vitamins that included beta-carotene, vitamin C, vitamin E, and other compounds. After 18 weeks, they saw a "great" improvement in their tinnitus, the study authors wrote.

Dr. Seidman and some other ear doctors suggest that you consider a smorgasbord of antioxidant nutrients: 400 IU of vitamin E daily, 250 milligrams of vitamin C twice daily, 50 to 200 micrograms of the mineral selenium daily, and about 50,000 IU of beta-carotene twice daily. Doses of selenium exceeding 400 micrograms daily can be toxic and should be taken only under medical supervision.

Dr. Seidman has received a patent on a series of ingredients that includes Acetyl-l-carnitine, alpha-lipoic acid, coenzyme Q10, and an absorbable form of L-glutathione. His studies show that the antioxidants not only slow age- and noise-related hearing loss but also reverse it in some cases. You can buy Dr. Seidman's specially formulated supplement, called the Anti-Age/Energy Formula, at www.bodylanguagevitamin.com. Dr. Seidman also recommends three other supplements from his product line for people with tinnitus: the Antioxidant Formula, the Multivitamin Formula, and the Essential Oils Formula.

"I've had hundreds of patients tell me that their tinnitus is better when they use the 'flagship' four supplements," Dr. Seidman says. Though they won't work for everyone, people have reported that their tinnitus improves while they're supplementing and gets worse if they stop, he says. It takes at least 4 months to experience the full effect.

Also, Dr. Seidman and other researchers have done studies showing that specific essential oils, such as phosphatidylcholine, phosphatidylserine, and omega-3 fatty acids, among others, can improve hearing.

Zinc Can Make a Difference

Some parts of the body have much higher concentrations of certain vitamins and minerals than other parts. That's the case with the inner ear, which, like the retina of the eye, has a high concentration of zinc. That finding has led some doctors to speculate that zinc deficiency may play a role in inner ear problems such as tinnitus.

Studies have found that people with low levels of zinc have a higher risk of hearing loss, while one study found that increasing zinc levels helped improve hearing. Zinc is involved in a wide array of functions, including helping to maintain healthy cell membranes and protecting cells from oxygen-related damage.

Zinc doesn't always help, however. In people who have normal hearing, zinc may not help with tinnitus. You can have your doctor test your zinc levels if you suspect they're the cause of your tinnitus.

Ear, nose, and throat specialists may initially give large doses of zinc, up to 150 milligrams a day, but it's important to take no more than about 15 milligrams a day without medical supervision. Doctors monitor blood levels of zinc when they prescribe higher amounts. That's because zinc can be toxic in large doses.

Zinc also interferes with copper absorption, so if you're taking high doses of zinc, you may need to take supplemental copper (the ratio that's generally recommended is 1 milligram of copper for every 10 milligrams of zinc). Copper, too, can be toxic, so follow your doctor's advice on this.

The Daily Value for zinc is 15 milligrams. However, many experts agree that most Americans don't get enough zinc. One study found that 30 percent of people who are elderly are deficient in zinc. Look to meats and shellfish for zinc; cooked oysters, beef, crab, and lamb all offer good amounts.

VARICOSE VEINS

WINNING AN UPHILL BATTLE

That marbled look might work well on a fireplace mantel or a coffee table, but when it's on your legs—no way! You'd prefer them without those blue squiggles, thank you very much.

Why is it that some people have those squiggles and others don't?

To understand that, it helps to look at how the veins function. The heart pumps blood to the lungs to pick up oxygen. Then the blood travels back to the heart to be pumped out through arteries, thus delivering oxygen throughout the body. The heart pushes blood out through the arteries with a great deal of force. And when blood is making its return trip to the heart from various parts of the body, it moves through veins.

But veins, particularly the ones in your legs, have a harder time pumping blood back to the heart because they have to overcome gravity. They rely on muscle contractions in the legs to pump blood through them while one-way valves in the veins allow blood to flow in only one direction. Inefficient? Well, send your complaints to Mother Nature.

Varicose veins, those blue bulges, develop when veins can't return blood to the heart efficiently. Over time veins lose their elasticity and stretch and their valves become weak, allowing blood to flow backward. Blood pools in the veins, making them dilate. That hinders the valves' ability to close tightly and stop backward blood flow. Eventually, veins may become permanently dilated and scarred and take on a torturous configuration similar to a road map of West Virginia.

Varicose veins are not just a cosmetic problem. They can contribute to swollen, tired legs and muscle cramps.

Some people develop varicose veins because they have inherited structural problems with the valves in the upper parts of their legs, says Joseph Pizzorno Jr., ND, president emeritus of Bastyr University in Seattle. "Even if just one or two valves fail, that can put enough pressure on the lower part of a vein so that it, too, has problems," Dr. Pizzorno says.

Other people have leaky valves because their veins are simply too weak to withstand the pressure of backflowing blood.

Varicose veins also tend to pop up or worsen during pregnancy. The volume of blood in your body rises when you're pregnant, but bloodflow from your legs to your pelvis decreases to help the growing fetus, which causes varicose veins. And as your pregnancy progresses, your uterus puts pressure on the veins in your legs. Hemorrhoids, a complication of pregnancy, are actually varicose veins.

Most doctors' nutritional advice for varicose veins is limited to "Lose weight, eat more fiber." Both of these dietary measures help reduce pressure in veins. The few doctors who go beyond this advice to recommend nutritional supplements say they're focusing on nutrients that help maintain the structural integrity of the vein wall and help reduce the possibility of blood clots in veins. Here's what these doctors recommend.

Vitamin C Helps Fragile Veins

Keeping vein walls strong is important when it comes to preventing varicose veins or keeping them from getting worse, according to medical experts. Strong vein walls can resist more pressure without dilating, which allows the veins' valves to work better.

That's where vitamin C comes in. The body needs it to manufacture two important connective tissues: collagen and elastin. Both of these fibers are used to repair and maintain veins to keep them strong and flexible, explains Dr. Pizzorno. Vitamin C, he says, may be especially important for you if you bruise easily or have broken capillaries, which may show up on your skin as tiny "spider veins."

Even more important to keeping veins and capillaries in tip-top shape may be vitamin C's first cousins, bioflavonoids. Bioflavonoids are chemical compounds often found in the same foods as vitamin C.

Dr. Pizzorno recommends 500 to 3,000 milligrams of vitamin C and 100 to 1,000 milligrams of bioflavonoids daily. These high amounts are easily obtained only with supplements. Some people experience diarrhea with as little as 1,200 milligrams of vitamin C a day, so you should discuss taking this much with your doctor.

Vitamin E Keeps Blood Flowing

While there are no studies to show that vitamin E heals varicose veins, people with varicose veins apparently do use it, hoping that it will help prevent the biggest potential complication: blood clots.

"Vitamin E helps keep platelets, blood components involved in clotting, from sticking together and from adhering to the sides of blood vessel walls," Dr. Pizzorno explains. Research shows that reducing platelet stickiness with vitamin E could help people at particularly high risk for blood-clotting problems, such as those with diabetes.

If you're going to take vitamin E, aim for 200 to 600 IU daily, suggests Dr. Pizzorno. Some research suggests that 200 IU a day is enough to reduce platelet adhesion. If you've had bleeding problems or a stroke, it's important that you talk to your doctor before starting vitamin E supplementation. If you are taking anticoagulants, you should not take vitamin E supplements.

Food Factors

In addition to getting exercise, not crossing your legs, elevating your feet, and avoiding sitting or standing for long periods of time, certain foods can help minimize clotting, reduce pressure, and strengthen vein walls. Spice up your menu with these suggestions.

Beef up on bioflavonoids. Deep-colored berries, such as cherries, blueberries, and blackberries, contain these chemical compounds, as do the white membranes of citrus fruits. They're also found in wine and grape juice.

"Bioflavonoids are thought to reduce capillary fragility," says Joseph Pizzorno Jr., ND, president emeritus of Bastyr University in Seattle. When fragile capillaries distend or break down, they can appear on the skin as red or blue "spider veins."

Reach for fiber foods. If you strain hard to move your bowels from constipation, you create pressure in your abdomen that can block the flow of blood back up your legs. Over time, the increased pressure may weaken vein walls and result in hemorrhoids, which are varicose veins.

So avoid constipation by eating plenty of fiber-containing foods. Besides those berries, try other fruits as well as vegetables, beans, and whole grains.

Pare down. Added body fat, especially around your middle, also creates pressure in your abdomen, making it harder for blood to return to your heart. Keep your weight down, and chances are you'll have fewer problems with bulging veins.

Lick the salt habit. Too much salt can make your legs swell and stress already damaged veins. Some experts suggest cutting back by loading your diet with fresh fruits and vegetables as well as whole grains. You'll also be upping your intake of other minerals that help reduce fluid retention: potassium, magnesium, and calcium.

A Trace Mineral Helps Keep Veins Strong

We all know that minerals help keep bones strong. Studies show that some minerals do the same for blood vessels, helping to build and maintain the layers of tissues that form blood vessel walls.

Copper, which we all need in small amounts, is used in the body to knit together collagen and elastin, the same connective tissues that require vitamin C.

"Copper is involved in the cross-linking between the molecules that make up these tissues," explains Leslie Klevay, MD, ScD, professor of internal medicine at the University of North Dakota School of Medicine and Health Sciences in Grand Forks. Research has shown that copper-deficient animals have weakened arteries and capillaries, two of the three types of blood vessels in our bodies (the third is veins), that can bulge out under pressure.

According to Dr. Klevay, little research has been done on copper's effect on veins. But because arteries and veins have similar structures, it is quite possible that the strength of veins depends on adequate copper levels, too. This is why everyone, including people with varicose veins, should make sure that they're getting adequate amounts of this trace mineral, Dr. Klevay says.

Copper is also needed to build and repair endothelial cells, the smooth protective cells lining the insides of blood vessels, Dr. Klevay explains. Getting adequate copper appears to help protect blood vessels against microscopic tears and rough spots, caused by high blood pressure and smoking, that can lead to the buildup of cholesterol-laden plaque and to blood clots.

The estimated average requirement for copper is 0.7 milligram and the Daily Value is 2 milligrams. Your best bet for getting enough? Include whole grains, nuts, and seeds, along with shellfish (especially cooked oysters), in your diet, recommends Dr. Klevay.

B Vitamins May Help Stop Clots

Endothelial cells are also damaged by high blood levels of an amino acid called homocysteine. The damage has been linked to early heart disease and, more recently, to increased risk of recurrent blood clots in veins.

That's where the three Bs come in. Researchers now know that folate

Prescriptions for Healing

Using supplements to treat varicose veins is not standard medical practice, but some doctors feel that certain nutrients are helpful. Here's what they recommend.

Nutrient	Daily Amount
Copper	0.7 milligram
Folic acid	2,500 micrograms
Vitamin B_6	25 milligrams
Vitamin B_{12}	2 micrograms
Vitamin C	500–3,000 milligrams
Vitamin E	200–600 IU

MEDICAL ALERT: *Folic acid in doses exceeding 400 micrograms daily can mask symptoms of pernicious anemia, a vitamin B_{12} deficiency disease, and should be taken only under medical supervision.*

Some people may experience diarrhea when taking vitamin C in doses of more than 1,200 milligrams daily.

If you've had bleeding problems or a stroke, it's important that you talk to your doctor before starting vitamin E supplementation. If you are taking anticoagulants, you should not take vitamin E supplements. (Though generally a dose of up to 1,500 IU of vitamin E a day is considered safe, some recent reports suggest that taking more than 400 IU a day could be harmful to people with cardiovascular or circulatory disease or with cancer. If you have such a condition, be sure to consult your doctor before you begin supplementation.)

(the naturally occurring form of folic acid) and vitamins B_6 and B_{12} help break down and clear homocysteine from the blood. In the United States, grains are fortified with folate, so people are getting enough of this important B vitamin from their diet, says J. David Spence, MD, professor of neurology and clinical pharmacology at the University of Western Ontario, director of the Stroke Prevention and Atherosclerosis Research Centre at Robarts Research Institute in London, Canada, and author of *How to Prevent Your Stroke*. Vitamin B_6 isn't a problem, either.

Vitamin B_{12}, on the other hand, is a special case because people lose the ability to absorb vitamin B_{12} as they get older, particularly after age 50. And some people are born not being able to absorb vitamin B_{12} adequately. However, a normal blood test won't necessarily identify a vitamin B_{12} deficiency. That's why Dr. Spence recommends asking your doctor for a test that measures methylmalonic acid, which is suppressed when you have adequate levels of vitamin B_{12}.

Dr. Spence advises people with a severe deficiency of B_{12} to take 1,200 micrograms of the vitamin twice a day. People with a less severe deficiency should take 1,000 micrograms of vitamin B_{12} once a day. If you're getting the vitamin through an injection rather than a pill, get it once a week because the vitamin is water-soluble and will elevate vitamin B_{12} levels for only about a week.

WATER RETENTION

BEATING THE BLOAT

Forget that "ashes to ashes, dust to dust" stuff. Water to water is more like it. Our aquatic ancestors brought the sea with them when they crawled on land, and human beings remain mostly fluid. We're 56 percent fluid, to be exact—but sometimes more, sometimes less, depending on the degree of bloat.

People who retain fluid know just how easy it is to swell up like a sponge. Extra water can add up to 5 extra pounds of weight.

Bloating occurs when fluid that normally flows through the body in blood vessels, lymph ducts, and tissues gets trapped in tissues in the interstitial spaces, the tiny channels between cells. The fluid flows through the membranes of tiny blood capillaries into the tissue cells because of osmotic pressure (cell wall pressure), which is controlled by electrolytes such as sodium. A high sodium level attracts more fluid from the blood into the cells, where the fluid gets trapped and the cells become overhydrated. This occurs more readily in women, because their tissues are designed to fluctuate or expand for pregnancy.

Food Factors

If you know that bag of salty chips is going to lead to water retention, then you pretty much know what you have to do to avoid the problem. Other dietary choices are not quite so obvious. Here's what many experts recommend.

Drink more water. If your fluid retention is caused by excess salt intake, cut back immediately and drink plenty of water, at least 8 glasses a day, to help flush out the salt.

Watch out for MSG. MSG, or monosodium glutamate, also contains sodium. MSG is found in lots more than Chinese food; it's a common ingredient in processed foods. Read your labels for "MSG" or "hydro-lyzed vegetable protein," which contains MSG, and avoid these foods as much as possible.

Avoid alcohol. Alcohol does act as a diuretic at first, making you lose excess water. But this loss of fluid can progress to the point of dehydration. And medical experts have another good reason for giving this advice: Alcohol depletes your body of important vitamins and minerals.

Try a natural diuretic. Several herbal teas have a mildly diuretic effect. Parsley tea is the best-known type. Brew 2 teaspoons of dried leaves per cup of boiling water and steep for 10 minutes. Drink up to 3 cups a day.

Lose weight if you need to. Overweight women have more estrogen in their systems because fat tissue produces estrogen. This puts them at higher than normal risk for retaining fluid in their tissues and for adding to their overall weight. Overweight women need lots of water and must drastically reduce salt intake.

Ferret out food allergies. If you wake up in the morning congested, with puffy eyes and a headache, suspect a food allergy, says Joseph Pizzorno Jr., ND, president emeritus of Bastyr University in Seattle. "In my opinion, wheat is by far the most common allergy-causing food, but it could be any food. So it's best to get tested," he says.

Lots of things can cause waterlogged tissues: allergic reactions to foods, heart and kidney problems, and prescription drugs such as hormones. In women, hormonal changes often cause bloating beginning 7 to 10 days prior to menstruation, as higher levels of estrogen and progesterone during that part of the cycle cause the body to retain salt (sodium) and therefore to retain fluid in tissues.

Usually, fluid retention is uncomfortable but not health-threatening. People who retain fluid because of heart or kidney problems, however, or who are taking diuretics (water pills) need to be under a doctor's care for their problems.

Nutritional changes for fluid retention are meant to counteract hormonal changes, balance the minerals that influence body fluid, and eliminate foods that trigger bloating in some people. Here's what doctors say helps.

The Salt Connection

Most of us know that too much salt in our bodies can lead to temporary swelling. An evening's overload on movie popcorn or ballpark franks can leave us puffy-eyed and headachy, with stiff, swollen hands and feet, the next morning. "That's because our kidneys retain fluid in our bodies so that the excess salt can be diluted," explains David McCarron, MD, visiting professor in the department of nutrition at the University of California, Davis, and president of Academic Network LLC, a health-care consulting and communications firm in Portland, Oregon.

Some people are particularly sensitive to sodium and will retain fluids more easily after ingesting too much sodium. This is a serious problem because retaining too much water can increase your blood pressure.

Contrary to what you might think, drinking more water will not worsen fluid retention and may even help.

And some researchers believe that too little salt in the diet can also cause fluid retention, Dr. McCarron says. "We speculate that too little salt may trigger the kidneys to secrete more of a hormone that conserves salt, in part by reducing urinary output," Dr. McCarron says. He recommends keeping salt intake at 2,400 milligrams (a little more than 1 teaspoon) a day, an amount thought to maintain optimum blood pressure.

For most people, this still means cutting back by about 1,000 milligrams (about a half teaspoon) a day. Since 77 percent of the sodium in the average American diet comes from processed foods, not from the shaker, the best way to cut back is to look for sodium-free or low-sodium versions of cheeses, nuts, crackers, lunchmeats, and canned soups and vegetables and integrate more fresh fruits and vegetables into your diet. Also, watch your condiments. Some, such as soy sauce, can add 1,005 milligrams of sodium to your meal when you use just one tablespoon.

Mix-and-Match Minerals

Getting too little potassium, calcium, or magnesium in your diet can also contribute to fluid retention, Dr. McCarron says. "These minerals all play important roles in the fluid balance in your body—your body's ability to move fluid into and out of cells and from the bloodstream or lymphatic system into tissues and back again," he says.

He recommends getting about 3,500 milligrams of potassium a day (the Daily Value), an amount you can obtain by eating at least five servings of fruits and vegetables. (Potassium is lost in cooking water, though, so don't count on boiled potatoes or greens for this mineral unless you consume the water that they're cooked in.)

Prescriptions for Healing

There are a number of nutrients that can help relieve some cases of water retention. Here's what some experts recommend.

Nutrient	Daily Amount
Calcium	1,000–1,500 milligrams
Magnesium	400 milligrams
Potassium	3,500 milligrams
Vitamin B$_6$	100 milligrams
Plus a B-complex supplement	

MEDICAL ALERT: Doctors recommend limiting your sodium intake to no more than 2,400 milligrams a day.

Some doctors advise against supplementing calcium, magnesium, or potassium without medical supervision if you have diabetes or heart, kidney, or liver problems or if you are taking diuretics.

Potassium supplements should not be taken by those with diabetes or kidney disease or by those using certain medications, including nonsteroidal anti-inflammatory drugs, potassium-sparing diuretics, ACE inhibitors, and heart medications such as heparin.

Vitamin B$_6$ can be toxic in large amounts. Do not take more than 100 milligrams a day without medical supervision.

For magnesium, aim for the Daily Value of 400 milligrams, Dr. McCarron suggests. Most people fall short of this amount, with men getting about 320 milligrams a day and women averaging 230 milligrams a day. Nuts, legumes, and whole grains supply the most magnesium; other good food sources are green vegetables and bananas.

And for calcium, doctors recommend striving for 1,000 to 1,500 milligrams a day. One quart of fat-free milk contains about 1,400 milligrams of calcium. On average, men between ages 30 and 70 get close to 1,000 milligrams a day, while women in the same age group consume only about 700 milligrams daily, at least 300 milligrams less than they need.

If you have heart, kidney, or liver problems or diabetes, or if you're taking a diuretic to relieve fluid retention or high blood pressure, you should supplement these minerals only under medical supervision to make sure you don't develop dangerously high blood levels, says Dr. McCarron. People who are taking nonsteroidal anti-inflammatory drugs, potassium-sparing diuretics, ACE inhibitors, or heart medications such as heparin should also check with their doctor before supplementing potassium.

Vitamin B_6 May Aid Hormone-Related Bloating

Most women don't need a calendar to tell them when that time of the month is imminent. Their tender breasts, swollen hands and feet, and tightening blue jeans from abdominal swelling—all signs of fluid retention—mark time as well as any calendar. Fluid retention is also a problem among women going through perimenopause, between ages 35 and 50. That's because rising and falling levels of estrogen have an impact on how much water your body retains.

In addition to the changes in mineral intake outlined earlier, some doctors recommend increases in the B vitamins, B_6 in particular. When researchers reviewed 25 studies that looked at vitamin B_6's effect on premenstrual syndrome, they found that doses of up to 100 milligrams of vitamin B_6 helped with symptoms, although high-quality studies weren't available.

In one study, 500 milligrams of vitamin B_6 daily relieved the breast tenderness, headaches, and weight gain associated with water retention in 215 women.

Vitamin B_6 can be toxic and can cause serious nerve damage in excessive amounts. For these reasons, it's best not to take more than 100 milligrams a day without checking with your doctor. Your doctor may tell you, however, that it's safe to take up to 200 milligrams daily for 5 days to relieve premenstrual bloating. If your hands or feet start to feel numb or clumsy, stop taking B_6 and tell your doctor.

WILSON'S DISEASE

NEUTRALIZED BY ZINC

At age 22, the woman weighed 69½ pounds, consumed 700 calories a day, appeared depressed, didn't menstruate, chattered incessantly, and worried constantly about everything and anything.

Her doctors suspected an eating disorder, so they admitted her to a hospital at the National Institutes of Health and began to run some tests.

Everything checked out normally until they looked at her liver. There the doctors found that the woman had almost 15 times the normal amount of copper tucked away, a sure sign that she had Wilson's disease, a condition in which various body tissues are slowly poisoned by copper.

Sunflower Eyes and Shaking Limbs

Copper is a nutrient that is required by all cells, most notably for the development of healthy nerves, connective tissue, and the dark pigment in hair and skin. Everyone needs a little copper. In someone with Wilson's disease, however, a genetic error allows the metal to build up to toxic levels in the brain, liver, kidneys, and eyes. The astronomical amounts that accumulate can result in impaired mental ability, dementia, and liver failure.

Fortunately, the disease is rare, preventable, and treatable. It occurs in one in every 40,000 people, generally somewhere between the ages of 10 and 40 and most often among Eastern European Jews and their descendants.

Depending on where toxic levels of copper are accumulating, symptoms can range from malaise, fatigue, tenderness over the liver, and perhaps lowgrade fever—which together may seem to indicate a viral infection or acute hepatitis—all the way to eating disorders, the cessation of menstruation, shaking limbs, and "sunflower cataracts," which are green, yellow, or brown rings around the corneas. A telltale sign of the disease is the Kayser-Fleischer ring, a rusty brown ring around the cornea of the eye, but it can only be seen during an eye exam.

"The biggest problem is recognition of the disease," says pioneering researcher George Brewer, MD, professor emeritus of human genetics and internal medicine at the University of Michigan Medical School in Ann Arbor. "Many cases go unrecognized because the disease masquerades as, say, hepatitis or cirrhosis of the liver caused by alcohol."

Complicating recognition is the fact that symptoms frequently evolve over time rather than appearing all at once. "Instead of developing obvious neurological complications, for example, many people will have behavioral abnormalities for several years," explains Dr. Brewer. "They can become depressed, and they usually lose the ability to focus mentally. So if they're in school, their grades will drop. Or if they have jobs, they'll start to not perform as well. They'll become temperamental. They may become suicidal, and they can become exhibitionists.

"Often these behaviors are attributed to drug abuse, because you have people who have been normal and they sort of go off the deep end. Their spouses often leave during this period," he says.

The Blessing of Zinc

Fortunately, Wilson's disease is both preventable and treatable with zinc, according to Dr. Brewer.

In a series of studies at the University of Michigan, Dr. Brewer and his colleagues found that zinc induces formation of metallothionein, a substance that grabs on to any copper it can find and holds the copper in intestinal cells until they are sloughed off and excreted with other intestinal waste.

"The intestinal cells, like cells on the surface of your skin, turn over fairly rapidly," explains Dr. Brewer. "They have about a six-day life span. So when they slough into the intestines, they take the copper with them. It then goes out into the stool."

Zinc is also a good choice over drugs that treat Wilson's disease, such as penicillamine and trientine, because it has fewer side effects. In 2006, Italian researchers followed 35 people who had Wilson's disease for 15 years. Some were treated with penicillamine, and others were treated with zinc sulfate. While both treatments were effective at removing copper from the body, they found that 75 percent of the patients treated with penicillamine saw a

Prescriptions for Healing

Zinc counteracts the toxic accumulation of copper that occurs in the brain, liver, kidneys, and eyes of a person with Wilson's disease. Here's the amount recommended by George Brewer, MD, professor emeritus of human genetics and internal medicine at the University of Michigan Medical School in Ann Arbor.

Nutrient	Daily Amount
Zinc	150 milligrams, taken as 3 doses spaced evenly throughout the day, each at least 1 hour before or after a meal

MEDICAL ALERT: Anyone with Wilson's disease should be under a doctor's care, especially since the amount of zinc recommended here can be toxic. Likewise, people who do not have Wilson's disease should not take this much zinc without the knowledge and consent of their doctor. Zinc can deplete copper in your body.

worsening of neurological symptoms and 26 percent stopped treatment because of side effects. Meanwhile, 90 percent of the people taking zinc sulfate saw an improvement in neurological symptoms.

Although the FDA has approved zinc for the treatment of Wilson's disease, it's not the first thing that doctors reach for when symptomatic Wilson's disease is diagnosed. "Zinc is kind of leisurely acting for somebody who is symptomatic," says Dr. Brewer. "So we've developed a new drug called tetrathiomolybdate, a compound that works very nicely in the initial treatment of people with brain symptoms. We use it for eight weeks, and then we transition to zinc.

"For people with liver disease," he continues, "we use a combination of another drug, trientine hydrochloride (Syprine), and zinc. The trientine helps flush out the copper fairly rapidly."

Once on zinc-only therapy, a person with Wilson's disease will not reaccumulate copper or develop new symptoms, as long as they keep taking the zinc. "You're not trying to get rid of all of the copper in your body," says Dr. Brewer. "Copper is an essential nutrient, and without copper, people die. So what you're doing with zinc therapy is reducing the excessive load of copper and preventing it from reaccumulating."

That's why you can eat a normal diet. "The only two foods we ask people not to eat are liver, which is loaded with copper, and shellfish, which have intermediately high amounts," adds Dr. Brewer.

Sopping Up Copper

How much zinc does it take to sop up the extra copper in your body?

A study conducted by Dr. Brewer at the University of Michigan indicated that 150 milligrams of zinc a day, taken as three separate 50-milligram doses, each at least an hour before or after a meal, provides optimum copper removal. Because zinc can be toxic in such a high amount, it's important that you be under medical supervision while using this therapy.

Taking zinc with meals negates the mineral's effect. "If zinc is taken with a food, it's almost like not taking it, because it gets bound with material in the food and doesn't do much," says Dr. Brewer. "But if you split it away from food, as little as 25 milligrams will have a detectable effect on copper balance."

And that's also why people who do not have Wilson's disease should not take large amounts of zinc, adds Dr. Brewer. Since it takes a fairly small amount of zinc to have an effect on copper levels in the body, taking more than the Daily Value of zinc (15 milligrams) could easily make you copper-deficient within a few months.

Preventing the Problem

Zinc also has the ability to prevent the onset of Wilson's disease symptoms in people who have inherited the aberrant gene but have not yet developed any symptoms. Unfortunately, the only way to detect the possibility that you might have Wilson's disease before symptoms appear is to have it hit a brother or sister.

That's why siblings of those with Wilson's disease should have their urine monitored by their family physicians on a regular basis for elevated levels of copper, says Dr. Brewer. The odds are one in four that they will develop the disease at some time in their lives.

"Wilson's disease is an autosomal recessive disease," Dr. Brewer says. "That means the affected person has two doses of the abnormal gene that triggers the disease. The parents are obligatory carriers, but since each parent has only one dose, they will be completely normal."

Fortunately, even children who have inherited the disease will be completely normal, too—once they're put on zinc, says Dr. Brewer.

WRINKLES

SMOOTHING OUT THE LINES

Skin is like brand-new underwear. In the beginning, the elastic is snug and resilient, stretching and snapping right back into place. But after years of wear and tear, pulling and tugging and exposure to the elements, that elastic gradually gives, until one day . . . well, it's time to get new underwear.

Would that we could get new skin, too. Because after years of our laughing, crying, rubbing, and, worst of all, sunning, our skin begins to give as well. In fact, if it weren't for sun exposure, say the experts, our skin would stay relatively smooth into our eighties. That's why a dermatologist's first recommendation for wrinkle prevention is "Get out of the sun."

Sun exposure damages skin inside and out. First it attacks the epidermis, the thin, outermost tier of skin, forming a layer of dead cells that give skin a leathery appearance. Then it progressively damages the upper layers of the dermis, or the bulk of the skin, leaving them thinner, less resilient, and more susceptible to wrinkling. Over time, the collagen and elastin fibers that form the dermis also break down, causing gradual drooping and sagging.

Of course, you can't avoid the sun altogether—nor should you, since it's an important source of vitamin D. That's where sunscreen comes in. Try one that has an SPF of 30 and that protects against both UVA and UVB rays. UVA rays are the ones that cause fine lines, wrinkles, and discoloration from age.

Fortunately, dermatologists say, the appearance of a few crow's-feet and laugh lines doesn't mean that you're on a slippery slope to Wrinkle City. By protecting yourself from the sun, shunning cigarettes, and eating right, you can prevent many new wrinkles from occurring. You can also do some wrinkle erasing as well. Star players in getting rid of wrinkles once they've formed are some vitamin-derived compounds that are applied topically.

An A-Plus for Retin-A

Aside from plastic surgery, the best thing for getting rid of wrinkles is tretinoin, a vitamin A compound better known as Retin-A. No, it can't iron out deep lines, lift droops, or undo severe damage, but Retin-A can erase the crow's-feet, fine lines, and crinkling left by aging and the sun.

Retin-A, originally developed as an acne medication to unplug clogged pores, works against wrinkles by stimulating cell turnover, explains Retin-A creator Albert Kligman, MD, PhD, professor emeritus of dermatology at the University of Pennsylvania School of Medicine in Philadelphia. "Retin-A stimulates collagen production and blood flow into the dermis," says Dr. Kligman. "It creates tissue and makes the dermis thicker. In short, it returns skin to a more youthful condition and prevents many wrinkles from occurring."

But having heard that promise a thousand times before, you may wonder: Are the results noticeable?

Investigators at the University of Michigan Health System in Ann Arbor say they are. After studying 29 people who had sun-damaged skin, they reported that those who were treated for 10 to 12 months with Retin-A experienced an 80 percent increase in collagen formation compared with a 14 percent decrease in collagen formation among those using a cream not fortified with vitamin A.

In another study involving 45 people with photodamaged skin, half were given a 0.1 percent Retin-A microsphere gel while the other half applied a placebo gel. After 6 months, the patients receiving Retin-A saw significant improvements in fine lines, sallowness, and discoloration compared with the placebo group.

Food Factors

Ask most dermatologists about the best foods for healthy skin, and their answer will likely be "just eat a good, nutritious diet." But here are two specific dietary measures that they recommend to help avoid wrinkles.

Go easy on the spirits. Making too much merry can make your skin . . . well, very unmerry. Not only does that morning-after puffiness contribute to wrinkles, but alcohol also dehydrates you, which is anything but good for your skin, especially if you're using topical vitamin A (Retin-A), says Albert Kligman, MD, PhD, professor emeritus of dermatology at the University of Pennsylvania in Philadelphia and the creator of Retin-A. "Like smoking or unprotected exposure to sunlight, too much drinking can cause skin irritation in people using Retin-A," he says.

Get plenty of water. You should drink 4 glasses of water a day, says Dr. Kligman, unless you are sweating heavily. If you are sweating a lot, of course, drink more water.

Just don't try to get the same results by upping your dietary intake of vitamin A, warns Dr. Kligman. "When people try to get the same effects by megadosing vitamin A supplements, the results are almost the opposite," he says. "Their skin becomes dry and itchy, and their hair starts to fall out from vitamin A toxicity."

Retin-A cream comes in a variety of strengths, from 0.025 to 0.1 percent. It's available by prescription only, so your dermatologist can help determine which concentration is best for you. Generally, people beginning Retin-A treatment apply the lowest-dosage cream nightly or every other night until their dermatologists instruct them otherwise.

Because Retin-A removes the dead top layer of skin and exposes an area previously sheltered from evaporation and the elements, a common side effect is dry, sun-sensitive skin that can be irritated and scaly. Though both of these side effects typically diminish with time, if you're using Retin-A, you'll likely need a moisturizer. And you'll definitely need a sunscreen; once you start taking Retin-A, your days in the sun are over. Also, ask about Renova, an "updated" Retin-A with built-in moisturizer that has been approved by the FDA as a prescription cream.

C Is for Collagen

Though not as well established in the antiwrinkle business as vitamin A, vitamin C, a nutrient known for its importance in the manufacture of collagen, is being touted by some experts as a key player in keeping the complexion smooth.

It's well known that people who eat a balanced diet keep a youthful glow, and vitamin C should get some of that credit. By helping to manufacture collagen, vitamin C plays a vital role in creating connective tissue in the body, including your skin.

The Daily Value of vitamin C is 60 milligrams, but because the Daily Values are set only to prevent deficiency diseases, you'll need to surpass that amount to help your skin. Some doctors recommend taking a supplement of 500 to 1,000 milligrams of vitamin C a day.

Topical vitamin C has also been shown to prevent the free radical skin damage that occurs following exposure to ultraviolet rays from the sun. Free radicals are unstable molecules that steal electrons from your body's healthy molecules to balance themselves. Unchecked, free radicals can cause significant tissue damage and contribute to premature wrinkling. In one study,

Prescriptions for Healing

Doctors agree that certain nutrients can not only diminish some of our fine lines but also provide a touch of "permanent press" to slow the formation of new ones. Here's what some doctors recommend.

Nutrient	Daily Amount/Application
Oral	
Selenium	50–200 micrograms (l-selenomethionine)
Vitamin C	500–1,000 milligrams
Vitamin E	400 IU (d-alpha-tocopherol)
Topical	
Idebenone	0.5%–1% lotion
Vitamin A	0.025%–0.1% cream, depending on skin type
Vitamin C	10%–17% lotion (Cellex-C)
Vitamin E	5%–100% ointment or oil, applied after sun exposure

MEDICAL ALERT: Selenium can be toxic in doses exceeding 400 micrograms daily. High amounts should be taken only under medical supervision.

If you are taking anticoagulant drugs, you should not take oral vitamin E supplements. (Though generally a dose of up to 1,500 IU of vitamin E a day is considered safe, some recent reports suggest that taking more than 400 IU a day could be harmful to people with cardiovascular or circulatory disease or with cancer. If you have such a condition, be sure to consult your doctor before you begin supplementation.)

topical vitamin C actually decreased the amount of sunburned cells and began to repair damaged skin when it was applied 30 to 60 minutes after skin was exposed to ultraviolet rays.

"It's possible that topical vitamin C, when used in conjunction with sunscreen, could prevent a significant amount of the wrinkling caused by sun exposure," says Douglas Darr, PhD, a biotechnology industry consultant in Research Triangle Park, North Carolina. Cellex-C, a topical vitamin C product available in 10 or 17 percent lotion or cream form, can be purchased without a prescription from dermatologists, plastic surgeons, and licensed aestheticians (full-service beauty salon operators) and by mail order from Cellex-C International (www.cellex-c.com). It should be applied 15 to 30 minutes prior to sun exposure, along with sunscreen, for best results.

For a burst of vitamin C in your diet, you can go the traditional orange juice and citrus route, or you can create a vegetable medley of broccoli, brussels sprouts, and red bell peppers. But take note: If you want sun damage protection, don't count on being able to eat enough vitamin C, says Dr. Darr. "You can't get enough into your skin without applying it topically," he says.

Stopping Wrinkles with Vitamin E

Vitamin E, another free radical-fighting antioxidant, can also prevent skin damage from sun exposure when used topically, say researchers. But they recommend it for postsun use rather than presun use. It's a powerful moisturizer and can prevent inflammation and skin damage.

But save it for after you come inside, as vitamin E itself can produce free radicals when exposed to ultraviolet light. Vitamin E oil can be bought over the counter in drugstores.

And although you'd want to put this on before going out in the sun, you can even get vitamins C and E in your sunscreen as added insurance that you're properly protected.

For additional sun damage protection, try taking vitamin E supplements, adds Karen E. Burke, MD, PhD, a dermatologic surgeon and dermatologist in private practice in New York City. Dr. Burke recommends 400 IU daily in the form of d-alpha-tocopherol. "Although studies of oral vitamin E and wrinkles still need to be done, the supplements can help reduce photodamage and keep skin healthier," says Dr. Burke.

Vitamin E-rich foods include wheat germ, spinach, and sunflower seeds.

The New Super Antioxidant

The most recent addition to wrinkle-fighting creams is idebenone. It's a topical antioxidant ingredient developed by cosmetic chemists that's touted as being more powerful than vitamins C and E. In a clinical trial, idebenone beat out vitamins C and E, coenzyme Q10, kinetin, and alpha-lipoic acid in its ability to fight against free radicals.

What makes idebenone unique are its small molecules that can penetrate the deepest layers of the skin and neutralize free radicals. It also decreases the breakdown of collagen in the skin, leading to fewer lines and wrinkles, and reduces inflammation. You'll find it in three face and neck lotions: Prevage from Allergan, and Youth Revealing Complex and Radiance Revealing Complex from True Cosmetics. They're available at spas, salons, dermatologists' offices, and plastic surgeons' offices. For best results, use these products with a sunscreen that protects against both UVA and UVB rays.

Selenium Wrinkle Prevention

Like vitamin E, the mineral selenium quenches free radicals caused by sun exposure and prevents skin damage, says Dr. Burke. But because selenium is found in the soil and its concentrations vary nationwide, some people may get adequate amounts, while others are deficient, she says. People in the Southeast in particular tend to have low selenium levels, she notes.

For optimum skin protection, Dr. Burke recommends daily supplements of 50 to 200 micrograms of selenium (preferably the l-selenomethionine form), depending on where you live and your family history of skin cancer. However, Dr. Burke doesn't advise taking more than 200 micrograms of selenium daily. It's best to supplement high amounts only under medical supervision.

For a big dietary boost of selenium, reach for tuna, as one 3-ounce can packs 99 micrograms. Other good sources include garlic, onions, and broccoli.

Dr. Burke has developed a selenium cream that reverses photoaging, but it's not yet available commercially. (For more details on using nutrients to protect yourself from sun damage, see page 525.)

YEAST INFECTIONS

DITCHING THE ITCH

Have itchy palms? Some would say that money is coming your way. A 7-year itch? Better have a heartfelt chat with your mate. An itch where . . . well, you'd rather not discuss it? Welcome to one of the most common of feminine struggles: woman versus the beast called yeast.

In fact, at some point during their childbearing years, three in four women will wonder what they did to deserve the itching, burning, odor, and unpleasant discharge that accompany vaginal yeast infections. They'll also want to know exactly what they can do to stop it from ever happening again.

The Nature of the Yeast

Fortunately, there are steps women can take to prevent these itchy episodes. But first, it helps to understand why a yeast infection happens at all.

The most likely culprit behind this maddening malady is a generally mild-mannered fungus known as *Candida albicans* that lives in the vagina, mouth, and intestines. Normally, candida is kept to its small, harmless colonies by the immune system and by *Lactobacillus acidophilus*, bacteria commonly found in the vagina that create an acidic environment that candida doesn't like. When something throws this ecosystem off balance, however, candida runs rampant, and yeast infections can result.

The most common offenders, things that upset this delicate ecosystem, include wet bathing suits, panty hose, skintight jeans, and leotards. All of these things foster a warm, moist environment that candida loves. Women are also prone to yeast infections during pregnancy, just before they get their periods, and during menopause. Candida also multiplies when women are taking antibiotics, because such medications often kill too many good bacteria, such as lactobacillus, along with the bad, leaving candida unchecked.

Because women's natural cycles may lead to an infection, douching with warm water (not vinegar) on the sixth or seventh day of your period will remove germs that tend to accumulate by the cervix and lead to an infection, says Satty Gill Keswani, MD, a physician at St. Barnabas Medical Center and director of Livingston Fertility in Livingston, New Jersey. She also recommends following the douche with a vaginal cream that contains proteins.

There are also a host of ways to fight the infections through nutrition. Here's how.

Be a Bad Host with Good Nutrition

Once candida has become a flaming yeast infection, doctors commonly recommend over-the-counter medications such as miconazole (Monistat) and clotrimazole (Gyne-Lotrimin) or the one-dose, prescription-only fluconazole (Diflucan), all of which can have you sitting comfortably again in less than

Food Factors

You probably already know that shedding a wet bathing suit or sweaty underclothes is a good preventive against moisture-loving yeast infections. But you may not know that doctors have found that adding certain foods to your diet, or removing others, might help fight these itchy occurrences as well. Here are their dietary recommendations for staying yeast-free.

Say yes to yogurt. Whoever developed the old home remedy of douching with yogurt to stop a yeast infection was close to being right. She was just putting it in the wrong place! You have to eat a cup of it a day, and it has to contain active *Lactobacillus acidophilus* cultures. (If the yogurt contains live cultures, it will say so on the label.)

In a study of 33 women at the Long Island Jewish Medical Center in Hyde Park, New York, researchers found that women with histories of yeast infection recurrence could decrease the incidence of recurrence threefold just by eating 8 ounces of yogurt a day.

Say no to sweets. *Candida albicans* (the medical term for the kind of yeast that causes vaginal infections) is a fungus with a real sweet tooth. Indulging in too many sweet, sugary foods can raise your blood sugar level and create the perfect candida breeding ground.

Have you ever thrown sugar on yeast and watched it multiply? When you eat a typical American high-glycemic diet, that's what you're doing, says nutritionist Shari Lieberman, PhD, president of the American Association for Health Freedom and author of *The Real Vitamin and Mineral Book,* who runs a private nutritional practice in New York City. If you want to keep yeast infections from returning, stay away from foods that are high on the glycemic index, such as flour, potatoes, sugary cereal, cookies, cake, and a host of others. Instead, eat more whole grains and fruits and vegetables.

Skip yeasty foods. Eating foods that contain yeast will increase your chances of having an overgrowth of yeast in the vagina, says Satty Gill Keswani, MD, a physician at St. Barnabas Medical Center and director of Livingston Fertility in Livingston, New Jersey. There's always some yeast in the vaginal canal, but it's when your immunity goes down that it becomes an infection.

If you have chronic yeast infections, it's a good idea to try to remove as many high-yeast foods as you can from your diet, such as bread made with yeast, pizza, beer, cheese, wine, and smoked meats. Instead, look for unleavened bread, which is made without yeast.

Ward off vampires. It's not just a folktale. Eating a clove of garlic every day or adding the spice turmeric to your food may help you avoid yeast infections, says Dr. Keswani. Garlic and turmeric work as anti-inflammatory agents to help prevent yeast infections.

a week. But since these medications won't kick candida out for good, and since yeast infection recurrence is common, doctors say you have to be a bad host if you want to stay yeast-free.

What you put in your body can help get at the source of the problem. According to the experts, that means boosting your immunity through good diet and nutritional supplements such as vitamins A, C, and E and the mineral zinc. Here's what they recommend.

Note: Although *Candida albicans* is the most common cause of vaginal infections, it isn't the only cause. So if you've never had a yeast infection before, see your doctor for a proper diagnosis before starting any treatment on your own.

Keep Yeast from Rising with Zinc

When it comes to fighting disease, the mineral zinc is often a heavyweight contender. It stimulates the production of T-lymphocytes, the cells in your immune system that are responsible for cleaning up cells that have been invaded by infection. According to medical research, this makes zinc a prize-fighter against *Candida albicans*.

In fact, zinc supplements are likely beneficial even if your body's zinc levels are normal, according to a study done in India. Researchers there worked with laboratory animals that were not deficient in zinc. They gave these animals high-dose zinc supplements and found that they were significantly more resistant to infection from *Candida albicans* than those not supplemented with zinc.

The Daily Value of zinc is 15 milligrams. Dr. Keswani recommends getting zinc from a multivitamin. And to get more zinc through your diet, try cooked oysters. They contain about 76 milligrams of zinc per half dozen.

Acidify with Vitamin C

When it comes to fighting *Candida albicans*, vitamin C does double duty.

First, research has shown that vitamin C boosts immunity by keeping disease-fighting white blood cells up and running, so the body is better able to stave off infections, especially opportunistic ones such as candida that take advantage of a weak immune system. As a bonus, vitamin C adds acidic zip to your vaginal environment, fighting candida where it grows.

Prescriptions for Healing

While medicated creams can give your most tender areas the quickest relief from an annoying yeast infection, you'll need some nutritional immunity builders if you want to prevent a recurrence. Here's what many experts suggest.

Nutrient	Daily Amount/Application
Vitamin A	5,000 IU
Vitamin C	5,000 milligrams, taken as 5 divided doses during an infection; 500 milligrams a day when you're not having an infection
Vitamin E	400-mg gelatin capsule twice a day, used as a suppository
Zinc	15 milligrams

MEDICAL ALERT: *If you've never had a yeast infection before, be sure to see a doctor for proper diagnosis before starting treatment on your own.*

Some people experience diarrhea from taking more than 1,200 milligrams of vitamin C daily. So check with your doctor before trying this higher dose.

If you are taking anticoagulants, you should not take vitamin E supplements.

When you're having an infection, Dr. Keswani recommends taking 1,000 milligrams of vitamin C every hour for 5 hours. Although such high amounts of vitamin C are considered safe, some people experience diarrhea from taking just 1,200 milligrams daily. If you want to try this higher dose to prevent yeast infections, discuss it with your doctor.

To keep yeast infections at bay when you're healthy, Dr. Keswani says to take 500 milligrams of vitamin C a day. "Better still, squeeze your own oranges and drink them within 30 minutes," she says, because it's always preferable to get vitamins and minerals from food.

Other ways to boost vitamin C in your diet: Have one cup of broccoli or brussels sprouts to get about 100 milligrams.

Build Immunity with A and E

For women who are having ongoing battles with candida, the antioxidant vitamins A and E are powerful players in fighting off the infection.

The problem is, most of us aren't reaping the benefits of these vitamins because our diets aren't healthy enough to keep our health and immunity at optimal levels. "A balanced meal is not happening for most Americans," Dr. Keswani says. Foods today are so processed that they've lost 80 percent of their nutrients by the time they reach our tables.

She recommends getting vitamin A from a multivitamin, which provides about 5,000 IU.

To keep your resistance up when you're not suffering from an infection, Dr. Keswani recommends using vitamin E as a suppository. Twice a day, puncture one capsule containing 400 milligrams of vitamin E and insert it into the vagina. Doing so will provide optimal protection.

If you are a frequent victim of the yeast beast and would like to increase these nutrients in your diet, try cooking with vegetable oils and eating whole-grain cereals for more vitamin E, drinking fortified fat-free milk for a burst of vitamin A, and upping your intake of bright orange and yellow vegetables to increase beta-carotene (a substance that turns to vitamin A in the body).

INDEX

Underscored page references indicate boxed text.

A

Acetretin, for psoriasis, 475–76
Acidic beverages, nicotine replacement
    products and, 519
Acidic foods
    avoiding, with psoriasis, 475
    scurvy from avoidance of, 506
Additives, aggravating tinnitus, 543
Adenocarcinoma, 513
Age spots, 61–65
Aging, 66–71
    bruising with, 123
    folate and, 150–51
AIDS. See also HIV
    slowing progression to, 318–20
Alcohol
    avoiding, with
        carpal tunnel syndrome, 162
        eating disorders, 228
        endometriosis, 235
        epilepsy, 243
        fatigue, 248
        fibrocystic breasts, 253
        gout, 276, 278
        heart arrhythmia, 287
        high blood pressure, 305
        infertility, 335
        insomnia, 340
        leg cramps, 356
        menopausal problems, 389
        migraines, 401
        osteoporosis, 431
        pregnancy, 116
        premenstrual syndrome, 462
        psoriasis, 475
        smoking, 519
        tinnitus, 543
        water retention, 555
    cancer risk from, 137, 150
    cataract risk from, 167
    in diabetes diet, 217
    for heart disease prevention, 293
    kidney stones and, 351
    magnesium excretion from, 11
    malnutrition from, 14
    wrinkles and, 564
Alcoholism, 72–78
    beriberi from, 113
    cardiomyopathy and, 156, 158–59
    Wernicke-Korsakoff syndrome from, 113–14
    zinc deficiency from, 76
Allergies, 44, 79–84. See also Food allergies
Allopurinol, for gout, 278
ALS, 359–61
Aluminum
    bone loss from, 431
    preventing phosphorus absorption, 16
    sleep problems from, 343
Alzheimer's disease, 13, 54, 84–91, 114
Amyotrophic lateral sclerosis (ALS), 359–61
Anemia, 91–97
    causes of
        alcoholism, 72
        eating disorders, 233
        excessive zinc, 53
        iron deficiency, 91, 92
    effects of
        fatigue, 249
        gallstones, 263
        hair loss, 281–82
    foods preventing, 96
    macrocytic, 41
    pernicious, 8, 41, 94, 95, 141, 151, 279
    symptoms of, 91, 257, 483

Angina, 98–102, 292, 537
Anorexia nervosa, 226–33
Antacids
  bone loss from, <u>431</u>
  interacting with nutrients, <u>56–57</u>
  preventing phosphorus absorption, 16
  sleep problems from, 343
Anti-Age/Energy Formula, for tinnitus, 547
Antibacterial agents, interacting with
    nutrients, <u>56–57</u>
Antibiotics
  interacting with nutrients, <u>56–57</u>
  for scleroderma, <u>500</u>, 503
  yogurt with, <u>500</u>
Anti-cancer drugs, interacting with
    nutrients, <u>56–57</u>
Anticoagulants
  fish oil supplements and, <u>141</u>
  interacting with nutrients, <u>56–57</u>
  vitamin E and, 50, <u>64</u>
  vitamin K and, 51
Anticonvulsants, interacting with nutrients,
    <u>56–57</u>
Antidepressants
  grapefruit juice and, <u>55</u>
  vitamin C and, 45, 46
Antihypertensive agents
  grapefruit juice and, <u>55</u>
  interacting with nutrients, <u>54</u>, <u>56–57</u>
Anti-inflammatory agents, interacting with
    nutrients, <u>56–57</u>
Antimalarials, interacting with nutrients,
    <u>56–57</u>
Antioxidant Formula, for tinnitus, 547
Antioxidants. *See also specific antioxidants*
  high blood pressure and, 309
  neutralizing free radicals, 18, 49, 63, 70,
    129, 138, 360, 440, 502
  for preventing
    cancer, 43
    cervical dysplasia, 175–77
    heart disease, 291, 293–94
  for protection from aging, 67–71
  in sunscreen, 527
  for treating
    alcoholism, 73
    allergies, 80–82

  chronic fatigue syndrome, <u>185</u>, 186
  endometriosis, 238–39
  multiple sclerosis, 414
  overweight, 440–41
  scleroderma, 502
  tinnitus, 547–48
Apples, for cancer prevention, <u>137</u>
Arches Tinnitus Relief formula, <u>543</u>
Arginine, avoiding, with
  cold sores, <u>194</u>
  genital herpes, <u>265</u>
  shingles, <u>509</u>
Arrhythmia, heart, 284–90
Arterial plaque
  angina from, 97, 98
  formation of, 291–92
Arthritis
  osteoarthritis, 421–26
  rheumatoid, 487–95
Aspartame
  migraines from, <u>401</u>
  seizures from, <u>242–43</u>
  tinnitus and, <u>543</u>
Aspirin
  avoiding, with gout, 280
  contributing to scurvy, 506
Asthma, 44, 102–8
Atherosclerosis
  heart disease from, 291–92
  from high homocysteine, 297
  impotence from, <u>337</u>
  preventing, 293, 537

B

Baldness, 280–84
Bananas, for leg cramps, <u>356</u>
Bedsores, 109–12
Beef, for preventing anemia, <u>96</u>
Benign prostatic hyperplasia (BPH), 467–72
Beriberi, 112–14, 156
Berries
  as anti-aging food, <u>68</u>
  for preventing memory loss, <u>374</u>
  for treating varicose veins, <u>551</u>

Beta-blockers, for angina, 98
Beta-carotene
    alcoholism and, 74–75
    controversy about, 148–49
    for HIV patients, 318, 320
    overview of, 3–4
    for preventing
        cancer, 140, 145–49
        cataracts, 166
        cervical cancer, 176–77, 178
        heart disease, 295–96
        macular degeneration, 369
    for smokers, 520–21
    smoking and, 3, 296–97, 520–21
    for treating
        asthma, 107, 108
        burns, 128, 131
        cancer, 141
        effects of aging, 70
        effects of smog exposure, 515, 516–17
        endometriosis, 236, 238
        fibrocystic breasts, 256, 256
        immune system, 327, 330
        lupus, 364
        prostate problems, 472
        rheumatoid arthritis, 492, 493, 494
        tinnitus, 545, 547
Bioflavonoids
    for preventing heart disease, 293
    for treating
        allergies, 82–83
        bruises, 124
        heavy menstrual bleeding, 390–91,
            398
        varicose veins, 551
Biotin
    hair loss and, 283
    overview of, 4–5
    for treating
        carpal tunnel syndrome, 164, 165
        diabetes, 220, 223
        endometriosis, 236, 238
        fingernail problems, 4, 258, 258
Birth control pills. See Contraceptives
Birth defects, 8, 114–19, 522
Bladder cancer, 119–23
Bladder infections, 119–23, 413

Bleeding, heavy menstrual, 389–91, 398
Bloating, from water retention, 554–59
Blood clots
    from phlebitis, 456–60
    from varicose veins, 550–51
Blood pressure. See also High blood
        pressure
    normal vs. abnormal levels of, 301–2
    potassium regulating, 16–17
    sodium and, 20
Blood pressure medications. See
        Antihypertensive agents
Blood sugar regulation, Vitamin B_6 for, 39
Blueberries, as anti-aging food, 68
Bone health
    boron for, 25
    calcium for, 5–6, 263, 390, 392
    flouride for, 30
    manganese and, 31–32
    vitamin D for, 46–47
Bone loss. See also Osteoporosis
    causes of
        alcoholism, 76
        corticosteroids, 367
        dieting, 444
        eating disorders, 230, 232
        smoking, 522, 524
        vitamin D deficiency, 47
Boron
    function of, 24
    overview of, 25–26
    for preventing osteoporosis, 434–35,
        437
BPH, 467–72
Bradycardia, 285
Brain function
    manganese for, 32
    Vitamin B_6 for, 39
Brain tumors, from cured meats, 116
B.R.A.T. diet, for diarrhea, 224, 225
Breast cancer
    factors increasing
        alcohol, 72, 150
        grilled or smoked meats, 136
        red meat, 136
    vs. fibrocystic breasts, 251, 254
    iodine for treating, 30–31

Breast cancer (*cont.*)
  preventing, with
    fiber, 136
    flavonoids, 134
    folate, 150
    monounsaturated fats, 134
    soy foods, 136
    vitamin C, 138
    vitamin E, 139
  vitamin C deficiency and, 133
Breasts, fibrocystic, 251–57
Bruises, 123–27
Buckwheat, for bruises, 124
Bulimia, 226–33
Burns, 127–32
B vitamins. *See also specific B vitamins*
  for preventing
    blood clots, 457–59
    cataracts, 169–70, 169
  for reducing homocysteine, 297–99, 457,
      553
  for smokers, 523, 524
  for treating
    chronic fatigue syndrome, 184, 185,
      186
    depression, 204–6
    diabetes, 220, 222–23
    endometriosis, 238
    fatigue, 250, 251
    gout, 279, 279
    menopausal problems, 390, 391
    varicose veins, 552–54, 553
    water retention, 557, 558–59

C

Caffeine
  avoiding, with
    chronic fatigue syndrome, 180
    endometriosis, 235
    epilepsy, 243
    fatigue, 248
    fibrocystic breasts, 252, 253
    insomnia, 340
    menopausal problems, 388–89
      migraines, 400–401
      mitral valve prolapse, 406
      osteoporosis, 430
      premenstrual syndrome, 462
      restless legs syndrome, 482
      tinnitus, 543
  depression and, 204–5
  heart arrhythmia and, 287
  rheumatoid arthritis and, 489
Calcium
  for bone health, 5–6, 47, 263, 390, 392
  magnesium and, 11
  manganese absorption and, 32
  overview of, 5–7
  phosphorus and, 6, 15–16, 269, 389, 430
  during pregnancy, 118, 119
  for preventing
    colon cancer, 144
    gallstones, 260–63, 262
    kidney stones, 350–52, 351, 353
    migraines, 404
    osteoporosis, 5–6, 263, 390, 392,
      428–32, 437, 461
  recommended intake of, 6
  for smokers, 523, 524
  for treating
    alcoholism, 76, 77, 78
    asthma, 108
    celiac disease, 173, 174
    eating disorders, 230, 231, 232
    endometriosis, 236, 239
    high blood pressure, 307, 308–9
    leg cramps, 486
    lupus, 366, 367
    Ménière's disease, 383, 383
    menstrual problems, 394–97, 396
    mitral valve prolapse, 408, 408
    premenstrual syndrome, 461, 463, 465
    water retention, 557, 558
  vitamin D and, 46–47
  vitamin K and, 51
  for weight loss, 441–44, 445
  zinc absorption and, 53
Calcium carbonate, 6–7
Calcium-channel blockers, for angina, 98
Calcium citrate, 6
Calcium formate, 7

Calories, for HIV patients, 317
Cancer. *See also specific types of cancer*
  alcohol increasing, 72, 150
  preventing, with
    antioxidants, 71
    beta-carotene, 3, 4, 145–49
    dietary changes, 132–33, 134–37
    folic acid, 7–8, 150–51
    riboflavin, 18
    selenium, 143–45
    vitamin C, 43, 133, 138–39
    vitamin D, 48
    vitamin E, 139–43
  selenium and, 65
  treating, with
    nutrients, 140–41, 146–47
    selenium, 34, 145
  vitamin E and, 64
Cancer medications, nutrients and, 149
Candida albicans, yeast infections from, 569, 570, 571
Canker sores, 151–55
Carbohydrates
  as folate source, 116
  gallstones and, 261
  glycemic index of, 216, 218
  refined, avoiding, with
    fatigue, 248
    premenstrual syndrome, 462
Cardiomyopathy, 155–61
Cardiovascular disease. *See also* Heart disease
  potassium preventing, 17
  vitamin E and, 64
Carotenoids, for preventing cervical dysplasia, 176
Carpal tunnel syndrome, 161–65, 478
Cast-iron cookware, for preventing anemia, 96
Cataracts, 18, 44, 166–71, 369
C E Ferulic
  for bruises, 126–27
  for sun protection, 529–30
Celiac disease, 171–74
Cellex-C
  for sun protection, 63
  for wrinkle prevention, 566–67

Cervical cancer, antioxidants preventing, 175–77
Cervical dysplasia, 8, 174–79
Chelation therapy, 301
Chemotherapy, nutrients and, 149
Cherries, for gout, 276–77
Chickenpox virus, shingles from, 507
Chicken soup, for colds, 188
Chocolate
  migraines from, 401
  for preventing blood clots, 458
Cholesterol, blood
  controlling, with
    niacin, 13
    riboflavin, 18
  high (*see* High cholesterol)
  LDL vs. HDL, 309–10
  vitamin E affecting, 49
  zinc affecting, 53
Cholesterol, dietary
  in heart disease prevention, 292
  reducing, for
    for gallstone prevention, 261
    for lowering blood cholesterol, 311
Cholesterol-lowering drugs
  for angina, 98
  grapefruit juice and, 55
  interacting with nutrients, 56–57
Choline, for memory loss, 378
Chromium, 23
  caution about, 220
  depletion of, 273
  overview of, 26–27
  sugar depleting, 442
  for treating
    diabetes, 218–19, 220
    glaucoma, 272–74, 274
  for weight loss, 444, 445, 446
Chronic fatigue syndrome, 179–86, 248, 249
Clotrimazole, for yeast infections, 569, 571
Cobalt, 23, 27
Cod liver oil, for rheumatoid arthritis, 488
Coenzyme Q10
  for detoxification, 14
  for treating
    chronic fatigue syndrome, 183
    gingivitis, 269, 270

Coenzyme Q10 (*cont.*)
  for treating (*cont.*)
    heart failure, <u>158–59</u>
    memory loss, <u>374</u>
    Parkinson's disease, 451–53, <u>452</u>
Coffee, kidney stones and, <u>351</u>
Cola. *See also* Soft drinks
  osteoporosis and, <u>430</u>
Colds, 44, 45, 106, 187–93
Cold sores, 193–97
Colon cancer
  factors increasing
    red meat, <u>136</u>
    saturated fat, <u>134</u>
  preventing, with
    calcium, <u>144</u>
    fiber, <u>136</u>
    selenium, 143
    soy foods, <u>136</u>
    vitamin E, 142
Concord grape juice, for preventing heart
    disease, <u>293</u>
Congestive heart failure, 23, 300
Constipation
  fiber for, <u>395</u>, <u>551</u>
  with multiple sclerosis, <u>413</u>
Contraceptives
  bladder infections from, 121–22
  depression and, 203, 206, 391
  folic acid and, <u>118</u>
  gallstones and, 260
Copper, 23
  Alzheimer's disease and, 85–86
  caution about, <u>266</u>
  overview of, 28–29
  for preventing osteoporosis, 436, <u>437</u>
  for treating
    anemia, 92–94, <u>95</u>
    asthma, 108
    infertility, 336, <u>338</u>
    insomnia, 341–42, 343, <u>344</u>
    rheumatoid arthritis, <u>493</u>, 495
    tinnitus, <u>545</u>, 548
    varicose veins, 552, <u>553</u>
  weight loss and, <u>445</u>, 446
  Wilson's disease and, 29, 54, 559–60, 562
  zinc and, 29, 53, 93, 154–55, <u>266</u>, 267, 548

Copper bracelets, for rheumatoid arthritis, 495
Coronary artery disease, 292
Coronary heart disease
  angina with, 97
  homocysteine and, 98–99
Corticosteroids, for lupus, 362, <u>363</u>, 367
Cramps, leg, 355–59, 486
Cramps, menstrual, 393–98
Cranberry juice, for preventing bladder
    infections, <u>120–21</u>
Crash diets
  avoiding, with mitral valve prolapse, <u>406</u>
  hair loss from, <u>281</u>
Creatine, for Parkinson's disease, 452, <u>452</u>
Cruciferous vegetables
  for cancer prevention, <u>137</u>, 466
  for premenstrual syndrome, 466
Curcumin, for preventing Alzheimer's
    disease, <u>87</u>
Cured meats
  avoiding, with lupus, <u>363</u>
  brain tumors from, <u>116</u>
Cystic fibrosis, 197–201, 496
Cysts, breast, 251–57

D

Dairy products
  for depression, <u>205</u>
  low-fat, for endometriosis, <u>235</u>
  worsening dermatitis, <u>210</u>
DASH diet, for high blood pressure, 302, <u>304</u>
Dehydration, from diarrhea, 225, 226
Depression, 202–8
  menopausal, 391
Dermatitis, 208–13
Detoxification, pantothenic acid for, 14, 15
Diabetes, 213–23
  effects of, 214–15
    bedsores, 111
    cardiomyopathy, 159–60
    glaucoma, 273–74
    intermittent claudication, <u>347</u>
  magnesium excretion and, 11
  potassium supplements and, 18

pregnancy and, 118
steroid-induced, from lupus, 363
treating, with
   biotin, 5
   B vitamins, 222–23
   chromium, 26, 27, 218–19
   diet, 214, 215–18
   magnesium, 221–22
   multivitamin/mineral supplement, 223
   thiamin, 23
   vitamin E, 219–21
types of, 214
vitamin C and, 44
vitamin D deficiency and, 47
Diagnostic tests, vitamin C and, 46
Diaphragm use, bladder infections from, 121
Diarrhea, 223–26
from vitamin C, 45, 46, 81, 82
Dieting. *See also* Crash diets; Fad diets
bone loss from, 444
Differin, for age spots, 61
Diflucan, for yeast infections, 569, 571
DIM, for premenstrual syndrome, 465,
   466–67
Dimethyl sulfoxide (DMSO), 22
Diuretics
   interacting with nutrients, 54, 56–57
   leg cramps from, 356
   magnesium deficiency from, 101
   for Ménière's disease, 384
   natural, for fibrocystic breasts, 253
   potassium supplements and, 17, 558
DMSO, 22
Douching, for preventing yeast infections, 569
Dovonex, for psoriasis, 474–75, 476
Drug-nutrient interactions, 54–57, 532, 532,
   538

E
———

Eating disorders, 226–33
Eczema, 208–13
Eggs, dermatitis from, 210
Eicosapentaenoic acid (EPA), for multiple
   sclerosis, 413

Electrolytes
   leg cramps and, 355–56
   for treating
      diarrhea, 225
      eating disorders, 230
      heart arrhythmia, 290
Endometriosis, 233–39
EPA, for multiple sclerosis, 413
Epilepsy, 240–47
Epsom salts, magnesium in, 11
Erectile dysfunction, 337
Esophageal cancer, riboflavin preventing, 18
Essential Oils Formula, for tinnitus, 547
Estrogen
   depression and, 391
   infertility and, 335
   menopausal problems and, 385–87
   from overweight, 555
Evening primrose oil, for fibrocystic breasts,
   253, 254
Eye problems
   cataracts, 18, 44, 166–71, 369
   glaucoma, 271–75
   macular degeneration, 53, 367–73
   night blindness, 72, 417–20
   retinitis pigmentosa, 418–19, 419, 420

F
———

Fad diets, nutrient deficiences from, 439–40
Fat, body, affecting hormones, 335
Fatigue, 247–51
Fats, dietary
   aging and, 69
   cancer prevention and, 134
   in diabetes diet, 217
   fatigue and, 248
   fibrocystic breasts and, 252–53, 253
   in heart disease prevention, 292
   premenstrual syndrome and, 461
   prostate problems and, 468
Fava beans, avoiding, with Parkinson's
   disease, 450
Ferrous sulfate, as iron supplement, 10
Fetal alcohol syndrome, 116

Fever blisters. *See* Cold sores
Fiber
  for preventing
    cancer, <u>136</u>
    prostate cancer, <u>469</u>
  after surgery, <u>534</u>
  for treating
    constipation, <u>395</u>, <u>551</u>
    diabetes, <u>216–17</u>
    fibrocystic breasts, <u>253</u>
    high cholesterol, <u>311</u>
    multiple sclerosis, <u>413</u>
  for weight loss, <u>443</u>
Fibrocystic breasts, 30, 251–57
Fingernail problems, 257–58
Fish
  for preventing
    Alzheimer's disease, <u>87</u>
    angina, <u>99</u>
    cancer, <u>135–36</u>
    gallstones, <u>261</u>
    glaucoma, <u>273</u>
    hair loss, <u>281</u>
    heart disease, <u>292</u>
    prostate cancer, <u>469</u>
  for treating
    asthma, <u>105</u>
    depression, <u>205</u>
    dermatitis, <u>211</u>
    fatigue, <u>248</u>
    heart arrhythmia, <u>286</u>
    high blood pressure, <u>305</u>
    high cholesterol, <u>311</u>
    intermittent claudication, <u>346</u>
    lupus, <u>365</u>
    Raynaud's phenomenon, <u>478</u>
    rheumatoid arthritis, <u>488</u>
    scleroderma, <u>500</u>
Fish oil supplements
  caution about, <u>141</u>
  for preventing
    cancer, <u>140</u>
    heart disease, <u>292</u>
  for treating
    cancer, <u>141</u>
    dermatitis, <u>211</u>

    gout, <u>277</u>
    heart arrhythmia, <u>286</u>
    high blood pressure, <u>305</u>
    intermittent claudication, <u>346</u>
    lupus, 364, <u>365</u>
    osteoarthritis, 423
    psoriasis, <u>474</u>
    Raynaud's phenomenon, <u>478</u>
Flavonoids, for cancer prevention, <u>134–35</u>
Flaxseed oil, for treating
  fibrocystic breasts, <u>253</u>
  prostate problems, <u>469</u>, <u>471</u>
Fluconazole, for yeast infections, 569, 571
Fluids. *See also* Water
  for colds, <u>188</u>
  for HIV patients, <u>317</u>
  after surgery, <u>534</u>
Fluoride
  overview of, 29–30
  for preventing osteoporosis, 30, 435–36,
    <u>437</u>
Folate. *See also* Folate deficiency; Folic acid
  for cancer prevention, 150–51
  food sources of, 117
Folate deficiency
  in alcoholics, 76
  anemia from, 95–97
  from low-carbohydrate diet, <u>116</u>
Folic acid
  caution about, <u>100</u>, <u>141</u>
  overview of, 7–9
  for preventing
    Alzheimer's disease, 89
    birth defects, 115–17, <u>118</u>
    blood clots, 457–59, <u>459</u>
    cancer, <u>140</u>, 150–51
    cervical dysplasia, 177–79, <u>178</u>
  for reducing homocysteine, 98–99, 298,
    299, <u>299</u>
  for smokers, <u>523</u>, 524
  for treating
    alcoholism, 76, <u>77</u>
    Alzheimer's disease, <u>88</u>
    anemia, 95–97, <u>95</u>
    angina, 98–100, <u>100</u>
    cancer, <u>141</u>

depression, 204–5, <u>207</u>
endometriosis, <u>236</u>, 238
epilepsy, <u>245</u>, 246–47
gout, 278–79, <u>279</u>
infertility, 337, <u>338</u>
lupus, 364
osteoarthritis, 422, <u>424</u>
restless legs syndrome, <u>484</u>, 485
varicose veins, 552–53, <u>553</u>
Food allergies
asthma and, <u>105</u>
with chronic fatigue syndrome, <u>181</u>
dermatitis and, <u>210</u>
epilepsy and, <u>243</u>
foods causing, <u>81</u>
menstrual problems and, <u>395</u>
with multiple sclerosis, <u>413</u>
rickets from, 496–97
water retention and, <u>555</u>
weight loss and, <u>443</u>
Food triggers, in rheumatoid arthritis,
<u>489</u>
Fractures
in alcoholics, 76
from osteoporosis, 427, <u>431</u>
from vitamin D deficiency, 47
vitamin K preventing, 52
Free radicals
aging from, 66–67
from alcohol, 73
from allergic reactions, 84
Alzheimer's disease and, 86
antioxidants neutralizing, 18, 49, 63, 70,
129, 138, 360, 440, 502
from burns, 129–30
cancer from, 43
cataracts from, 166
from dietary fat, <u>69</u>
heart disease from, 291
Lou Gehrig's disease and, 360, 361
multiple sclerosis and, 414
rheumatoid arthritis and, 490–91
skin damage from, 63, 65
from smoking, 518
from UVA/UVB rays, 525–26
wrinkles from, 565

Fruits
citrus, avoiding, with canker sores,
<u>152</u>
for preventing
cancer, <u>134–35</u>, 145, 147–48, <u>513</u>
heart disease, <u>293</u>
menopausal problems, <u>389</u>
for smokers, <u>519</u>

G

Gallstones, 259–63
Gamma-linolenic acid (GLA), for multiple
sclerosis, <u>413</u>
Garlic
for preventing
angina, <u>99</u>
cancer, <u>135</u>
heart disease, <u>293</u>
yeast infections, <u>570</u>
for treating
colds, <u>188</u>
diarrhea, <u>224</u>
lupus, <u>363</u>
Gazpacho, as anti-aging food, <u>68</u>
Genital herpes, 263–68
Ginger
for preventing angina, <u>99</u>
for treating morning sickness, <u>410</u>
Gingivitis, 268–71
Ginkgo, for tinnitus, <u>543</u>
GLA, for multiple sclerosis, <u>413</u>
Glaucoma, 271–75
Glucose intolerance, from chromium
deficiency, 26
Glucose tolerance factor (GTF), 27
Glutathione, for preventing macular
degeneration, <u>370</u>
Gluten-free diet
for celiac disease, <u>172</u>, 173
for multiple sclerosis, <u>413</u>
Gluten sensitivity
with celiac disease, 171–74
dermatitis from, <u>210–11</u>

Glycemic index and load, diabetes diet and, 216, 218

Gout, 275–80

Grapefruit juice, interacting with drugs, 55

Grape juice, for preventing heart disease, 293

GTF, 27

Gum problems, 268–71

Gyne-Lotrimin, for yeast infections, 569, 571

H

Hair, biotin strengthening, 4

Hair care products, for hair loss, 283–84

Hair loss, 280–84

Headaches. *See* Migraines

Heart arrhythmia, 284–90

Heart attacks, 97, 98, 292, 293

Heart disease, 290–301. *See also* Cardiovascular disease; Coronary heart disease

beta-carotene supplements and, 3

B vitamins and, 457–58, 459

cardiomyopathy, 155–61

causes of, 291–92

copper deficiency and, 28

incidence of, 290

iron and, 301

with lupus, 363, 363

preventing, with

  antioxidants, 291, 293–94

  beta-carotene, 3, 4, 295–96

  B vitamins, 297–99

  diet, 292–93

  folic acid, 7, 99–100

  homocysteine reduction, 39, 41

  magnesium, 300

  niacin, 12–13

  selenium, 100–101, 299, 300

  thiamin, 23

  vitamin B6, 39

  vitamin C, 43–44, 297

  zinc, 299, 300

vitamin E and, 49, 294–95

Heart failure, coenzyme Q10 for, 158–59

Heart health

chromium for, 26

selenium for, 34

Heart-healthy diet, for heart arrhythmia, 287

Heart surgery, vitamin E and, 537–38

Herpes, genital, 263–68

Herpes simplex virus

cold sores from, 193, 194

genital herpes from, 264

Herpes zoster, 507–12

High blood pressure, 301–9

antioxidants and, 309

intermittent claudication with, 347

from potassium deficiency, 17

pregnancy and, 118

sodium and, 20–21

treating, with

  calcium, 307, 308–9

  DASH diet, 302, 304

  diet, 304–5

  drugs, 54, 56–57, 302

  magnesium, 306–8, 307

  potassium, 306, 307

  salt restriction, 302–5, 304

  vitamin C, 44

High cholesterol, 309–14

inner ear damage from, 380

treating, with

  diet, 311

  mucilage, 99

  niacin, 312, 313

  omega-3 fatty acids, 99

  vitamin C, 310, 312–13, 312

  vitamin E, 49, 312, 313

zinc and, 314

Histamine, allergies from, 79–80

HIV, 314–24

dietary considerations with, 317

nutrient deficiencies with, 315–17

nutrient support with, 23, 34, 44, 318–24

shingles and, 507

Homocysteine

atherosclerosis from, 297

blood clots and, 457, 458

memory loss and, 375, 376

reducing, with
 B vitamins, 297–99, 457, 553
 folic acid, 7, 98–99, 298, 299, _299_
 riboflavin, 18
 vitamin B_{12,} 41
Hormone replacement therapy, depression
 and, 203, 206, 391
Hormones, effects on
 depression, 203, 206
 fibrocystic breasts, 252–53
 gallstones, 260
 infertility, _335_
Hospital food, _533_
Hot flashes, menopausal, _386_, 387–89, _388_,
 _389_
HPV, cervical cancer and, 175
H_2 receptor antagonists, interacting with
 nutrients, _56–57_
Human papillomavirus (HPV), cervical
 cancer and, 175
Hypertension. _See_ High blood pressure
Hysterectomy, menopause from, 391–92

I

Icaps, for eye health, 369
Idebenone, for wrinkles, _566_, 567–68
Immune system. _See also_ Immunity
 food intolerances and, _443_
 in HIV, 322–23
 nutritional deficiencies affecting, 324–26
 in scleroderma, 499
 vitamin C for, 206
 vitamin D for, 48
 zinc and, 52–53
Immunity, 324–32. _See also_ Immune system
 boosting, in shingles patients, 511–12
 of overweight people, 440, 441
Immunomax, for cancer treatment, _146_
Impotence, _337_
Infections, bladder. _See_ Bladder infections
Infections, yeast, 568–73
Infertility, 332–39, 522
Inner ear damage, from Ménière's disease,
 380–84

Inositol nicotinate, for Raynaud's
 phenomenon, 479, _480_
Insomnia, 339–44
Insulin, effect of chromium on, 26
Intermittent claudication, 345–49
Iodine
 for fibrocystic breasts, 255, _256_
 overview of, 30–31
Iodoral, as iodine supplement, 31
Iron. _See also_ Iron deficiency
 caution about, _95_
 copper and, 29
 heart disease and, 301
 overview of, 9–10
 poisoning from, 10
 during pregnancy, _118_, 119
 for preventing
  gallstones, 263
  hair loss, 281–82, _281_, _282_
 for treating
  anemia, 92, _95_
  eating disorders, _231_, 233
  endometriosis, _236_, 239
  fatigue, 249, _250_
  heavy menstrual bleeding, 389–90, _390_,
   391, _396_, 398
  immune system, _330_, 331
  insomnia, 342–43, _344_
  memory loss, _377_, 379
  restless legs syndrome, 483–85, _484_
 vitamin C and, _281_, 282, _282_, _325_, 391
 weight loss and, _445_, 446, 447
Iron deficiency
 anemia from, 91, 92
 restless legs syndrome from, 9, 483–85
 symptoms of, 9

K

Ketogenic diet, for epilepsy, _242_, 243–44
Kidney disease, potassium supplements and,
 18
Kidneys, magnesium excretion and, 11
Kidney stones, 17, 19, 349–55
Kiwifruit, for preventing blood clots, _458_

L

—

Lactose intolerance, with celiac disease, 172
Laxatives, interacting with nutrients, 56–57
L-carnitine, for treating depression, 205
Lecithin, for treating memory loss, 378
Leg cramps, 355–59, 486
Levodopa, for Parkinson's disease, 450
Liver damage
    from alcoholism, 72, 73, 78
    from niacin, 13
Lou Gehrig's disease, 359–61
Low-acid diet, for preventing bladder
        infections, 121
Low-carbohydrate diet, folate deficiency
        from, 116
Low-fat diet
    for preventing impotence, 337
    for treating
        angina, 98, 99
        chronic fatigue syndrome, 181
        depression, 205
        fatigue, 248
        fibrocystic breasts, 252–53, 253
        high cholesterol, 311
        intermittent claudication, 347
        leg cramps, 356
        overweight, 442
        rheumatoid arthritis, 488–89
        scleroderma, 500
L-tyrosine, aggravating restless legs
        syndrome, 481
Lung cancer
    beta-carotene supplements and, 3,
        520–21
    preventing, with
        diet, 513
        selenium, 143
    from smog exposure, 513
    supplement use with, 149
    vitamin E and, 142, 514
Lupus, 362–67
Lutein, for preventing
    cataracts, 167
    glaucoma, 273
    macular degeneration, 370

Lycopene, for preventing
    macular degeneration, 370
    prostate cancer, 135, 470–71
Lysine, for treating
    cold sores, 194
    genital herpes, 265
    shingles, 509

M

—

Macrocytic anemia, 41
Macular degeneration, 53, 367–73
Magnesium. See also Magnesium deficiency
    caution about, 77, 83, 102
    overview of, 10–12
    for preventing
        kidney stones, 352, 353
        leg cramps, 357–59, 358
        migraines, 401–4, 403
        osteoporosis, 390, 392, 433–34, 437
    for treating
        alcoholism, 76, 77
        allergies, 82, 83
        angina, 100, 101–2
        asthma, 103–5, 107
        cardiomyopathy, 160–61, 160
        chronic fatigue syndrome, 183–84
        congestive heart failure, 300
        diabetes, 220, 221–22
        eating disorders, 230, 231
        endometriosis, 236, 239
        fatigue, 249–50, 250
        heart arrhythmia, 285–87, 288–89,
            288
        high blood pressure, 306–8, 307
        insomnia, 343–44, 344
        Ménière's disease, 382–83, 383
        menstrual problems, 394–97, 396
        mitral valve prolapse, 405–8, 408
        premenstrual syndrome, 463–64, 465
        prostate problems, 472
        restless legs syndrome, 484, 486
        tinnitus, 545, 546–47
        water retention, 557, 558
    weight loss and, 445, 446–47

Magnesium deficiency
  from alcoholism, 76
  drugs causing, 101
  heart arrhythmia from, 286, 287–88
  seizures from, 241
  symptoms of, 11
  treating, 102
Magnesium gluconate, 12, 403–4
Malabsorption, with scleroderma, 503
Malnutrition, pantothenic acid deficiency
      with, 14
Manganese, 23
  overview of, 31–32
  for preventing osteoporosis, 436, 437
  for treating
    menstrual problems, 394–97, 396
    premenstrual syndrome, 463, 465
Meats
  avoiding, for kidney stone prevention, 350–51
  cured
    avoiding, with lupus, 363
    brain tumors from, 116
  grilled or smoked, cancer risk from, 136
  premenstrual syndrome and, 462
  red
    cancer risk from, 136
    iron in, 233
    menstrual cramping and, 395
    for preventing anemia, 96
    prostate problems and, 468
  for treating depression, 205
Mediterranean diet, for preventing
    Alzheimer's disease, 87
Memory loss, 72, 373–79. *See also* Alzheimer's
    disease
Ménière's disease, 380–84
Menopausal problems, 385–92
Menstrual bleeding, heavy, 389–91, 398
Menstrual problems, 393–98
  heavy bleeding, 389–91, 398
  premenstrual syndrome, 460–67
Methylsulfonylmethane (MSM), 22
Miconazole, for yeast infections, 569, 571
Migraines, 399–404
  preventing, with
    calcium, 404
    diet, 400–401

    magnesium, 401–4, 403
    riboflavin, 18, 399–401, 403
    vitamin B$_6$, 39
  symptoms of, 399
Milk, worsening dermatitis, 210
Milk allergy, rickets from, 496–97
Minimeals, for weight loss, 442
Mitral valve prolapse, 404–8
Molybdenum, 23
  overview of, 33–34
Monistat, for yeast infections, 569, 571
Monounsaturated fats
  for cancer prevention, 134
  in diabetes diet, 217
Morning sickness, 409–11
MRI contrasting agent, scleroderma from,
    501
MSG
  aggravating tinnitus, 543
  migraines from, 400
  water retention from, 555
MSM, 22
Mucilage, for angina prevention, 99
Mucous membranes, allergies and, 84
Multiple sclerosis, 411–16
Multivitamin Formula, for tinnitus, 547
Multivitamin/mineral supplements
  for preventing
    birth defects, 119
    cancer, 140
    canker sores, 153, 154
    cataracts, 167, 169, 369
    macular degeneration, 369, 372
    osteoporosis, 437, 438
  for slowing aging, 71
  for smokers, 523, 524
  trace minerals in, 24, 27, 29, 32, 34, 36
  for treating
    alcoholism, 77
    allergies, 82, 84
    bedsores, 111, 111
    cancer, 141, 146
    cardiomyopathy, 160
    diabetes, 220, 223
    eating disorders, 229, 231
    epilepsy, 245
    fingernail problems, 258, 258

Multivitamin/mineral supplements (*cont.*)
  for treating (*cont.*)
    hair loss, <u>282</u>, 283
    immune system, 332
    infertility, <u>338</u>, 339
    Ménière's disease, <u>383</u>, 384
    osteoarthritis, <u>424</u>, 426
    overweight people, 439–40, 441, <u>445</u>
    Parkinson's disease, <u>452</u>, 453
    psoriasis, 476
    tinnitus, <u>545</u>
Muscles, magnesium for, 11

N

Nail problems, 257–58
Nails, biotin strengthening, 4, 248, <u>258</u>
Nephrogenic fibrosing dermopathy, 501
Nerve damage, from Vitamin B$_6$ deficiency, 39
Nerve function, vitamin B$_{12}$ for, 40–41
Neural tube defects, folic acid preventing, 8,
    115–17
Neuropathy, peripheral, biotin and, 5
Niacin
  avoiding, with gout, 280
  for HIV patients, 319
  overview of, 12–14
  for preventing cataracts, 169–70
  for treating
    endometriosis, <u>236</u>, 238
    high cholesterol, <u>312</u>, 313
    insomnia, 341, <u>344</u>
    menopausal problems, <u>390</u>, 391
    menstrual problems, <u>396</u>, 398
    pellagra, 455–56
    Raynaud's phenomenon, 479
Niacinamide, 14
  for treating
    osteoarthritis, <u>424</u>, 426
    pellagra, 455–56, <u>455</u>
Nicotine replacement products, <u>519</u>
Nicotinic acid, for treating
  Ménière's disease, <u>383</u>, 384
  pellagra, 455–56
  Raynaud's phenomenon, 479, <u>480</u>
Niferex, for hair loss, 282

Night blindness, 72, 417–20
Night sweats, menopausal, <u>386</u>, 387
Nitrates, vitamin C neutralizing, 43
Nitrites
  brain tumors from, <u>116</u>
  migraines from, <u>400</u>
  vitamin C neutralizing, 43
Nitroglycerin, for angina, 98
Nutrition, drugs affecting, <u>54–57</u>

O

Obesity. *See also* Overweight
  asthma and, <u>104</u>
  carpal tunnel syndrome and, 163
Ocuvite, for eye health, 369
Oils, in cancer prevention, <u>134</u>
Omacor, for heart arrhythmia, <u>286</u>
Omega-3 fatty acids
  for preventing
    angina, <u>99</u>
    cancer, <u>135–36</u>
    gallstones, <u>261</u>
    glaucoma, <u>273</u>
    hair loss, <u>281</u>
    heart disease, <u>292</u>, <u>298</u>
    macular degeneration, 370
    prostate cancer, <u>469</u>
  for treating
    depression, <u>205</u>
    dermatitis, <u>211</u>
    diabetes, <u>217</u>
    fatigue, <u>248</u>
    gout, <u>277</u>
    heart arrhythmia, <u>286</u>
    high blood pressure, <u>305</u>
    high cholesterol, <u>311</u>
    intermittent claudication, <u>346</u>
    lupus, <u>365</u>
    osteoarthritis, 423
    psoriasis, <u>474</u>
    Raynaud's phenomenon, <u>478</u>
    rheumatoid arthritis, <u>488</u>
Onions, for preventing
  angina, <u>99</u>
  cancer, <u>135</u>

Orange peels, for preventing skin cancer, 526
Oregano, for cancer prevention, 136–37
Organic foods, for endometriosis, 235
Osteoarthritis, 421–26
Osteomalacia, 46, 496, 498, 499. *See also*
    Rickets
Osteoporosis, 427–38
  causes of
    alcohol, 72, 76
    bone loss, 427–28, 522
    copper deficiency, 28
    corticosteroids, 367
    phosphorus imbalance, 15–16, 389
    proton-pump inhibitors, 54
  manganese deficiency and, 31–32
  preventing, with
    boron, 434–35, 437
    calcium, 5–6, 263, 390, 392, 428–32,
      437, 461
    copper, 436, 437
    diet, 430–31
    fluoride, 30, 435–36, 437
    magnesium, 433–34, 437
    manganese, 436, 437
    multivitamin/mineral supplement, 437,
      438
    vitamin D, 46, 47, 432–33, 437
    vitamin K, 437–38, 437
    zinc, 436, 437
  vitamin K deficiency and, 51
Overeating, insomnia from, 340
Overweight, 438–47, 555. *See also* Obesity
Oxalates, kidney stones and, 351

P

Pancreatic digestive enzymes, for cystic
    fibrosis patients, 199, 200, 201
Pantothenic acid
  overview of, 14–15
  for treating
    endometriosis, 236, 238
    fatigue, 251
Parkinson's disease, 447–53
Pauling, Linus, 43, 189
Peanuts, dermatitis from, 211

Pellagra, 453–56
  in alcoholics, 72
  cardiomyopathy from, 156
  niacin preventing, 13
Perimenopause, 385, 389, 558. *See also*
    Menopausal problems
Periodontal disease, 268
Peripheral neuropathy, biotin and, 5
Pernicious anemia, 8, 41, 94, 95, 141, 151, 279
Phenylketonuria, seizures from, 242
Phlebitis, 456–60
Phosphorus
  calcium and, 6, 15–16, 269, 389, 430
  overview of, 15–16
  vitamin D and, 46–47
Phytoestrogens, for menopausal problems,
    386
Pineapple, for gout, 277
Plaque, arterial
  angina from, 97, 98
  formation of, 291–92
PMS. *See* Premenstrual syndrome
Polyunsaturated fats, 134
Postpartum depression, 203
Potassium. *See also* Potassium deficiency
  caution about, 231
  overview of, 16–18
  for preventing
    kidney stones, 353, 354–55
    leg cramps, 357, 358
  sodium and, 16, 20
  for treating
    eating disorders, 230, 231
    fatigue, 249–50, 250
    heart arrhythmia, 288, 289–90
    high blood pressure, 306, 307
    leg cramps, 356, 486
    Ménière's disease, 383–84, 383
    osteoporosis, 431
    water retention, 557, 557
Potassium deficiency
  from diuretics, 101
  symptoms of, 17
Pregnancy
  carpal tunnel syndrome and, 163, 164
  leg cramps during, 356
  morning sickness during, 409–11
  nutrient deficiency after, 461

Pregnancy (*cont.*)
  preventing birth defects during, 8, 114–19
  varicose veins from, 549–50
Premenstrual depression, 203, 206
Premenstrual syndrome (PMS), 39, 460–67,
      558–59
Propolis, for canker sores, 152
Prostate cancer
  from excessive zinc, 54–55
  preventing, with
    fiber, 136, 469
    fish, 135–36, 469
    lycopene, 135, 470–71
    selenium, 143
    soy foods, 136
    vitamin E, 139
  saturated fat increasing, 134
Prostate problems, 53, 467–72. *See also*
      Prostate cancer
Protein
  animal, premenstrual syndrome and, 462
  as anti-aging food, 69
  for HIV patients, 317
  Parkinson's disease and, 450
  for preventing bedsores, 100
  after surgery, 534
  for treating
    bedsores, 100
    burns, 131
    osteoporosis, 431
Protein powders, glaucoma and, 273
Proton-pump inhibitors, interacting with
      nutrients, 54, 56–57
Psoralens, sun sensitivity from, 526
Psoriasis, 472–76
Purines, avoiding, with gout, 276–77, 276,
      278
Pyridoxine. *See* Vitamin B$_6$

Raynaud's phenomenon, 477–81
Renova, for wrinkles, 565
Restless legs syndrome (RLS), 9, 343,
      481–86

Retin-A
  alcohol and, 564
  for treating
    age spots, 61
    wrinkles, 563–65
Retinitis pigmentosa, 418–19, 419, 420
Retinoic acid, for age spots, 61–63, 64
Rheumatoid arthritis, 487–95
Riboflavin
  overview of, 18–19
  for preventing
    cataracts, 169–70, 169
    migraines, 18, 399–401, 403
  symptoms of deficiency of, 19
  for treating
    carpal tunnel syndrome, 164, 165
    depression, 205, 206, 207
    endometriosis, 236, 238
    HIV patients, 319, 320
    immune system, 327, 330
Rickets, 46, 47, 496–99. *See also*
      Osteomalacia
RLS. *See* Restless legs syndrome
Rutin, for bruises, 124

Salt. *See* Sodium
Salt restriction. *See* Sodium restriction
Saturated fat
  cancer risk from, 134
  fibrocystic breasts and, 252–53
  lung cancer risk from, 513
  reducing
    for gallstone prevention, 261
    for lowering blood cholesterol, 311
    with lupus, 363
    with Ménière's disease, 380
Saw palmetto, for prostate problems, 471–72,
      471
Scleroderma, 499–503
Scurvy, 503–6
  in alcoholics, 72
  depression with, 206
  from vitamin C deficiency, 45, 503–6

R

S

Seizures, epileptic, 240–47
Selenium
  cardiomyopathy from deficiency of,
      156–57
  caution about, _64_, 65, _77_
  for mucous membrane protection, 84
  overview of, 34–36
  Parkinson's disease and, 453
  for preventing
    cancer, _140_, 143–45
    cataracts, _169_, 171
    heart disease, _299_, 300
    macular degeneration, _372_, 373
    wrinkles, _566_, 568
  for sun protection, _529_, 530
  for treating
    age spots, _64_, 65
    alcoholism, _77_
    angina, 100–101, _100_
    asthma, _107_, 108
    cancer, _141_, 145
    cardiomyopathy, 157, _160_
    colds, _190_, 193
    depression, _207_, 208
    effects of aging, 70, _70_
    effects of smog exposure, _515_, 517
    endometriosis, _236_, 239
    epilepsy, _245_, 246
    HIV patients, _321_, 322–24
    infertility, 336, _338_
    lupus, 364, _366_
    multiple sclerosis, 414, _415_
    osteoarthritis, 424–25, _424_
    prostate problems, 472
    rheumatoid arthritis, 491–92, _493_
    tinnitus, _545_, 547
Shellfish, dermatitis from, _211_
Shingles, 507–12
Silicon, 24
Skin cancer, 61
  preventing, _526_
  selenium and, 143
Skin problems. _See also_ Skin cancer
  age spots, 61–65
  bedsores, 109–12
  bruises, 123–27
  burns, 127–32

dermatitis, 208–13
  psoriasis, 472–76
  sunburn, 525–31
  wrinkles, 563–68
Sleep problems
  insomnia, 339–44
  restless legs syndrome, 343, 481–86
Smell and taste problems, 539–42
Smog exposure, 512–17
Smokers, vitamins C and E for,
      141–42
Smoking, 517–24
  alcohol and
    avoiding, _519_
    increasing cancer risk, _137_
  beta-carotene supplements and, 3,
      296–97, 520–21
  sperm abnormalities from, 521–22
  vitamin C deficiency from, 506
  vitamin E and, 142
Soda. _See_ Soft drinks
Sodium. _See also_ Sodium restriction
  for leg cramps, _356_
  overview of, 20–21
  potassium and, 16, 20
Sodium restriction
  with premenstrual syndrome, _462_
  for preventing kidney stones, _350_
  for treating
    asthma, _105_
    fibrocystic breasts, _253_
    high blood pressure, 302–5, _304_
    intermittent claudication, _347_
    Ménière's disease, _381_, 382
    menopausal problems, _388_
    menstrual problems, _395_
    osteoporosis, _431_
    tinnitus, _543_
    varicose veins, _551_
    water retention, _555_, 556
Soft drinks
  phosphorus imbalance from, 15–16
Soft drinks, avoiding, with
  gingivitis, _269_
  leg cramps, _356_
  menopausal problems, _389_
  osteoporosis, _430_

Soy foods
  dermatitis from, 211
  for preventing
    cancer, 136
    heart disease, 293
    menopausal problems, 386
  for treating high cholesterol, 311
Sperm health, 333–36
  smoking and, 521–22
Spermicidal jellies, bladder infections from,
    122
Spicy foods, for colds, 188
Sports drinks, for diarrhea, 225, 226
Statins, vitamin C and, 46
Stomach cancer, vitamin C deficiency and, 133
Stress, magnesium deficiency and, 343–44
Stroke
  B vitamins and, 457–58, 459
  preventing, with
    folic acid, 7
    potassium, 17
    vitamin C, 44
Subscurvy, 505–6, 505
Sugar
  avoiding, for
    glaucoma prevention, 273
    kidney stone prevention, 350
    weight loss, 442
  avoiding, with
    chronic fatigue syndrome, 180
    fatigue, 248
    gingivitis, 269
    high blood pressure, 305
    leg cramps, 356
    lupus, 363
    Ménière's disease, 380–81
    mitral valve prolapse, 406
    premenstrual syndrome, 462
    tinnitus, 543
    yeast infections, 570
  depression and, 204
  immunity and, 325
  increasing cancer risk, 137
  worsening premenstrual syndrome, 461
Sulfites
  as asthma trigger, 104–5
  sensitivity to, 33

Sulfur, overview of, 21–22
Sunburn, 525–31
Sun damage, nutrients preventing, 63, 64,
    65
Sun exposure
  skin damage from, 525–26, 563
  vitamin D from, 47, 563
Sunscreen
  antioxidants in, 527
  for preventing wrinkles, 563
  used with anti-bruising formula, 126–27
  used with Cellex-C, 63
Sun sensitivity, foods increasing, 62
Supplements, drug interactions with, 532,
    532, 538
Surgery, 531–38

T

Tachycardia, 284–85
Taste and smell problems, 539–42
Tea
  for cancer prevention, 135
  for treating
    bruises, 124
    high blood pressure, 305
    infertility, 335
    water retention, 555
Thiamin. *See also* Thiamin deficiency
  caution about, 88
  overview of, 22–23
  for preventing cataracts, 169–70, 169
  for treating
    alcoholism, 75, 77
    Alzheimer's disease, 88, 90–91
    beriberi, 113, 114
    cardiomyopathy, 158–60, 160
    depression, 205–6, 207
    endometriosis, 237, 238
    HIV patients, 319, 320
    insomnia, 341, 344
    menopausal problems, 390, 391
Thiamin deficiency
  Alzheimer's disease from, 114
  beriberi from, 113–14

seizures from, 241
symptoms of, 23
Thrombophlebitis, 456–57
Tinnitus, 542–48
Tomato sauce, for cancer prevention, 135
Tooth health, flouride for, 29
Toxic exposure, scleroderma from, 500–501
Trace minerals, 23–36. *See also specific trace minerals*
Tranquilizers, interacting with nutrients, 56–57
Trans fats, cancer risk from, 134
Tretinoin. *See* Retin-A
Tryptophan, for insomnia, 342
Turmeric, for preventing
  cancer, 137
  yeast infections, 570
Tyramine, migraines from, 401

U

Ulcers, vitamin C and, 506
Urinary tract infections. *See* Bladder infections
UVA/UVB rays, from sun exposure, 525–26, 563

V

Valtrex, for genital herpes, 264
Vanadium, 24
  avoiding, for glaucoma prevention, 273
Varicella virus vaccine, 507
Varicose veins, 549–54
Vegans, vitamin B_{12} deficiency in, 93
Vegetables
  cruciferous
    for cancer prevention, 137, 466
    for premenstrual syndrome, 466
  for preventing
    anemia, 96
    cancer, 134–35, 145, 147–48
    heart disease, 293

lung cancer, 513
menopausal problems, 389
for smokers, 519
Vegetarian diet
  for treating
    premenstrual syndrome, 462
    psoriasis, 475
  vitamin B_{12} deficiency from, 27, 41, 93, 95
Vertigo, from Ménière's disease, 380–84
Vitamin A
  alcoholism and, 73–75
  birth defects from, 119
  caution about, 419
  deficiency of, 37
  excessive, effects of, 565
  for mucous membrane protection, 84
  overview of, 36–38
  for treating
    age spots, 64
    alcoholism, 77
    cancer, 145
    eating disorders, 231, 232–33
    effects of aging, 70
    effects of smog exposure, 515, 517
    endometriosis, 239
    fibrocystic breasts, 255–56
    HIV patients, 319, 320, 321
    immune system, 326–27, 330
    night blindness, 417–18, 419
    overweight people, 440, 441, 445
    prostate problems, 472
    psoriasis, 475–76
    surgical healing, 535–36
    yeast infections, 572, 573
Vitamin B_1. *See* Thiamin
Vitamin B_2. *See* Riboflavin
Vitamin B_5. *See* Pantothenic acid
Vitamin B_6
  deficiency of, 39, 241
  overview of, 38–40
  for preventing
    blood clots, 457–59, 459
    kidney stones, 352–54, 353
  for reducing homocysteine, 298, 299
  for treating
    alcoholism, 75–76, 77
    carpal tunnel syndrome, 163–65, 164

Vitamin B$_6$ (*cont.*)
  for treating (*cont.*)
    depression, 206, <u>207</u>
    diabetes, 222–23
    endometriosis, <u>237</u>, 238
    fibrocystic breasts, <u>256</u>, 257
    HIV patients, 319, 320, <u>321</u>
    insomnia, 341, <u>344</u>
    memory loss, 375–76, <u>377</u>, 379
    menopausal problems, <u>390</u>, 391
    menstrual problems, <u>396</u>, 397–98
    mitral valve prolapse, <u>408</u>
    morning sickness, 409–10, <u>411</u>
    premenstrual syndrome, <u>465</u>, 466
    prostate problems, 472
    varicose veins, 553, <u>553</u>
    water retention, <u>557</u>, 558–59
Vitamin B$_{12}$. *See also* Vitamin B$_{12}$ deficiency
  cobalt in, 27
  overview of, 40–42
  for preventing
    blood clots, 457–59, <u>459</u>
    cancer, <u>140</u>
  for treating
    anemia, 94–95, <u>95</u>
    cancer, <u>141</u>, 151
    diabetes, 222
    endometriosis, <u>237</u>, 238
    HIV patients, <u>321</u>, 322
    insomnia, 341, <u>344</u>
    memory loss, 375–77, <u>377</u>
    multiple sclerosis, 414–16, <u>415</u>
    osteoarthritis, 422, <u>424</u>
    shingles, 508, <u>510</u>
    tinnitus, 544–46, <u>545</u>
    varicose veins, 553, <u>553</u>, 554
Vitamin B$_{12}$ deficiency
  effects of, 40–41, 94, 375
  vs. folate deficiency, 96
  from food-bound malabsorption, 41–42
  treating, 94–95
  in vegetarians, 27, 41, <u>93</u>, 95
Vitamin C
  avoiding, with
    gout, 280
    kidney stones, <u>351</u>

copper and, 29
deficiency of, 45, 269–70
iron and, <u>281</u>, 282, <u>282</u>, <u>325</u>, 391
overview of, 42–46
for preventing
  anemia, <u>96</u>
  cancer, 133, 138–39
  cataracts, 166, 168–69, <u>169</u>
  cervical cancer, 175–76, <u>178</u>
  genital herpes recurrences, 265–67,
    266
  heart disease, 297, <u>298</u>
  macular degeneration, 369, 370–71, <u>372</u>
  wrinkles, 565–67, <u>566</u>
scleroderma and, 503
for smokers, 521–22, <u>523</u>
sun protection from, 527–28, <u>529</u>
for treating
  age spots, 63, <u>64</u>
  alcoholism, <u>77</u>
  allergies, 80–82, <u>82</u>
  asthma, 106–7, <u>107</u>
  bedsores, 111–12, <u>111</u>
  bladder infections, 122–23, <u>122</u>
  bruises, 125–27, <u>126</u>
  burns, <u>128</u>, 130–31
  cancer, <u>141</u>
  canker sores, 153, <u>154</u>
  colds, 189–91, <u>190</u>, 192
  cold sores, 195, <u>196</u>
  depression, 206–8, <u>207</u>
  dermatitis, 212–13, <u>212</u>
  effects of aging, 70, <u>70</u>
  effects of smog exposure, <u>515</u>, 516
  endometriosis, <u>237</u>, 238, 239
  fatigue, 250–51, <u>250</u>
  gingivitis, 269–71, <u>270</u>
  glaucoma, <u>274</u>, 275
  hair loss, <u>282</u>, 283
  heavy menstrual bleeding, 390–91, <u>390</u>,
    <u>396</u>, 398
  high cholesterol, 310, 312–13, <u>312</u>
  HIV patients, 319, <u>321</u>, 322
  immune system, 328, <u>330</u>
  infertility, 333–34, <u>338</u>
  intermittent claudication, 345–46, <u>348</u>

lupus, 363, 364, 366, <u>366</u>
multiple sclerosis, 414, <u>415</u>
osteoarthritis, 425
overweight people, 440, 441, <u>445</u>
Parkinson's disease, 449
prostate problems, 472
rheumatoid arthritis, 490–91, <u>493</u>
scurvy, <u>505</u>, 506
shingles, 508–11, <u>510</u>
subscurvy, <u>505</u>, 506
surgical healing, 533, 535
tinnitus, <u>545</u>, 547
varicose veins, 550, <u>553</u>
yeast infections, 571–72, <u>572</u>
vitamin E and, 50
Vitamin D
deficiency of, 46, 47–48, 496–97
overview of, 46–48
for preventing
osteoarthritis, <u>424</u>, 425–26
osteoporosis, 432–33, <u>437</u>
rickets, 498, <u>498</u>
for treating
alcoholism, 76, <u>77</u>, 78
asthma, 108
celiac disease, <u>173</u>, 174
effects of smog exposure, 514–15, <u>515</u>
immune system, 328–29, <u>330</u>
lupus, <u>366</u>, 367
multiple sclerosis, <u>415</u>, 416
psoriasis, 473–75
rickets, 498–99, <u>498</u>
Vitamin E
caution about, <u>64</u>, 82, <u>502</u>, 514
diabetes and, 219–21, <u>220</u>
heart disease and, 294–95, <u>298</u>
lung cancer and, 142, 514
overview of, 48–50
Parkinson's disease and, 449–51
for preventing
Alzheimer's disease, 87–89
cancer, 139–43, <u>140</u>
cataracts, 166, <u>169</u>, 170–71
cervical dysplasia, 175, <u>178</u>
genital herpes recurrences, <u>266</u>, 267–68

Lou Gehrig's disease, 361
macular degeneration, 369, 371, <u>372</u>
phlebitis, <u>459</u>, 460
for smokers, 518, 520, <u>523</u>
sun protection from, 528, <u>529</u>
for treating
age spots, 64–65, <u>64</u>
alcoholism, <u>77</u>
allergies, 80–81, <u>82</u>
Alzheimer's disease, <u>88</u>
asthma, <u>107</u>, 108
bruises, 126
burns, <u>128</u>, 129–30
cancer, <u>141</u>
cold sores, <u>196</u>, 197
dermatitis, 211–12, <u>212</u>
eating disorders, <u>231</u>, 232–33
effects of aging, 70, <u>70</u>
effects of smog exposure, 514, <u>515</u>, 516
endometriosis, <u>237</u>, 238–39
epilepsy, 244, <u>245</u>
gout, 279–80, <u>279</u>
heart surgery patients, 537–38
high cholesterol, <u>312</u>, 313
HIV patients, <u>321</u>
hot flashes, 387–89, <u>390</u>
immune system, 329–31, <u>330</u>
infertility, 336, <u>338</u>
intermittent claudication, 345–49, <u>348</u>
lupus, 363, 364, 366, <u>366</u>
memory loss, 377–78, <u>377</u>
multiple sclerosis, 414, <u>415</u>
night blindness, 420
osteoarthritis, 423–24, <u>424</u>
overweight people, 440, 441, <u>445</u>
premenstrual syndrome, 464–65, <u>465</u>
prostate problems, 472
Raynaud's phenomenon, 479–81, <u>480</u>
restless legs syndrome, <u>484</u>, 486
rheumatoid arthritis, 492, <u>493</u>
shingles, <u>510</u>, 511
tinnitus, <u>545</u>, 547
varicose veins, 550–51, <u>553</u>
wrinkles, <u>566</u>, 567
yeast infections, <u>572</u>, 573

Vitamin K
    deficiency of, 51
    overview of, 50–52
    for preventing osteoporosis, 437–38, 437
    for treating bruises, 124–25, 126
    vitamin E and, 50

W

Water
    for preventing
        bladder infections, 120
        kidney stones, 350
        wrinkles, 564
    for treating
        gout, 277
        mitral valve prolapse, 406
        multiple sclerosis, 413
        prostate problems, 468
        water retention, 555
    for weight loss, 442–43
Water retention, 554–59
Weight, fertility and, 335
Weight control, for gallstone prevention,
        260, 261
Weight loss
    calcium for, 441–44
    diet for, 442–43
    hair loss from, 281
    nutrients supporting, 444–47
    slow, with mitral valve prolapse, 406
    for treating
        carpal tunnel syndrome, 162, 163
        diabetes, 216
        gout, 277
        high blood pressure, 305
        osteoarthritis, 422
        prostate problems, 468
        varicose veins, 551
        water retention, 555
Wernicke-Korsakoff syndrome, 113–14
Wheat germ, for preventing memory loss, 374
Wheat sensitivity
    in celiac disease, 171–74
    menstrual problems and, 395

Wilson's disease, 29, 54, 559–62
Wrinkles, 525, 563–68

Y

Yeast infections, 568–73
Yeasty foods, avoiding, with yeast infections,
        570
Yogurt
    with antibiotic use, 500
    for canker sores, 152
    for yeast infections, 570

Z

Zeaxanthin
    for preventing
        cataracts, 167
        glaucoma, 273
        macular degeneration, 370
Zinc. See also Zinc deficiency
    AIDS and, 319, 320–22
    Alzheimer's disease and, 85–86
    anemia and, 93–94
    caution about, 154
    copper and, 29, 53, 93, 154–55, 266, 267,
        548
    high cholesterol and, 314
    for mucous membrane protection, 84
    overview of, 52–55
    for preventing
        genital herpes recurrences, 266, 267
        heart disease, 299, 300
        macular degeneration, 369, 371–72, 372
        osteoporosis, 436, 437
    for treating
        alcoholism, 76, 77
        asthma, 108
        bedsores, 111, 112
        bruises, 124, 126, 127
        burns, 128, 132
        canker sores, 154–55, 154
        colds, 190, 191–93

cold sores, 195–97, <u>196</u>
dermatitis, 210–11, <u>212</u>
eating disorders, <u>231</u>, 232
hair loss, <u>282</u>, 283
immune system, <u>330</u>, 331–32
infertility, 334–36, <u>338</u>
insomnia, 341, <u>344</u>
lupus, <u>366</u>
memory loss, <u>377</u>, 379
prostate problems, 469–70, <u>471</u>
rheumatoid arthritis, <u>493</u>, 494–95
surgical healing, 536–37
taste and smell problems, <u>539</u>, 540–42
tinnitus, <u>545</u>, 548

Wilson's disease, 560–62, <u>561</u>
  yeast infections, 571, <u>572</u>
  weight loss and, <u>445</u>, 446
Zinc deficiency
  from alcoholism, 76
  effects of
    dermatitis, 209–10
    hair loss, 283
    seizures, 241
    taste and smell problems, 540, 541
  after surgery, 537
Zinc oxide, for sun protection, 526, <u>529</u>, 531
Zostavax, for shingles prevention, 507
Zyloprim, for gout, 278